Hepatology and Transplant Hepatology: A Case-Based Approach

Hepatology and Transplant Hepatology: A Case-Based Approach

Editor: Dylan Long

AMERICAN
MEDICAL PUBLISHERS
www.americanmedicalpublishers.com

AMERICAN
MEDICAL PUBLISHERS
www.americanmedicalpublishers.com

Cataloging-in-Publication Data

Hepatology and transplant hepatology : a case-based approach / edited by Dylan Long.
p. cm.
Includes bibliographical references and index.
ISBN 979-8-88740-181-2
1. Hepatology. 2. Liver--Transplantation. 3. Liver--Diseases. 4. Gastroenterology. I. Long, Dylan.
RC845 .H47 2023
616.362--dc23

American Medical Publishers,
41 Flatbush Avenue,
1st Floor, New York,
NY 11217, USA

ISBN 979-8-88740-181-2 (Hardback)

Contents

Preface

Over the recent decade, advancements and applications have progressed exponentially. This has led to the increased interest in this field and projects are being conducted to enhance knowledge. The main objective of this book is to present some of the critical challenges and provide insights into possible solutions. This book will answer the varied questions that arise in the field and also provide an increased scope for furthering studies.

Transplant hepatology is a subspecialty of gastroenterology that focuses on the treatment of chronic liver disease. The liver performs a variety of crucial functions, such as producing bile to aid in digestion, converting food into energy and eliminating toxins from the body. Transplant hepatology is the study of diseases that lead to transplantation, the assessment of patients prior to transplantation, the assessment and treatment of patients following transplantation, and management of transplant-related complications. It involves a thorough understanding of hepatopathology and the diagnostic methods required to assess and treat individuals in need of liver transplants. This medical specialty is also concerned with the management of issues like infectious diseases associated with transplant and immunosuppression. This book unravels the recent studies in hepatology and transplant hepatology. It presents researches and studies performed by experts across the globe. For all readers who are interested in these areas of study, the case studies included in this book will serve as an excellent guide to develop a comprehensive understanding.

I hope that this book, with its visionary approach, will be a valuable addition and will promote interest among readers. Each of the authors has provided their extraordinary competence in their specific fields by providing different perspectives as they come from diverse nations and regions. I thank them for their contributions.

Editor

1

Vitamin D receptor gene polymorphisms and risk of hepatocellular carcinoma in hepatitis C-related liver cirrhosis

Ghada M. Galal[1], Ahmad Abudeif[1], Nagwa Sayed Ahmed[2], Nahed Fathallah Fahmy[3], Abeer Sheneef[3], Elsayed Mostafa Ali[4], Usama M. Abdelaal[5*] and Asmaa Naser Mohammad[1]

Abstract

Background: HCV is a major risk factor for HCC; however, the exact mechanism of hepatocarcinogenesis is still not fully understood. Host genetic factors have been reported to play a significant role. Experimental studies support the tumor inhibitory effect of vitamin D on HCC cells. Several single nucleotide polymorphisms (SNPs) have been depicted in the vitamin D receptor (VDR) gene. We aimed to assess whether any of these polymorphisms could be significantly associated with increased risk of HCC.

Results: This study was conducted on 76 patients with HCV-related liver cirrhosis (48 patients had HCC on top of cirrhosis, and the other 28 had liver cirrhosis only). All patients underwent full medical history assessment, clinical examination, laboratory investigations, abdominal ultrasonography, and genotyping of the VDR gene. HCC patients had a significantly higher frequency of ApaI CC genotype compared with those patients without HCC. There is no statistically significant difference between the studied groups at any TaqI genotypes but the carriage of the ApaI CC genotype had a significant association with liver disease severity in both patients groups compared with ApaI CA/AA genotypes. The carriage of the ApaI CC genotype was an independent predictor for HCC in HCV-related liver cirrhosis.

Conclusions: VDR ApaI polymorphism is significantly associated with the development of HCC; thus, ApaI CC genotype could be used as an important molecular marker to predict the risk of HCC in patients with HCV-related liver cirrhosis.

Keywords: Vitamin D receptor, Gene polymorphism, Hepatocellular carcinoma, Hepatitis C virus, Liver cirrhosis

Background

HCV is a major worldwide health problem. Globally, estimates indicate that about 71 million people are chronically infected [1]. The major complications of chronic HCV are hepatic fibrosis, cirrhosis, and hepatocellular carcinoma (HCC) [2].

HCC is considered to be the 6th common cancer all over the world, and it is accounting for 75 to 85% of primary liver cancers. HCC is in the fourth place as a cause of cancer death [3]. Besides HCV, there are a number of other risk factors that are suspected to cause HCC, including chronic HBV, non-viral cirrhosis, alcohol, nonalcoholic fatty liver disease (NAFLD), aflatoxin, hemochromatosis, Wilson's disease, family history or genetic factors, and smoking [4].

The relationship between HCV and HCC is well known; however, the exact mechanism of carcinogenesis, including the host and viral factors, is not fully understood [5]. Different genetic factors are accused as a contributing factor for HCC in patients with chronic HCV, particularly gene polymorphisms of diverse inflammatory cytokines [6].

* Correspondence: osamelaal74@yahoo.com
[5]Department of Internal Medicine, Sohag University, Sohag, Egypt
Full list of author information is available at the end of the article

Table 1 Size of DNA fragments following digestion with ApaI and TaqI restriction enzymes

Restriction enzyme	Size of restriction fragments and genotypes		
	Homozygous polymorphism	Heterozygous polymorphism	No polymorphism
ApaI	531, 214 bp (CC genotype)	745, 531, 214 bp (CA genotype)	745 bp (AA genotype)
TaqI	290, 245, 205 bp (GG genotype)	495, 290, 245, 205 bp (GA genotype)	495, 245 bp (AA genotype)

Vitamin D is a systemic hormone which is involved in the bone metabolism, but it also has a significant role in immunoregulation and cellular differentiation. Additionally, it has different anti-inflammatory and anticancer mechanisms through the vitamin D receptor (VDR) [7]. Studies have attributed the anticancer effect of vitamin D to its induction of cellular differentiation, proliferation, and angiogenesis inhibition, and hindering the progression of apoptosis as well [8].

The VDR is a nuclear hormone receptor that combines with the active form of vitamin D ($1,25(OH)_2D_3$; calcitriol) and reacts with characteristic nucleotide sequences of target genes to perform its final biologic effects. The VDR gene is quite polymorphic and located on the 12q13.11 chromosome. Single nucleotide polymorphisms (SNPs) are frequently determined, and some of them are linked to carcinogenesis [9, 10].

Currently, data on VDR polymorphisms and their relationship with HCC are limited and extremely discordant [11]. As far as we know, there are a few published articles that have addressed such a relationship in Egyptian patients with HCV-related liver cirrhosis.

Table 2 Baseline patient characteristics

Parameter	Group		*P* value
	HCC− (*n* = 28)	HCC+ (*n* = 48)	
Age			
Mean ± SD	57.5 ± 7.29	56.94 ± 6.82	0.736
Median (range)	56.5 (41–70)	55.5 (42–75)	
Sex			
Male (M)	20 (71.4%)	36 (75%)	0.733
Female (F)	8 (28.6%)	12 (25%)	
Smoking	3 (10.7%)	4 (8.3%)	0.704
Hypertension	8 (28.6%)	10 (20.8%)	0.444
Diabetes mellitus	9 (32.1%)	17 (35.4%)	0.772
Child class			
A	4 (14.3%)	8 (16.6%)	0.78
B	10 (35.7%)	20 (41.7%)	
C	14 (50%)	20 (41.7%)	
MELD score			
Mean ± SD	16.82 ± 4.99	16.02 ± 5.35	0.521
Median (range)	17.5 (8–25)	16 (6–31)	

HCC hepatocellular carcinoma
P value < 0.05 is statistically significant

Methods

Seventy-six patients with HCV-related cirrhosis (56 males and 20 females, with age range 41–75 years) were included during the period from May 2017 to December 2018 in a cross-sectional study.

Forty-eight patients had HCC on top of liver cirrhosis [single or multiple more than 1 cm] (group HCC+) (36 males (75%), mean age 56.94 ± 6.82 years), while 28 patients had no HCC (group HCC−) (20 males (71.4%), mean age 57.5 ± 7.29 years). The study protocol was approved by the ethics committee of our institute. Informed written consent was obtained from all patients before inclusion in the study.

The exclusion criteria were the presence of other factors that could cause hepatocellular injury such as HBV co-infection (HBsAg-negative), history of alcoholism, autoimmune hepatitis (normal autoimmune markers; smooth muscle antibodies (SMA), anti-nuclear antibodies (ANA), and liver-kidney microsomal type 1 antibodies (LKM-1)), primary cholangitis (serum bilirubin and alkaline phosphatase levels, and MRCP in suspected cases), and primary biliary cirrhosis (negative anti-mitochondrial antibodies (AMA)).

All patients underwent complete medical history assessment, clinical examination, laboratory investigations, and abdominal ultrasonography. Abdominal triphasic CT scan was done if a hepatic focal lesion was detected on ultrasonography for the diagnosis of HCC.

The criteria for HCC diagnosis by CT were arterial phase enhancement pattern with rapid washout in the portal venous phase [12], liver disease severity estimated by Child-Turcotte-Pugh (CTP) classification [13], and model for end-stage liver disease (MELD) score [14].

Table 3 Distribution of frequencies of VDR genotypes at ApaI and TaqI loci among the two groups

Parameter	Group		*P* value
	HCC− (*n* = 28)	HCC+ (*n* = 48)	
ApaI genotype			
CC (*n* = 44)	6 (21.4%)	38 (79.1%)	**< 0.001**
CA (*n* = 19)	12 (42.9%)	7 (14.6%)	
AA (*n* = 13)	10 (35.7%)	3 (6.3%)	
TaqI genotype			
GA (*n* = 12)	6 (21.4%)	6 (12.5%)	0.341
AA (*n* = 64)	22 (78.6%)	42 (87.5%)	

P value < 0.05 is statistically significant

Detection of VDR polymorphisms

PCR (polymerase chain reaction)

Genomic DNA was obtained from the buffy coat collected from EDTA blood using the QIAamp DNA Mini Kits (QIAGEN, Milan, Italy). The Ap fragment of the VDR gene containing the ApaI and TaqI restriction sites was amplified by PCR assay by using 200 ng of the genomic DNA in a total reaction volume of 50 μL. The PCR mix according to the manufacturer's instructions consisted of 25 μL of master mix (Bioline, England) and 2.5 μL of each primer (10 pmol): forward (5′-CAGAGC ATGGACAGGGAGCAA) and reverse (5′-GCAACTCC TCATGGCTGAGGTCTC)[5]. Thirty-five cycles of amplification were performed in a thermal cycler (T Gradient - Biometra). After the initial denaturation of DNA at 95 °C for 2 min, each cycle consisted of a denaturation step at 94 °C for 45 s, optimization of the primer annealing step modified to be at 58 °C for 1 min, an extension step at 72 °C for 1 min, and a final extension step at 72 °C for 7 min following the last cycle [15].

PCR products were analyzed on 2% agarose gel stained with ethidium bromide. The stained gels were visualized and analyzed with a gel documentation system to assess the size of PCR amplicon 745 bp.

RFLP assay (restriction fragment length polymorphism)

The amplified PCR products were then digested with the restriction endonucleases (ApaI and TaqI). For each endonuclease digestion reaction, 21.5 μL of the PCR product was digested with 1 μL (10 U) of the restriction enzyme ApaI (Jena Bioscience, Germany) or TaqI (Jena Bioscience, Germany), and 2.5 μL of restriction enzyme buffer "1×." The resulting reaction solution (25 μL) was incubated at 37 °C for 1 h, then electrophoresed on 2% ethidium bromide-stained agarose gel, and visualized under UV illumination through a gel documentation system. Through a direct comparison with 100-bp DNA ladder (Jena Bioscience, Germany), the size of the DNA fragments was assessed. The restriction fragments generated after digesting the target gene by ApaI and TaqI restriction endonucleases are shown in Table 1.

Statistical analysis

Data were analyzed using the IBM SPSS Statistics for Windows, version 25 (IBM Corp., Armonk, NY, USA). Quantitative data were expressed as mean ± standard deviation, median, and range. Qualitative data were expressed as number and percentage. Quantitative data were tested for normality by the *Shapiro–Wilk test.* The

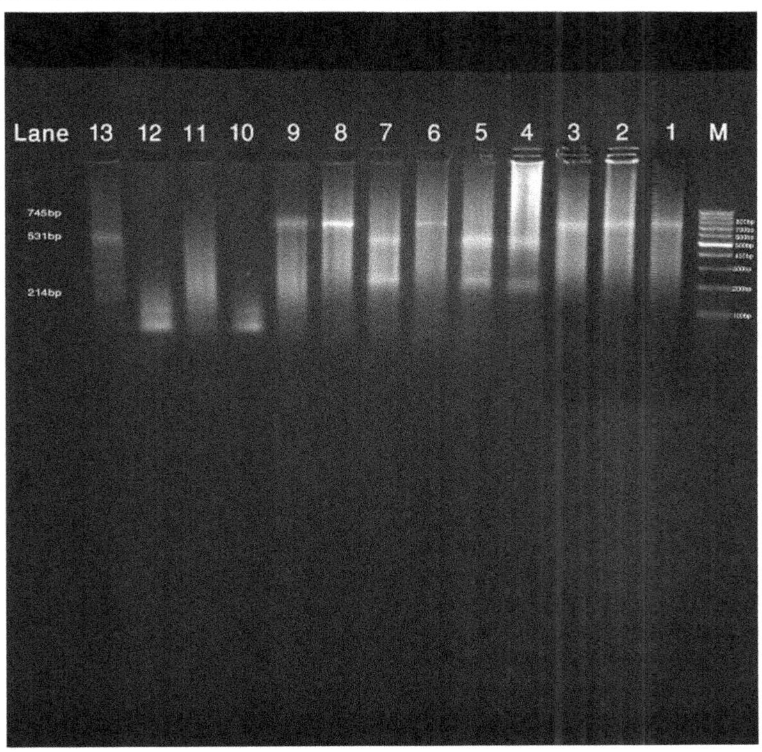

Fig. 1 Representative gel picture showing the PCR-RFLP analysis of ApaI VDR gene polymorphism on ethidium bromide-stained 2% agarose gel. M, marker (100 bp DNA ladder); lanes 4, 5, and 7 represent homozygous polymorphism (CC genotype; 531 and 214 bp bands); lanes 1, 2, 3, 6, 8, 9, and 13 represent no polymorphism (AA genotype; 745 bp band)

Mann–Whitney U test and *Kruskal–Wallis H test* were used for data which were not normally distributed. Independent samples *t* test and *one-way ANOVA* test were used for normally distributed data. The *chi-square* (χ^2) test and *Fisher's exact t*est were used for the comparison of qualitative variables as appropriate. *Univariate and multivariate binary logistic regression* analyses were used to determine the predictor variables of HCC. A 5% level was chosen as a level of significance in all statistical tests used in the study.

Results

The demographic variables, smoking status, comorbid illness, some laboratory data, Child class, and MELD score of the patient groups are summarized in Table 2.

The frequency distribution of VDR genotypes at ApaI and TaqI loci was summarized in Table 3. The HCC+ group had a statistically significant higher frequency of ApaI CC genotype compared to the HCC– group ($P < 0.001$). However, no statistically significant difference was found between the studied groups and any TaqI genotypes.

The digestion products of the VDR gene by ApaI and TaqI restriction enzymes were shown in Figs. 1, 2, 3, and 4.

The relation between the different ApaI genotypes and the severity of the liver disease among both groups is demonstrated in Table 4. In HCC– group, the carriage of the ApaI CC genotype was associated with a more severe liver disease (100% were Child C; MELD 20.33 ± 1.37; $P = 0.011$ and 0.01, respectively), compared to ApaI CA genotype (58.4% were Child C; MELD 17.92 ± 4.85) and ApaI AA genotype (10% were Child C; MELD 13.4 ± 4.69). Additionally, in the HCC+ group, the carriage of the ApaI CC genotype had a significant association with severe liver disease (52.6% were Child C vs. 0% for ApaI CA and AA genotypes; $P = 0.003$), ApaI CC carriers had the highest MELD score ($P = 0.001$). There is no significant difference between TaqI genotypes and liver disease severity among the studied groups.

Both univariate and multivariate binary logistic regression analyses confirmed that the carriage of the ApaI CC genotype (odds ratio (OR) 37.71, 95% confidence interval ($CI_{95\%}$) 5.83–244.12, $P < 0.001$) and platelet count (OR 1.02, $CI_{95\%}$ 1.002–1.04, $P = 0.01$) were independent predictors for HCC development in patients with HCV-related liver cirrhosis (Table 5).

Discussion

The development of HCC is a complicated and multifactorial process, in which both environmental and genetic factors play a role in carcinogenesis. The association

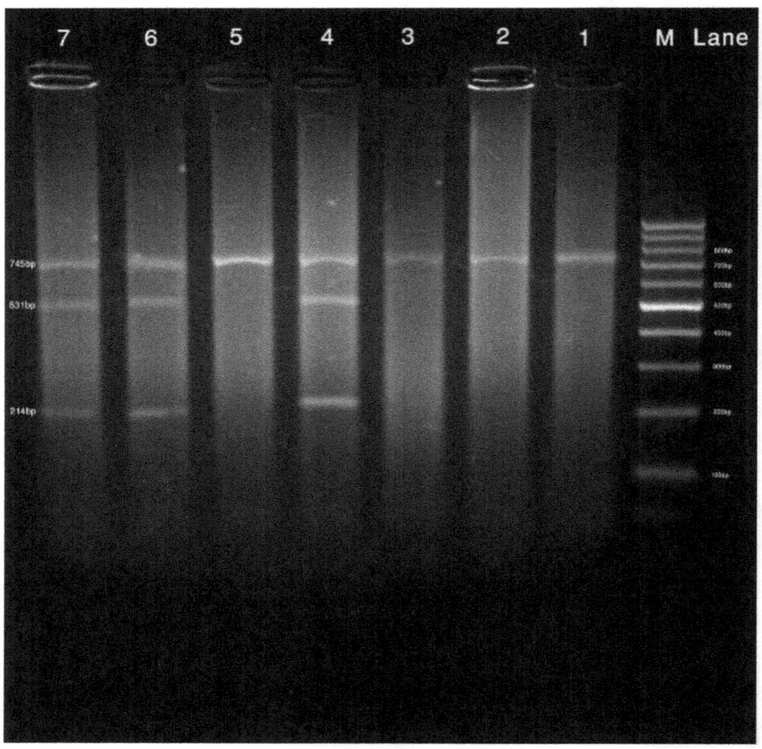

Fig. 2 Representative gel picture showing the PCR-RFLP analysis of ApaI VDR gene polymorphism on ethidium bromide-stained 2% agarose gel. M, marker (100 bp DNA ladder); lanes 4, 6, and 7 represent heterozygous polymorphism (CA genotype; 745, 531, and 214 bp bands); lanes 1, 2, 3, and 5 represent no polymorphism (AA genotype; 745 bp band)

between SNPs and HCC has been reported by numerous studies. These genetic traits may alter the natural history of cirrhosis and explain to some extent the observed differences in the risk of HCC development [16].

Interestingly, SNPs in the VDR gene are implicated in carcinogenesis in different organs such as the breast, prostate, skin, colon and rectum, and kidneys [17].

Here, we investigated the relationship between ApaI and TaqI VDR gene polymorphisms and HCC in patients with HCV-related liver cirrhosis.

We demonstrated that cirrhotic patients with HCC on top had a significantly higher frequency of VDR ApaI CC genotype compared to those patients who do not have HCC. Our results agree with previous studies [5, 15, 18, 19]. Some studies are matching us; they did not find a significant association between HCC and TaqI polymorphism [5, 15].

We investigated the implication of VDR ApaI and TaqI polymorphisms on the liver disease severity in both liver cirrhosis and HCC patients. The carriage of the ApaI CC genotype had significantly more severe liver disease (Child C and higher MELD score) compared to ApaI CA/AA genotypes, while the carriage of TaqI genotypes was not related to disease severity. These results came in agreement with Hung et al. [5] and Mohammed et al. [15].

On the contrary, Triantos et al. [20] reported that the carriage of VDR ApaI AA and TaqI AA genotypes was associated with more severe liver disease compared to ApaI CC/CA and TaqI GG/GA genotypes, respectively. This conflict could be simply explained by the difference in the inclusion criteria as Triantos et al. [20] investigated patients with chronic liver disease whatever the cause (viral, autoimmune, cryptogenic, etc.) and not complicated by HCC on top, while in our study, we selected only the HCV-related cirrhotic patients.

On addressing the risk factors for the development of HCC among HCV-related liver cirrhosis patients in this study, univariate binary logistic regression analysis was performed on age, sex, smoking, diabetes mellitus, Child and MELD scores, platelet count, and VDR ApaI and TaqI genotypes. Only platelet count and the carriage of the ApaI CC genotype were the factors significantly associated with HCC development; this was confirmed by multivariate binary logistic regression analysis.

The present study reported that the carriage of the ApaI CC genotype was an independent risk factor, proposing that the ApaI CC polymorphism may be a good molecular marker to predict the risk of HCC in patients with HCV-related liver cirrhosis. This agrees with Asal

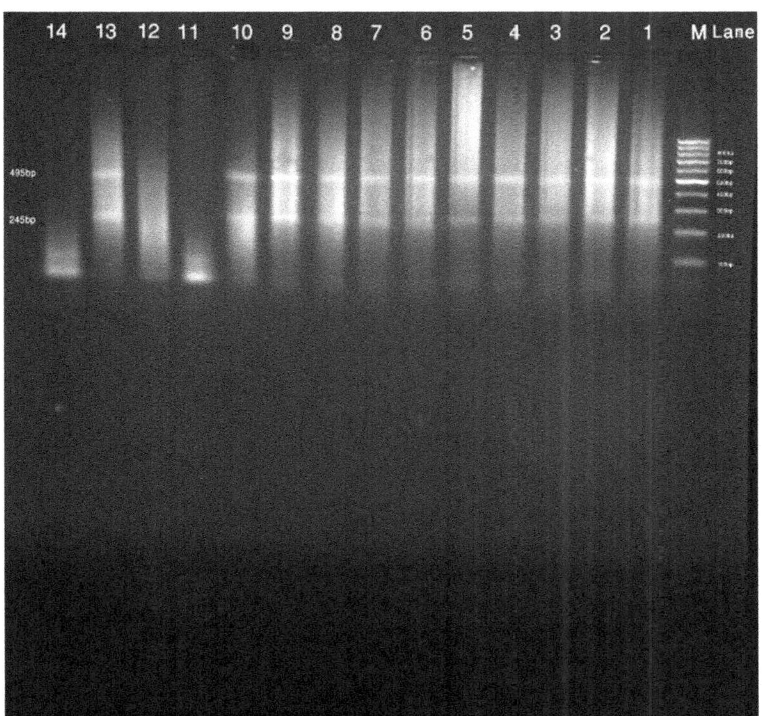

Fig. 3 Representative gel picture showing the PCR-RFLP analysis of TaqI VDR gene polymorphism on ethidium bromide-stained 2% agarose gel. M, marker (100 bp DNA ladder); lanes 1, 2, 3, 4, 5, 6, 7, 8, 9, 10, and 13 represent no polymorphism (AA genotype; 495 and 245 bp bands)

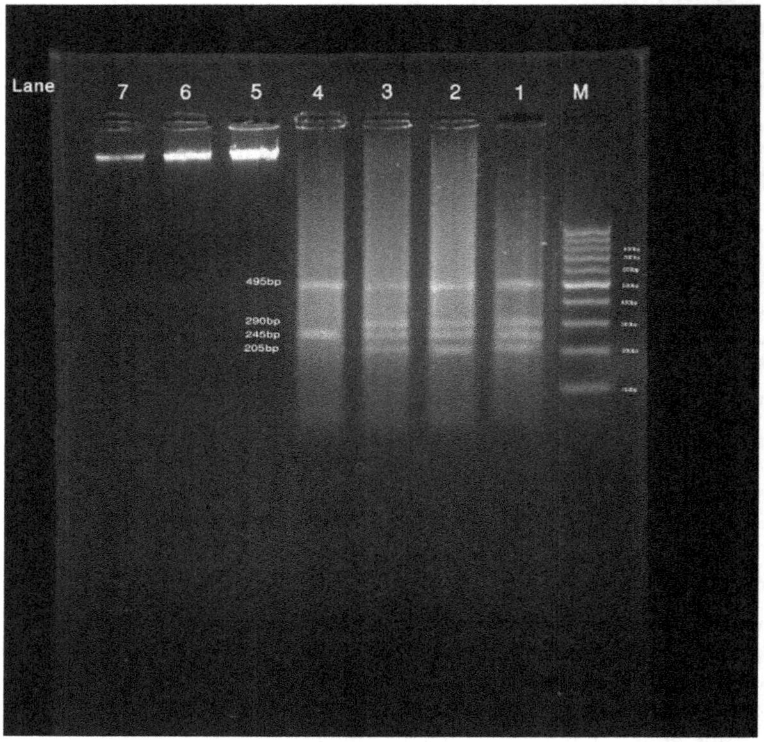

Fig. 4 Representative gel picture showing the PCR-RFLP analysis of TaqI VDR gene polymorphism on ethidium bromide-stained 2% agarose gel. M, marker (100 bp DNA ladder); lanes 1, 2, and 3 represent heterozygous polymorphism (GA genotype; 495, 290, 245, and 205 bp bands); lane 4 represents no polymorphism (AA genotype; 495 and 245 bp bands)

Table 4 Relationship between the individual ApaI genotypes and severity of liver disease among the two groups

Parameter		ApaI genotype			*P* value
HCC− group		**CC (*n* = 6)**	**CA (*n* = 12)**	**AA (*n* = 10)**	
	Child class				
	A	0 (0.0%)	1 (8.3%)	3 (30%)	**0.011**
	B	0 (0.0%)	4 (33.3%)	6 (60%)	
	C	6 (100%)	7 (58.4%)	1 (10%)	
	MELD score				
	Mean ± SD	20.33 ± 1.37	17.92 ± 4.85	13.4 ± 4.69	**0.01**
	Median (range)	20.5 (18–22)	17.5 (9–25)	12.5 (8–21)	
HCC+ group		**CC (*n* = 38)**	**CA (*n* = 7)**	**AA (*n* = 3)**	
	Child class				
	A	4 (10.5%)	4 (57.1%)	0 (0.0%)	**0.003**
	B	14 (36.9%)	3 (42.9%)	3 (100%)	
	C	20 (52.6%)	0 (0.0%)	0 (0.0%)	
	MELD score				
	Mean ± SD	17.37 ± 4.92	9.57 ± 3.26	14 ± 2.65	**0.001**
	Median (range)	17 (8–31)	8 (6–16)	15 (11–16)	

Table 5 Univariate and multivariate binary logistic regression analysis of predictor variables of HCC in patients with HCV-related liver cirrhosis

Characteristics	Univariate analysis		Multivariate analysis	
	OR ($CI_{95\%}$)	*P* value	OR ($CI_{95\%}$)	*P* value
Age	0.99 (0.92–1.06)	0.732		
Sex				
Male	1.2 (0.42–3.42)	0.733		
Female	1			
Smoking				
No	1			
Yes	0.76 (0.16–3.66)	0.73		
Diabetes mellitus				
No	1			
Yes	1.16 (0.43–3.11)	0.772		
Child class				
A	1			
B	1 (0.24–4.14)	1		
C	0.71 (0.18–2.84)	0.633		
MELD score	0.97 (0.89–1.06)	0.516		
Platelets	1.02 (1.002–1.04)	**0.024**	1.02 (1.002–1.04)	**0.01**
ApaI genotype				
AA	1		1	
CA	1.94 (0.39–9.55)	0.413	1.96 (0.29–12.94)	0.486
CC	21.11 (4.48–99.58)	**< 0.001**	37.71 (5.83–244.12)	**< 0.001**
TaqI genotype				
AA	1			
GA	0.524 (0.15–1.82)	0.308		

OR odds ratio, $CI_{95}\%$ 95% confidence interval

et al. [18] and El-Edel et al. [19]. Additionally, the ApaI CC genotype was reported to be associated with HCC development in non-cirrhotic patients with chronic HCV [5, 15].

Related studies of several polymorphisms in the VDR gene have been done to investigate their implication on the risk of HCC, although with different results. Falleti and his colleagues [21] demonstrated that the carriage of the BsmI GG and TaqI TT genotypes were significantly associated with HCC development in post-liver transplantation patients. However, this study was performed more particularly on patients with alcoholic cirrhosis, not other etiology of liver cirrhosis, where the carriage of the BAT [ATC] and [GTT] haplotypes was independently associated with an increased risk of HCC. This discrepancy could be explained by the low number of patients in the subgroup analysis of virus cirrhotic patients.

Peng et al. [10] reported that the carriage of the FokI TT/CT genotypes was associated with increased HBV-related HCC risk as compared to the FokI CC genotype. Some investigators in previous researches [15, 22–24] have reported that the carriage of the FokI TT genotype had a significantly higher risk for HCC after adjustment of other associated risk factors in those chronically infected with viral hepatitis. In addition, it was found that the FokI TT genotype was associated with advanced tumor stage and lymph node involvement.

On the contrary, Huang et al. [25] reported that VDR polymorphisms could influence the distinct clinical phenotypes in HBV carriers, but are not associated with HCC proposing a limited role of the VDR gene polymorphisms in carcinogenesis. However, a biochemical evidence obviously reported the inhibitory effect of vitamin D and its analogs on HCC cells [26]. Moreover, it had been described that the antiproliferative effect of vitamin D against malignant cells depends on the intracellular VDR level [27, 28].

Conclusions

In our country, the increasing HCC incidence is a result of the high prevalence of HCV, estimated to be around 14% in the general population [29, 30]. However, HCC is usually asymptotic, and diagnosis is usually made on an accidental basis. We suggested that the ApaI CC genotype may be used as a molecular marker to predict the risk of HCC in patients with HCV-related liver cirrhosis particularly in thrombocytopenic patients.

Abbreviations
HCV: Hepatitis C virus; HCC: Hepatocellular carcinoma; SNPs: Several single nucleotide polymorphisms; VDR: Vitamin D receptor; NAFLD: Non-alcoholic fatty liver disease; HBV: Hepatitis B virus; SMA: Smooth muscle antibodies; ANA: Anti-nuclear antibodies; LKM-1: Liver-kidney microsomal type 1 antibodies; MRCP: Magnetic resonance cholangiopancreatography; AMA: Anti-mitochondrial antibodies; CTP: Child-Turcotte-Pugh; MELD: Model for end-stage liver disease; PCR: Polymerase chain reaction

Acknowledgements
Not applicable

Authors' contributions
GMG, AA, and ANM collected, analyzed, and interpreted the data. NSA, NFF, and AS shared and helped in the designing and conceptualization of the study. EMA and UMA helped in the designing, editing, writing, and publishing of the study. All authors read and approved the final manuscript.

Ethics approval and consent to participate
The study protocol was approved by the Sohag University Faculty of Medicine Ethical Committee (date 2018/2019; No. 1), and written informed consents were obtained from all participants. The procedures followed are in accordance with the institutional guidelines.

Competing interests
The authors declare that they have no competing interests.

Author details
[1]Department of Tropical Medicine and Gastroenterology, Sohag University Hospital, Sohag, Egypt. [2]Medical Biochemistry, Sohag Faculty of Medicine, Sohag University Hospital, Sohag, Egypt. [3]Microbiology and Immunology, Sohag Faculty of Medicine, Sohag University Hospital, Sohag, Egypt. [4]Clinical Oncology Department, Sohag Faculty of Medicine, Sohag University Hospital, Sohag, Egypt. [5]Department of Internal Medicine, Sohag University, Sohag, Egypt.

References
1. The Polaris Observatory HCV Collaborators (2017) Global prevalence and genotype distribution of hepatitis C virus infection in 2015: a modelling study. Lancet Gastroenterol Hepatol 2(3):161–176
2. Hajarizadeh B, Grebely J, Dore GJ (2013) Epidemiology and natural history of HCV infection. Nat Rev Gastroenterol Hepatol 10(9):553–562
3. Bray F, Ferlay J, Soerjomataram I, Siegel RL, Torre LA, Jemal A (2018) Global cancer statistics 2018: GLOBOCAN estimates of incidence and mortality worldwide for 36 cancers in 185 countries. CA Cancer J Clin 68(6):394–424
4. Tang A, Hallouch O, Chernyak V, Kamaya A, Sirlin CB (2018) Epidemiology of hepatocellular carcinoma: target population for surveillance and diagnosis. AbdomRadiol (NY). 43(1):13–25
5. Hung CH, Chiu YC, Hu TH, Chen CH, Lu SN et al (2014) Significance of vitamin d receptor gene polymorphisms for risk of hepatocellular carcinoma in chronic hepatitis C. Transl Oncol 7(4):503–507
6. Bataller R, North KE, Brenner DA (2003) Genetic polymorphisms and the progression of liver fibrosis: a critical appraisal. Hepatology 37(3):493–503
7. Raimondi S, Johansson H, Maisonneuve P, Gandini S (2009) Review and meta-analysis on vitamin D receptor polymorphisms and cancer risk. Carcinogenesis 30(7):1170–1180
8. Bikle D (2009) Nonclassic actions of vitamin D. J Clin Endocrinol Metab 94(1):26–34
9. Whitfield GK, Remus LS, Jurutka PW, Zitzer H, Oza AK, Dang HT et al (2001) Functionally relevant polymorphisms in the human nuclear vitamin D receptor gene. Mol Cell Endocrinol 177(1-2):145–159
10. Peng Q, Yang S, Lao X, Li R, Chen Z, Wang J et al (2014) Association of single nucleotide polymorphisms in VDR and DBP genes with HBV-related hepatocellular carcinoma risk in a Chinese population. PLoS One 9(12): e116026
11. Louka ML, Fawzy AM, Naiem AM, Elseknedy MF, Abdelhalim AE, Abdelghany MA (2017) Vitamin D and K signaling pathways in hepatocellular carcinoma. Gene 629:108–116
12. Lencioni R, Cioni D, Della Pina C, Crocetti L, Bartolozzi C (2005) Imaging diagnosis. Semin Liver Dis. 25(2):162–170
13. Pugh RN, Murray-Lyon IM, Dawson JL, Pietroni MC, Williams R (1973) Transection of the oesophagus for bleeding oesophageal varices. Br J Surg 60(8):646–649
14. Kamath PS, Wiesner RH, Malinchoc M, Kremers W, Therneau TM, Kosberg CL et al (2001) A model to predict survival in patients with end-stage liver disease. Hepatology 33(2):464–470
15. Mohammed M, Omar N, Mohammed S, Deiab A (2017) The significance of vitamin D receptor gene polymorphisms for susceptibility to hepatocellular carcinoma in subjects infected with hepatitis C virus. Gastroenterol Hepatol Open Access 7(4):00246
16. Nahon P, Zucman-Rossi J (2012) Single nucleotide polymorphisms and risk of hepatocellular carcinoma in cirrhosis. J Hepatol 57(3):663–674
17. Vaughan-Shaw PG, O'Sullivan F, Farrington SM, Theodoratou E, Campbell H, Dunlop MG et al (2017) The impact of vitamin D pathway genetic variation and circulating 25-hydroxyvitamin D on cancer outcome: systematic review and meta-analysis. Br J Cancer 116(8):1092–1110
18. Asal FES, El Bendary AS, El Khalawany WA, Abd-Elsalam S, Sheta BM (2017) The role of the vitamin D receptor gene polymorphisms in hepatocarcinogenesis in cirrhotic patients infected with chronic hepatitis C virus. Nat Sci 15(12):172–175
19. El-Edel RH, Mostafa MS, Montaser BA, Ali YAE-H (2017) Study of Apa-I vitamin D receptor gene polymorphism in patients with hepatocellular carcinoma. Menoufia Med J 30:619
20. Triantos C, Aggeletopoulou I, Kalafateli M, Spantidea PI, Vourli G, Diamantopoulou G et al (2018) Prognostic significance of vitamin D receptor (VDR) gene polymorphisms in liver cirrhosis. Sci Rep 8(1):14065
21. Falleti E, Bitetto D, Fabris C, Cussigh A, Fontanini E, Fornasiere E et al (2010) Vitamin D receptor gene polymorphisms and hepatocellular carcinoma in alcoholic cirrhosis. World J Gastroenterol. 16(24):3016–3024
22. Yao X, Zeng H, Zhang G, Zhou W, Yan Q, Dai L et al (2013) The associated ion between the VDR gene polymorphisms and susceptibility to hepatocellular carcinoma and the clinicopathological features in subjects infected with HBV. Biomed Res Int 2013:953974
23. Nada HA, Elsamanoudy AZ, Elalfy HA, Mogahed RE (2016) Study of vitamin D receptor-FOK-I gene polymorphism in chronic hepatitis C induced hepatocellular carcinoma patients: a case control study. Int J Innov Res Sci Eng Technol 5:4645–4655
24. Mohapatra S, Saxena A, Gandhi G, Koner BC, Ray PC (2013) Vitamin D and VDR gene polymorphism (FokI) in epithelial ovarian cancer in Indian population. J Ovarian Res. 6(1):37
25. Huang YW, Liao YT, Chen W, Chen CL, Hu JT, Liu CJ et al (2010) Vitamin D receptor gene polymorphisms and distinct clinical phenotypes of hepatitis B carriers in Taiwan. Genes Immun 11(1):87–93
26. Pourgholami M, Akhter J, Lu Y, Morris D (2000) In vitro and in vivo inhibition of liver cancer cells by 1, 25-dihydroxyvitamin D3. Cancer Lett 151(1):97–102
27. Dalhoff K, Dancey J, Astrup L, Skovsgaard T, Hamberg KJ, Lofts FJ et al (2003) A phase II study of the vitamin D analogue seocalcitol in patients with inoperable hepatocellular carcinoma. Br J Cancer 89(2):252–257

28. Merchan BB, Morcillo S, Martin-Nunez G, Tinahones FJ, Macías-González M (2017) The role of vitamin D and VDR in carcinogenesis: through epidemiology and basic sciences. J Steroid Biochem Mol Biol 167:203–218
29. El-Serag HB (2002) Hepatocellular carcinoma: an epidemiologic view. J Clin Gastroenterol. 35(5 Suppl 2):S72–S78
30. Hassany SM, Moustafa EFA, El Taher M, Abdeltawab AA, Blum HE (2015) Screening for hepatocellular carcinoma by Egyptian physicians. World J Gastrointest Oncol. 7(9):161–171

2

Crossroad of infection and autoimmunity in acute liver failure

Akash Roy[1], Sunil Taneja[1*], Arka De[1], Ashim Das[2], Ajay K. Duseja[1] and Virendra Singh[1]

Abstract

Background: Acute liver failure (ALF) is a syndromic diagnosis, consisting of jaundice, coagulopathy, and any degree of encephalopathy in a patient without pre-existing liver disease within 26 weeks of the onset of symptoms. Autoimmune hepatitis has a wide range of presentations and can rarely present as ALF, which frequently tends to be autoantibody negative. Tropical infections like dengue, malaria, and leptospirosis, which present as mimickers of ALF, always remain a differential diagnosis of ALF and mandate an etiology specific management. In rare cases, such infections themselves act as a trigger for autoimmunity. We report a case of diagnostic crossroads of infection and autoimmunity, presenting as acute liver failure and describe the challenges in management.

Case presentation: A 25-year-old female presented with a syndromic diagnosis of acute liver failure with possibility of tropical illness-related ALF mimic on account of positive Leptospira serology. After initial improvement, there was a rebound worsening of liver functions which prompted a liver biopsy. Biopsy narrowed the differential to Leptospira-associated hepatitis and severe auto-immune hepatitis. Trial of low dose steroid was given which led to dramatic improvement.

Conclusion: Tropical infections can present as ALF mimics and can themselves act as triggers for autoimmunity. Distinguishing such cases from de-novo acute severe autoimmune hepatitis is difficult and requires therapeutic brinksmanship. An early trial of steroid is mandated but comes with its own challenges.

Keywords: Leptospira, Autoimmune hepatitis, Acute liver failure; Case report

Background

Acute liver failure (ALF) is a syndromic diagnosis characterized acute onset (< 4 weeks) of jaundice, coagulopathy, and encephalopathy in a patient without pre-existing liver disease. Tropical infections like dengue, malaria, enteric fever, and leptospirosis often present as mimickers of ALF [1, 2]. Another etiology of ALF is autoimmune hepatitis, which differs from its classical presentation in being frequently seronegative in such cases [3]. Infections have been associated with AIH and can serve as a trigger for autoimmunity, thus leading to a grey zone in diagnosis. We report a case of ALF with a diagnostic crossroads between leptospirosis and autoimmunity

* Correspondence: drsuniltaneja@hotmail.com
[1]Department of Hepatology, Post Graduate Institute of Medical Education and Research (PGIMER), Chandigarh, India
Full list of author information is available at the end of the article

Case presentation

A 25-year-old female presented with complaints of fever for 2 weeks, jaundice for 1 week, and altered sensorium for 2 days. There was no history of headache, trauma, vision abnormalities, retro-orbital pain, conjunctival suffusion, rashes, or seizures. On examination, she was febrile, normotensive, maintained oxygen saturation, pale, icteric, and had grade II hepatic encephalopathy. Per abdominal examination was unremarkable. There was no significant history of any previous medical comorbidities. Her investigations revealed presence of anemia, leucocytosis deranged liver functions and coagulopathy. On etiological workup, viral markers including IgM hepatitis A, IgM hepatitis E, HBsAg, and anti-HCV were negative, while the IgM antibody for leptospirosis came out to be positive (titers 27.7 NTU). There was no definite history of potential exposure to Leptosira.

Abdominal ultrasonography showed a normal liver with a span of 12 cm and a normal spleen, with no free fluid. A syndromic diagnosis of acute liver failure (ALF) with the possibility of Leptospira associated ALF-mimicker was kept. She was managed as per standard ALF protocol along with intravenous doxycycline in view of positive Leptospira serology. The fever subsided, and hepatic encephalopathy improved; however, as liver functions and coagulogram failed to improve, she was given five sessions of plasmapheresis. However, 5 days after plasmapheresis, there was a worsening of liver functions and coagulation [Bilirubin (Total/direct) 35 mg/dl/24 mg/dl, AST/ALT/ALP 734/656/128 U/L, INR 1.9). The trend in the biochemical parameters is shown in Table 1. The further etiological workup including autoimmune (ANA, SMA, AMA, LKM, PCA ANCA, SLA), total immunoglobulin G levels, viral serologies for cytomegalovirus, Epstein–Barr virus, herpes simplex virus, and Wilson's disease workup were all negative. A transjugular liver biopsy was done, which showed centrizonal necrosis with lymphohistiocytic cell infiltrate with canalicular and intracellular cholestasis with multiple foci of lobular inflammation. The portal tracts showed minimal irregular portal tract expansion, minimal portal tract inflammation, and minimal interface hepatitis (Fig. 1). A histological possibility of Leptospira-associated-acute hepatitis versus acute severe autoimmune hepatitis was kept. She was started on low dose prednisolone (20 mg/day), which led to a gradual improvement of liver functions. Subsequently, the steroids were tapered after normalization of LFTs, and presently she is on 5 mg of prednisolone on regular follow.

Discussion

Tropical febrile syndromes mimicking as ALF is a frequently encountered challenge. The most common etiologies are falciparum malaria, dengue, Leptospirosis, and rickettsial fevers [1]. Identification and differentiation of these specific etiologies is essential to ensure a specific therapy. Features like high-grade fever, persistent febrile spikes after the onset of jaundice, overt bleeding manifestations, and splenomegaly serve as possible indicators of a tropical illness-related ALF. Similarly, laboratory indices like higher AST or LDH than ALT and INR < 1.5, thrombocytopenia, and early-onset hemodynamic instability and renal failure is more common in ALF mimickers [1, 2]. The clinical indicators of an initial suspicion of Leptospira-associated ALF in our case were persistent febrile spikes and positive serological tests. However, features like an absence of renal dysfunction, lack of hemorrhagic manifestations, and markedly elevated liver enzymes questioned the possibility of a Leptospira related ALF.

After an initial improvement post five sessions of plasmapheresis, there was enzyme elevation and worsening liver function. A detailed workup of possible etiology of acute liver failure was however inconclusive. At this crossroads, the patient was taken up for a transjugular liver biopsy, which was suggestive of acute hepatitis with a diagnostic possibility of Leptospira-associated-acute hepatitis versus acute autoimmune hepatitis. Acute severe AIH (AS-AIH) is an acute presentation (≤ 26 weeks) with an INR of ≥ 1.5 without any histological evidence of cirrhosis [3]. It is of importance to note that patients with an acute severe AIH frequently tend to be seronegative for

Table 1 Hematological and biochemical parameters

Investigations	Index presentation	Pre-plasmapharesis	Post-plasmapharesis	Post-steroids
Hemoglobin (g/dl)	8.9	8.3	8 1	8.6
Total leucocyte count(/mm^3)	11900	10200	7300	10200
Platelet count (/mm^3)	290000	275000	134000	204000
International normalized ratio (INR)	2.8	2	1 3	1.1
Liver function tests (LFT)				
• **Bilirubin (mg/dl)**	22	51	19	3
• **AST (IU)**	1161	530	212	45
• **ALT (IU)**	913	127	239	44
• **Protein (g/dl)**	6.6	6.8	6 9	7
• **Albumin(g/dl)**	3.4	3.3	3 2	3.3
• **SAP (IU)**	109	127	120	97
Renal function tests				
• **Urea (mmol/L)**	28	31	23	21
• **Creatinine(mg/dl)**	1.0	1.1	0 9	0.9

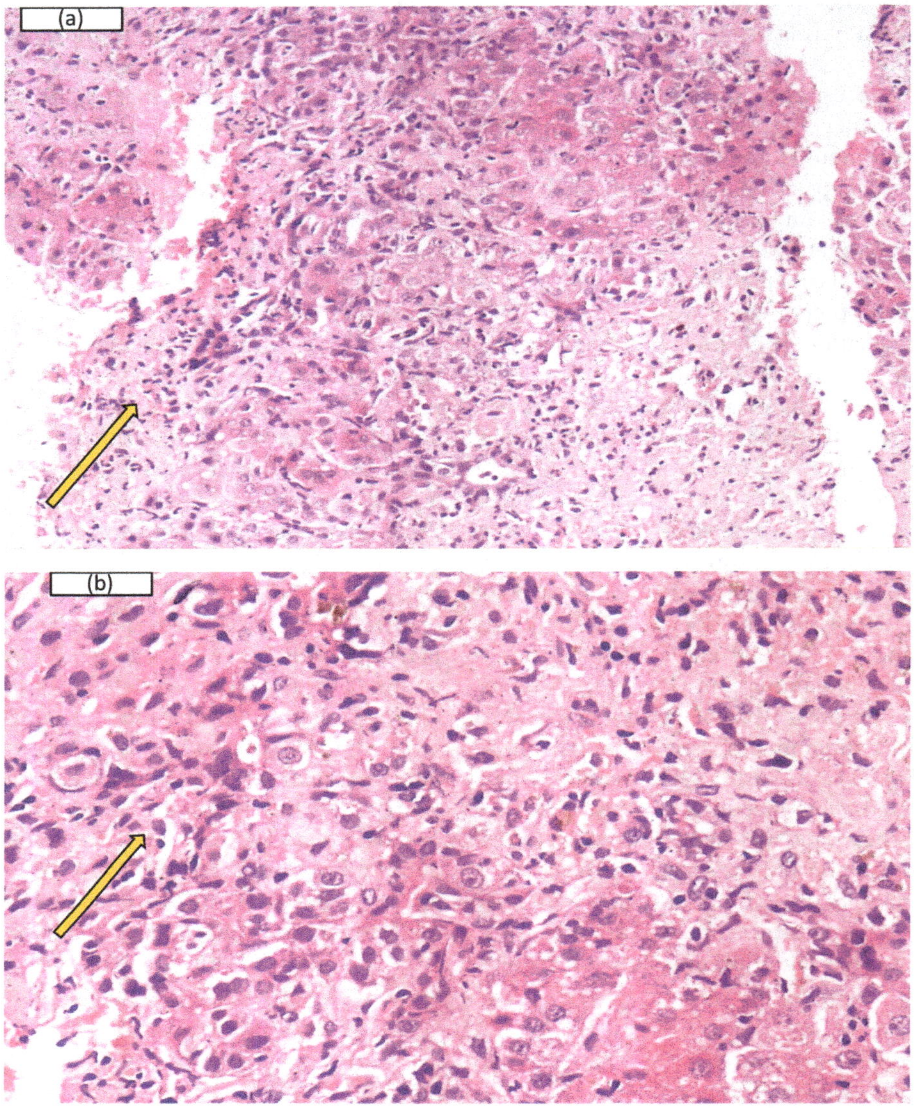

Fig. 1 a H& E stain showing extensive centrizonal necrosis. **b** H&E stain showing necrotic hepatocytes surrounded by lymphohistiocytic infiltrate

autoimmune markers. ANA antibodies are negative or weakly positive in 29–39% of patients whereas gamma-globulin levels may be normal in 25–39% thus adding to the diagnostic challenge [4, 5]. Our patient was started on a steroid trial, to which she responded, although literature suggests that such patients frequently tend to be steroid non-responders and end up requiring liver tranplantation [6].

The two primary differentials in our case were tropical illness-related ALF and AS-AIH. While the diagnosis of AS-AIH itself becomes a challenge due to frequent seronegativity, the other possibility of an infection itself triggering an autoimmune phenomenon adds to the diagnostic puzzle. Pathogens like HAV, HCV, EBV, CMV, HIV, and *Leishmania* have been postulated to trigger autoimmune hepatitis. However, the literature with Leptsopira as a trigger of autoimmune hepatitis presenting as ALF is scarce with only a single case report in a pediatric patient [7, 8]. Thus, management of such cases entails an element of therapeutic brinksmanship to closely balance the two contrasting entities of infection and autoimmunity.

Conclusion

Tropical infections may present as ALF mimics and can themselves act as triggers for autoimmunity. Distinguishing such cases from de-novo acute severe autoimmune hepatitis is difficult and requires therapeutic brinksmanship. An early trial of steroid is mandated in such cases and can alter the course of the disease.

Key learning

- Tropical infections can present as ALF mimics
- Clinical pointers and biochemical signatures should be carefully looked for to determine the etiology of an ALF mimicker
- Acute severe AIH can be seronegative in up to one-third of the cases
- Infections can serve as a trigger for autoimmunity and the interplay needs further understanding
- Acute severe AIH with early grades of HE may benefit from a trial of steroids

Abbreviations

AIH: Autoimmune hepatitis; ALF: Acute liver failure; HAV: Hepatitis A virus; HBV: Hepatitis B virus; HCV: Hepatitis C virus; EBV: Epstein-Barr virus; HIV: Human immunodeficiency virus; ANA: Antinuclear antibodies; AMA: Antimitochondrial antibodies; AST: Aspartate transaminase; ALT: Alanine transaminase; ALP: Alkaline phosphatase; LKM: Liver kidney microsome antibodies; PCA: Parietal cell antibodies; SAP: Serum alkaline phosphatase; SMA: Smooth muscles antibodies; SLA: Soluble liver antigen antibodies; INR: International normalized ratio

Acknowledgements

Nil

Authors' contributions

AR: data compilation and writing; ST: critical revision; AD: critical revision; AD: histopathological support; AKD critical revision; VS: critical revision. All authors have read and approved the manuscript.

Ethics approval and consent to participate

Written informed consent was obtained from patient.

Competing interests

The authors declare that they have no competing interests.

Author details

[1]Department of Hepatology, Post Graduate Institute of Medical Education and Research (PGIMER), Chandigarh, India. [2]Department of Pathology, Post Graduate Institute of Medical Education and Research (PGIMER), Chandigarh, India.

References

1. Patel ND, Amrapurkar D (2006) Differential diagnosis of acute liver failure in India. Ann Hepatol 5(3):150–156
2. Murthy GL, Sahay RK, Sreenivas DV, Sundaram C, Shantaram V (1998) Hepatitis in falciparum malaria. Trop Gastroenterol 19:152–154
3. Czaja AJ (2013) Acute and acute severe (fulminant) autoimmune hepatitis. Dig Dis Sci 58:897–914
4. Yasui S, Fujiwara K, Yonemitsu Y, Oda S, Nakano M, Yokosuka O (2011) Clinicopathological features of severe and fulminant forms of autoimmune hepatitis. J Gastroenterol 46:378–390
5. Fujiwara K, Fukuda Y, Yokosuka O (2008) Precise histological evaluation of liver biopsy specimen is indispensable for diagnosis and treatment of acute-onset autoimmune hepatitis. J Gastroenterol 43:951–958
6. Anand L, Choudhury A, Bihari C, Sharma BC, Kumar M, Maiwall R et al (2018) Flare of autoimmune hepatitis causing acute on chronic liver failure: diagnosis and response to corticosteroid therapy. Hepatology 70(2):587 596
7. Christen L, Hintermann E (2019) (2019). Pathogens and autoimmune hepatitis. Clin Exp Immunol 195(1):35–51
8. Urganci N Kalyoncu D, Cayonu N, Erdem E, Yildirmak Y, Yilmaz B (2011) Acute live- failure, autoimmune hepatitis, and Leptospirosis: a case report. Pediatr Emerg Care 27(10):963–965

3

Melatonin-primed ADMSCs elicit an efficacious therapeutic response in improving high-fat diet induced non-alcoholic fatty liver disease in C57BL/6J mice

Aliasgar Hatimbhai Vohra[1], Kapil Kumar Upadhyay[2], Apeksha Suhas Joshi[1], Hitarthi Swetang Vyas[1], Jaymesh Thadani[3] and Ranjitsinh Vijaysinh Devkar[1*]

Abstract

Background: Stem cells are widely used for therapy including treatment of liver damage. Adipose-derived mesenchymal stem cells (ADMSCs) administered to treat fatty liver are known to improve liver function but their use is restricted due to a poor success rate. This study investigates efficacy of melatonin-primed ADMSCs (Mel. MSCs) in experimentally induced non-alcoholic fatty liver disease (NAFLD).

Results: MSCs treated with LPS showed prominent DCFDA fluorescence as compared to the untreated cells. Also, the JC-1 staining had accounted for higher intensity of green monomer and a weak fluorescence of red dimer indicating weaker mitochondrial membrane potential. But melatonin co-treatment could make necessary corrective changes as evidenced by reverse set of results. The overall cell survival was also found to be improved following melatonin treatment as evidenced by the MTT assay. Also, the antioxidant (*Nrf2* and *Ho-1*) and anti-inflammatory genes (*Il-4* and *Il-10*) showed a decrement in their mRNA levels following LPS treatment whereas the pro-inflammatory genes (*Tnf-α*, *Il-6*, *Tlr-4*, and *Lbp*) showed a reciprocal increment in the said group. Melatonin co-treatment accounted for an improved status of antioxidant and anti-inflammatory genes as evidenced by their mRNA levels. High-fat high-fructose diet (HFFD) fed C57BL/6J mice recorded higher serum AST and ALT levels and fatty manifestation in histology of liver along with lowered mRNA levels of antioxidant (*Nrf2*, *Catalase*, and *Gss*) genes and Hgf. These set of parameters showed a significant improvement in HFFD + Mel.MSC group.

Conclusion: A significant improvement in viability of MSCs was recorded due to lowered intracellular oxidative stress and improves mitochondrial membrane potential. Further, melatonin-primed MSCs accounted for a significant decrement in fatty manifestations in liver and an improved physiological status of NAFLD in HFFD fed C57BL/6J mice. Taken together, it is hypothesized that melatonin priming to MSCs prior to its use can significantly augment the success of stem cell therapy.

Keywords: Melatonin, Non-alcoholic fatty liver disease, Stem cell therapy, Adipose-derived mesenchymal stem cells, NAFLD

Background

The ability of mammalian liver to undergo reparative regeneration in condition of hepatotoxic manifestations by a single or multiple factors is well established. Non-alcoholic fatty liver disease (NAFLD) is characterized by

*Correspondence: rv.devkar-zoo@msubaroda.ac.in
[1] Division of Metabolic Physiology and Endocrinology, Department of Zoology, Faculty of Science, The Maharaja Sayajirao University of Baroda, Vadodara, Gujarat 390002, India
Full list of author information is available at the end of the article

fat accumulation and resultant inflammation in hepatocytes [1]. These early symptoms may progress from NAFLD to Non-alcoholic steatohepatitis (NASH); a transition that gets compounded by comorbidity such as type 2 diabetes, dyslipidemia and obesity [2]. Early detection and lack of single therapeutics are major challenges faced by clinicians for treating NAFLD. Current therapeutic strategy comprises of synthetic drugs used for treatment of hyperglycemia and/or hypertriglyceridemia [3]. A variety of herbal extracts and phytopharmaceuticals have also been reported to be effective against experimentally induced NAFLD owing to their antioxidant and free radical scavenging potential but due to a limited success their clinical use is restricted [4].

Stem cell-based therapies have been widely explored as an alternative to conventional therapeutic strategy wherein, mesenchymal stem cells (MSCs) have emerged as a viable option for treating NAFLD. MSCs are known for their immunomodulatory, anti-inflammatory and immunosuppressive properties in degenerative diseases [5]. MSCs are responsive to several signaling molecules such as hormones, growth factors, chemotactic molecules and cytokines [6]. Bone marrow, umbilical cord blood, and adipose tissue-derived MSCs exhibits easy acceptance as an isograft [7]. In mouse model of CCL4-induced liver fibrosis, bone marrow-derived MSCs administered via tail vein prevent liver scarring and stimulate liver regeneration [8]. Also, these MSCs could reverse high-fat diet (HFD) induced NAFLD in mice by suppressing CD4+ T lymphocytes [9]. Further, MSCs with upregulated levels of SOD and CAT could effectively reduce systemic inflammation and improve diet induced fatty liver [10]. In pre-clinical and clinical trials, MSCs are known to readily differentiate into hepatocytes [11] but a poor success rate of stem cell therapy was attributed to an inflamed microenvironment in NAFLD [12]. Subtle modifications in stem cell therapy had resulted in an improvement in ischemic acute renal failure [13], inflammatory bowel diseases [12], heart [14], lungs [7], brain [15], rheumatoid arthritis [16], periodontal ligament [17] or knee cartilage [18], and liver function in CCL4 induced liver fibrosis [19]. Hence, it is imperative to appropriately modify the stem cell therapy for a higher efficacy and success rate.

Melatonin (N-acetyl-5-methoxytryptamine), a lipophilic indoleamine tryptophan derivative is synthesized by the pineal gland, skin, retina, gastrointestinal tract and immune cells [20] and is known for regulating circadian rhythm. Also, anti-oxidant [21], anti-neoplastic, anti-inflammatory, neuroprotective [22], and anti-apoptotic properties [23] of melatonin have been reported till date. Further, melatonin induced decrement in body weight gain, increased insulin sensitivity, homeostasis of lipid and glucose metabolism and an improvement in HFD-induced NAFLD in obese mice were reported [24]. Neural stem cells treated with melatonin had lowered expression of pro-inflammatory markers [25] whereas; ADMSCs treated with melatonin underwent proliferation, stemness and self-renewal [26]. Overall, melatonin priming is known to improve the viability of a variety of transformed cells [27] including the mesenchymal stem cells [28].

In liver disorders including NASH, the anti-inflammatory potential of melatonin has been pinned as the reason for its therapeutic potential [29, 30]. Bone marrow derived MSCs have been reported to improve function of steatotic liver albeit with limited success [31]. But the merits of adipose derived MSCs in treating NAFLD and possible advantages of prior melatonin priming are not known [32]. This study is designed to evaluate the merits of melatonin priming, to adipose derived MSCs and their possible improvement in their efficacy in treating experimentally induced NAFLD.

Methods

Chemicals

Melatonin, hematoxylin, eosin, collagenase type 1, and lipopolysaccharide (LPS) were purchased from Sigma Aldrich (St. Louis, MO, USA). Methanol, ethanol, dimethyl sulphoxide (DMSO) and 3-(4, 5-dimethylthiazol-2-yl)-2, 5-diphenyl tetrazolium bromide (MTT) were purchased from Sisco Research Laboratory Pvt. Ltd. (Mumbai, India). Molecular biology reagents except iScriptcDNA synthesis kit (Bio-Rad, CA, USA) and all other reagents such as TRIzol, DreamTaq Green master mix, and SYBR select master mix were procured from Invitrogen (CA, USA). Chemicals for cell culture like Dulbecco's modified Eagle's medium (DMEM), fetal bovine serum (FBS), trypsin phosphate versene glucose (TPVG), and antibiotic-antimycotic solution were purchased from Hi-media Laboratories (Mumbai, India). ENZOPAK aspartate aminotransferase (AST), alanine transaminase (ALT), alkaline phosphatase (ALP), total lipids (TL), total cholesterol (TC), triglycerides (TG), low-density lipoprotein (LDL), very low-density lipoprotein (VLDL), high-density lipoprotein (HDL), and glucose kits were purchased from Reckon Diagnostics (Vadodara, Gujarat). RNA-later was purchased from Ambion Inc. (USA).

ADMSCs isolation, characterization, and melatonin priming

Adipose derived mesenchymal stem cells (MSCs) were isolated from 8-week-old male C57BL/6J mice (20 ± 2 g) as per Yu et al. [33]. Briefly, bilateral fat pads in retroperitoneal cavity were collected, minced in small pieces using sterile scissors, and digested (45 min in water bath at 37 °C) in equal amount of collagenase-1 in incomplete media. After the digestion, tubes were centrifuged (300 g for 5 min) and mixed vigorously for 5–10 s. This step was repeated three times to obtain a dark red cells pellet. That was resuspended in complete media and seeded in T25 flask. Media was changed once daily till the cells were 80–90% confluent. At the 4th passage cells were fixed with freshly prepared 2% Paraformaldehyde (PFA) for 10 minutes at room temperature and permeabilized with 0.1% Triton X-100 for 3–5 min on ice. AD-MSCs were examined for expression of surface markers (CD34, CD44, CD45, and CD105) by flow-cytometry. Briefly, the cultured cells were suspended in cold DPBS at the dilution of 10^6 cells/ml. Incubation with primary antibodies (CD34, CD44, CD45, and CD105) was followed by exposure to secondary conjugated antibody at 4 °C for 30 min, and the complex was analyzed by flow-cytometry. MSCs were cultured in T-25 flask and, at passage 4, were incubated in presence of 5 μM melatonin (dissolved in ethanol and diluted in saline to 5%) for 24 h [34, 35].

Cell viability (MTT) assay

Mesenchymal stem cells (6×10^3 cells/ well) were maintained in 96-well culture plates (Tarson India Pvt. Ltd.) for 24 h with or without LPS (1 and 3 μg/ml) and melatonin (5 μM). Later, 10 μl of 3-(4, 5-dimethylthiazol-2-yl)-2, 5-diphenyltetrazolium bromide (MTT, 5 mg/ml) was added to the wells and plates were incubated at 37 °C for 4 h [36]. Subsequently, the culture media was discarded and wells were washed with PBS. The resultant formazan formed was dissolved in 150 μl of DMSO and absorbance was read at 540 nm using a Synergy HTX Multimode reader (BioTek, USA).

Intracellular oxidative stress

MSCs were maintained for 24 h as mentioned above with or without LPS (1 and 3 μg/ml for 24 h) and melatonin (5μM). ROS mediated intracellular oxidative stress in MSCs was studied using 7.5 μM 2,7-dichlorodihydrofluoroscein diacetate (CM-H2-DCFDA) stain (37 °C for 30 min) [37]. Cells were photographed using Floid cell imaging station (Invitrogen, USA) and their fluorescent intensity was quantified using ImageJ (NIH, Bethesda, USA) software.

Mitochondrial membrane potential

MSCs were maintained for 24 h as mentioned above with or without LPS (1 and 3 μg/ml) and melatonin (5 μM). Mitochondrial membrane potential was assessed using 5,5′,6,6′-tetrachloro-1,1′,3,3′-tetraethylbenzimidazolcarbocyanine iodide JC-1 stain (5 μg/ml) in pre-warmed 1× PBS for 30 min at 37 °C [38, 39]. Cells were observed and photographed using Floid cell imaging station (Invitrogen, USA) and fluorescent intensity was quantified using ImageJ (NIH, Bethesda, USA) software [40].

mRNA studies of key marker genes in MSCs and liver of C57BL/6J mice

Total RNA was isolated from the MSCs and liver of control and various experimental groups using TRIzol reagent and quantified using a nanodrop spectrophotometer (Thermo scientific, Ltd.). Later, samples (A_{260}/A_{280} > 1.9) were processed for cDNA synthesis using iScript cDNA Synthesis kit (Bio-Rad, CA, USA) at 37 °C for 1 h (using a T 100 Bio-Rad 96-well thermal cycler; Bio-Rad, CA, USA). mRNA levels of key genes in MSCs (*Tlr-4, Lbp, Nrf2, Ho-1, Tnf-α, Il-6, Il-4, Il-10*) and in liver (*Nrf2, Sod, Catalase, Gss, Il-4,* and *Hgf*) were quantified by qPCR analysis (Quant-Studio-3, Life Technologies, CA, USA) using SYBR Select Master Mix [40] using primers sequences shown in Table 1. The following two steps thermal cycling profile was used for qPCR analysis, step I (cycling step): 95 °C for 10 min, 95 °C for 15 s, 60 °C for 1 min and 95 °C for 15 s for 40 cycles. step II (melt curve step): 60 °C for 15 s, 60 °C 1 min and 95 °C for 30 s.

The data obtained was normalized to the *Gapdh* (internal control) and analyzed using 2−ΔΔCT method.

Experimental animals and their treatment with MSCs

C57BL/6J mice (24 male mice; 6–8 weeks of age; 18–22 g) were procured (Zydus Research Centre) Ahmadabad, India, housed in clean polypropylene cages with laboratory chow diet and water ad libitum in Committee for the Purpose of Control and Supervision of Experiments on Animals (CPCSEA), India, approved animal house facility of Department of Zoology, The Maharaja Sayajirao University of Baroda, Vadodara, Gujarat, India (Approval No. 827/GO/Re/S/04/CPCSEA). After an acclimatization of 10 days, mice were randomly divided into 4 groups of 6 mice per group viz. Group I (fed with laboratory chow diet), groups II, III, and IV were fed with HFFD (high-fat diet + 20% Fructose through water) and water ad libitum for 16 weeks [40]. At the end of 13th week group III was treated with (1×10^6 cells in 0.2 ml) MSCs and group IV with 5 μM melatonin-primed MSCs via tail vein [19]. The experimental protocol was carried out according to the guidelines of the Committee for the Purpose of Control and Supervision of Experiments on Animals (CPCSEA), India, and approved by the Institutional Animal Ethical Committee (IAEC). Our previous study had revealed that results obtained in groups fed with normal chow diet and injected MSCs or melatonin-primed MSCs (MSC + NCD or Mel.MSC+NCD respectively) were comparable to that of control; hence they are not showcased herein (Unpublished observations).

Table 1 PCR primers sequences of the genes analyzed

Sr. no.	Gene	Forward primer	Reverse primer
1	GAPDH	5′-TGTGAACGGATTTGGCCGTA-3′	5′-ACTGTGCCGTTGAATTTGCC-3′
2	TLR-4	5′-TTTGCTGGGGCTCATTCACT-3′	5′-GACTCGGCACTTAGCACTGT-3′
3	LBP	5′-TGTTACCACATGACTCCGGC-3′	5′-AGGTGGGCAGGATCACAAAG-3′
4	NRF2	5′-CGAGATATACGCAGGAGAGGTAAGA-3′	5′-GCTCGACAATGTTCTCCAGCTT-3′
5	HO-1	5′-ACATCGACAGCCCCACCAAGTTCAA-3′	5′-CTGACGAAGTGACGCCATCTGTGAG-3′
6	TNF-α	5′-GTGGAACTGGCAGAAGAG-′	5′-AATGAGAAGAGGCTGAGAC-3′
7	IL-6	5′-TGGATGCTACCAAACTGGAT-3′	5′-CCTCAAAGCCAAGATGAGAA-3′
8	IL-4	5′-GTAGGGCTTCCAAGGTGCTT-3′	5′-GGCATCGAAAAGCCCGAAAG-3′
9	IL-10	5′-AAGGGTTACTTGGGTTGCCA-3′	5′-TTCAGCTTCTCACCCAGGGA-3′
10	HGF	5′-TGAGTTATGTGCTGGGGCTG-3′	5′-CACATCCACGACCAGGAACA-3′
11	CAT	5′-CTGGATGGATTCTCCCCCGC-3′	′-TCAGGAAACGGCATCAAAAGC-3′
12	GSS	5′-AACGAGCGAGTTGGGATG-3′	5′-TATGTCACCACGTCGGAGGA-3′
13	SOD	5′-TTGGCCTGTGGAGTGATTGG-3′	5′-AGCCCAGTCAAAGGAGTCAC-3′

Experimental procedure

At the end of 16 weeks, animals were fasted overnight and whole blood was collected by retro-orbital sinus puncture under mild isoflurane anesthesia [41–44]. Isoflurane is the most frequently used halogenated anesthetic in animal research and does not produce any significant differences in liver injury, inflammation, and regeneration [41, 44]. Whole blood was centrifuged (at 4 °C and 3000 rpm for 10 min) and serum was collected and stored. Later, mice were sacrificed using isoflurane under minimum stress and liver was collected and stored in 10% formalin (for histopathology) and in RNAlater (for mRNA studies). No mortality was observed in any of the experimental groups during the period of study.

Serum biochemical parameters

Circulating titers of enzymes indicative of liver function (AST, ALT, and ALP), fasting blood glucose [45] and serum lipid profile (TL, TC, TG, LDL, VLDL, and HDL) [46] were estimated using commercially available kits (Reckon Diagnostic kits, Vadodara, Gujarat, India).

Microscopic evaluations

Liver samples were fixed in 10% formalin for 48 h, and then embedded in paraffin. Tissues sections (5 µm thick) were deparaffinized and stained with hematoxylin and eosin (HXE) [37, 40].

Quantification of cellular immunofluorescence

Immunofluorescent images were captured using Floid cell imaging station and were analyzed using ImageJ (NIH, Bethesda, USA). Cell area, integrated density and mean gray value were measured for each selected cell. Also, mean gray values (fluorescence intensities) of four different background areas were measured in every image for normalization of background auto fluorescence. The resultant values were normalized with the background fluorescence of 4 areas. The corrected total cell fluorescence (CTCF) for each cell was calculated as [47]:

$$\text{CTCF} = \text{Integrated density} - (\text{area of cell} \times \text{mean of background flourescence})$$

Fluorescent intensities of about 70 cells from 5 to 8 different images were recorded for each experimental group for statistical analysis.

Statistical analysis

Results were expressed as means ± standard deviation (SD) and analyzed by one-way analysis of variance (ANOVA) with Bonferroni's multiple comparison tests using Graph Pad Prism 5 (CA, USA). $^{*}p < 0.05$, $^{**}p < 0.01$, and $^{***}p < 0.001$ is when LPS treated or HFFD is compared with control. $\#p < 0.05$, $\#\#p < 0.01$, and $\#\#\#p < 0.001$ is when LPS + Mel is compared with LPS-treated group.

Results

Characterization of MSCs, intracellular oxidative stress, and cell viability assay

Adipose derived mesenchymal stem cells (MSCs) were isolated from the perirenal and visceral fat pads of healthy C57BL/6J mice and were characterized using positive (CD44 and CD105) and negative (CD34 and CD45) surface markers (Figure S1). Flow cytometric studies had shown 98.18% of CD44 and 97.05% of CD105 (positive) cells. Lipopolysaccharide (LPS; 1 and 3 µg/ml) treatment accounted for a dose-dependent decrement (~

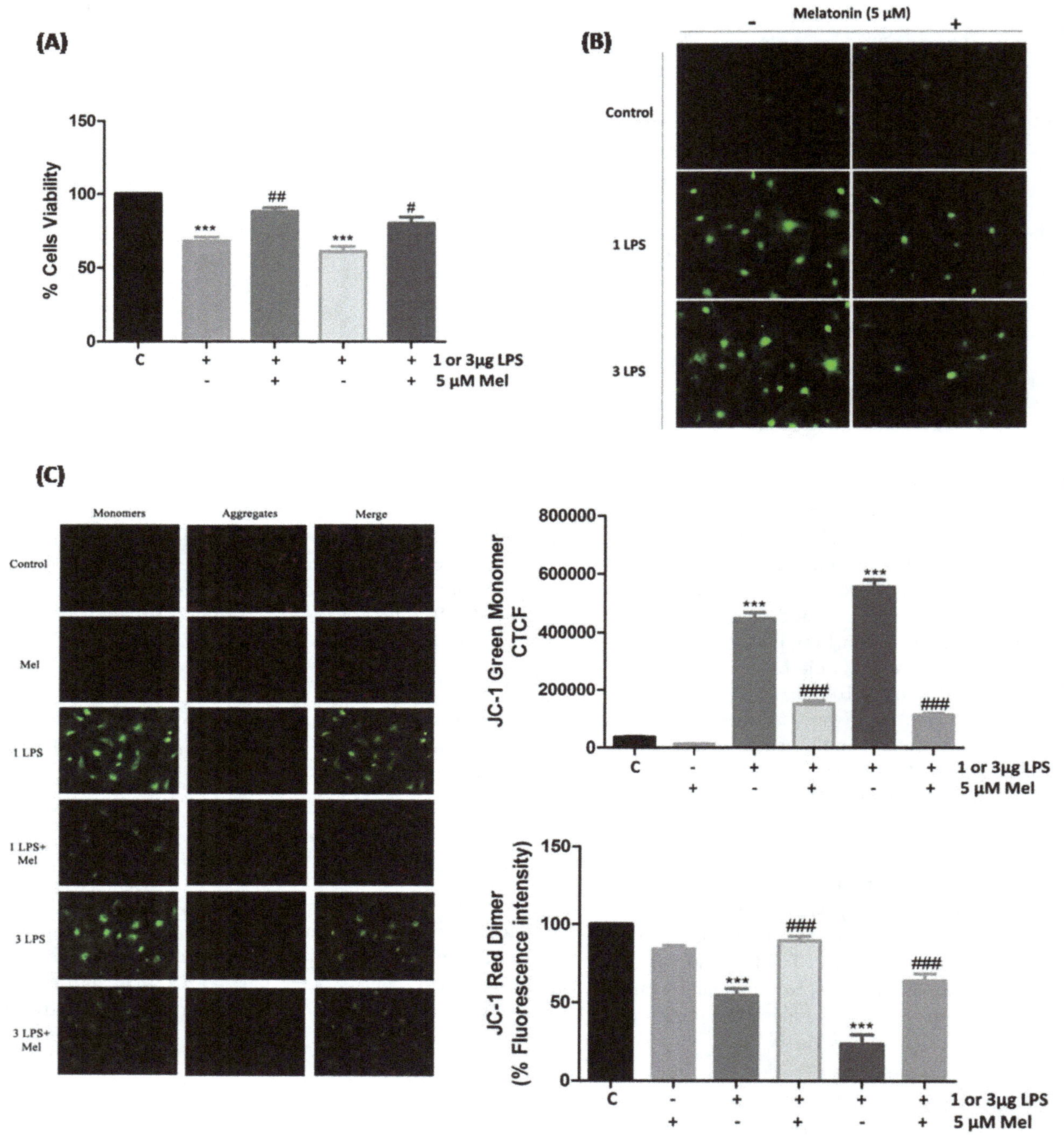

Fig. 1 Adipose-derived MSCs treated with lipopolysaccharide (LPS) and/or melatonin (Mel). Mel alleviates LPS-induced (**A**) cytotoxicity; MTT assay, (**B**) intracellular oxidative stress; DCFDA staining and (**C**) mitochondrial membrane potential; JC-1 staining. Data expressed as mean ± S.E.M. for $n = 3$. *$p < 0.05$, **$p < 0.01$, and ***$p < 0.001$ is when LPS treated is compared with control. #$p < 0.05$, ##$p < 0.01$ and ###$p < 0.001$ is when LPS + Mel is compared with LPS-treated group

25% and ~ 40% respectively; $p < 0.001$) in cell viability in MSCs as evidenced by the (MTT) assay (Fig. 1A). Also, a prominent green fluorescence in these cells was observed following DCFDA staining that implied towards a heightened intracellular oxidative stress (Fig. 1B). LPS + 5 μM melatonin co-treatment accounted for ~ 20–25%

improvement in cell viability ($p < 0.05$) and relatively weaker DCFDA fluorescence as compared to LPS-treated MSCs.

Mitochondrial membrane potential (JC-1 staining)

MSCs were stained with JC-1 to assess the changes in mitochondrial membrane potential (ΔΨm). MSCs treated with LPS (1 and 3 μg LPS doses) recorded prominent green (monomer) and weak red (dimer) fluorescence implying towards a significant decrement ($p < 0.001$) in mitochondrial membrane potential. Improvement in the fluorescence following co-treatment with 5 μM melatonin suggested an improvement ($p < 0.001$) in mitochondrial membrane potential as compared to LPS-treated groups (Fig. 1C).

mRNA levels of pro, anti-inflammatory, and antioxidant genes in MSCs

Tlr4 and *Lbp* are key genes for assessing LPS induced inflammation and, in our study, LPS treated MSCs (for 24 h) recorded a significant increase in the mRNA levels of the said genes as compared to control ($p < 0.001$) (Fig. 2A). Further, mRNA levels of *Nrf2* were non-significantly decreased following LPS treatment (Fig. 2B) thus implying towards a compromised cellular antioxidant status. LPS + Mel group accounted for lower *Tlr-4* ($p < 0.001$), *Lbp* ($p < 0.05$), and higher *Nrf2* as compared to LPS-treated group. However, *HO-1* levels were found to be elevated in all the experimental groups (Fig. 2B). Further, LPS treated MSCs recorded a significant increment in mRNA levels *Tnf-α* ($p < 0.01$) and *Il-6* ($p < 0.05$) and a decrement in *Il-4* ($p < 0.01$) and *Il-10* ($p <0.05$). Melatonin co-treatment to these cells accounted for a significant decrement in *Tnf-α* and *Il-6* mRNAs ($p < 0.01$) and; a significant increment in *Il-4* ($p < 0.001$). *Il-10* mRNA levels were found to be non-significantly higher in this group (Fig. 3A, B).

Serum AST, ALT, and lipid profile

Food and water intake of C57BL/6J mice was monitored (16 weeks) during the period of study. HFFD treatment accounted for a significant increment in body weight gain ($p < 0.001$), liver weight ($p < 0.001$), and liver:body weight ratio ($p < 0.05$) as compared to control (Figure S2, A, B).

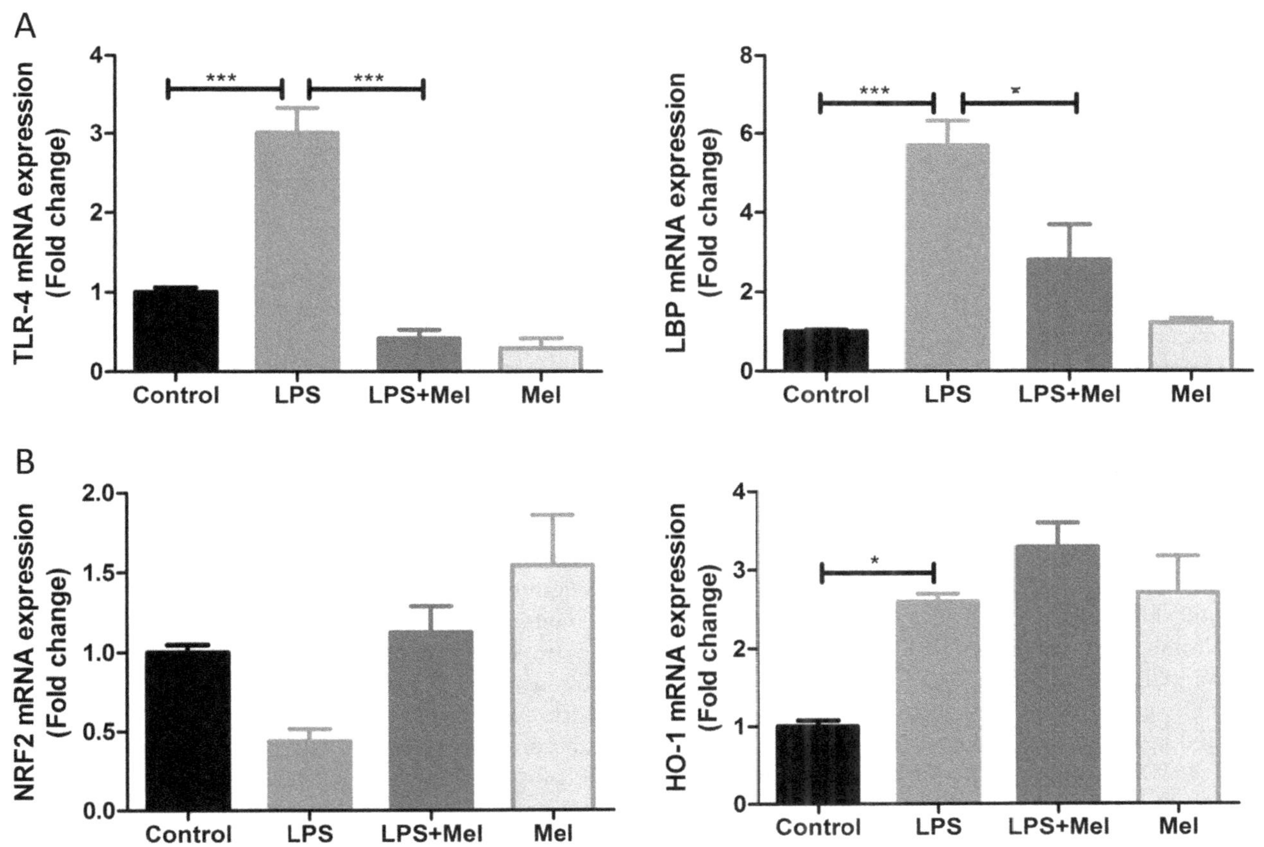

Fig. 2 mRNA levels of **a** *Tlr-4* and *Lbp* and **b** *Nrf2* and *Ho-1* following lipopolysaccharide (LPS) and/or melatonin (Mel) treatments to adipose-derived MSCs. Data expressed as mean ± S.E.M. for $n = 3$. *$p < 0.05$, **$p < 0.01$, and ***$p < 0.001$

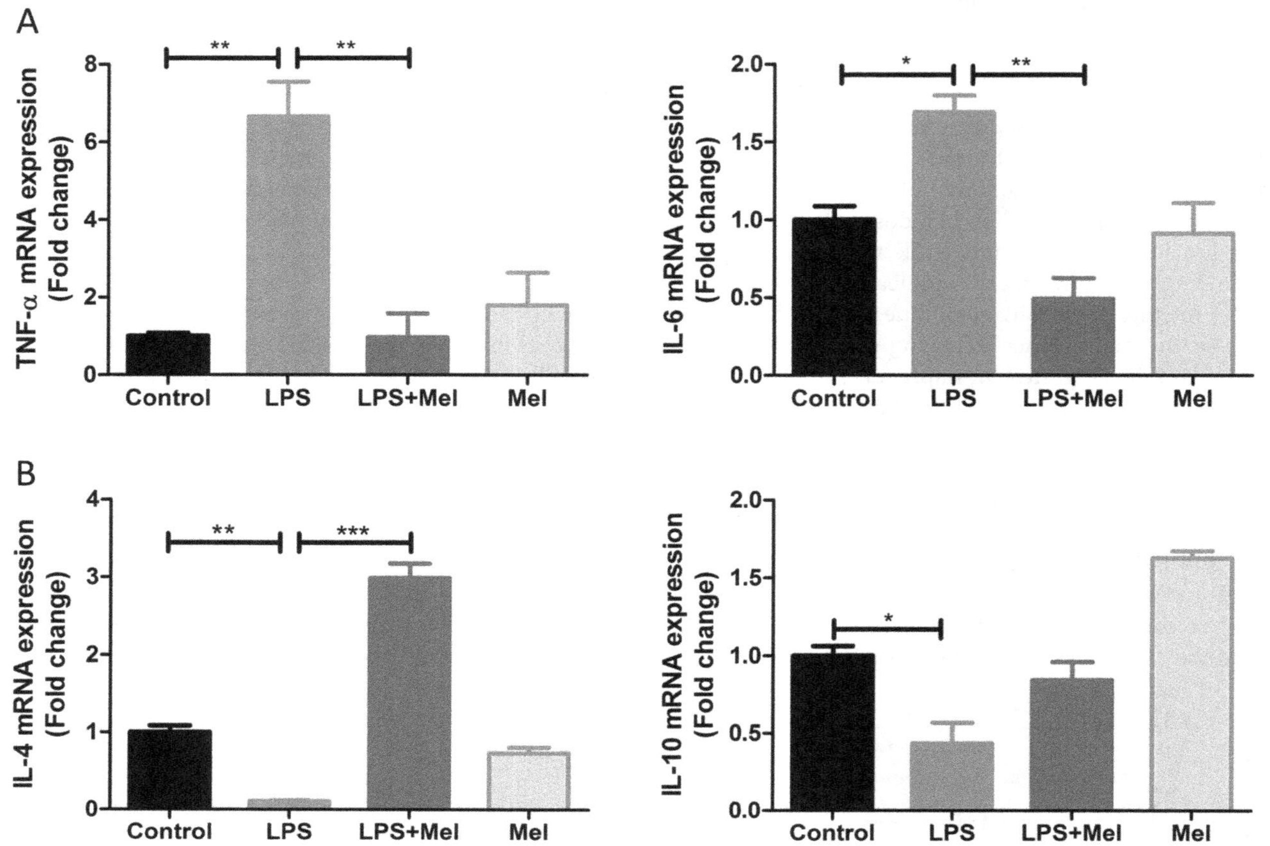

Fig. 3 m-RNA levels of **a** pro-inflammatory *Tnf-α* and *Il-6* and **b** anti-inflammatory *Il-4* and *Il-10* cytokines in adipose derived MSCs treated with lipopolysaccharide (LPS) and/or Melatonin (Mel). Data expressed as mean ± S.E.M. for $n = 3$. *$p < 0.05$, **$p < 0.01$, and ***$p < 0.001$

Significant hyperglycemia was recorded in serum ($p < 0.001$) of HFFD group but HFFD + MSCs had recorded a significantly decrement ($p < 0.001$). Also, non-significant hyperglycemia was recorded in HFFD + melatonin-primed MSCs (Mel.MSC) group. Circulating titers of serum AST and ALT were significantly elevated in the HFFD group ($p < 0.001$) but, MSC and Mel.MSC groups accounted for a significant decrement in titers of the ALT ($p < 0.01$) and AST ($p < 0.05$). ALP levels did not show any significant alterations in all the experimental groups (Fig. 4).

Significantly higher levels of serum total lipids ($p < 0.01$), total cholesterol ($p < 0.001$), triglycerides ($p < 0.01$), and LDL cholesterol ($p < 0.001$) were recorded in HFFD group whereas; significant decrement was recorded in serum HDL-cholesterol ($p < 0.05$). Though, HFFD + MSC group had recorded non-significant decrements in total lipids, total cholesterol, triglycerides, LDL cholesterol, and VLDL cholesterol, a significant increment in HDL cholesterol ($p < 0.05$) was recorded in this group. A similar trend was witnessed in HFFD + Mel.MSC group with respect to the said parameters wherein, decrements in total lipids ($p < 0.05$), total cholesterol ($p < 0.01$), and LDL cholesterol ($p < 0.01$) were significant (Fig. 5).

Histological assessment of liver tissue

The liver tissue sections showed normal hepatic cords radiating from the central vein and a preserved hepatic architecture. Also, the hepatocytes were polygonal and of uniform size with granular cytoplasm. The cells in vicinity of the portal vein showed healthy cellular characteristics. Liver of HFFD group showed distorted hepatic cords, ballooning hepatocytes with rarefied cytoplasm and macrovesicular steatosis. Also, the infiltration of inflammatory cells was evident in the said tissue. Treatment of HFFD fed mice with MSCs or Mel.MSCs led to a visible decrement in the fatty hepatocytes and macrovesicular steatosis. Overall, a normal cellular architecture could be observed in these groups with minimal infiltration of cells due to inflammation (Fig. 6).

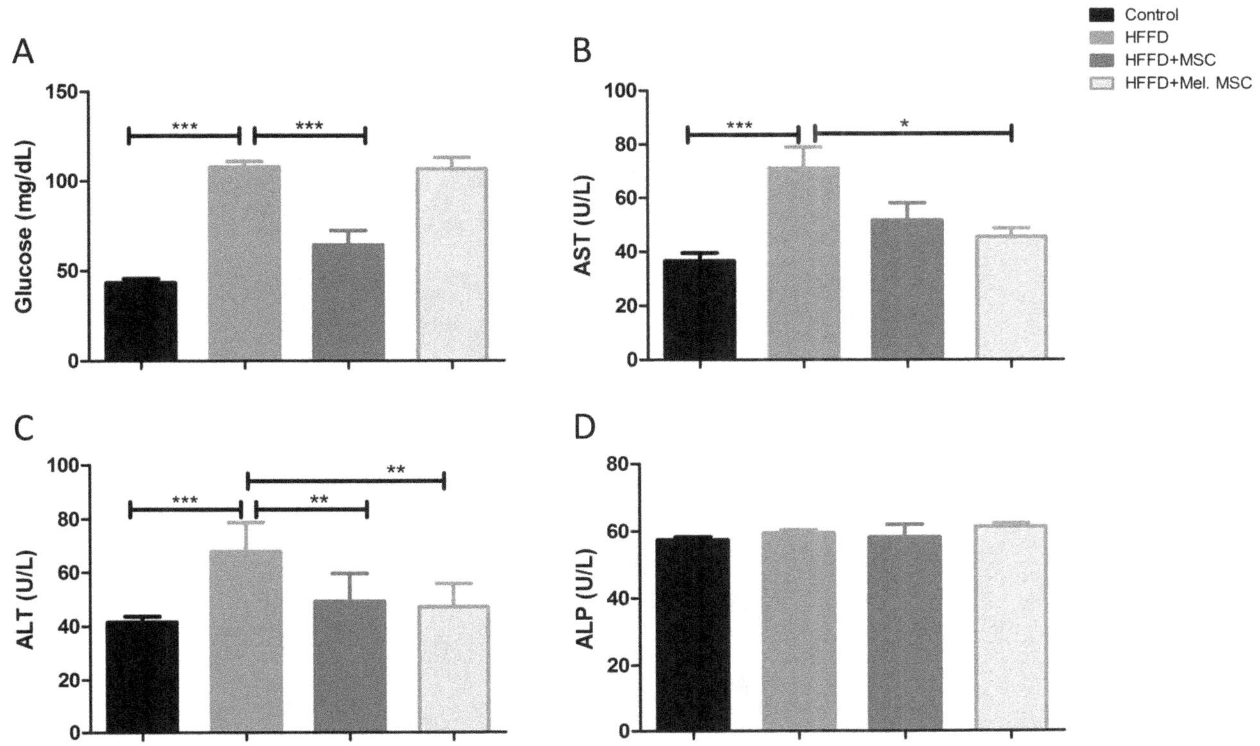

Fig. 4 Alterations in serum (**A**) glucose and liver markers (**B**), AST (**C**), ALT (**D**) ALP on high-fat high-fructose diet (HFFD), HFFD + adipose-derived mesenchymal stem cell (MSC) therapy (HFFD + MSC) and HFFD + melatonin (Mel) primed MSC therapy (HFFD + Mel.MSC). Data expressed as mean ± S.E.M. for $n = 6$. *$p < 0.05$, **$p < 0.01$, and ***$p < 0.001$

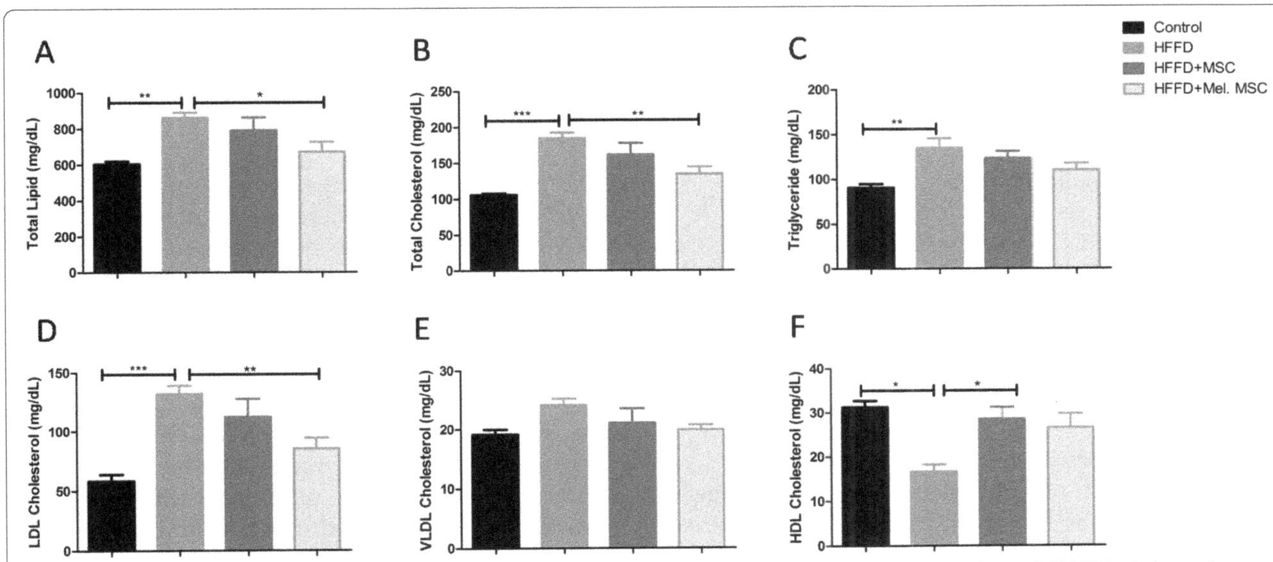

Fig. 5 Alterations in lipid markers (**A**) total lipids; TL (**B**) total cholesterol; TC (**C**) triglyceride; TG (**D**) LDL cholesterol; LDL-C (**E**) VLDL cholesterol; VLDL-C (**F**) HDL cholesterol; HDL-C. Data expressed as mean ± S.E.M. for $n = 6$. *$p < 0.05$, **$p < 0.01$, and ***$p < 0.001$

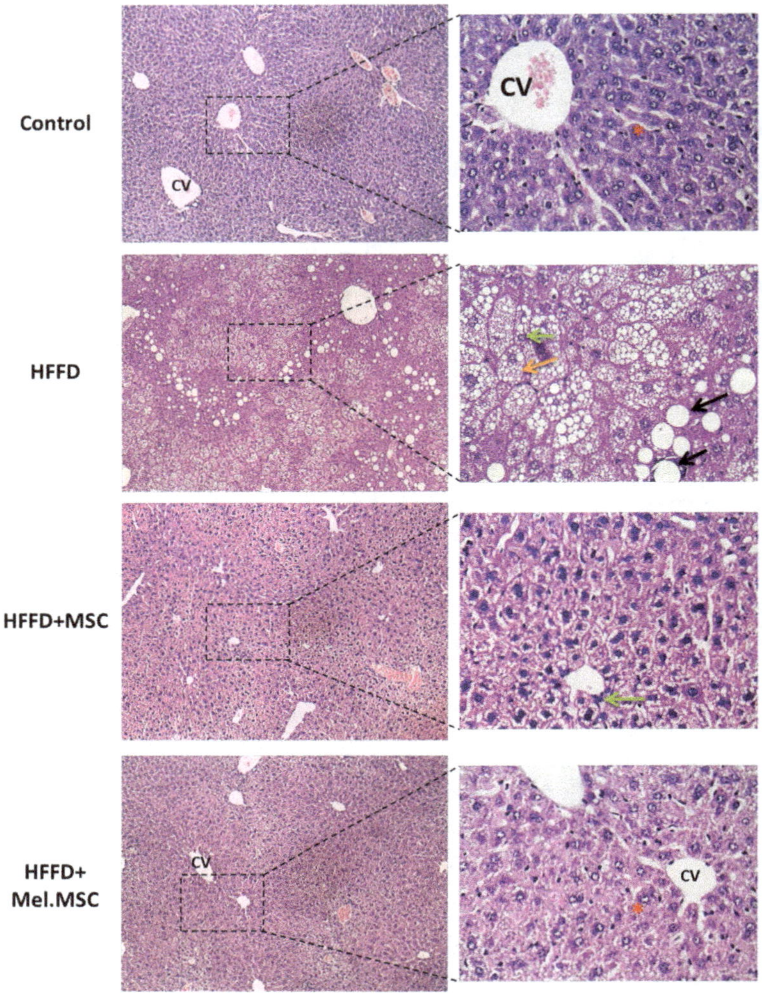

Fig. 6 Photomicrographs of liver: Control group showing normal of hepatic cords (orange star) radiating from the central vein (CV). HFFD group showing macrovesicular steatosis (black arrow), ballooning degeneration with rarefied cytoplasm (orange arrow) and infiltration of inflammatory cells (green arrow). HFFD + MSC and HFFD + Mel.MSC groups showing normal hepatic cords, moderate infiltration of inflammatory cells without any fatty manifestations

mRNA levels of hepatic *Nrf2*, *Sod*, *Catalase*, and *Gss*

HFFD group had recorded a decrement in mRNA levels of *Catalase* and *Gss* whereas; the *Nrf2* and *Sod* levels were unchanged. However, *Nrf2* ($p < 0.01$), *catalase* ($p < 0.01$), and *Gss* ($p < 0.01$) mRNA were higher in HFFD + MSC and HFFD + Mel.MSC groups. The mRNA levels of *Sod* showed non-significant changes in all these experimental groups (Fig. 7).

mRNA levels of hepatic *Il-4* and *Hgf*

The mRNA levels of anti-inflammatory marker gene *Il-4* was found to be lowered in HFFD group. However, both HFFD + MSC ($p < 0.01$) and HFFD + Mel.MSC ($p < 0.001$) groups had recorded significant increment in mRNA levels of *Il-4*. *Hgf* has a mitogenic property in liver and accounts for its regeneration. In our study, all the three experimental groups had recorded an increment in mRNA levels of *Hgf* with the most significant increase recorded in HFFD + Mel.MSC group ($p < 0.05$) (Fig. 7).

Discussion

The observations made in this study suggest that administration of MMSCs in HFFD-fed mice results in improvement in functional status and histological features of liver. Currently there is no single US-FDA-approved pharmacological drug for treatment of NAFLD or NASH. The complications associated with liver transplantation create the earnest need for alternative

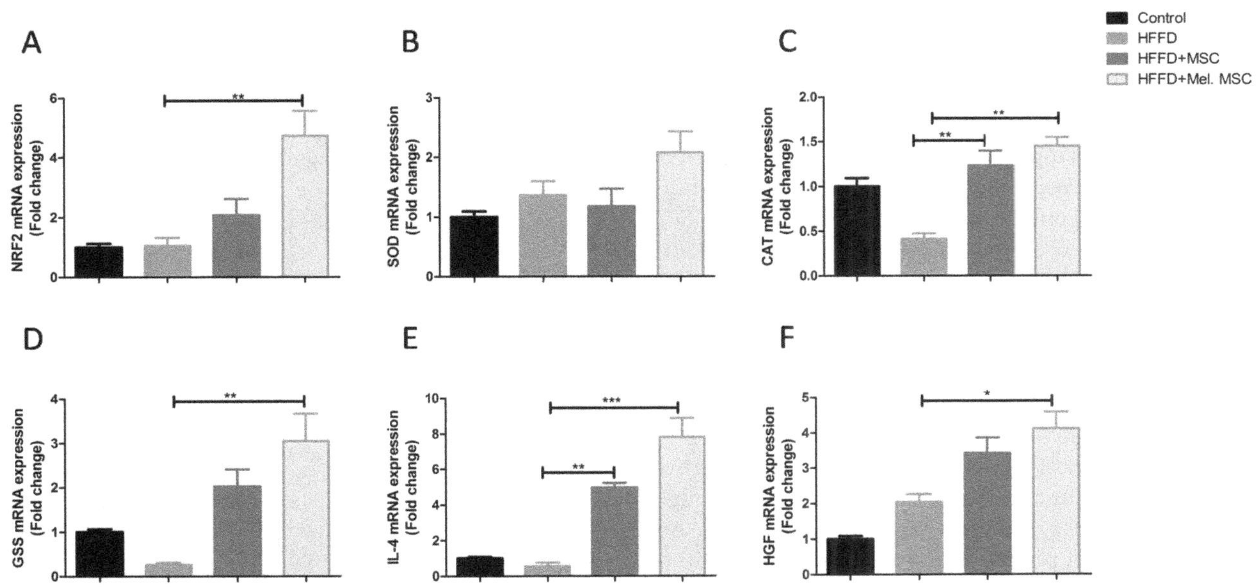

Fig. 7 m-RNA expression of markers **A** *Nrf2*, **B** *Sod*, **C** *Cat*, **D** *Gss*, **E** *Il-4*, and **F** *Hgf* in hepatic tissue of control, HFFD, HFFD + MSC, and HFFD + Mel. MSC. Data expressed as mean ± S.E.M. for $n = 6$. $^{*}p < 0.05$, $^{**}p < 0.01$, and $^{***}p < 0.001$

therapeutic options. Stem cell therapy had shown varying degrees of success in treating liver diseases but an inflamed hepatic microenvironment often results in low survival ratio of transplanted cells [48]. In the present study, melatonin-primed adipose derived mesenchymal stem cells (MSCs) were administered to high-fat high-fructose diet (HFFD) fed mice and the possible improvement in success rate of transplant with respect to liver function was put to scrutiny. Based on the anti-oxidant attributes of melatonin we had hypothesized that melatonin primed MSCs can possibly improve the functional status of a fatty liver. Intracellular oxidative stress and mitochondrial dysfunction plays a crucial role in various cellular activities including cell growth, survival and death. Research groups had shown that exogenous stressors such as tert-butyl hydroperoxide (t-BHP), hydrogen peroxide (H_2O_2), tumor necrosis factor alpha (TNF-α), or lipopolysaccharides (LPS) produced an heightened intracellular oxidative stress in a variety of cell lines [49]. Also, LPS treatment causing mitochondrial ROS production in microglial cells with an upregulation of pro-inflammatory mediators [50]. In bone marrow-derived macrophages, LPS induced ROS signaling has been reported to be downregulated in the inner mitochondrial membrane UCP2 (uncoupling protein 2) [51]. Also, LPS mediated production of nitric oxide (NO) and ROS that leads to nuclear translocation of NF-κB in murine macrophages. In our study, LPS-treated MSCs symbolize an inflamed microenvironment in a fatty liver. Hence, an improvement in toxicity indices, intracellular oxidative stress, and mitochondrial membrane potential of LPS + melatonin-treated MSCs generates the 'proof of concept' and forms the basis of our study.

LPS-mediated activation of SIRT1/NRF2 pathway and the resultant oxidative stresses have been reported to be attenuated following melatonin treatment [52]. Also, studies with human ADMSCs had reported an upregulation of cellular prion protein (PrPC) and lowered ER stress in ADMSCs treated with melatonin [53]. Melatonin is also known to prevent senescence of canine ADMSCs by activating *Nrf2* via MT1/MT2 receptors [54]. Hence, the observed upregulation of *Nrf2* mRNA following melatonin treatment recorded in our study is in agreement with the published reports. LPS mediated inflammatory changes in kupffer cells and upregulation of TLR4 and LBP has reported [55]. In our study, melatonin treatment could successfully alleviate changes in the said parameters and further had accounted for a decrement in mRNA levels of pro-inflammatory markers (*Tnf-α* and *Il-6*) and increment in anti-inflammatory markers (*Il-4* and *Il-10*). These observations corroborate with reported upregulation of anti-inflammatory markers that inhibit synthesis and release of pro-inflammatory markers [56]. Overall, this part of the study had justified the use of melatonin in alleviating LPS induced inflammation and had accounted for an improved survival status of MSCs.

Mesenchymal stem cells have been reported to differentiate into hepatocyte like cells and contributing towards an improved liver function [11]. Also BMMSCs have been reported to improve CCL-4 induced liver fibrosis in mice [8]. Melatonin pre-treatment to ADMSCs had reduced apoptosis in an ischemic diseases model [57] and had improved homing of MSCs in liver of CCL4 treated rats [19]. Hepatocellular injury like apoptosis and ballooning or enlarged hepatocytes with a clear reticular cytoplasm are characteristic features of NAFLD and have been reported in HFD fed [40], MCD diet fed [58], and gene knockout mouse models [59, 60]. The said changes occur in correlation with higher circulating titers of total cholesterol and triglycerides [40, 61]. In our study, the liver of HFFD fed mice showed fatty changes in hepatocytes, macrovesicular steatosis, infiltration of inflammatory cells and elevated parameters of serum lipid profile. However, an improvement in the said histological parameters is attributable to the administration of MSCs that are known to improve hepatic histoarchitecture and liver function through an autocrine and/or paracrine mechanism [62, 63]. An improved status of serum lipid profile and higher titers of HDL-c in melatonin primed MSC treated group are indicative of improved systemic lipid load and metabolism. An improvement in physiological status of fatty liver (lower AST and ALT) observed in experimental group treated with melatonin primed MSCs are the highlight of our study.

The mechanism of repair of fatty liver is yet unclear but study by Domingues et al. (2019) had reported that antioxidant-upregulated MSCs have lower oxidative stress, systemic inflammation and an improved liver function in high-fat diet induced obesity in [10]. Also, UC-MSCs could ameliorate NAFLD and regulate lipid metabolism by increasing the expression of fatty acid oxidation genes in *db/db* mice [60]. Further, upregulation of SOD and downregulation of apoptotic markers in melatonin primed MSCs had resulted in lowering of ROS production. In our study, an increment in the expression of *Sod*, *Gss*, and *Nrf2* in Mel.MSC group is in agreement with these reports. A recent study from our lab had shown that carbon monoxide releasing molecule A-1 had led to an improved oxidative stress and mitochondrial function in a steatotic liver of C57BL/6J mice via activation of NRF2-ARE pathway [40]. Hence, the observed improvement in fatty changes in liver of Mel.MSC mice is possibly mediated via an improved intracellular antioxidant status orchestrated by NRF-ARE pathway that needs further scrutiny. Reports of an improved homing of stem cells following melatonin priming have been reported in experimentally induced liver toxicity in rats [19] and the same can also be assumed to be responsible for an improvement in the therapeutic response and status of HFFD-fed NAFLD mice following Mel.MSC treatment.

Conclusions

Therapeutic response of ADMSCs shows an improvement in HFFD-mediated NAFLD in C57BL/6J mice by priming the cells with melatonin. Overall, melatonin priming of MSCs is an effective therapeutic strategy that can be scaled-up for bench-to-bedside studies involving lifestyle disorders.

Abbreviations

ALT: Alanine aminotransferase; AST: Aspartate aminotransferase; CM-H2-DCFDA: 2,7-dichlorodihydrofluoroscein diacetate; CTCF: Corrected total cell fluorescence; DMEM: Dulbecco's; : modified Eagle's medium; DMSO: Dimethyl sulphoxide; FBS: Fetal bovine serum; HDL-C: High-density lipoprotein cholesterol; HFD: High-fat diet; HFFD: High-fat high-fructose diet; HXE: Hematoxylin and eosin; JC-1: 5,5′,6,6′-tetrachloro-1,1′,3,3′-tetraethylbenzim idazolcarbocyanine iodide; LPS: Lipopolysaccharide; Mel.MSC: Melatonin-primed MSCs; Mel: Melatonin; MSCs: Mesenchymal stem cells; MTT: 3-(4, 5-dimethylthiazol-2-yl)-2, 5-diphenyl tetrazolium bromide; NAFLD: Non-alcoholic fatty liver disease; NASH: Non-alcoholic steatohepatitis; NO: Nitric oxide; PrPC: Cellular prion protein; RT-PCR: Reverse transcriptase polymerase chain reaction; TC: Total cholesterol; TG: Triglycerides; TL: Total lipids; TPVG: Trypsin phosphate versene glucose; UCP2: Uncoupling protein 2; VLDL: Very low-density lipoprotein.

Acknowledgements

Authors acknowledge Prof. Rajesh Singh, Department of Biochemistry, MSU Baroda for use of thermal cycler and Dr. Kishore Rajput, Department of Botany, MSU Baroda for microscopy. Valuable inputs by Ms. Kavita Shirsath are also duly acknowledged.

Authors' contributions

Study was conceptualized and executed by AHV and RVD. ASJ performed the animal experimentation and biochemical studies. HSV and JT performed stem cell isolation and in vitro experimentation. AHV and KKU performed the microscopy studies. Manuscript was written by AHV and RVD. All authors have read and approved the final manuscript.

Declarations

Ethics approval and consent to participate

All animal experiments were in compliance with the ethical standards of the Committee for the Purpose of Control and Supervision of Experiments on Animals (CPCSEA), India, with prior approved by Institutional Animal Ethical Committee (IAEC), Department of Zoology, The Maharaja Sayajirao University of Baroda (MSU/Z/IAEC/05-2017).

Competing interests

The authors declare that they have no competing interests.

Author details

[1]Division of Metabolic Physiology and Endocrinology, Department of Zoology, Faculty of Science, The Maharaja Sayajirao University of Baroda, Vadodara, Gujarat 390002, India. [2]Department of Internal Medicine, Division of Gastroenterology & Hepatology, University of Michigan Medical School, Ann Arbor, Michigan, USA. [3]Total Potential Cells (P) Ltd., 1st floor Parimal Majumdar Wada, Pratap road, Raopura, Vadodara, Gujarat 390001, India.

References

1. Rakha M, Saleh O, Abdelgawad MS, El Baiomy A (2021) Helicobacter pylori infection in patients with metabolic syndrome, with or without nonalcoholic fatty liver disease. Egypt Liver J 11:1–9
2. Awaad AK, Kamel MA, Mohamed MM, Helmy MH, Youssef MI, Zaki EI, Essawy MM, Hegazy MGA (2020) The role of hepatic transcription factor cAMP response element-binding protein (CREB) during the development of experimental nonalcoholic fatty liver: a biochemical and histomorphometric study. Egypt Liver J 10:1–13
3. Oni ET, Agatston AS, Blaha MJ, Fialkow J, Cury R, Sposito A, Erbel R, Blankstein R, Feldman T, Al-Mallah MH (2013) A systematic review: burden and severity of subclinical cardiovascular disease among those with nonalcoholic fatty liver; should we care? Atherosclerosis 230:258–267
4. Jadeja R, Devkar RV, Nammi S (2014) Herbal medicines for the treatment of nonalcoholic steatohepatitis: current scenario and future prospects. Evid-Based Complement Altern Med 2014:1–19
5. Bulut O, Gürsel İ (2020) Mesenchymal stem cell derived extracellular vesicles: promising immunomodulators against autoimmune, autoinflammatory disorders and SARS-CoV-2 infection. Turk J Biol 44:273–282
6. Bolamperti S, Guidobono F, Rubinacci A, Villa I (2019) The role of growth hormone in mesenchymal stem cell commitment. Int J Mol Sci 20:5264
7. Ortiz LA, Gambelli F, McBride C, Gaupp D, Baddoo M, Kaminski N, Phinney DG (2003) Mesenchymal stem cell engraftment in lung is enhanced in response to bleomycin exposure and ameliorates its fibrotic effects. Proc Natl Acad Sci 100:8407–8411
8. Sakaida I, Terai S, Yamamoto N, Aoyama K, Ishikawa T, Nishina H, Okita K (2004) Transplantation of bone marrow cells reduces CCl4-induced liver fibrosis in mice. Hepatology 40:1304–1311
9. Wang H, Zhang H, Huang B, Miao G, Yan X, Gao G, Luo Y, Chen H, Chen W, Yang L (2018) Mesenchymal stem cells reverse high-fat diet-induced non-alcoholic fatty liver disease through suppression of CD4+ T lymphocytes in mice. Mol Med Rep 17:3769–3774
10. Domingues CC, Kundu N, Kropotova Y, Ahmadi N, Sen S (2019) Antioxidant-upregulated mesenchymal stem cells reduce inflammation and improve fatty liver disease in diet-induced obesity. Stem Cell Res Ther 10:1–10
11. Ju S, Teng G-J, Lu H, Jin J, Zhang Y, Zhang A, Ni Y (2010) In vivo differentiation of magnetically labeled mesenchymal stem cells into hepatocytes for cell therapy to repair damaged liver. Investig Radiol 45:625–633
12. Tsuchiya A, Kojima Y, Ikarashi S, Seino S, Watanabe Y, Kawata Y, Terai S (2017) Clinical trials using mesenchymal stem cells in liver diseases and inflammatory bowel diseases. Inflamm Regen 37:1–15
13. Togel F, Hu Z, Weiss K, Isaac J, Lange C, Westenfelder C (2005) Administered mesenchymal stem cells protect against ischemic acute renal failure through differentiation-independent mechanisms. Am J Physiol Physiol 289:F31–F42
14. Wang X-J, Li Q-P (2007) The roles of mesenchymal stem cells (MSCs) therapy in ischemic heart diseases. Biochem Biophys Res Commun 359:189–193
15. Harting MT, Jimenez F, Xue H, Fischer UM, Baumgartner J, Dash PK, Cox CS (2009) Intravenous mesenchymal stem cell therapy for traumatic brain injury. J Neurosurg 110:1189–1197
16. Liu Y, Mu R, Wang S, Long L, Liu X, Li R, Sun J, Guo J, Zhang X, Guo J (2010) Therapeutic potential of human umbilical cord mesenchymal stem cells in the treatment of rheumatoid arthritis. Arthritis Res Ther 12:1–13
17. Nisa GÜL, Gökmen K, Yandim MK, Aysun A, Baran Y (2018) A minimally invasive transfer method of mesenchymal stem cells to the intact periodontal ligament of rat teeth: a preliminary study. Turk J Biol 42:382–391
18. Westminster CO, Westminister CO, Vail CO, Busse D (2008) Increased knee cartilage volume in degenerative joint disease using percutaneously implanted, autologous mesenchymal stem cells. Pain Physician 11:343–353
19. Mortezaee K, Pasbakhsh P, Kashani IR, Sabbaghziarani F, Omidi A, Zendedel A, Ghasemi S, Dehpour AR (2016) Melatonin pretreatment enhances the homing of bone marrow-derived mesenchymal stem cells following transplantation in a rat model of liver fibrosis. Iran Biomed J 20:207
20. Lynch HJ, Ozaki Y, Shakal D, Wurtman RJ (1975) Melatonin excretion of man and rats: effect of time of day, sleep, pinealectomy and food consumption. Int J Biometeorol 19:267–279
21. Rodriguez C, Mayo JC, Sainz RM, Antolín I, Herrera F, Martín V, Reiter RJ (2004) Regulation of antioxidant enzymes: a significant role for melatonin. J Pineal Res 36:1–9
22. Alghamdi BS (2018) The neuroprotective role of melatonin in neurological disorders. J Neurosci Res 96:1136–1149
23. Sainz RM, Mayo JC, Reiter RJ, Antolín I, Esteban MM, Rodríguez C (1999) Melatonin regulates glucocorticoid receptor: an answer to its antiapoptotic action in thymus. FASEB J 13:1547–1556
24. Sun H, Wang X, Chen J, Song K, Gusdon AM, Li L, Bu L, Qu S (2016) Melatonin improves non-alcoholic fatty liver disease via MAPK-JNK/P38 signaling in high-fat-diet-induced obese mice. Lipids Health Dis 15:1–8
25. Li H, Zhang Y, Liu S, Li F, Wang B, Wang J, Cao L, Xia T, Yao Q, Chen H (2019) Melatonin enhances proliferation and modulates differentiation of neural stem cells via autophagy in hyperglycemia. Stem Cells 37:504–515
26. Heo JS, Pyo S, Lim J, Yoon DW, Kim BY, Kim J, Kim GJ, Lee SG, Kim J (2019) Biological effects of melatonin on human adipose-derived mesenchymal stem cells. Int J Mol Med 44:2234–2244
27. Shah SA, Khan M, Jo M, Jo MG, Amin FU, Kim MO (2017) Melatonin stimulates the SIRT 1/Nrf2 signaling pathway counteracting lipopolysaccharide (LPS)-induced oxidative stress to rescue postnatal rat brain. CNS Neurosci Ther 23:33–44
28. Rodríguez-Lozano FJ, García-Bernal D, de los Ángeles Ros-Roca M, del Carmen Algueró M, Onate-Sánchez RE, Camacho-Alonso F, Moraleda JM (2015) Cytoprotective effects of melatonin on zoledronic acid-treated human mesenchymal stem cells in vitro. J Cranio-Maxillofacial Surg 43:855–862
29. Solís-Muñoz P, Solís-Herruzo JA, Fernández-Moreira D, Gómez-Izquierdo E, García-Consuegra I, Muñoz-Yagüe T, García Ruiz I (2011) Melatonin improves mitochondrial respiratory chain activity and liver morphology in ob/ob mice. J Pineal Res 51:113–123
30. Stacchiotti A, Grossi I, García-Gómez R, Patel GA, Salvi A, Lavazza A, De Petro G, Monsalve M, Rezzani R (2019) Melatonin effects on non-alcoholic fatty liver disease are related to microRNA-34a-5p/Sirt1 axis and autophagy. Cells 8:1053
31. Wang H, Wang D, Yang L, Wang Y, Jia J, Na D, Chen H, Luo Y, Liu C (2017) Compact bone-derived mesenchymal stem cells attenuate nonalcoholic steatohepatitis in a mouse model by modulation of CD4 cells differentiation. Int Immunopharmacol 42:67–73
32. Mishra A, Paul S, Swarnakar S (2011) Downregulation of matrix metalloproteinase-9 by melatonin during prevention of alcohol-induced liver injury in mice. Biochimie 93:854–866
33. Yu G, Wu X, Kilroy G, Halvorsen Y-DC, Gimble JM, Floyd ZE (2011) Isolation of murine adipose-derived stem cells. In: Adipose-Derived Stem Cells. Springer, pp 29–36
34. Ara C, Kirimlioglu H, Karabulut AB, Coban S, Hascalik S, Celik O, Yilmaz S, Kirimlioglu V (2005) Protective effect of melatonin against oxidative stress on adhesion formation in the rat cecum and uterine horn model. Life Sci 77:1341–1350
35. Uz T, Giusti P, Franceschini D, Kharlamov A, Manev H (1996) Protective effect of melatonin against hippocampal DNA damage induced by intraperitoneal administration of kainate to rats. Neuroscience 73:631–636
36. Thounaojam MC, Jadeja RN, Valodkar M, Nagar PS, Devkar RV, Thakore S (2011) Oxidative stress induced apoptosis of human lung carcinoma (A549) cells by a novel copper nanorod formulation. Food Chem Toxicol 49:2990–2996
37. Upadhyay KK, Jadeja RN, Thadani JM, Joshi A, Vohra A, Mevada V, Patel R, Khurana S, Devkar RV (2018) Carbon monoxide releasing molecule A-1 attenuates acetaminophen-mediated hepatotoxicity and improves survival of mice by induction of Nrf2 and related genes. Toxicol Appl Pharmacol 360:99–108
38. Cai B, Li X, Wang Y, Liu Y, Yang F, Chen H, Yin K, Tan X, Zhu J, Pan Z (2013) Apoptosis of bone marrow mesenchymal stem cells caused by homocysteine via activating JNK signal. PLoS One 8:e63561
39. Huang D, Yin L, Liu X, Lv B, Xie Z, Wang X, Yu B, Zhang Y (2018) Geraniin protects bone marrow-derived mesenchymal stem cells against hydrogen peroxide-induced cellular oxidative stress in vitro. Int J Mol Med 41:739–748
40. Upadhyay KK, Jadeja RN, Vyas HS, Pandya B, Joshi A, Vohra A, Thounaojam MC, Martin PM, Bartoli M, Devkar RV (2020) Carbon monoxide releasing

molecule-A1 improves nonalcoholic steatohepatitis via Nrf2 activation mediated improvement in oxidative stress and mitochondrial function. Redox Biol 28:101314

41. Janssen BJA, De Celle T, Debets JJM, Brouns AE, Callahan MF, Smith TL (2004) Effects of anesthetics on systemic hemodynamics in mice. Am J Physiol Circ Physiol 287:H1618–H1624
42. Dardai E, Heavner JE (1987) Respiratory and cardiovascular effects of halothane, isoflurane and enflurane delivered via a Jackson-Rees breathing system in temperature controlled and uncontrolled rats. Methods Find Exp Clin Pharmacol 9:717–720
43. Njoku D, Laster MJ, Gong DH, Eger EI, Reed GF, Martin JL (1997) Biotransformation of halothane, enflurane, isoflurane, and desflurane to trifluoroacetylated liver proteins: association between protein acylation and hepatic injury. Anesth Analg 84:173–178
44. He S, Atkinson C, Qiao F, Chen X, Tomlinson S (2010) Ketamine–xylazine–acepromazine compared with isoflurane for anesthesia during liver transplantation in rodents. J Am Assoc Lab Anim Sci 49:45–51
45. Andersson U, Bränning C, Ahrné S, Molin G, Alenfall J, Önning G, Nyman M, Holm C (2010) Probiotics lower plasma glucose in the high-fat fed C57BL/6J mouse. Benefic Microbes 1:189–196
46. Shirsath K, Joshi A, Vohra A, Devkar R (2021) Chronic photoperiodic manipulation induced chronodisruption upregulates HSP60 during early pro-atherogenic remodeling in thoracic aorta of C57BL/6J mice. J Basic Appl Zool 82:1–10
47. Shirsath K, Joshi A, Vohra A, Devkar R (2021) HSP60 knockdown exerts differential response in endothelial cells and monocyte derived macrophages during atherogenic transformation. Sci Rep 11:1–17
48. Kuo TK, Hung S, Chuang C, Chen C, Shih YV, Fang SY, Yang VW, Lee OK (2008) Stem cell therapy for liver disease: parameters governing the success of using bone marrow mesenchymal stem cells. Gastroenterology 134:2111–2121
49. Menon D, Coll R, Board PG (2014) Glutathione transferase omega 1 is required for the lipopolysaccharide-stimulated induction of NADPH oxidase 1 and the production of reactive oxygen species in macrophages. Free Radic Biol Med 73:318–327
50. Wang J, Li L, Wang Z, Cui Y, Tan X, Yuan T, Liu Q, Liu Z, Liu X (2018) Supplementation of lycopene attenuates lipopolysaccharide-induced amyloidogenesis and cognitive impairments via mediating neuroinflammation and oxidative stress. J Nutr Biochem 56:16–25
51. Emre Y, Hurtaud C, Nübel T, Criscuolo F, Ricquier D, Cassard-Doulcier A-M (2007) Mitochondria contribute to LPS-induced MAPK activation via uncoupling protein UCP2 in macrophages. Biochem J 402:271–278
52. Arioz BI, Tastan B, Tarakcioglu E, Tufekci KU, Olcum M, Ersoy N, Bagriyanik A, Genc K, Genc S (2019) Melatonin attenuates LPS-induced acute depressive-like behaviors and microglial NLRP3 inflammasome activation through the SIRT1/Nrf2 pathway. Front Immunol 10:1511
53. Lee JH, Yoon YM, Han Y, Jung SK, Lee SH (2019) Melatonin protects mesenchymal stem cells from autophagy-mediated death under ischaemic ER-stress conditions by increasing prion protein expression. Cell Prolif 52:e12545
54. Fang J, Yan Y, Teng X, Wen X, Li N, Peng S, Liu W, Donadeu FX, Zhao S, Hua J (2018) Melatonin prevents senescence of canine adipose-derived mesenchymal stem cells through activating NRF2 and inhibiting ER stress. Aging (Albany NY) 10:2954
55. Su GL, Klein RD, Aminlari A, Zhang HY, Steinstraesser L, Alarcon WH, Remick DG, Wang SC (2000) Kupffer cell activation by lipopolysaccharide in rats: role for lipopolysaccharide binding protein and toll-like receptor 4. Hepatology 31:932–936
56. Cassatella MA, Meda L, Bonora S, Ceska M, Constantin G (1993) Interleukin 10 (IL-10) inhibits the release of proinflammatory cytokines from human polymorphonuclear leukocytes. Evidence for an autocrine role of tumor necrosis factor and IL-1 beta in mediating the production of IL-8 triggered by lipopolysaccharide. J Exp Med 178:2207–2211
57. Lee JH, Han Y, Lee SH (2017) Potentiation of biological effects of mesenchymal stem cells in ischemic conditions by melatonin via upregulation of cellular prion protein expression. J Pineal Res 62:e12385
58. Jung Y-A, Choi Y-K, Jung G-S, Seo H-Y, Kim H-S, Jang BK, Kim J-G, Lee I-K, Kim M-K, Park K-G (2014) Sitagliptin attenuates methionine/choline-deficient diet-induced steatohepatitis. Diabetes Res Clin Pract 105:47–57
59. Wortham M, He L, Gyamfi M, Copple BL, Wan Y-JY (2008) The transition from fatty liver to NASH associates with SAMe depletion in db/db mice fed a methionine choline-deficient diet. Dig Dis Sci 53:2761–2774
60. Li B, Cheng Y, Yu S, Zang L, Yin Y, Liu J, Zhang L, Mu Y (2019) Human umbilical cord-derived mesenchymal stem cell therapy ameliorates nonalcoholic fatty liver disease in obese type 2 diabetic mice. Stem Cells Int 2019:1-12
61. Jadeja RN, Thounaojam MC, Dandekar DS, Devkar RV, Ramachandran AV (2010) Clerodendron glandulosum. Coleb extract ameliorates high fat diet/fatty acid induced lipotoxicity in experimental models of non-alcoholic steatohepatitis. Food Chem Toxicol 48:3424–3431
62. Driscoll J, Patel T (2019) The mesenchymal stem cell secretome as an acellular regenerative therapy for liver disease. J Gastroenterol 54:763–773
63. Zhang S, Chen L, Liu T, Zhang B, Xiang D, Wang Z, Wang Y (2012) Human umbilical cord matrix stem cells efficiently rescue acute liver failure through paracrine effects rather than hepatic differentiation. Tissue Eng part A 18:1352–1364

4

Role of bile acids in the prediction of hepatocellular carcinoma in HCV-induced liver cirrhosis

Ashraf Khalil[1*], Azza Elsheashaey[1,2], Eman Abdelsameea[3], Manar Obada[1], F. F. Mohamed Bayomy[1,2] and Hala El-Said[1]

Abstract

Background: Bile acids are essential organic molecules synthesized from cholesterol in the liver and regarded as indicators of hepatobiliary impairment; however, their role in the pathogenesis of hepatocellular carcinoma (HCC) is still unclear. The study aimed to examine the feasibility of bile acids in distinguishing HCC from post hepatitis C virus liver cirrhosis. A UPLC/MS was used to measure 14 bile acids in patients with noncirrhotic HCV disease ($n = 50$), cirrhotic HCV disease ($n = 50$), hepatocellular carcinoma ($n = 50$), and control group ($n = 50$).

Results: The progression of liver cirrhosis to HCC was associated with a significant increase in serum bile acids compared to the normal or the noncirrhotic HCV disease ($p < 0.05$). The fold changes in bile acids concentrations showed a trend that HCC > cirrhotic HCV disease > noncirrhotic HCV disease. Four conjugated acids GCA, GCDCA, GUDCA, and TCDCA steadily increased across the different groups. ROC curves analysis revealed that these bile acids discriminated noncirrhotic liver patients from HCC (AUC 0.850–0.963), with a weaker potential to distinguish chronic liver cirrhosis from HCC (AUC 0.414–0.638).

Conclusion: The level of serum bile acid was associated primarily with liver cirrhosis, with little value in predicting the progress of chronic liver cirrhotic disease into hepatocellular carcinoma.

Keywords: Cirrhosis, Hepatocellular carcinoma (HCC), Liquid chromatography-mass spectrometry; Metabolic profiling

Background

Bile acids constitute more than 20 molecules synthesized by the liver as primary bile acids cholic acid (CA) and chenodeoxycholic acid (CDCA) then modified by intestinal bacteria into secondary bile acids deoxycholic acid (DCA), lithocholic acid (LCA), and ursodeoxycholic acid (UDCA). Conjugation of the bile acids through the enterohepatic circulation results in more water-soluble bile acids and thus protecting against hepatic cellular damage from the toxic hydrophobic bile acids, which can induce oxidative stress and cell death signaling [1].

Numerous studies related liver cirrhosis to the changes in bile acid metabolism, and high serum bile acids can distinguish liver cirrhosis with higher sensitivity than the traditional liver function tests [2–4]. Bile acids metabolism has a role in cellular processes related to carcinogenesis, e.g., elevated intracellular concentrations of bile acids were associated with oxidative stress and DNA damage both in adult and fetal liver [5, 6]. Bile acid may trigger apoptosis by directly activating the Fas death receptor or through mitochondrial dysfunction secondary to oxidative damage. Therefore, the disturbance in bile acid metabolism could be an early clue in the development of HCC, which is aggressive cancer, with around 90% of cases developing from pre-existing liver cirrhosis [7–10]. Early detection of HCC remains a challenge as it is typically diagnosed at advanced stages [11, 12], and

* Correspondence: ashkalil2010@gmail.com
[1]Department of Biochemistry and Molecular Diagnostics, National Liver Institute, Menoufia University, Shebeen El kom, Egypt
Full list of author information is available at the end of the article

there are no clinically approved alternatives to alpha-fetoprotein (AFP) that could form a noninvasive test for early detection of HCC. AFP had a low sensitivity as 40% of HCC patients have normal AFP levels, and only 20% of patients with early HCC have elevated AFP levels [13]. Des-gamma-carboxyprothrombin and lectin-bound AFP (AFP-L3), glypican-3, Osteopontin, or high c-met expression were hypothesized as alternatives, but their sensitivity for HCC remains unsatisfactory especially, for small lesions [14–18]. In this study, a metabolomics approach applying, ultra-performance liquid chromatography coupled with mass spectrometry was conducted to characterize 14 bile acids profiles in the serum of patients with post HCV noncirrhotic liver disease, in HCV cirrhotic liver disease, and post HCV complicating HCC patients, as potential markers for HCC.

Patients

The study was carried out in the Departments of Biochemistry and Molecular diagnostics of the National Liver Institute hospital, Menouffia University, Egypt, from October 2017 to August 2018 and included three groups. The HCV-noncirrhotic liver disease (NCLD) group (n = 50) enrolled patients with a documented HCV infection for ≥ 6 months without any clinical or imaging (ultrasound and fibro scan) evidence of liver cirrhosis. The post hepatitis C cirrhotic liver disease (CLD) group (n = 50) enrolled patients with liver cirrhosis secondary to previous HCV infection. The post hepatitis C liver cirrhosis complicated with HCC group (n = 50) enrolled patients whose HCC developed on the existing liver cirrhosis complicating chronic HCV infection. The NHC group (n = 50) enrolled normal, healthy subjects, matching the age and the gender of the other groups with no clinical, laboratory, or imaging sign of liver cirrhosis or focal hepatic lesions. NHC subjects were also free from any other cancers, diabetes mellitus, and obesity and were abstinent from drug abuse and alcohol consumption.

Inclusion criteria

Liver cirrhosis based on the established clinical findings, liver function tests, and positive serological tests (anti-HCV antibody and HCV- RNA PCR tests), fibro scan ≥ 14.5kPa, and liver ultrasound confirming the characteristic echogenic pattern of liver cirrhosis. The noncirrhotic patients had a history of HCV infection ≥ 6 months with positive serological tests without evidence of liver cirrhosis by fibro scan and ultrasound examination of the liver [19]. HCC diagnosis by imaging consisting of single or multiple focal hepatic lesion(s) associated with elevated serum AFP > 200 ng/ml and or detection of HCC by histological examination of the liver biopsy. The study used the standard Child-Pugh classification in CLD and HCC groups [20] and the Barcelona Clinic Liver Cancer (BCLC) staging system to stage HCC [21]. No history of alcohol intake or illicit drug abuse in all patients enrolled in the study.

Exclusion criteria

Patients having both HCV and HBV infection, chronic cholestasis, and obstructive gall bladder diseases, liver disease associated with severe renal or systemic diseases as cardiovascular, DM, and obesity were excluded.

Ethical considerations

The research ethics committees of the National Liver Institute (IRB00003425), Menouffia University, approved the research proposal and the protocols to comply with national research guidelines. Patients provided informed written consent for the use of tissue for research purposes.

Methods

Chemicals and reagents

HPLC grade methanol, acetonitrile, and formic acid were purchased from Fisher Scientific (Daytona plus, Randox laboratories limited, UK). Bile acid standards are as follows: cholic acids (CA), chenodeoxycholic acid CDCA, deoxycholic acid DCA, lithocholic acid LCA, ursodeoxycholic acid UDCA, glycocholic acid (GCA), glycochenodeoxycholic acid (GCDCA), glycodeoxycholic acid (GDCA), glycoursodeoxycholic acid (GUDCA), taurocholic acid (TCA), taurochenodeoxycholic acid (TCDCA), taurodeoxycholic acid (TDCA), tauroursodeoxycholic acid (TUDCA), and taurolithocholic acid (TLCA) from Sigma Chemical Sigma-Aldrich (Sysmex KX-21, Sysmex Inc., Japan). HPLC grade water from Millipore pure water purification system (Diamond TII, USA).

Serum sample collection

Five milliliters of blood were collected from patient and control subjects after overnight fasting about 8–12 h, under a sterile venipuncture, and the extracted serum was stored at − 80 °C until UPLC analysis. Blood chemistry was measured by an automatic biochemical analyzer (Bachman Ltd, London, UK).

Serum sample preparation and bile acid detection

Serum bile acids were prepared for UPLC/MS/MS as described in [22]. One hundred microliters of the serum sample mixed with 400 µl of ice-cold methanol were centrifuged at 12500 *rpm* for 20 min, and then 50 µl of the supernatant was added to 100 µl of the mobile phase A (0.001% formic acid) where 5 µl was injected into a C18 column (1.7 µm, 100 mm × 2.1 mm internal dimensions) of the ultra-performance liquid chromatography at 50 °C (Waters ACQUITY, Milford, MA). The mass spectrometer had an electrospray source operated in the negative ion mode using the multiple reactions monitoring (MRM). Each bile acid was eluted by gradient at a flow rate of 0.5 ml/min, for 2 min with 80% mobile phase A (0.001 formic acid in water) and 20% mobile phase B (acetonitrile), then with a linear gradient of 20% mobile phase B over 5 min followed by mobile phase B at (80%) for 8 min. At the end of each cycle, the column was equilibrated with 80% mobile phase A for 2 min. UPLC-MS raw data obtained with MRM mode were analyzed using Target Lynx application manager version 4.1 (Waters Corp., Milford, MA) to get the quantitative concentration of each bile acid.

Calibration curves and method assessment

Seven serially diluted standard calibration points, ranging from 0.125 to 20 μmol/l, and three quality control (QC) standards points 0.2, 2, and 20 μmol/l were prepared from the 14 bile acids mixture and the QC standard in charcoal-stripped serum. Calibrators and QC standards underwent the sample preparation process described before and were used to calibrate the machine. Calibration curves confirmed that bile acids had a linear response, with a coefficient of determination (R2) ≥ 0.99. The recovery was evaluated by comparing the mean detector response of the extracted QC samples at 0.2, 2, and 20 μmol/l in triplicates to the mean detector response of the post-extracted serum blanks spiked at equal concentrations. The accuracy and precision were checked regularly before any assay using three replicates of freshly prepared QC standard samples at 0.2, 2, and 20 μmol/l. Accuracy was calculated from the formula % relative error (RE) [% (measured-theoretical)/theoretical concentration]. Precision was calculated from the formula relative standard deviation (%RSD = % standard deviation/mean). The developed UPLC-MS/MS assay

Table 1 Demographic, clinical, and hematological parameter of the enrolled groups

	NHC	NCLD	CLD	HCC
Age, mean (range)	45 (34–73)	46 (36–69)^{NS}	46 (37–70)^{NS}	46 (37–69)^{NS}
BMI (kg/m^2)	23.5 ± 0.4	23.6 ± 0.3^{NS}	22.9 ± 0.3^{NS}	23.4 ± 0.3^{NS}
Sex				
Male	25 (50%)	19 (38%)	29 (58%)	15 (30%)
Female	25 (50%)	31 (62%)	21 (42%)	35 (70%)
AFP ng/ml, median (IQR)	1.7 (0.8)	2.3 (1.2) ^{NS}	3.7 (4.4)*	68.4 (877)*
Child-Pugh class, A/B/C			38 (76%)/8 (16%)/4 (8%)	18 (36%)/17 (34%)/15 (30%)
HFL, single/multiple				19 (38%)/31 (62%)
Metastasis, No/Yes				46 (92%)/4 (8%)
Lymph node, No/yes				43 (86%)/7 (14%)
PV invasion, No/yes				50 (100%)/0 (0%)
Barcelona, HCC stage A/B/C				36 (72%)/10 (20%)/4 (8%)
AST (IU/L)	20.7 ± 6.5	39.8 ± 34.4*	56.6 ± 35*	55.4 ± 29.2*
ALT (IU/L)	20.2 ± 8.6	41.3 ± 36.7*	41.9 ± 44.2*	31.9 ± 18.5*
GGT (IU/ml)	23 ± 13	35 ± 22*	71 ± 53*	73 ± 61*
ALP (IU/ml)	60.3 ± 22.6	74.5 ± 47 ^{NS}	113.5 ± 57*	117.2 ± 49.2*
TBil (mg/dl)	0.5 ± 0.2	0.6 ± 0.3*	1.5 ± 1.6*	1.5 ± 1.2*
DBil (mg/dl)	0.2 ± 0.1	0.2 ± 0.1 ^{NS}	1.2 ± 1.7*	0.8 ± 0.7*
ALB (g/dl)	4 ± 0.2	4.7 ± 0.3	3.5 ± 0.8*	3.3 ± 0.7*
TP (mg/dl)	7 ± 0.9	8 ± 0.4 ^{NS}	8 ± 0.7 ^{NS}	7 ± 0.7*
Hb (g/l)	134 ± 12	131 ± 15 ^{NS}	119.8 ± 20*	120 ± 20*
Platelets x (10^9/l)	290.9 ± 72.2	259 ± 91 ^{NS}	132.3 ± 63.8*	128.7 ± 63.1*
WBCs x (10^9/l)	7.3 ± 1.4	6.9 ± 1.5 ^{NS}	5.4 ± 2.3*	5 ± 1.9*

NHC normal healthy control, *CLD* cirrhotic liver diseases, *HCC* hepatocellular carcinoma. *N* = 50 for each group, value = mean ± standard deviation, median; *IQR* interquartile range, **P* value < 0.05 indicates significance when NHC compared to NCLD, CLD, and HCC. ^{NS}*P* value > 0.05 indicates non significance when NHC compared to NCLD, CLD, and HCC. *BMI* body mass index, *HFL* hepatic focal lesion, *PV* portal vein, *AST* aspartate transaminase, *ALT* alanine transaminase, *GGT* gamma-glutamyl transferase, *ALP* alkaline phosphatase, *TBil* total bilirubin, *DBiL* direct bilirubin, *TP* total protein, *Alb* albumin, *Hb* hemoglobin, *WBCs* white blood cells

method had the capability of quantitation of all the 14 bile acids included in the study. The assay performance was accurate and precise for bile acid analysis in the human serum [22].

Statistical analysis

Data were analyzed using SPSS 23 (SPSS Inc., CA, USA). The nonparametric Kruskal Wallis test and the Mann-Whitney test were used to detect the significance in multiple comparisons. The receiver operating characteristic (ROC) curve was used to assess the ability of bile acids to distinguish healthy subjects from patients with liver diseases. AUC ≥ 0.8 was considered as a significant test result to discriminate between two groups. Youden's index or J obtained from equation J = [(sensitivity + specificity) − 1] was applied to select a cutoff, where the sensitivity and the specificity are maximal. Pearson correlation analysis was used to assess relationships between the serum bile acids and AFP. Multivariate analysis was used to detect the predictive potential of bile acids to HCC [23, 24].

Results

Clinical characteristics and laboratory parameters of study groups

Table 1 presents the anthropometric and clinical parameters of the NCLD, CLD, and HCC groups. Patients were matched by age, gender, and body mass index (BMI) to control the biological and lifestyle confounders. These parameters did not show any significant differences across groups, all $P > 0.05$. In the NCLD group, all 50 patients had a well-compensated liver function. In the CLD group, the patients were Child-Pugh A (n = 38), Child-Pugh B (n = 8), and Child-Pugh C (n = 4). The HCC patients were Child-Pugh A (n = 18), Child-Pugh B (n = 17), and Child-Pugh C (n = 15). According to Barcelona staging system HCC group were stage A (n = 13), stage B (n = 10), and stage C (n = 7). HCC patients had either single focal lesion (n = 19) or multiple focal lesions (n = 31), lymph node involvement (n = 7), or distant metastasis (n = 4), but none had portal vein invasion. The laboratory parameters showed that CLD and HCC groups had a significant increase in AST, ALT, TBil, DBil, GGT, ALP, and AFP with a significant decrease in total protein TP, Alb, Hb, WBCs, and platelets relative to the control group, (all $P < 0.05$). However, there was no statistically significant difference between the NCLD group and the NHC regarding DBil, TP, Hb, and WBCs (all $P > 0.05$). The levels of DBil, GGT, and ALP increased while the level of Alb, TP, Hb, and platelets decreased in cirrhotic patients compared to NCLD or NHC (all $P < 0.05$).

Serum bile acid patterns in different stages of liver impairments

Table 2 presents the comparison of serum bile acids across the four groups. The progress of liver disease was associated with an increase in the serum level of bile acids. The serum bile acids were significantly higher in CLD and HCC groups than either NCLD or NHC groups. Eight bile

Table 2 Serum bile acids and fold changes in the studied groups

BA	NHC	NCLD	CLD	HCC	F, NCLD	F, CLD	F, HCC
CA	0.20 ± 0.3	0.6 ± 1.7 NS	0.5 ± 0.86*	1.7 ± 4*	3*	3*	9*
CDCA	0.38 ± 0.51	0.73 ± 1.2 NS	1.45 ± 1.91*	5.1 ± 14*	2*	4*	13*
DCA	0.15 ± 0.16	0.19 ± 0.11*	0.31 ± 0.40 NS	0.25 ± 0.39 NS	1	2*	2*
LCA	0.01 ± 0.03	0.03 ± 0.05*	0.05 ± 0.09*	0.11 ± 0.20*	3*	4*	9*
UDCA	0.04 ± 0.1	0.04 ± 0.08 NS	1.56 ± 5.01*	1.99 ± 6*	1	38*	48*
GCA	0.24 ± 0.33	0.43 ± 0.77 NS	3.77 ± 4.06*	8.4 ± 13*	2*	16*	35*
GCDCA	0.45 ± 0.66	0.86 ± 1.04*	7.7 ± 11.5*	12.5 ± 17*	2*	17*	29*
GDCA	0.24 ± 0.36	0.26 ± 0.33 NS	1.48 ± 2.9*	1.72 ± 7.2 NS	1	6*	7*
GUDCA	0.15 ± 0.2	0.07 ± 0.12*	5.2 ± 12.9*	9.4 ± 30*	0.5	35*	38*
TCA	0.01 ± 0.05	0.04 ± 0.09*	1.7 ± 2.7*	7.05 ± 16*	3*	113*	473*
TCDCA	0.11 ± 0.18	0.07 ± 0.15 NS	4.77 ± 13.8*	9.1 ± 16*	0.7	44*	83*
TDCA	0.07 ± 0.15	0.02 ± 0.03 NS	0.19 ± 0.36 NS	1.6 ± 6 NS	0.3	3*	24*
TLCA	0.006 ± 0.028	0.001 ± 0.002*	0.02 ± 0.07*	0.08 ± 0.3*	0.3	4*	13*
TUDCA	0.04 ± 0.12	0.01 ± 0.02NS	0.09 ± 0.37 NS	0.90 ± 5.17 NS	0.3	2*	18*

NHC normal healthy control, *NCLD* noncirrhotic liver disease, *CLD* cirrhotic liver diseases, *HCC* hepatocellular carcinoma. N = 50, number of each group, values: mean ± standard deviation of bile acids (μM/L); F, fold changes relative to NHC. *P value < 0.05 indicates significance when NHC compared to either NCLD, CLD, or HCC. NSP value > 0.05 indicates significance when NHC compared to either NCLD, CLD, or HCC

CA cholic acid, *CDCA* chenodeoxycholic acid, *DCA* deoxycholic acid, *LCA* lithocholic acid, *UDCA* ursodeoxycholic acid, *GCA* glycholic acid, *GCDCA* glycochenodeoxycholic acid, *GDCA* glycodeoxycholic acid, *GUDCA* glycoursodeoxycholic acid, *TCA* taurocholic acid, *TCDCA* taurochenodeoxycholic acid, *TDCA* taurodeoxycholic acid, *TLCA* taurolithocholic acid, *TUDCA* tauroursodeoxycholic acid

acids (CA, CDCA, UDCA, TCA, GCA, GUDCA, TCDCA, and GCDCA) were significantly higher in CLD and HCC than in NHC or NCLD (all $P < 0.05$). The fold change of bile acids relative to the NHC showed a pattern that HCC > CLD > NCLD, and the increase in the fold was mainly prominent in conjugated bile acids.

Serum bile acids as potential marker of chronic liver impairment

ROC analysis of the 14 serum bile acids evaluated the ability of bile acids to discriminate HCC from liver cirrhosis. Figure 1 displayed the results of the ROC curves of the 14 bile acids and their diagnostic performance. Five conjugated bile acids (GCA, GCDCA, GUDCA, TCA, and TCDCA) had the best diagnostic performance to separate HCC from NHC with AUC ranging from (0.792–0.963, all $p < 0.05$) and to separate HCC from NCLD with AUC ranging from (0.795–0.966, all $p < 0.05$). Bile acids did not discriminate HCC from CLD with AUC ranged from (0.414–0.638, *all* $p > 0.05$). Table 3 summarizes the AUC, sensitivity, and specificity of the 14 bile acids at the cutoff points detected by Youden's index of the ROC curves.

The interaction of the serum bile acids with the clinicopathological aspect of HCC

Table 4 presents the correlation between AFP and bile acids and multivariate analysis between bile acids and the clinicopathological parameter of HCC. Correlation analysis showed that among the 14 bile acids, CA, $r = 0.285$ $p < 0.001$; LCA, $r = 0.126$ $p < 0.033$; TCA, $r = 0.117$ $p < 0.048$; TLCA, $r = 0.128$ $p < 0.031$; and TUDCA, $r = 0.656$ $p < 0.001$ were positively correlated with AFP.

Multivariate analysis of the clinicopathological feature of HCC (number of the focal lesion, lymph node involvement, metastasis, Child-Pugh score, and Barcelona stage of the disease) revealed that TLCA correlated with three of these clinical parameters, namely, lymph node involvement, number of focal lesions, and the Barcelona stage of HCC. GDCA is associated with metastasis. DCA, TDCA, and TLCA correlated with the Barcelona stage. Five bile acids, one primary and four conjugated bile acids (CDCA, GCA, GDCA, GUDCA, and TUDCA), are associated with the Child-Pugh score. Five bile acids (CA, GCDCA, LCA, TCDCA, and UDCA) did not correlate with any of these clinical parameters and were statistically insignificant ($P > 0.05$).

Discussion

The study characterized the metabolic profile of 14 bile acids associated with different stages of liver diseases complicating chronic HCV infection in matched groups of patients with NCLD, LCD, and HCC utilizing a metabolomics approach employing ultrahigh-performance liquid chromatography-tandem mass spectrometry. The

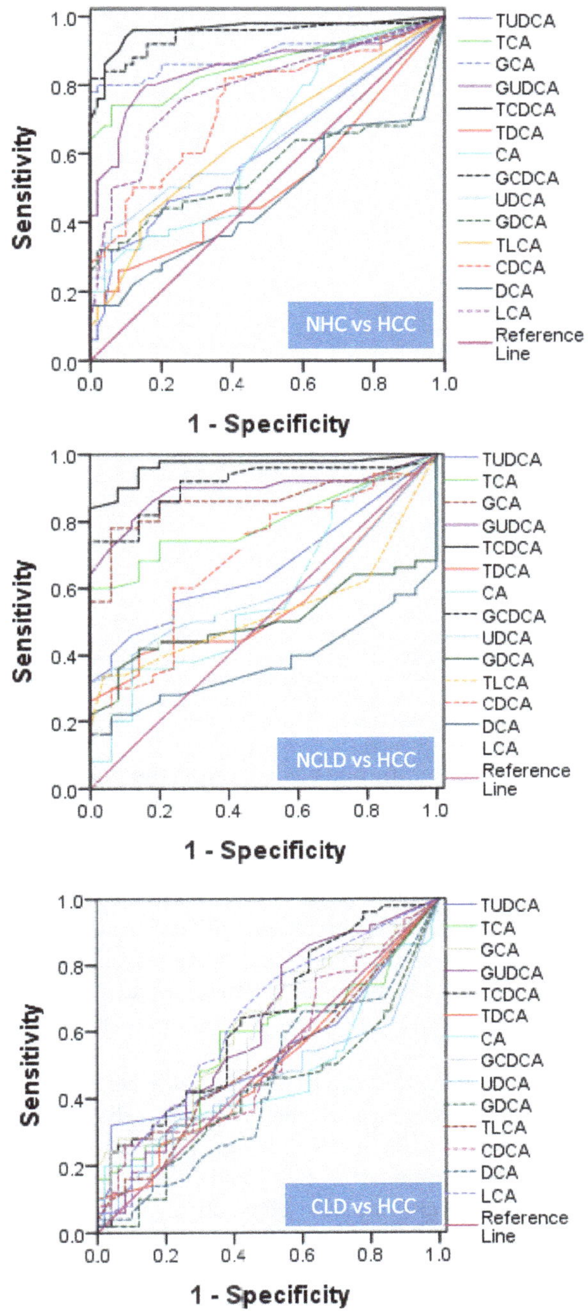

Fig. 1 Receiver operating characteristic curves for the 14 bile acids in the NHC, NCLD, and HCC: the corresponding analytical data obtained from ROC curve analysis including AUC, the cutoff point at the Youden's index, the sensitivity, and the specificity of each bile acid are summarized in Table 3. NHC, normal healthy control; NCLD, noncirrhotic liver disease; CLD, cirrhotic liver diseases; HCC, hepatocellular carcinoma; TUDCA, tauroursodeoxycholic acid; TCA, taurocholic acid; GCA, glycholic acid; GUDCA, glycoursodeoxycholic acid; TCDCA, taurochenodeoxycholic acid; TDCA, taurodeoxycholic acid; CA, cholic acid; GCDCA, glycochenodeoxycholic acid; UDCA, ursodeoxycholic acid; GDCA, glycodeoxycholic acid; TLCA, taurolithocholic acid; CDCA, chenodeoxycholic acid; DCA, deoxycholic acid; LCA, lithocholic acid

Table 3 Analytical data obtained from ROC curve analysis of 14 Bile acid. The AUC, the cutoff point at the Youden's index, the sensitivity, and the specificity of each bile acid

BA	NHC vs. HCC				NCLD vs. HCC				CLD vs HCC			
	AUC	Cutoff	Sen%	Spe%	AUC	Cutoff	Sen%	Spe%	AUC	Cutoff	Sen%	Spe%
CA	0.640	0.005	88	34	0.577	0.35	36	88	0.469	2.9	20	98
CDCA	0.743	0.215	82	62	0.684	0.51	60	76	0.532	3.35	26	92
DCA	0.470	0.55	16	100	0.375	0.365	22	94	0.442	0.045	66	40
LCA	0.792	0.001	76	74	0.614	0.035	50	80	0.638	0.001	76	48
UDCA	0.643	0.12	38	94	0.594	0.325	32	100	0.447	0.325	32	78
GCA	0.889	1.55	78	100	0.859	1.35	78	94	0.626	1.45	78	46
GCDCA	0.948	1.705	84	96	0.910	3.15	74	100	0.584	3.1	74	48
GDCA	0.558	1.015	32	98	0.502	0.405	42	86	0.414	32.2	2	100
GUDCA	0.850	0.22	80	84	0.891	0.15	86	82	0.612	0.215	80	46
TCA	0.859	0.025	74	94	0.795	0.475	60	100	0.563	0.435	60	64
TCDCA	0.963	0.21	96	88	0.966	0.55	84	100	0.635	0.55	84	38
TDCA	0.516	0.375	20	96	0.559	0.11	26	100	0.496	1.025	10	100
TLCA	0.648	0.002	40	86	0.533	0.007	34	96	0.508	0.002	40	70
TUDCA	0.611	0.125	32	94	0.662	0.055	46	88	0.536	0.115	32	96

NHC normal healthy control, *NCLD* noncirrhotic liver disease, *CLD* cirrhotic liver diseases, *HCC* hepatocellular carcinoma, *BA* bile acid, $N = 50$, number of each group, *ROC* receiver operator characteristic, *AUC* Area under curve, *Sen.* sensitivity, *Spe.* specificity. AUC > 0.8 indicates significant relation
CA cholic acid, *CDCA* chenodeoxycholic acid, *DCA* deoxycholic acid, *LCA* lithocholic acid, *UDCA* ursodeoxycholic acid, *GCA* glycholic acid, *GCDCA* glycochenodeoxycholic acid, *GDCA* glycodeoxycholic acid, *GUDCA* glycoursodeoxycholic acid, *TCA* taurocholic acid, *TCDCA* taurochenodeoxycholic acid, *TDCA* taurodeoxycholic acid, *TLCA* taurolithocholic acid, *TUDCA* tauroursodeoxycholic acid

changes in the serum bile acids level in the noncirrhotic patients compared to healthy controls were trivial, indicating that the liver can handle the insult without compromising the pool of the bile acids. Four conjugated bile acids, namely GCA, GCDCA, GUDCA, and TCDCA, significantly increased in cirrhotic patients compared with noncirrhotic and were consistent with the clinical and biochemical parameters and thus could be observed as biomarkers of the progress of the liver cirrhosis disease.

In agreement with Zhao et al., this study also found an increase in the conjugated bile acids more than the unconjugated bile acids in cirrhotic and HCC patients, suggesting that conjugated bile acids may reflect the progress of the chronic liver cirrhosis to HCC [25]. Abnormal metabolism of bile acids and oxidative stress are early metabolic changes observed during the progression of liver cirrhosis to early stages of HCC as they can trigger DNA damage and induce apoptosis [26, 27]. An increase in conjugated bile acids has long been recognized in patients with hepatobiliary diseases such as viral hepatitis, cirrhosis, and cholangiocarcinoma [28]. Bile acid conjugation results in less toxic and more water-soluble bile acid types, thus protecting against cellular damage from such toxic compound that triggers oxidative stress and stimulates cell death signaling [22]. Yang et al. found upregulation of bile acids GCDCA, GDCA, and GCA in patients with hepatitis B compared to healthy control s[25]. Yin Wan et al. detected upregulation of

Table 4 Bile acids correlation analysis with AFP and their multivariate analysis with HCC clinical parameters

BA	Pearson Correlation	Multivariate analysis, F test				
	AFP	# FL	LN	Met	CHP-S	B. stage
CA	0.29*	0.40 ^{NS}	0.07 ^{NS}	1.03 ^{NS}	2.39 ^{NS}	0.71 ^{NS}
CDCA	0.01 ^{NS}	0.07 ^{NS}	0.13 ^{NS}	1.27 ^{NS}	3.21*	0.12 ^{NS}
DCA	− 0.04 ^{NS}	1.82 ^{NS}	3.88 ^{NS}	0.39 ^{NS}	1.62 ^{NS}	4.02*
LCA	0.13*	1.40 ^{NS}	1.75 ^{NS}	1.34 ^{NS}	0.46 ^{NS}	0.45 ^{NS}
UDCA	− 0.02 ^{NS}	1.53 ^{NS}	0.16 ^{NS}	0.91 ^{NS}	2.34 ^{NS}	0.03 ^{NS}
GCA	0.04 ^{NS}	0.76 ^{NS}	0.10 ^{NS}	0.26 ^{NS}	28.15*	0.45 ^{NS}
GCDCA	0.08 ^{NS}	0.01 ^{NS}	0.00 ^{NS}	0.11 ^{NS}	2.38 ^{NS}	0.37 ^{NS}
GDCA	− 0.01 ^{NS}	0.29 ^{NS}	0.34 ^{NS}	5.07*	1.33 ^{NS}	0.58
GUDCA	0.06 ^{NS}	0.77 ^{NS}	0.14 ^{NS}	0.48 ^{NS}	2.67*	0.29 ^{NS}
TCA	0.10*	0.12 ^{NS}	0.41 ^{NS}	0.31 ^{NS}	14.90*	2.49 ^{NS}
TCDCA	0.07 ^{NS}	0.08 ^{NS}	0.30 ^{NS}	0.20 ^{NS}	0.61 ^{NS}	0.62 ^{NS}
TDCA	− 0.01 ^{NS}	1.63 ^{NS}	0.02 ^{NS}	0.13 ^{NS}	0.18 ^{NS}	18.14*
TLCA	0.13*	4.46*	7.14*	1.26 ^{NS}	1.38 ^{NS}	4.44*
TUDCA	0.66*	0.00^{NS}	0.00 ^{NS}	0.00 ^{NS}	4.11*	0.00 ^{NS}

BA bile acid, *HCC* hepatocellular carcinoma, $N = 50$; *FL* number of focal lesions, *LN* lymph node, *Met* metastasis, *CHP-S* Child-Pugh Score, *B. stage* Barcelona stage of HCC, * indicates P value < 0.05 and presence of a significant correlation. ^{NS} indicates P value > 0.05 and absence of a significant correlation
CA cholic acid, *CDCA* chenodeoxycholic acid, *DCA* deoxycholic acid, *LCA* lithocholic acid, *UDCA* ursodeoxycholic acid, *GCA* glycholic acid, *GCDCA* glycochenodeoxycholic acid, *GDCA* glycodeoxycholic acid, *GUDCA* glycoursodeoxycholic acid, *TCA* taurocholic acid, *TCDCA* taurochenodeoxycholic acid, *TDCA* taurodeoxycholic acid, *TLCA* taurolithocholic acid, *TUDCA* tauroursodeoxycholic acid

four bile acids, GCA, GCDCA, TCA, and TCDCA in cirrhotic patients [23].

In the current study, bile acids profiles did not distinguish HCC from liver cirrhosis, although, GCDCA, GCA, GUDCA, and TCDCA tended to be higher in HCC but without evident statistical significant difference. Several metabolomics studies have identified metabolite expression profile differences between HCC and healthy controls [2, 29], however, as HCC is usually present in patients with liver cirrhosis, it is more relevant to consider cirrhotic patients as a control rather than healthy subjects. The current study had the privilege of including both the NCLD and CLD groups to reflect the progress of liver cirrhosis. Fewer studies reported metabolomics profile differences between HCC and liver cirrhosis [30, 31]. Ressom et al. characterized the metabolic changes relating to HCC in patients with liver cirrhosis and found that bile acids reduced in HCC relative to cirrhosis [32]. Xiao et al. detected a downregulation of three bile acids, GCA, GDCA, and GCDCA, in HCC compared to liver cirrhosis [33]. Chen et al. identified four bile acids CA, GCA, DCA, and GCDCA, altered differently in HCC from liver cirrhosis [2]. The interaction of the bile acids with the clinicopathological features of HCC showed that five bile acids, one primary (CDCA) and four conjugated (GCA, GDCA, GUDCA, TUDCA), correlated with the Child-Pugh score with a predominance of the glycoconjugates form of bile acids. Another three bile acids, one primary (DCA) and two taurine-conjugated (TDCA, TLCA), bile acid correlated with the Barcelona stage of the disease. Therefore, the metabolic profile of these bile acids may predict the progress of liver cirrhosis to HCC [34]. As this study lacks the HCC group without cirrhosis, therefore, the effect of the associated background cirrhosis as a confounding factor could not be ignored, and further studies with noncirrhotic HCC are required to confirm these findings. The limitation of the study is as follows: although patients groups were matched by demographic and clinical characteristics to control factors that may confound interpretation of the bile acids data yet, other diseases such as diabetes, obesity, metabolic syndrome, cardiovascular disease, and gastrointestinal microbiota are related to bile acids metabolism. Therefore, the coexisting of these diseases with liver cirrhosis adds layers of complexity to metabolomics profiling of bile acids [35–38]. The primary objective of this work was to examine the disturbance of bile acids in HCV-induced liver cirrhosis complicated by HCC. Further studies integrating HCC metabolomics data and the relationship of serum bile acid to the direct-acting antiviral agents (DAAs) are needed to delineate the complicated relationship with the other diseases that might confound the result.

Conclusion

This study characterized the metabolic profile of 14 bile acids in serum in patients with post HCV liver dysfunction ranging from non cirrhosis, cirrhosis, and hepatocellular carcinoma using UPLC-MS/MS methods. The level of conjugated bile acids GCA, GCDCA, GUDCA, and TCDCA were consistently higher in HCC than in NCLD and showed a tendency to be higher in HCC than CLD but without evident statistical significant difference. The increase in the serum bile acids level in patients with HCV-induced liver cirrhosis might serve as warring biomarkers for the progress of liver cirrhosis disease but not HCC.

Abbreviations

NHC: Normal healthy control; NCLD: Noncirrhotic liver disease; CLD: Cirrhotic liver diseases; HCC: Hepatocellular carcinoma; CA: Cholic acid; CDCA: Chenodeoxycholic acid; DCA: Deoxycholic acid; LCA: Lithocholic acid; UDCA: Ursodeoxycholic acid; GCA: Glycholic acid; GCDCA: Glycochenodeoxycholic acid; GDCA: Glycodeoxycholic acid; GUDCA: Glycoursodeoxycholic acid; TCA: Taurocholic acid; TCDCA: Taurochenodeoxycholic acid; TDCA: Taurodeoxycholic acid; TLCA: Taurolithocholic acid; TUDCA: Tauroursodeoxycholic acid; AST: Aspartate transaminase; ALT: Alanine transaminase; GGT: Gamma-glutamyl transferase; ALP: Alkaline phosphatase; TBil: Total bilirubin; DBiL: Direct bilirubin; TP: Total protein; Alb: Albumin; Hb: Hemoglobin; WBCs: White blood cells; HBV: Hepatitis B virus; HCC: Hepatocellular carcinoma; HCV: Hepatitis C virus; AASLD: American Association for the Study of Liver Diseases; AFP: Alpha-fetoprotein; ECLC: Barcelona Clinic Liver Cancer; CT: Computed tomography; ESAL: European Association for the Study of the Liver; NMR: Nuclear magnetic resonance; TNM (T) tumor, (N) nodes, (M), metastases; FL: Focal lesions; LN: Lymph node; Met: Metastasis; CHP: Child-Pugh; HFL: Hepatic focal lesion; PV: Portal vein

Acknowledgements

We would like to express our deep appreciation to all departments and personnel of the National Liver Institute, Menoufia University, for their continuous help and support of the research.

Authors' contributions

A.S: optimized the UPLC/MS/MS method and performed the experiments. E.A: collection of clinical data and gaining ethical approval. M.O: study design and involved in protocol development. H.S: study concept and contributed reagents, materials, and analysis tools. M.B: help in UPLC/MS/MS method. A.K: corresponding author, analyzed the data, wrote and edited the manuscript. All authors reviewed and edited the manuscript and approved the final version of the manuscript.

Declarations

Ethics approval and consent to participate

The research ethics committees of the National Liver Institute (IRB00003413), Menouffia University, approved the research proposal and the protocols to comply with national research guidelines. Patients provided informed written consent for the use of tissue for research purposes.

Competing interests

The authors declare they do not have any conflict of interest.

Author details
[1]Department of Biochemistry and Molecular Diagnostics, National Liver Institute, Menoufia University, Shebeen El kom, Egypt. [2]Department of Zoology, Faculty of Science, Menoufia University, Shebeen El kom, Egypt; Misr University for Science and Technology (MUST), 6th of October City, Giza, Egypt. [3]Department of Hepatology and Gastroenterology, National Liver Institute, Menoufia University, Shebeen El kom, Egypt.

References

1. Altekruse SF, McGlynn KA, Reichman ME (2009) Hepatocellular carcinoma incidence, mortality, and survival trends in the United States from 1975 to 2005. J Clin Oncol **27**(9):1485–1491. https://doi.org/10.1200/JCO.2008.20.7753
2. Chen T et al (2011) Serum and urine metabolite profiling reveals potential biomarkers of human hepatocellular carcinoma. Mol Cell Proteomics 10(7): M110 004945
3. Greco AV, Mingrone G (1993) Serum bile acid concentrations in mild liver cirrhosis. Clin Chim Acta 221(1-2):183–189. https://doi.org/10.1016/0009-8981(93)90032-Y
4. Mannes GA et al (1986) Prognostic significance of serum bile acids in cirrhosis. Hepatology 6(1):50–53. https://doi.org/10.1002/hep.1840060110
5. Baptissart M, Vega A, Maqdasy S, Caira F, Baron S, Lobaccaro JM, Volle DH (2012) Bile acids: from digestion to cancers. Biochimie 95(3):504–517. https://doi.org/10.1016/j.biochi.2012.06.022
6. Davila JA, Morgan RO, Richardson PA, du XL, McGlynn KA, el-Serag HB (2010) Use of surveillance for hepatocellular carcinoma among patients with cirrhosis in the United States. Hepatology 52(1):132–141. https://doi.org/10.1002/hep.23615
7. Moustafa T, Fickert P, Magnes C, Guelly C, Thueringer A, Frank S, Kratky D, Sattler W, Reicher H, Sinner F, Gumhold J, Silbert D, Fauler G, Höfler G, Lass A, Zechner R, Trauner M (2012) Alterations in lipid metabolism mediate inflammation, fibrosis, and proliferation in a mouse model of chronic cholestatic liver injury. Gastroenterology 142(1):140–151 e12. https://doi.org/10.1053/j.gastro.2011.09.051
8. Chiang JYL, Ferrell JM (2018) Bile acid metabolism in liver pathobiology. Gene Expr 18(2):71–87. https://doi.org/10.3727/105221618X15156018385515
9. Barr DC, Hussain HK (2014) MR imaging in cirrhosis and hepatocellular carcinoma. Magn Reson Imaging Clin N Am 22(3):315–335. https://doi.org/10.1016/j.mric.2014.04.006
10. van den Bos IC et al (2007) MR imaging of hepatocellular carcinoma: relationship between lesion size and imaging findings, including signal intensity and dynamic enhancement patterns. J Magn Reson Imaging 26(6): 1548–1555. https://doi.org/10.1002/jmri.21046
11. Chayanupatkul M et al (2017) Hepatocellular carcinoma in the absence of cirrhosis in patients with chronic hepatitis B virus infection. J Hepatol 66(2): 355–362
12. El-Serag HB et al (2013) Hepatocellular carcinoma screening practices in the Department of Veterans Affairs: findings from a national facility survey. Dig Dis Sci 58(11):3117–3126. https://doi.org/10.1007/s10620-013-2794-7
13. Zhao ZH, Lai JKL, Qiao L, Fan JG (2019) Role of gut microbial metabolites in nonalcoholic fatty liver disease. J Dig Dis 20(4):181–188. https://doi.org/10.1111/1751-2980.12709
14. Kondo S et al (2013) Clinical impact of c-Met expression and its gene amplification in hepatocellular carcinoma. Int J Clin Oncol 18(2):207–213
15. Khalil A et al (2013) Plasma osteopontin level as a diagnostic marker of hepatocellular carcinoma in patients with radiological evidence of focal hepatic lesions. Tumori 99(1):100–107
16. Taura N et al (2013) Frequency of elevated biomarkers in patients with cryptogenic hepatocellular carcinoma. Med Sci Monit 19:742–750
17. Hu K-Q, Kyulo NL, Lim N, Elhazin B, Hillebrand DJ, Bock T (2004) Clinical significance of elevated alpha-fetoprotein (AFP) in patients with chronic hepatitis C, but not hepatocellular carcinoma. Am J Gastroenterol 99(5):860–865. https://doi.org/10.1111/j.1572-0241.2004.04152.x
18. Tameda M et al (2013) Des-gamma-carboxy prothrombin ratio measured by P-11 and P-16 antibodies is a novel biomarker for hepatocellular carcinoma. Cancer Sci 104(6):725–731
19. Schutte K et al (2014) Characterization and prognosis of patients with hepatocellular carcinoma (HCC) in the non-cirrhotic liver. BMC Gastroenterol 14(1):117. https://doi.org/10.1186/1471-230X-14-117
20. Pugh RN, Murray-Lyon IM, Dawson JL, Pietroni MC, Williams R (1973) Transection of the oesophagus for bleeding oesophageal varices. Br J Surg 60(8):646–649. https://doi.org/10.1002/bjs.1800600817
21. de Freitas LBR, Longo L, Santos D, Grivicich I, Álvares-da-Silva MR (2019) Hepatocellular carcinoma staging systems: Hong Kong liver cancer vs Barcelona clinic liver cancer in a Western population. World J Hepatol 11(9): 678–688. https://doi.org/10.4254/wjh.v11.i9.678
22. Luo L, Aubrecht J, Li D, Warner RL, Johnson KJ, Kenny J, Colangelo JL (2018) Assessment of serum bile acid profiles as biomarkers of liver injury and liver disease in humans. PLoS One 13(3):e0193824. https://doi.org/10.1371/journal.pone.0193824
23. Akobeng AK (2007) Understanding diagnostic tests 3: receiver operating characteristic curves. Acta Paediatr 96(5):644–647. https://doi.org/10.1111/j.1651-2227.2006.00178.x
24. Fischer JE, Bachmann LM, Jaeschke R (2003) A readers' guide to the interpretation of diagnostic test properties: clinical example of sepsis. Intensive Care Med 29(7):1043–1051. https://doi.org/10.1007/s00134-003-1761-8
25. Yang J, Zhao X, Liu X, Wang C, Gao P, Wang J, Li L, Gu J, Yang S, Xu G (2006) High performance liquid chromatography-mass spectrometry for metabonomics: potential biomarkers for acute deterioration of liver function in chronic hepatitis B. J Proteome Res 5(3):554–561. https://doi.org/10.1021/pr050364w
26. Agosti P, Sabba C, Mazzocca A (2018) Emerging metabolic risk factors in hepatocellular carcinoma and their influence on the liver microenvironment. Biochim Biophys Acta Mol Basis Dis 1864(2):607–617. https://doi.org/10.1016/j.bbadis.2017.11.026
27. Gowda GA (2010) Human bile as a rich source of biomarkers for hepatopancreatobiliary cancers. Biomark Med 4(2):299–314. https://doi.org/10.2217/bmm.10.6
28. Neale G, Lewis B, Weaver V, Panveliwalla D (1971) Serum bile acids in liver disease. Gut 12(2):145–152. https://doi.org/10.1136/gut.12.2.145
29. Patterson AD, Maurhofer O, Beyoğlu D, Lanz C, Krausz KW, Pabst T, Gonzalez FJ, Dufour JF, Idle JR (2011) Aberrant lipid metabolism in hepatocellular carcinoma revealed by plasma metabolomics and lipid profiling. Cancer Res 71(21):6590–6600. https://doi.org/10.1158/0008-5472.CAN-11-0885
30. Wang B, Chen D, Chen Y, Hu Z, Cao M, Xie Q, Chen Y, Xu J, Zheng S, Li L (2012) Metabonomic profiles discriminate hepatocellular carcinoma from liver cirrhosis by ultraperformance liquid chromatography-mass spectrometry. J Proteome Res 11(2): 1217–1227. https://doi.org/10.1021/pr2009252
31. Zhou L, Ding L, Yin P, Lu X, Wang X, Niu J, Gao P, Xu G (2012) Serum metabolic profiling study of hepatocellular carcinoma infected with hepatitis B or hepatitis C virus by using liquid chromatography-mass spectrometry. J Proteome Res 11(11): 5433–5442. https://doi.org/10.1021/pr300683a
32. Ressom HW et al (2012) Utilization of metabolomics to identify serum biomarkers for hepatocellular carcinoma in patients with liver cirrhosis. Anal Chim Acta 743:90–100
33. Xiao JF, Varghese RS, Zhou B, Nezami Ranjbar MR, Zhao Y, Tsai TH, di Poto C, Wang J, Goerlitz D, Luo Y, Cheema AK, Sarhan N, Soliman H, Tadesse MG, Ziada DH, Ressom HW (2012) LC-MS based serum metabolomics for identification of hepatocellular carcinoma biomarkers in Egyptian cohort. J Proteome Res 11(12):5914–5923. https://doi.org/10.1021/pr300673x
34. Kimhofer T, Fye H, Taylor-Robinson S, Thursz M, Holmes E (2015) Proteomic and metabonomic biomarkers for hepatocellular carcinoma: a comprehensive review. Br J Cancer 112(7):1141–1156. https://doi.org/10.1038/bjc.2015.38
35. Hrncir T, Hrncirova L, Kverka M, Tlaskalova-Hogenova H (2019) The role of gut microbiota in intestinal and liver diseases. Lab Anim 53(3):271–280. https://doi.org/10.1177/0023677218818605
36. Kolodziejczyk AA et al (2019) The role of the microbiome in NAFLD and NASH. EMBO Mol Med 11(2):e9302. https://doi.org/10.15252/emmm.201809302
37. Tang WW, Hazen SL (2016) Dietary metabolism, gut microbiota and acute heart failure. Heart 102(11):813–814. https://doi.org/10.1136/heartjnl-2016-309268
38. Zhao ZH et al (2019) Role of gut microbial metabolites in nonalcoholic fatty liver disease. J Dig Dis 20(4):181–188

5

Hepatic steatosis: a risk factor for increased COVID-19 prevalence and severity—a computed tomography study

Asmaa Ali*, Mona Hasan, Shaimaa Hamed and Amir Elhamy

Abstract

Background: Around 25% of the world population was affected by the metabolic-related fatty liver disorder. Hepatic steatosis is frequently observed in conjunction with hypertension, obesity comorbidities, and diabetes. We evaluate the hepatic steatosis frequency found in chest CT exams of COVID-19-positive cases compared to non-infected controls and evaluate the related increased prevalence and severity of COVID.

Results: Our research includes 355 subjects, 158 with positive PCR for COVID-19 (case group) and 197 with negative PCR and negative CT chest (control group). The mean age in the positive group was 50.6 ± 16 years, and in the control, it was 41.3 ± 16 years ($p < 0.001$). Our study consists of 321 men (90.5%) and 34 women (9.5%). The number of males in both cases and control groups was greater. In the case group, 93% men vs. 6.9% women, while in controls, 88.3% men vs.11.6% women, $p < 0.001$. CT revealed normal results in 55.5% of individuals (i.e., CORADs 1) and abnormal findings in 45.5% of participants (i.e., CORADs 2–5). In abnormal scan, CO-RADs 2 was 13.92%, while CO-RADs 3–4 were 20.89% of cases. CO-RADs 5 comprised 65.19% of all cases. Approximately 42.6% of cases had severe disease (CT score ≥ 20), all of them were CO-RADs 5. The PCR-positive class had a greater prevalence of hepatic steatosis than controls (28.5% vs.12.2%, $p < 0.001$). CO-RADs 2 represented 11.1%, CO-RADs 3–4 represented 15.6%, and CO-RADs 5 represented 73.3% in the hepatic steatosis cases. The mean hepatic attenuation value in the case group was 46.79 ± 12.68 and in the control group 53.34 ± 10.28 ($p < 0.001$). When comparing patients with a higher severity score (CT score ≥ 20) to those with non-severe pneumonia, it was discovered that hepatic steatosis is more prevalent (73.2% vs. 26.8%).

Conclusions: Steatosis was shown to be substantially more prevalent in COVID-19-positive individuals. There is a relation among metabolic syndrome, steatosis of the liver, and obesity, as well as the COVID-19 severity.

Keywords: Fatty liver, Computed tomography, COVID-19

Key points

- High-resolution computed tomography aids clinicians in evaluating lung affection in COVID-positive cases.
- Fatty liver and obesity are rising globally.
- Fatty liver and metabolic syndrome are significant predisposing parameters for COVID-19 infection and increase disease's severity.

Background

The World Health Organization declared coronavirus disease 2019 (COVID-19) as a pandemic on March 11, 2020 [1]. By May 2021, around 165,772,430 reported cases and 3,437,545 mortalities had occurred (https://www.who.org). COVID-19 is symptomatized by fever and dry cough, and the infection is diagnosed by a real-

* Correspondence: asmaa_monir@hotmail.com
Theodor Bilharz Institute, Kornish Elnil, Embaba, Giza, Egypt

time reverse transcription-polymerase chain reaction (RT-PCR) test [2, 3]. Due to the rise in global cases, other symptoms like constipation, diarrhea, abdominal pain, and vomiting have risen; these are associated with abnormal renal and liver functions, and D-Dimer levels [4, 5]

COVID-19 can impact other organs besides the respiratory system, like the cardiovascular system, kidneys, liver, and coagulation system [6–10].

Diabetes, age, metabolic syndrome, hypertension, and obesity are all risk parameters for severe/critical illness and death [11–13].

People with obesity and type 2 diabetes are at greater risk for non-alcoholic fatty liver disease NAFLD, that worsen these disorders. It has been linked to an inflammatory response (increased neutrophil-to-lymphocyte ratio [NLR]) and subsequent poor outcomes in COVID-19-infected cases [14].

NAFLD has risen over the last two decades, affecting around 24% of the individual [15, 16]. NAFLD is a complex process with hepatic and extrahepatic pathophysiology and clinical symptoms. It leads to ectopic fatty substrate deposits in the liver, ranging from simple steatosis without inflammation to steatohepatitis, which causes cirrhosis and fibrosis [15].

CT affects the care of COVID-19 individuals because it aids in the early discovery and diagnosis, particularly in cases when the RT-PCR result is false-negative [16].

COVID-19 chest CT results are typically multifocal bilateral, mostly peripheral subpleural round, ground-glass opacities with or without patchy consolidations affecting mostly the posterior lower lobes [17]. Additionally, airway changes, reversed halo sign, and crazy paving patterns can be detected [18]. The Radiological Society of North America (RSNA) defined four categories on reporting chest CT findings in COVID-19 pneumonia: (1) typical features that are usually reported in COVID-19, (2) indeterminate features that are not characteristic of COVID-19 pneumonia, (3) atypical features that are uncommon in COVID-19 pneumonia but can occur with other infections, and (4) negative for lung inflammation with no lung results denoting infection. Chest CT may be negative in the early stages of COVID-19 infection [19].

We frequently include the upper abdomen in the regular CT scan of the chest conducted to assess cases with COVID-19 pneumonia, so that most of the liver and spleen can be viewed and examined [20].

The regular liver appears slightly more attenuated on non-contrast CT than the blood and spleen, and the intrahepatic arteries present as hypo-attenuated structures. Although histopathological analysis and liver biopsy are the gold measure for determining hepatic steatosis, they are invasive procedures. As a result, numerous studies have examined non-invasive alternatives to liver biopsy utilizing CT imaging [21].

Unenhanced CT liver attenuation alone is highly specific for moderate to severe hepatic steatosis, obviating the requirement for verification by biopsy [22].

Numerous approaches have been used for evaluating hepatic steatosis by computed tomography; the most important of which is determining the liver's attenuation value. In the non-enhanced phase, the region of interest is set in the right hepatic lobe; if it is less than 40 HU, this indicates moderate hepatic steatosis with a fat liver percentage greater than 30% [23, 24]. Another way for assessing hepatic steatosis is to compare the area of interest in the splenic parenchyma to the liver, when we find the attenuation of liver is at least 10 HU less than that of the spleen. Several studies have demonstrated that non-enhanced CT has a great sensitivity (from 43 to 95%) and a great specificity (from 90 to 100%) for detecting hepatic steatosis [25–27].

Methods

This retrospective study was conducted at our institution's Radiology Department from May 1, 2020, to June 1, 2020. Approval was acquired from the Institution's Ethics and Research Committee. Informed consent was taken.

Inclusion criteria

Our research included 355 subjects who presented with flu-like symptoms and were suspected of being infected with COVID-19. They underwent PCR checking and chest CT for COVID-19. For all, we utilize the same 64-slice CT scanner (Siemens Healthcare, Germany).

The case group included 158 subjects (PCR positive for COVID-19), while the control group consisted of 197 subjects with a negative PCR test. It is widely established that false-negative RT-PCR can happen in infected individuals, but CT chest may reveal disease signs (positive CT). Therefore, to ensure the control group's negativity, we checked their CT chest and retained only those who had a negative CT chest (PCR-negative and chest CT-negative pattern).

Two radiologists with over 10 years of expertise interpreted the CT chest.

CT evaluation involved identifying the areas of ground-glass opacities, crazy-paving patterns (ground-glass opacities with interlobular septal thickening), atelectatic bands, and consolidations. CT results were divided into five classes using the RSNA Expert Consensus Criteria [28], as well as the COVID-19 Reporting and Data System (CO-RADs) from the COVID-19 Working Group of the Dutch Radiological Society [29]. CT results are graded according to these grading methods as normal, inconsistent, or typical of COVID-19 pneumonia.

The severity of lung affection (CT severity index) was measured as per Yang et al. A CT score of more than 20/40 indicates serious illness and is typically related to a poor prognosis [30].

We assess hepatic steatosis in our research by determining the attenuation of liver value. The area of interest (with an average area of 10 cm^2) was located in the right hepatic lobe (between segments VI and VII), chosen area away from the biliary tree, vessels, or focal lesions. We examine one slice and define the liver as fatty if the HU reading is less than 40.

Statistical analysis

SPSS (Statistical Package for the Social Sciences; SPSS Inc., Chicago, IL, USA) release 25 was utilized for all statistical calculations. Standard deviations and means are used to describe quantitative data, while percentages are used to indicate qualitative data. Per the variable distribution, we employed the t-Student and chi-square checks. A p-value below 0.05 was considered significant.

Results

Characteristics of study group (Table 1)

- Our research includes 355 subjects, 158 with positive PCR for COVID-19 (case group) and 197 with negative PCR and negative CT chest (control group). The mean age in the positive group was 50.6 ± 16 years, and in the control, it was 41.3 ± 16 years ($p < 0.001$).
- Our study comprised 321 men (90.5%) and 34 women (9.5%). The number of males in both cases and control groups was greater. In the case group, 93% men vs. 6.9% women, while in controls, 88.3% men vs.11.6% women, $p < 0.001$.
- CT demonstrated normal results in 55.5% of individuals (i.e., CORADs 1) and abnormal findings in 45.5% of participants (i.e., CORADs 2–5). In abnormal scan, CO-RADs 2 was 13.92%, while CO-RADs 3–4 were 20.89% of cases. CO-RADs 5 comprised 65.19% of all cases. Approximately 42.6% of cases had severe disease (CT score ≥ 20); all of them were CO-RADs 5.

Association with steatosis (Figs. 1, 2, 3, 4, and 5)

- The PCR-positive group had a greater prevalence of hepatic steatosis than controls (28.5% vs.12.2%, $p < 0.001$). CO-RADs 2 represented 11.1%, CO-RADs 3–4 represented 15.6%, and CO-RADs 5 represented 73.3% in the hepatic steatosis cases.
- The mean hepatic attenuation value in the case group was 46.79 ± 12.68, and in the control group, 53.34 ± 10.28 ($p < 0.001$).
- When comparing patients with a higher severity score (CT score ≥ 20) to those with non-severe pneumonia, it was discovered that hepatic steatosis is more prevalent (73.2% vs. 26.8%).

Discussion

In 2016, the World Health Organization reported that 1.9 billion adults were overweight, with over 650 million being obese [31]. Obesity is the most major and significant risk factor in developing hepatic steatosis in adults and children [32].

Obesity is thought to be a condition of low-grade systemic inflammation that has been linked to a variety of metabolic diseases like type 2 diabetes mellitus and dyslipidemia. It can alter immunological responses, causing the immune system more sensitive to infection development [33].

Due to its endocrine roles and the release of various adipokines and proinflammatory cytokines like leptin, interleukin 6, C-reactive protein, visceral adipose tissue, and TNF are more metabolically active than subcutaneous adipose tissue [34, 35]. It is well documented that raised IL-6 levels are related to chronic inflammatory airway disorder. Numerous studies have discovered

Table 1 Demographic comparison parameters and statistics between the two groups

Parameter	Case group Positive PCR N = 158	Control group Negative PCR/negative chest CT N = 197
Age	50.6 ± 16 years	41.3 ± 16 years
Sex		
Male	N = 147 (93%)	N = 174 (88.3%)
Female	N = 11 (6.9%)	N = 23 (11.6%)
Steatosis	28.5%	12.2%
HU	46.79 ± 12.68	53.34 ± 10.28
CO-RADs	CO-RADs 2, N = 22 (13.92%)	CO-RADs 1, N = 197 (55.5%)
	CO-RADs 3–4, N = 33 (20.89%)	
	CO-RADs 5, N = 103 (65.19%)	

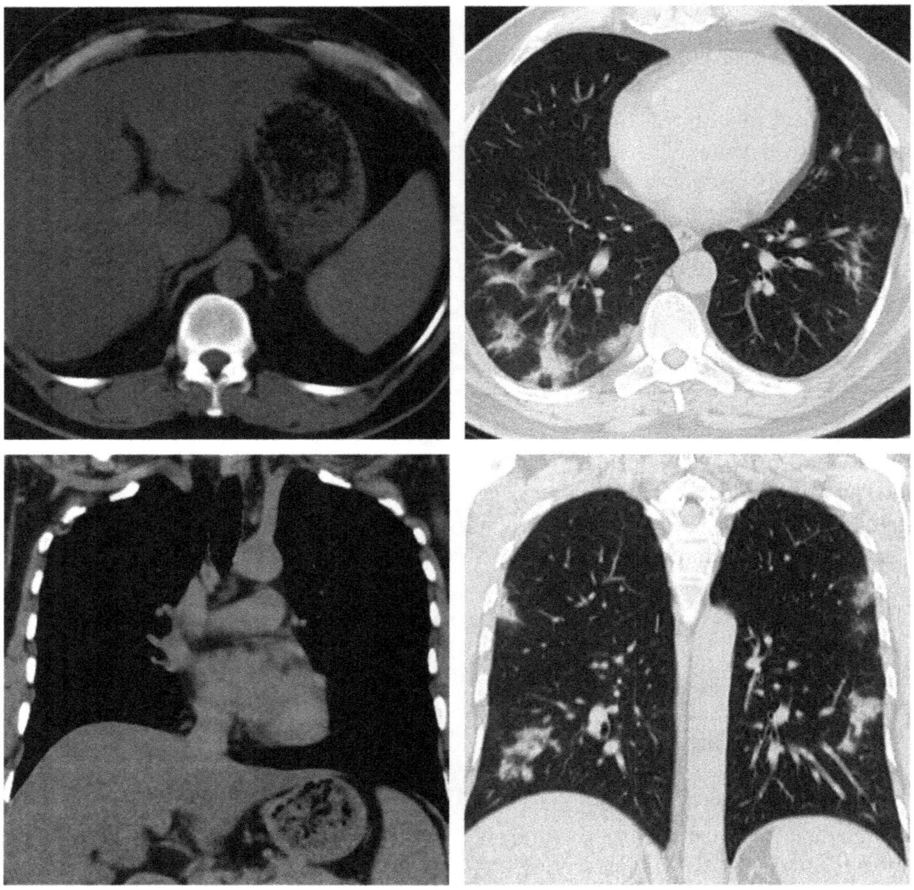

Fig. 1 Male patient, 45 years old. CT chest shows multiple bilateral pulmonary patchy ground-glass opacities, reported as CORADs 5. Upper abdominal cuts show hepatic steatosis

greater IL-6 concentrations in post-mortem specimens from COVID-19 cases [36, 37]. Leptin has been linked with airway reactivity, and current research indicates that leptin concentrations are increased in COVID-19 cases with significant pulmonary inflammation [38, 39].

COVID-19 invades human cells through binding with angiotensin-converting enzyme 2, and some research shows that the renin-angiotensin-aldosterone system's imbalanced activity in obese individuals contributes to this pathogenesis. Because ACE2 expression is greater in adipose tissue than in lung tissue, and because ACE2 in

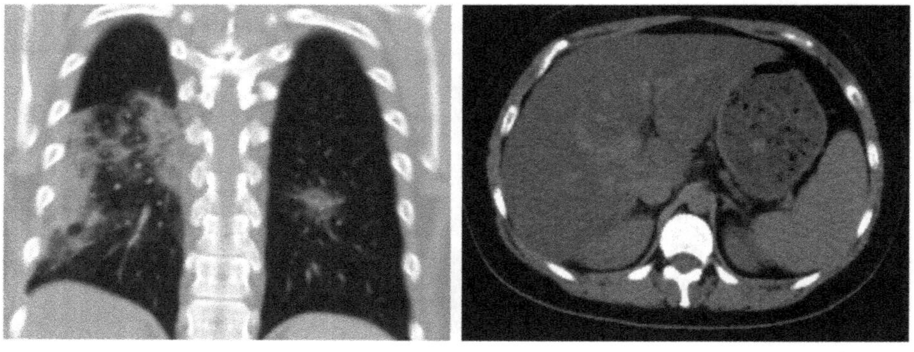

Fig. 2 Female patient, 28 years old. CT chest shows multiple pulmonary ground-glass opacities mounting to consolidative patches, reported as CORADs 5. Upper abdominal cuts show diffuse low parenchymal attenuation of the liver denoting fatty infiltration

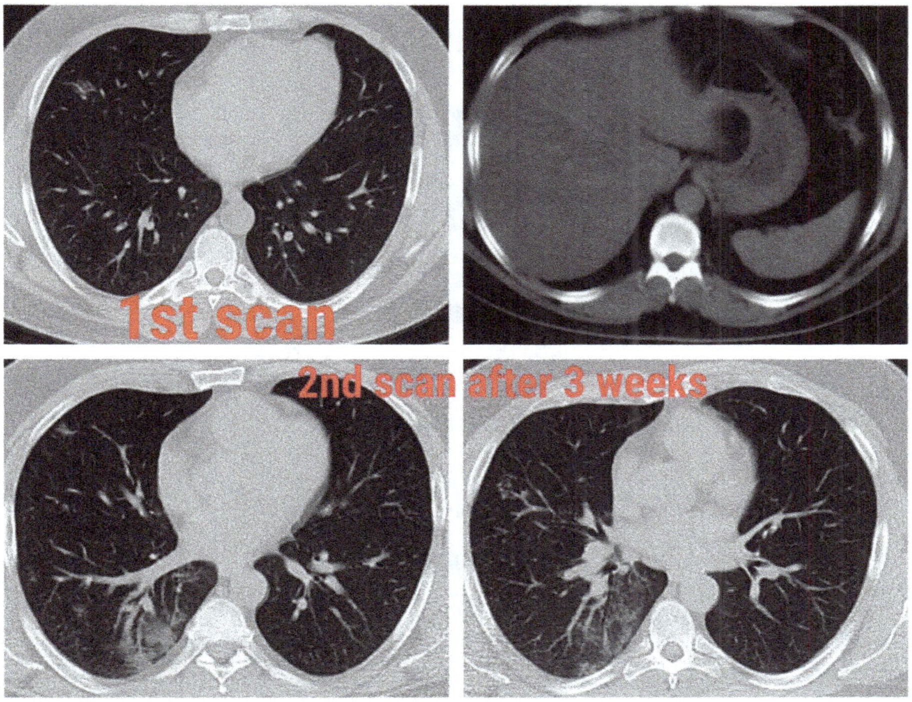

Fig. 3 Male patient, 36 years old. The first scan after few days of symptoms shows just a small patchy ground-glass opacity in the middle lobe. The second scan after 3 weeks for follow-up shows a progressive course with multiple pulmonary ground-glass opacities. CT cuts of the upper abdomen show a fatty liver

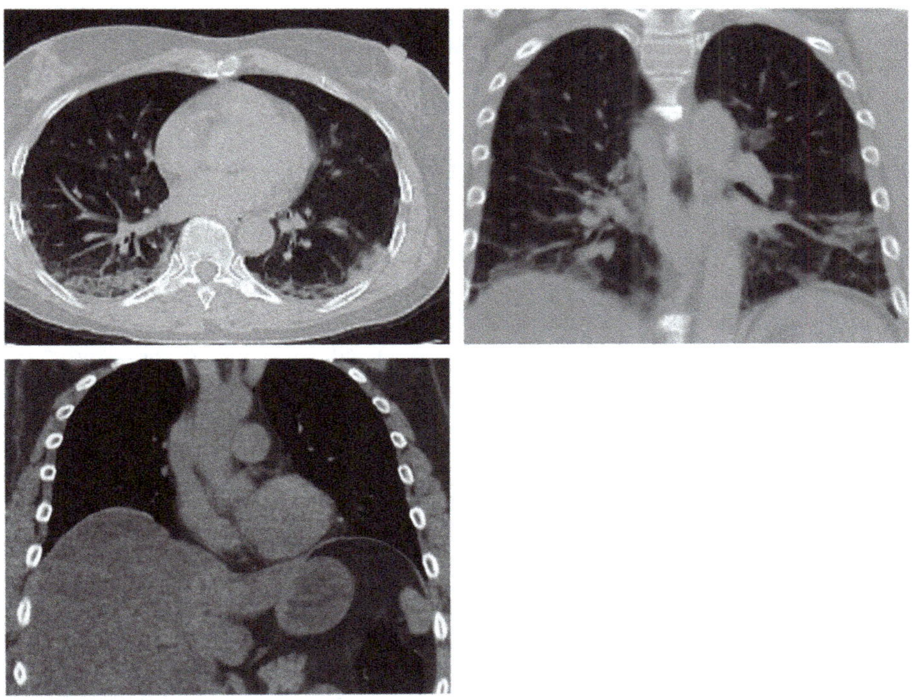

Fig. 4 Male patient, 64 years. CT chest shows bilateral lower lobar subpleural patchy ground-glass opacities with underlying interlobular septal thickening and atelectatic bands, reported as CORADs 5. Upper abdominal cuts show fatty hepatomegaly

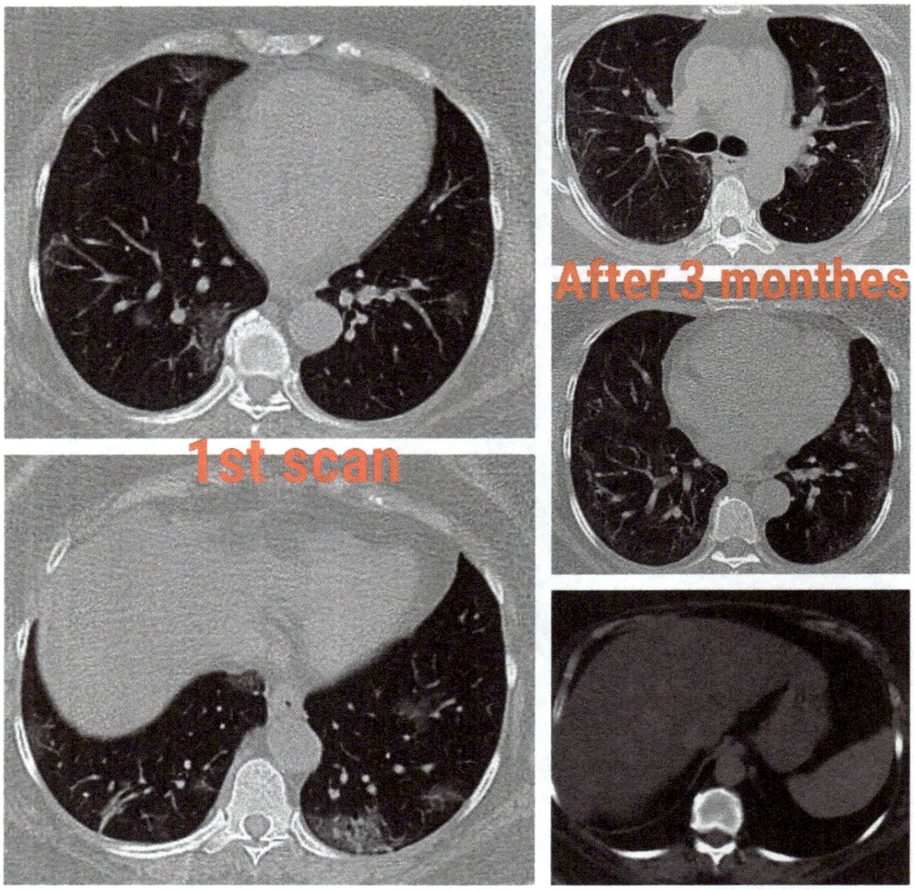

Fig. 5 Female patient, 58 years old. The first scan shows multiple subpleural ground-glass opacities on follow-up after 3 months. CT shows multiple subpleural parenchymal bands. Upper abdominal cuts show fatty hepatomegaly

lung tissue is known to be the primary entry point for SARS-CoV-2, this increases the sensitivity of obese patients to infection [40].

Additionally, obese individuals have impaired B and T cell responses due to changes in the quantity and function of lymphocytes, resulting in an increased vulnerability to viral infection. In virally infected obese individuals, the inflammatory response is dysregulated, resulting in a reduction and delay in macrophage activation [41]. Obesity can promote antiviral resistance as well [42].

NLR, a measure of systemic inflammation, was considerably elevated and related to poorer results in cases infected with COVID-19 [43]. There is a substantial correlation between this ratio and the severity of liver fibrosis in people with NAFLD. Current research has established that this association affects the COVID-19-induced inflammatory storm, which is associated with raised death and morbidity. In cases infected with COVID-19, liver injury occurs following lung injury [44]. This destruction could be caused by the overactivation of Kupffer cells, the production of a cytotoxic T cell response produced by the virus, or the production of a dysregulated innate immune response [45]. In these cases, post-mortem liver biopsies revealed microvascular steatosis [44].

According to Zheng et al., individuals with metabolic-associated fatty liver disease and obesity had a sixfold raised chance of developing severe COVID-19 infection [46]. Another research indicated that populations with metabolically related fatty liver disease (MAFLD) have a fourfold greater risk of developing severe forms of COVID-19 [47].

Per Palomar-Lever et al.'s findings, the combination of obesity and hepatic steatosis led to a significant relationship with serious illness, implying a synergic connection between both [20].

Medeiros et al. concluded that the steatosis prevalence on CT was greater in confirmed COVID pneumonia cases than in the control. This is important for radiologists because liver steatosis can be easily assessed and verified by any radiologist reading a chest CT. Moreover, this data can be added to the clinical data available to clinicians [48].

In research conducted in New York, cases with a body mass index (BMI) of ≥ 30 had a higher chance of acute care hospitalization, and those with a BMI of ≥ 35 had a higher risk of intensive care unit admission [49].

Additionally, it was observed that cases with NAFLD had a greater rate of progression to severe illness and poorer findings in COVID19 [44, 50, 51].

Ji et al. studied NAFLD in 202 cases with COVID-19 using the hepatic steatosis index based on ALT, AST, body mass index, gender, presence of diabetes, and/or an ultrasound examination. They discovered that preexisting comorbidities and NAFLD were linked with COVID-19 progression [44].

According to Zhou et al., the risk of severe COVID-19 increases fourfold when metabolic-related fatty liver disease is present [52].

As with the previous research, univariate and multivariate analyses suggested that individuals with NAFLD had an increased risk of disease progression. Comorbidities like diabetes mellitus, hypertension, coronary artery disease, and COPD are identified as additional risk parameters for COVID-19 progression [44, 53].

Petersen et al. used low-dose computed tomography and post-processing software to measure body fat distribution particularly visceral adipose tissue and upper abdominal circumference in COVID patients and found that these two parameters significantly increase the likelihood of COVID-19 severe courses [54].

Parlak et al. found that chest CT, which is critical for diagnosing COVID-19, can provide data about the disease's prognosis and that fatty liver is a significant indicator of a bad prognosis and may be easily spotted on chest CT used for COVID-19 diagnosis [55].

Limitations

Other significant variables like hypertension, lipid profile, diabetes, weight, obesity, body mass index, and liver function were not evaluated. Hence, a correlation between these variables and hepatic steatosis could not be established.

Conclusion

In confirmed COVID-19 cases, our research demonstrates a considerably greater frequency of hepatic steatosis by CT as compared to controls. There is a correlation among metabolic syndrome, steatosis of the liver, and obesity, as well as the severity of COVID-19.

Abbreviations

RT-PCR: Real-time reverse transcription polymerase chain reaction; COVID-19: Coronavirus disease of 2019; MAFLD: Metabolic fatty liver disease; NLR: Neutrophil-to-lymphocyte ratio; NAFLD: Non-alcoholic fatty liver disease; IL-6: Interleukin 6; HU: Hounsfield unit; SARS-CoV-2: Severe acute respiratory syndrome coronavirus 2; ACE2: Angiotensin-converting enzyme 2; HS: Hepatic steatosis

Acknowledgements

Not applicable

Authors' contributions

AA wrote the manuscript and was responsible for the correspondence to the journal. MH collected the patient data and participated in its design. SH contributed to the image processing and collection of the patient's images. AE participated in the design of the study, performed the statistical analysis and participated in its design and coordination, and helped to draft the manuscript.All authors have read and approved the final manuscript.

Declarations

Ethics approval and consent to participate

The study was approved by the ethical committee of "Theodor Bilharz Institute" institutional review board with ethical committee approval number FWA 10609. An informed written consent was taken from all patients.

Competing interests

The authors declare that they have no competing interests.

References

1. Watanabe M, Risi R, Tuccinardi D, Baquero CJ, Manfrini S, Gnessi L (2020) Obesity and SARS-CoV-2: a population to safeguard. Diabetes Metab Res Rev. https://doi.org/10.1002/dmrr.3325
2. Kanne JP (2020) Chest CT findings in 2019 novel coronavirus (2019-nCoV) infections from Wuhan, China: key points for the radiologist. Radiology 295(1):16–17. https://doi.org/10.1148/radiol.2020200241
3. Yoon SH, Lee KH, Kim JY, Lee YK, Ko H, Kim KH, Park CM, Kim YH (2020) Chest radiographic and CT findings of the 2019 novel coronavirus disease (COVID-19): analysis of nine patients treated in Korea. Korean J Radiol 21: 494–500. https://doi.org/10.3348/kjr.2020.0132
4. Cholankeril G, Podboy A, Aivaliotis VI, Tarlow B, Pham EA, Spencer SP, Kim D, Hsing A, Ahmed A (2020) High prevalence of concurrent gastrointestinal manifestations in patients with SARS-CoV-2: early experience from California. Gastroenterology. 159(2):775–777. https://doi.org/10.1053/j.gastro.2020.04.008
5. Luo S, Zhang X, Xu H (2020) Don't overlook digestive symptoms in patients with 2019 novel coronavirus disease (COVID-19). Clin Gastroenterol Hepatol 18(7):1636–1637. https://doi.org/10.1016/j.cgh.2020.03.043
6. Han H, Xie L, Liu R et al (2020) Analysis of heart injury laboratory parameters in 273 COVID-19 patients in one hospital in Wuhan, China [published online ahead of print, 2020 march 31]. J Med Virol https://doi.org/10.1002/jmv.25809
7. Ammirati E, Wang DW (2020) SARS-CoV-2 inflames the heart. The importance of awareness of myocardial injury in COVID-19 patients [published online ahead of print, 2020 April 6]. Int J Cardiol S0167-5273(20)31669-7. https://doi.org/10.1016/j.ijcard.2020.03.086
8. Zhang C, Shi L, Wang FS (2020) Liver injury in COVID-19: management and challenges. Lancet Gastroenterol Hepatol 5(5):428–430. https://doi.org/10.1016/S2468-1253(20)30057-1
9. Durvasula R, Wellington T, McNamara E, Watnick S (2020) COVID-19 and kidney failure in the acute care setting: our experience from Seattle [published online ahead of print, 2020 April 7]. Am J Kidney Dis S0272-6386(20)30618-1. https://doi.org/10.1053/j.ajkd.2020.04.001
10. Dolhnikoff M, Duarte-Neto AN, de Almeida Monteiro RA et al (2020) Pathological evidence of pulmonary thrombotic phenomena in severe COVID-19 [published online ahead of print, 2020 April 15]. J Thromb Haemost. https://doi.org/10.1111/jth.14844

11. Wu Z, McGoogan JM (2020) Characteristics of and important lessons from the coronavirus disease 2019 (COVID-19) outbreak in China: summary of a report of 72314 cases from the Chinese Center for Disease Control and Prevention. JAMA. 323(13):1239–1242. https://doi.org/10.1001/jama.2020.2648
12. Mantovani A, Byrne CD, Zheng MH, Targher G (2020) Diabetes as a risk factor for greater COVID-19 severity and in-hospital death: a meta-analysis of observational studies. Nutr Metab Cardiovasc Dis 30(8):1236–1248. https://doi.org/10.1016/j.numecd.2020.05.014
13. Targher G, Mantovani A, Wang XB, Yan HD, Sun QF, Pan KH, Byrne CD, Zheng KI, Chen YP, Eslam M, George J, Zheng MH (2020) Patients with diabetes are at higher risk for severe illness from COVID-19. Diabetes Metab 46(4):335–337. https://doi.org/10.1016/j.diabet.2020.05.001 In press
14. Targher G, Mantovani A, Byrne CD, Wang XB, Yan HD, Sun QF, Pan KH, Zheng KI, Chen YP, Eslam M, George J, Zheng MH (2020) Detrimental effects of metabolic dysfunction-associated fatty liver disease and increased neutrophil-to-lymphocyte ratio on severity of COVID-19. Diabetes Metab 46(6):505–507. https://doi.org/10.1016/j.diabet.2020.06.001 In press
15. Angulo P (2002) Nonalcoholic fatty liver disease. N Engl J Med 346(16): 1221–1231. https://doi.org/10.1056/NEJMra011775
16. Yang W, Sirajuddin A, Zhang X, Liu G, Teng Z, Zhao S et al (2020) The role of imaging in 2019 novel coronavirus (COVID-19). Eur Radiol. https://doi.org/10.1007/s00330-020-06827-4
17. Zu ZY, Jiang MD, Xu PP, Chen W, Ni QQ, Lu GM, Zhang LJ (2020) Coronavirus disease 2019 (COVID-19): a perspective from China. Radiology 296(2):E15–E25. https://doi.org/10.1148/radiol.2020200490
18. Ye Z, Zhang Y, Wang Y, Huang Z, Song B (2020) Chest CT manifestations of new coronavirus disease 2019 (COVID-19): a pictorial review. Eur Radiol 30(8):4381–4389. https://doi.org/10.1007/s00330-020-06801-0
19. Simpson S, Kay FU, Abbara S, Bhalla S, Chung JH, Chung M, Henry TS, Kanne JP, Kligerman S, Ko JP, Litt H (2020) Radiological Society of North America expert consensus statement on reporting chest CT findings related to COVID-19. Endorsed by the Society of Thoracic Radiology, the American College of Radiology, and RSNA. Radiol Cardiothoracic Imaging 2(2):e200152
20. Palomar-Lever A, Barraza G, Galicia-Alba J, Echeverri-Bolaños M, Escarria-Panesso R, Padua-Barrios J, Halabe-Cherem J, Hernandez-Molina G, Chargoy-Loustaunau TN, Kimura-Hayama E (2020) Hepatic steatosis as an independent risk factor for severe disease in patients with COVID-19: a computed tomography study. JGH Open 4(6):1102–1107. https://doi.org/10.1002/jgh3
21. Hamer OW, Aguirre DA, Casola G, Sirlin CB (2005) Imaging features of perivascular fatty infiltration of the liver: initial observations. Radiology 237: 159–169. https://doi.org/10.1148/radiol.2371041580
22. Pickhardt PJ, Park SH, Hahn L, Lee SG, Bae KT, Yu ES (2012) Specificity of unenhanced CT for non-invasive diagnosis of hepatic steatosis: implications for the investigation of the natural history of incidental steatosis. Eur Radiol 22(5):1075–1082. https://doi.org/10.1007/s00330-011-2349-2
23. Lawrence DA, Oliva IB, Israel GM (2012) Detection of hepatic steatosis on contrast-enhanced CT images: diagnostic accuracy of identification of areas of presumed focal fatty sparing. Am J Roentgenol 199:44–47. https://doi.org/10.2214/AJR.11.7838
24. Wells MM, Li Z, Addeman B, Mckenzie CA, Mujoomdar A, Beaton M et al (2016) Computed tomography measurement of hepatic steatosis: prevalence of hepatic steatosis in a Canadian population. Can J Gastroenterol Hepatol 2016:4930987. https://doi.org/10.1155/2016/4930987
25. Monjardim RDF, Costa DMC, Romano RFT, Salvadori PS, dos Santos J, de VC VAAC et al (2013) Diagnosis of hepatic steatosis by contrast-enhanced abdominal computed tomography. Radiol Bras 46:134–138. https://doi.org/10.1590/S0100-39842013000300005
26. Ma X, Holalkere NS, Avinash KR, Mino-Kenudson M, Hahn PF, Sahani DV (2009) Imaging-based quantification of hepatic fat: methods and clinical applications. Radiographics 29:1253–1277. https://doi.org/10.1148/rg.295085186
27. Boyce CJ, Pickhardt PJ, Kim DH, Taylor AJ, Winter TC, Bruce RJ et al (2010) Hepatic steatosis (fatty liver disease) in asymptomatic adults identified by unenhanced low-dose CT. Am J Roentgenol 194:623–628. https://doi.org/10.2214/AJR.09.2590
28. Simpson S, Kay FU, Abbara S, Bhalla S, Chung JH, Chung M (2020) Radiological Society of North America expert consensus statement on reporting chest CT findings related to COVID-19. Endorsed by the Society of Thoracic Radiology, the American College of Radiology, and RSNA. Radiology 2:2. https://doi.org/10.1148/ryct.2020200152
29. Prokop M, van Everdingen W, van Rees VT, Jet Quarles van Ufford JT, Stöger L et al (2020) CO-RADS - a categorical CT assessment scheme for patients with suspected COVID-19: definition and evaluation. Radiology. https://doi.org/10.1148/radiol.2020201473
30. Yang R, Li X, Liu H et al (2020) Chest CT severity score: an imaging tool for assessing severe COVID-19. Radiology 2:2. https://doi.org/10.1148/ryct.2020200047
31. Hill JJ (2018) Obesity: an emerging threat. J Natl Black Nurses Assoc 29(2): 36–39
32. Festi D, Colecchia A, Sacco T, Bondi M, Roda E, Marchesini G (2004) Hepatic steatosis in obese patients: clinical aspects and prognostic significance. Obes Rev 5:27–42. https://doi.org/10.1111/j.1467-789x.2004.00126.x
33. Dhurandhar NV, Bailey D, Thomas D (2015) Interaction of obesity and infections. Obes Rev 16(12):1017–1029. https://doi.org/10.1111/obr.12320
34. Muscogiuri G, Pugliese G, Barrea L, Savastano S, Colao A (2020) Comentary: obesity: the "Achilles heel" for COVID-19? Metabolism. 108:154251. https://doi.org/10.1016/j.metabol.2020.154251
35. Ritter A, Friemel A, Fornoff F, Adjan M, Solbach C, Yuan J, Louwen F (2015) Characterization of adipose-derived stem cells from subcutaneous and visceral adipose tissues and their function in breast cancer cells. Oncotarget. 6(33):34475–34493. https://doi.org/10.18632/oncotarget.5922
36. Zhou F, Yu T, Du R, Fan G, Liu Y, Liu Z et al (2020) Clinical course and risk parameters for mortality of adult inpatients with COVID-19 in Wuhan, China: a retrospective cohort study. Lancet. 395(10229):1054–1062. https://doi.org/10.1016/S0140-6736(20)30566-3
37. Park YS, Kwon HT, Hwang SS, Choi SH, Cho YM, Lee J, Yim JJ (2011) Impact of visceral adiposity measured by abdominal computed tomography on pulmonary function. J Korean Med Sci 26(6):771–777. https://doi.org/10.3346/jkms.2011.26.6.771
38. Sideleva O, Suratt BT, Black KE, Tharp WG, Pratley RE, Forgione P, Dienz O, Irvin CG, Dixon AE (2012) Obesity and asthma: an inflammatory disease of adipose tissue not the airway. Am J Respir Crit Care Med 186(7):598–605. https://doi.org/10.1164/rccm.201203-0573OC
39. Bourgonje AR, Abdulle AE, Timens W, Hillebrands JL, Navis GJ, Gordijn SJ et al (2020) Angiotensin-converting enzyme 2 (ACE2), SARS-CoV-2 and the pathophysiology of coronavirus disease 2019 (COVID-19). J Pathol Ahead of print
40. Lavie CJ, Sanchis-Gomar F, Henry BM, Lippi G (2020) COVID-19 and obesity: links and risks. Expert Rev Endocrinol Metab. https://doi.org/10.1080/17446651.2020.1767589
41. Kim J, Nam JH (2020) Insight into the relationship between obesity induced low-level chronic inflammation and COVID-19 infection. Int J Obes 44(7): 1541–1542. https://doi.org/10.1038/s41366-020-0602-y
42. Petrakis D, Margină D, Tsarouhas K, Tekos F, Stan M, Nikitovic D et al (2020) Obesity - a risk factor for increased COVID-19 prevalence, severity and lethality (review). Mol Med Rep 22:9–19. https://doi.org/10.3892/mmr.2020.11127
43. Lagunas-Rangel FA (2020) Neutrophil-to-lymphocyte ratio and lymphocyteto-C-reactive protein ratio in patients with severe coronavirus disease 2019 (COVID-19): a meta-analysis. J Med Virol 92(10):1733–1734. https://doi.org/10.1002/jmv.25819 In press
44. Ji D, Qin E, Xu J et al (2020) Non-alcoholic fatty liver diseases in patients with COVID-19: a retrospective study. J Hepatol 8:451–453
45. Wieckowska A, Papouchado BG, Li Z, Lopez R, Zein NN, Feldstein AE (2008) Increased hepatic and circulating interleukin-6 levels in human non-alcoholic steatohepatitis. Am J Gastroenterol 103(6):1372–1379. https://doi.org/10.1111/j.1572-0241.2007.01774.x
46. Zheng KI, Gao F, Wang XB, Sun QF, Pan KH, Wang TY et al (2020) Obesity as a risk factor for greater severity of COVID-19 in patients with metabolic associated fatty liver disease. Metabolism. 2020;108:154244.
47. Gao F, Zheng KI, Wang X-B, Yan H-D, Sun Q-F, Pan K-H et al (2020) Metabolic associated fatty liver disease increases COVID-19 disease severity in non-diabetic patients. J Gastroenterol Hepatol. https://doi.org/10.1111/jgh.15112
48. Medeiros AK, Barbisan CC, Cruz IR, Araújo EM, Libânio BB, Albuquerque KS, Torres US (2020) Higher frequency of hepatic steatosis at CT among COVID-19-positive patients. Abdom Radiol (NY) 45(9):2748–2754. https://doi.org/10.1007/s00261-020-02648-7 Epub 2020 July 18

49. Lighter J, Phillips M, Hochman S, Sterling S, Johnson D, Francois F et al (2020) Obesity in patients younger than 60 years is a risk factor for Covid-19 hospital admission. Clin Infect Dis 15:2019–2020. https://doi.org/10.1093/cid/ciaa4
50. Cai Q, Huang D, Ou P, Yu H, Zhu Z, Xia Z, Su Y, Ma Z, Zhang Y, Li Z, He Q, Liu L, Fu Y, Chen J (2020) COVID-19 in a designated infectious diseases hospital outside Hubei Province, China. Allergy 75(7):1742–1752. https://doi.org/10.1111/all.14309
51. Garrido I, Liberal R, Macedo G (2020) Review article: COVID-19 and liver disease-what we know on may 1 2020. Aliment Pharmacol Ther 52(2):267–275. https://doi.org/10.1111/apt.15813
52. Zhou YJ, Zheng KI, Wang XB, Sun QF, Pan KH, Wang TY, Ma HL, Chen YP, George J, Zheng MH (2020) Metabolic-associated fatty liver disease is associated with severity of COVID-19. Liver Int 40(9):2160–2163. https://doi.org/10.1111/liv.14575
53. Portincasa P, Krawczyk M, Smyk W, Lammert F, Di Ciaula A (2020) COVID-19 and non-alcoholic fatty liver disease: two intersecting pandemics. Eur J Clin Investig 50:e13338
54. Petersen A, Bressem K, Albrecht J, Thieß H, Vahldiek J, Hamm B, Makowski M, Niehues A, Niehues S, Adams L (2020) The role of visceral adiposity in the severity of COVID-19: highlights from a unicenter cross-sectional pilot study in Germany. Metabolism. 110:154317. https://doi.org/10.1016/j.metabol.2020.154317
55. Parlak S, Çıvgın E, Beşler MS, Kayıpmaz AE (2021) The effect of hepatic steatosis on COVID-19 severity: chest computed tomography findings. Saudi J Gastroenterol 27(2):105–110. https://doi.org/10.4103/sjg.sjg_540_20

6

Reversion to regular diet with alternate day fasting can cure grade-I non-alcoholic fatty liver disease (NAFLD) in high-fructose-intake-associated metabolic syndrome

Nehal Mohamed Bahgat Gamil[1,2*], Sahar Mohamed El Agaty[1], Gehan Khalaf Megahed[1], Rania Salah Mansour[1] and Marwa Saad Abdel-Latif[1]

Abstract

Background: Non-alcoholic fatty liver disease (NAFLD) is an emerging global health problem that accompanied the obesity epidemic and is considered as the hepatic component of metabolic syndrome (MetS). Modification of lifestyle of MetS patients remains the focus to reverse and prevent progression of hepatic steatosis to NAFLD and its worsening to severe forms. The present study investigates the possible curability of metabolic syndrome -associated grade-1 NAFLD merely by alternate day fasting with or without reversion to regular diet in adult male rats. The present study was performed on 66 local strain male rats aged (6–10 m.) distributed randomly into C group (n = 12), on regular rat diet; and M group (n = 54) on high fructose- intake. On the 8th week, then rats were subjected to measurement of BW, BMI, WC, FBG, IPGTT, HDL-C, TGs, and liver histopathology, to include MetS rats randomly into four experimental groups for 4 weeks as follows: MS (n = 14); MSRD (n = 12); MSF (n = 13); and MSRDF (n = 12). On the 12th week, all rats were subjected to measurements of BW, BMI, WC, LW, LW/BW, VFW, VFW/BW, FBG, IPGTT, Ins., HOMA-IR, HbA1C, TGs, TC, LDL-C, HDL-C, CRP, Alb., bilirubin, ALT, L-MDA, and liver histopathology.

Results: On the 8th week, M group developed MerS and grade-I NAFLD with score-4 hepatosteatosis (69%). On the 12th week, MS group had grade-1 NAFLD with score-4 hepatosteatosis (82%) with significantly increased Ins., HOMA-IR, HDL-C, LW, LW/BW, L-MDA, ALT, CRP, and significantly decreased Alb. than C rats. Both MSRD and MSF groups had grade-1 NAFLD with score-3 hepatosteatosis (42%) with significantly decreased Ins., HOMA-IR, TC, LDL-C, LW, LW/BW, L-MDA, ALT, CRP, and significantly increased HDL-C and Alb. than MS group. MSRDF rats showed cure of grade-1 NAFLD and significantly decreased LW than other groups and normalized HOMA-IR, HbA1C TC, LDL-C, ALT, and CRP.

Conclusion: One month of alternate-day fasting and regular rat diet could cure grade-I NAFLD associated with Mets due to high fructose intake possibly by attenuating metabolic disorders. These two interventions might be recommended in the management of MetS patients with grade 1-NAFLD disease.

Keywords: Metabolic syndrome, Non-alcoholic fatty liver disease, Hepatic steatosis, Alternate day fasting, Insulin resistance

* Correspondence: dr_nehalgamil@med.asu.edu.eg
[1]Medical Physiology Department, Faculty of Medicine, Ain Shams University, Cairo, Egypt
[2]Histology and Cell Biology Department, Faculty of Medicine, Ain Shams University, Cairo, Egypt

Background

The metabolic syndrome (MetS) is a cluster of risk factors for cardiovascular disease and type 2 diabetes mellitus [1]. The diagnosis of MetS is based on presence of 3 of 5factors, which include TGs 150 mg/dL or greater, high-density lipoprotein cholesterol (HDL-C) of less than 40 mg/dL in men and less than 50 mg/dL in women, hypertension defined as systolic blood pressure 130 mmHg or greater or diastolic blood pressure 85 mmHg or greater, hyperglycemia defined as fasting glucose 100 mg/dL or greater, and increased waist circumference, defined by country and population-specific criteria [1].

The incidence of non-alcoholic fatty liver disease (NAFLD) has been increasing in concert with the rising rates of MetS [2]. Epidemiological data shows that global prevalence of NAFLD in different populations is around 30% [3]. NAFLD is the most common cause of chronic liver disease worldwide [4]. NAFLD is comprised of non-alcoholic fatty liver (NAFL) and nonalcoholic steatohepatitis (NASH) [5]. NAFL is characterized by steatosis of the liver, involving greater than 5% of parenchyma, with no evidence of hepatocyte injury [6]. Whereas NASH is a necroinflammatory process whereby the liver cells become injured in a background of steatosis [6]. NASH may progress to fibrosis, cirrhosis, and hepatocellular carcinoma (HCC) [7, 8]. According to the guidelines of the American Association for the Study of Liver Diseases (AASLD), the definition of NAFLD requires the presence of primary hepatic steatosis diagnosed either by imaging or by histology and no other reasons for secondary hepatic fat accumulation [9]. Within the next 20 years, it is expected that NAFLD will be the major cause of liver-related morbidity and mortality as well as a leading indication for liver transplantation [10].

The development of NAFLD (i.e., steatosis) results from an increased inflow of free fatty acids (FFA) derived from insulin-resistant adipose tissue, altered hepatic processing of dietary lipids delivered by lipoproteins, increased hepatic de novo lipogenesis, or impaired lipid export out of the hepatocytes [4]. Also, alterations in the production and secretion of adipokines and inflammatory cytokines due to adipose tissue dysfunction because of insulin resistance are involved [11]. Moreover, the production of reactive oxygen species, endoplasmic reticulum stress coupled with mitochondrial dysfunction, and the gut microbiota had been recognized as key players in the pathogenesis of NAFLD [2, 12].

NAFLD remains asymptomatic in a significant proportion of patients, and the diagnosis is often suspected when liver functions are found abnormal on biochemical testing or hepatic imaging (ultrasonography, computed tomography [CT], or magnetic resonance imaging [MRI] of liver) suggest fatty liver, when performed for other purposes [13]. Liver biopsy remains the gold standard for diagnostic evaluation of NAFLD [13]. Biopsy not only confirms the diagnosis but provides information on extent of fibrosis and steatosis, necro-inflammation, and architectural distortion [13].

Human fructose consumption is largely driven by added sugars, and the intake of sugar-sweetened beverages generally corresponds to total fructose intake [14]. Several epidemiological studies have evaluated the association between average daily fructose intake and hepatic steatosis [15]. Several factors may potentially contribute to fructose-induced NAFLD, including the induction of the MetS [16].

There is no single intervention that is proven to be fully effective in the treatment and cure of NAFLD [13]. The main goals of treatment are to improve steatosis and to prevent progression of the disease [13]. Intense lifestyle modification and treatment of the risk factors are the cornerstones of disease management [13]. Medical and surgical interventions serve as second-line treatments, or as adjuvants [13]. Both exercise and dietary interventions in isolation or in combination have been shown to improve biochemical and histological parameters of NAFLD [13].

There are two methods of dietary restriction, which are caloric restriction (CR) and intermittent fasting (IMF) [17]. IMF protocols can be grouped into alternate-day fasting (ADF), whole-day fasting, and time-restricted feeding like one-meal-per-day [18]. ADF regimens consist of a "feed day" (ad libitum food intake for 24 h) alternated with a "fast day" (complete fast for 24 h), but the overall energy intake is not limited [19]. IMF is a nutritional intervention with significant metabolic effects on the liver that are not yet fully understood.

Methods

Experimental animals

This study was approved by the Research Ethics Committee at the Faculty of Medicine, Ain Shams University (The FMASU REC) that operates under Federal Wide Assurance No. FWA 000017585.

The present study was performed on 66 local strain male rats, initially weighing 120–180 g. Rats were purchased from VACSERA (EGY VAC) (Helwan, Cairo) and were housed in Medical Ain Shams Research Institute (MASRI) Animal House, Faculty of Medicine, Ain Shams University, under standard conditions of boarding at room temperature 22 ± 4 °C. Rats were kept in plastic cages (3–5 rats/cage) for 2 weeks for acclimatization. Animals were randomly allocated into the following two groups:

Group I; control rat group (C, n = 12): Rats in this group were fed the control diet for 8 weeks. At the end of the 8th week, two rats were scarified for histopathological study of the liver; the other 10 rats were continued on the control diet for additional 4 weeks and were studied by the end of the 12th week.

Group II; metabolic syndrome with liver steatosis rat group (M, n = 54): Metabolic syndrome was induced by high fructose diet besides additional fructose solution (4 g fructose dissolved in 4 ml distilled water/rat/day) introduced daily by gavage. The high fructose diet and solution was given for 8 weeks. At the end of the 8th week, three rats were scarified for histopathological study of the liver. Blood samples were withdrawn from all rats for laboratory examination, then the proven metabolic syndrome rats (n = 51) were randomly allocated into the following four experimental groups:

A. Untreated metabolic syndrome group (MS, n = 14): Rats in this group were continued on high fructose diet and the fructose solution by gavage similar to M group for additional 4 weeks and were studied at the end of the 12th week.
B. Metabolic syndrome group reverted to regular rat chow (MSRD, n = 12): Rats in this group were reverted to control diet for 4 weeks.
C. Metabolic syndrome group on alternate-day fasting (MSF, n = 13) according to Varady et al. [20]: Rats in this group underwent alternate-day fasting regimen in the form of alternating 24-h periods of ad libitum feeding and fasting (100% calorie restriction on fast day, ad libitum high fructose diet on feed day with the fructose solution by gavage similar to the M group) for 4 weeks.
D. Metabolic syndrome group reverted to regular rat chow and on alternate-day fasting (MSRDF, n = 12): Rats in this group underwent alternate-day fasting regimen in the form of alternating 24-h periods of ad libitum feeding and fasting (100% calorie restriction on fast day, ad libitum control diet on feed day) for 4 weeks.

Control diet: Rats were fed rat chow consisting of corn starch (61%), Kareish cheese (casein, 20%), wheat bran (9.5%), butter (5%), mineral mixture (3.5%), and vitamin mixture (1%) according to Patel et al. [21]. Food was prepared weekly and was kept in the refrigerator and was administrated ad libitum.

High fructose diet: This diet was prepared as the control diet except for corn starch, which was replaced by fructose powder (Fructofin C, manufactured by Danisco Sweeteners Oy, Kotka, Finland), according to Patel et al. [21] to be 61% fructose powder, 20% casein, 9.5% wheat bran, 5% butter, 3.5% mineral mixture, and 1% vitamin mixture; however, the route of administration was modified, where fructose content in the formula was reduced to 40% instead of 60% to avoid food aversion and the remaining 20% was given by gavage according to Bahgat et al. [22]. Adult rats on high fructose diet showed average food intake ~ 20 g/rat/day by the 2nd–4th week. Thus, 61% fructose content in the diet formula is ≈12 g/rat, 2/3 of it was given in the diet and the remaining 1/3 (4 g fructose/4 ml distilled water/rat/day) was given by gavage. Food was prepared weekly and was kept in the refrigerator.

At the end of the accommodation period, all rats in the present study were subjected to basal assessment of body weight (BW), body mass index (BMI), waist circumference (WC), fasting blood glucose level (FBG), and intraperitoneal glucose tolerance test (IPGTT). Retro-orbital blood samples were taken for determination of serum levels of HDL-C and TGs. Throughout the experiment, all rats were subjected to weekly assessment of BW. At the end of the induction period of metabolic syndrome (8th week), all rats were re-assessed for the same parameters mentioned before. Five randomly selected rats from C and M rat groups were scarified for histopathological study of the liver to prove the presence of steatosis.

At the end of the study on the 12th week, 1 day before sacrifice, rats were subjected to estimation of FBG by using GlucoDr SuperSensor™ test strips and the GlucoDr Super Sensor™ Meter apparatus (model name AGM-2200, manufactured by All Medicus Co., Ltd., KOREA). Glucose tolerance testing was performed according to Zhang et al. [23], using D-glucose stock (Anhydrous glucose A.R) supplied by El-Nasr Pharmaceutical Chemicals; area under the curve (AUC) was calculated according to Matthews et al. [24].

On the day of sacrifice, overnight fasted rats were weighed, placed on its back, fixed on the dissecting table, and the length of the rat was measured from the tip of the nose (while the neck is extended) to the anus to calculate the BMI according to the following equation: Body mass index (BMI) = Body weight (g) / length (cm^2) [25], then the measuring tape was carefully placed under the rat and around the transverse plane, directly below the bottom rib of the rib-cage to measure the WC according to Panchal et al. [26].

The rats were anesthetized by intraperitoneal injection of phenobarbitone in a dose of 40 mg/kg body weight, blood samples were taken in two separate tubes, one containing EDTA for estimation of glycosylated hemoglobin (HbA1C) and the other was centrifuged at 4000 rpm for 20 min to separate the serum, that was then stored frozen at − 80 °C for subsequent determination of the other biochemical studies. Visceral fat and liver were excised, washed with 0.9% saline solution, and dried by filter paper, then they were freshly weighed in the same day using 5-digit precision Metler balance (AE163).The results were expressed as absolute values

(g) and relative values to the body weight (absolute tissue weight / body weight, g/g).

Biochemical measurements

HbA1C (BioSystems S.A. Costa Brava, 30.08030 Barcelona (Spain), colorimetric method). Serum TGs (BioMed laboratory, Badr City, Egypt, colorimetric method) according to Fassati and Prencipe [27]. Serum TC (BioMed laboratory, Badr City, Egypt, colorimetric method) according to Tietz [28]. Serum HDL-C (BioMed laboratory, Badr City, Egypt, colorimetric method) according to Young [29]. Serum fasting insulin and C-reactive protein (CRP) (MyBiosource, Inc., USA, enzyme immunoassay (ELISA)). Serum albumin (BioMed laboratory, Badr City, Egypt, colorimetric method) according to Doumas and Biggs [30]. Serum total bilirubin (BioMed laboratory, Badr City, Egypt, colorimetric method) described by Rand and Di Pasqua [31] automated by Golub [32]. Serum alanine transferase (ALT) (BioMed laboratory, Badr City, Egypt, colorimetric method) according to Henry [33]. Liver tissue malondialdehyde (MDA) (Biodiagnostic, Egypt, colorimetric method) according to Satoh [34] and Ohkawa et al. [35]. Calculation of low-density lipoprotein cholesterol (LDL-C) according to the following equation: $C_{LDL} = C_{Total}-C_{HDL}-TG/5$ [36].

Calculation of insulin resistance (HOMA-IR) score: insulin resistance was calculated by the Homeostasis Model Assessment Score = (fasting insulin (μIU/mL) × fasting glucose (mmol/L) / 22.5) [37]. Serum insulin was converted from ng/mL, to μIU/mL by dividing it by 0.0347 [38]. To convert blood glucose to plasma glucose, the values were multiplied by 1.12 [39]. As blood glucose was measured in mg/dl, it was converted to mmol/L by dividing by 18.016. Biochemical analysis was carried out blindly by an expert clinical pathologist.

Histopathological study

The liver specimens were collected and fixed in 10% buffered formalin and embedded in paraffin. Five micrometer sections was cut and stained with hematoxylin and eosin (H&E), periodic acid–Schiff (PAS), and Maison Trichome. Diagnosis and grading of nonalcoholic fatty liver disease (NAFLD) was done according to Mendler et al. [40] in control (C) and metabolic syndrome (M) groups at the end of 8th week of the study; and in all studied groups 4 weeks later at the end of the study. Histopathology was carried out blindly by an expert histopathologist.

Statistical analysis

All statistical data and significance tests were performed by using Statistical program for Social Science (SPSS Inc.) version 20 according to Armitage and Berry [41]. Differences in the same group were determined by Student's "*t*" test for paired data, differences between 2 groups were compared by independent sample "*t*" test, and differences between all 5 groups were compared by one-way ANOVA with least significant difference test (LSD), a probability of $P < 0.05$ was considered statistically significant. Correlation coefficients were calculated by linear regression analysis (ranking data directly or indirectly) using the least square method. A probability of $P < 0.05$ was considered statistically significant. All results were expressed as mean ± SEM.

Results

Eighth week versus initial results of metabolic syndrome (M) and control (C) groups:

The 8th week values of BW, BMI, and WC were significantly higher than their corresponding initial values in both C ($P < 0.001$, $P < 0.005$, $P < 0.005$ respectively) and M groups ($P < 0.001$) (Table 1)

Eighth week values of the blood glucose levels during IPGTT at 60 min, 90 min, and 120 min, and AUC were significantly increased in C rats compared to their corresponding initial values ($P < 0.05$, $P < 0.05$, $P < 0.01$, $P < 0.05$ respectively). For M group, the 8th week values of FBG, blood glucose levels during IPGTT at 30 min, 60 min, 90 min, and 120 min, PG and AUC were significantly increased in M group compared to their corresponding initial values ($P < 0.001$) (Fig. 1); both C and M groups presented a significantly higher serum level of TGs ($P < 0.005$, $P < 0.001$ respectively) along with a significantly lower HDL-C ($P < 0.001$) in the 8th week compared to their corresponding initial values.

The initial values of BW, BMI, WC, FBG, IPGTT, PG, AUC, and serum levels of TGs and HDL-C were insignificantly different between C and M groups. After 8 weeks of high fructose diet, M rats exhibited a significantly higher values of WC; blood glucose levels (measured during IPGTT) at 30 min, and 120 min; PG, AUC associated with a significant lower serum levels of HDL-C in comparison to C group ($P < 0.05$) (Figs. 1 and 2).

Final versus 8th week results of C, MS, MSRD, MSF, and MSRDF

BW and BMI were not significantly changed, whereas WC was significantly increased in the C and MS groups in comparison to their corresponding 8th week's values ($P < 0.05$, $P < 0.01$, respectively). BW and WC were significantly increased in metabolic syndrome group reverted to regular rat chow (MSRD) group compared to their corresponding 8th week's values ($P < 0.05$). However, BW, BMI, and WC were significantly decreased in metabolic syndrome group on alternate-day fasting (MSF) group ($P < 0.001$, $P < 0.001$, $P < 0.005$ respectively) and MSRDF ($P < 0.001$) groups (Table 2).

Table 1 The initial and 8th week anthropometric and lipid parameters in control and metabolic syndrome groups

	BW (gm)		BMI (gm/cm^2)		WC (cm)		TGs (mg/dl)		HDL-C (mg/dl)	
	Initial	8th week	Initial	8th week	Initial	8th week	Initial	8th week	Initial	8th week
(C)	140.83 ±2.18 (12)	188.33* ±6.63 (12)	0.42 ±0.00 (12)	0.48* ±0.01 (12)	11.00 ±0.16 (12)	11.79* ±0.18 (12)	100.09 ±3.27 (11)	120.82* ±3.89 (11)	61.09 ±1.70 (11)	37.70* ±1.97 (10)
(M)	142.44 ±1.84 (54)	179.93* ±3.05 (54)	0.43 ±0.00 (54)	0.49* ±0.01 (54)	10.63 ±0.09 (54)	12.25*a ±0.09 (54)	93.78 ±1.72 (51)	119.33* ±2.77 (51)	58.14 ±1.09 (51)	30.84*a ±1.32 (51)

M, metabolic syndrome group; C, control group; BW, body weight; BMI, body mass index; WC, waist circumference; TGs, triglycerides; HDL-C, high density lipoprotein cholesterol
In the parenthesis is the number of observations
Data are expressed as mean ± SEM
*: Significance from initial value, by Student's "t" test for paired data, at P ≤0.05
a: Significance from control group, by Student's "t" test for un-paired data, at P ≤0.05

Compared to 8th week values, serum TGs were significantly decreased in C group ($P < 0.001$), but significantly increased in MS group ($P < 0.05$), but showed significant decrease in MSF group ($P < 0.01$) and insignificant change in MSRD and MSRDF groups. On the other hand, HDL-C showed significant increase in C, MSRD, MSF, and MSRDF groups ($P < 0.001$, $P < 0.05$, $P < 0.01$, $P < 0.005$ respectively) with insignificant change in MS group (Table 2).

Compared to 8th week values, final FBG, blood glucose levels during IPGTT at 30 min, 60 min, 90 min, and 120 min; PG; and AUC; all were not significantly changed in the C group. The MS group exhibited a significantly lower final levels of blood glucose during IPGTT at 60 min, 90 min, and 120 min, along with a significant decrease in AUC versus their corresponding 8th week's values ($P < 0.05$, $P < 0.001$, $P < 0.005$, $P < 0.005$ respectively). Although, alternate day fasting alone

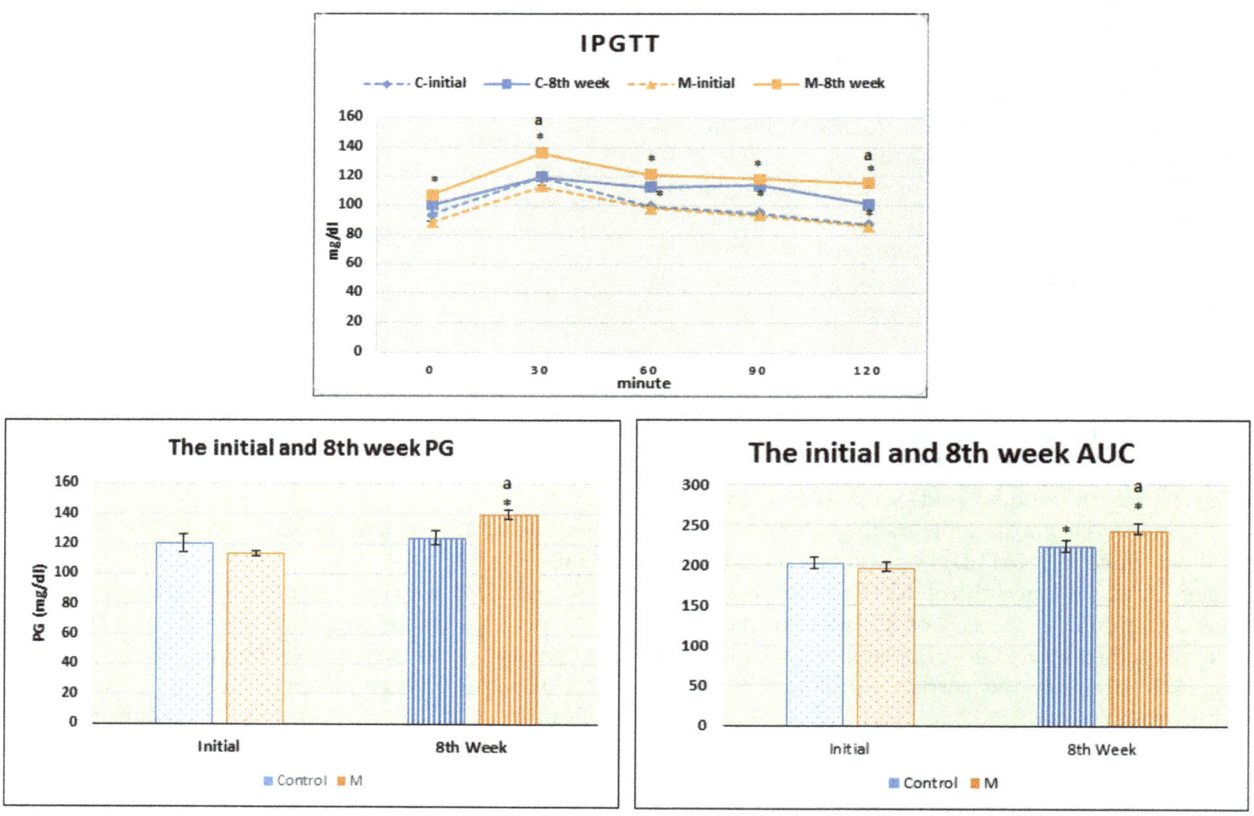

Fig. 1 The initial and 8th week glucose homeostasis parameters in control and metabolic syndrome groups. *M* metabolic syndrome group, *IPGTT* intraperitoneal glucose tolerance test, *PG* peak glycemia, *AUC* area under the curve. Data are expressed as mean ± SEM. * Significance from initial value, by Student's "*t*" test for paired data, at *P* ≤ 0.05. a: Significance from control group, by Student's "*t*" test for un-paired data, at *P* ≤ 0.05

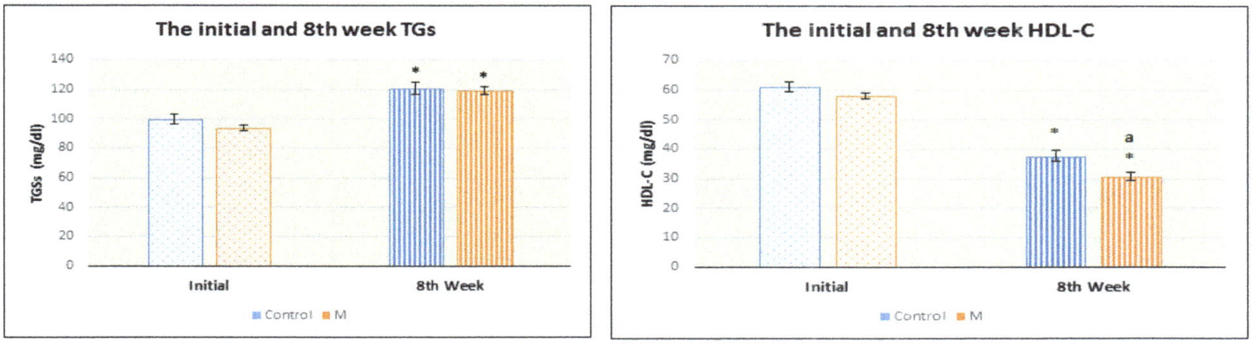

Fig. 2 The initial and 8th week lipid parameters, in control and metabolic syndrome groups. *M* metabolic syndrome group, *TGs* triglycerides, *HDL-C* high density lipoprotein cholesterol. Data are expressed as mean ± SEM. * Significance from initial value, by Student's "*t*" test for paired data, at $P \leq 0.05$. a: Significance from control group, by Student's "*t*" test for un-paired data, at $P \leq 0.05$

significantly decreased the final FBG only in MSF rats ($P < 0.05$); reversion to regular rat chow, whether alone or in combination with alternate day fasting, resulted in a significant decrease in FBG and blood glucose levels at 30 min, 60 min, 90 min, and 120 min; PG; and AUC) in both MSRD ($P < 0.05$, $P < 0.001$, $P < 0.005$, $P < 0.001$, $P < 0.01$, $P < 0.001$, $P < 0.001$ respectively) and MSRDF ($P < 0.001$, $P < 0.01$, $P < 0.001$, $P < 0.001$, $P < 0.005$, $P < 0.005$, $P < 0.001$ respectively) groups compared to their corresponding 8th week's values (Fig. 3).

Final results of C, MS, MSRD, MSF, and MSRDF

BW, BMI, WC, VFW, and VFW/BW

MS group demonstrated non-significant changes in the final values of BW, BMI, WC, visceral fat weight (VFW), and VFW/BW compared to those of the C group; similarly, MSRD group had no significant difference in these parameters compared to MS and C rat groups. On the other hand, these parameters were significantly decreased in MSF group compared to MS group ($P < 0.001$), MSRD group ($P < 0.001$, $P < 0.001$, $P < 0.005$, $P < 0.001$, $P < 0.001$ respectively) as well as C group ($P < 0.001$, $P < 0.005$, $P < 0.005$, $P < 0.001$, $P < 0.001$ respectively), and as well as C group ($P < 0.001$, $P < 0.005$, $P < 0.005$, $P < 0.001$, $P < 0.001$ respectively). Similarly, MSRDF group demonstrated significant decrease in all these parameters compared to MS ($P < 0.001$, $P < 0.005$, $P < 0.001$, $P < 0.001$, $P < 0.001$ respectively), MSRD ($P < 0.001$) groups, as well as those of C ($P < 0.001$, $P < 0.05$, $P < 0.001$, $P < 0.001$, $P < 0.001$ respectively) (Fig. 4).

Table 2 The 8th week and final anthropometric and lipid parameters in the five study groups

	BW (gm)		BMI (gm/cm^2)		WC (cm)		TGs (mg/dl)		HDL-C (mg/dl)	
	8th week	Final	8th week	Final	8th week	Final	8th week	Final	8th week	Final
C	186.80 ±7.93 (10)	197.20 ±8.06 (10)	0.48 ±0.01 (10)	0.47 ±0.01 (10)	11.90 ±0.19 (10)	12.90* ±0.41 (10)	122.22 ±3.35 (9)	83.11* ±3.93 (9)	38.38 ±2.40 (8)	57.88* ±1.66 (8)
MS	183.50 ±5.97 (14)	194.50 ±7.77 (14)	0.49 ±0.02 (14)	0.48 ±0.02 (14)	11.96 ±0.18 (14)	12.93* ±0.30 (14)	116.10 ±8.28 (10)	136.30* ±4.70 (10)	27.50 ±3.69 (10)	27.40 ±1.55 (10)
MSRD	181.58 ±7.20 (12)	198.00* ±8.26 (12)	0.48 ±0.01 (12)	0.49 ±0.01 (12)	12.17 ±0.14 (12)	12.88* ±0.26 (12)	118.67 ±6.53 (9)	107.56 ±3.22 (9)	34.78 ±2.74 (9)	45.11* ±1.62 (9)
MSF	176.85 ±4.65 (13)	151.31* ±5.59 (13)	0.48 ±0.01 (13)	0.41* ±0.01 (13)	12.35 ±0.17 (13)	11.46* ±0.23 (13)	121.11 ±4.43 (9)	103.22* ±3.67 (9)	31.22 ±2.68 (9)	48.22* ±2.60 (9)
MSRDF	172.08 ±7.18 (12)	148.92* ±5.85 (12)	0.50 ±0.02 (12)	0.42* ±0.01 (12)	12.54 ±0.21 (12)	11.17* ±0.20 (12)	114.75 ±7.32 (8)	96.25 ±3.24 (8)	31.00 ±2.90 (8)	50.25* ±2.46 (8)

C, control group, MS, untreated metabolic syndrome group, MSRD, metabolic syndrome group reverted to regular rat chow, MSF, metabolic syndrome group on alternate day fasting, MSRDF, metabolic syndrome group reverted to regular rat chow and on alternate day fasting;
BW, body weight; BMI, body mass index; WC, waist circumference; TGs, triglycerides; HDL-C, high density lipoprotein cholesterol
In the parenthesis is the number of observations
Data are expressed as mean ± SEM
*: Significance from 8th week value, by Student's "t" test for paired data, at $P \leq 0.05$

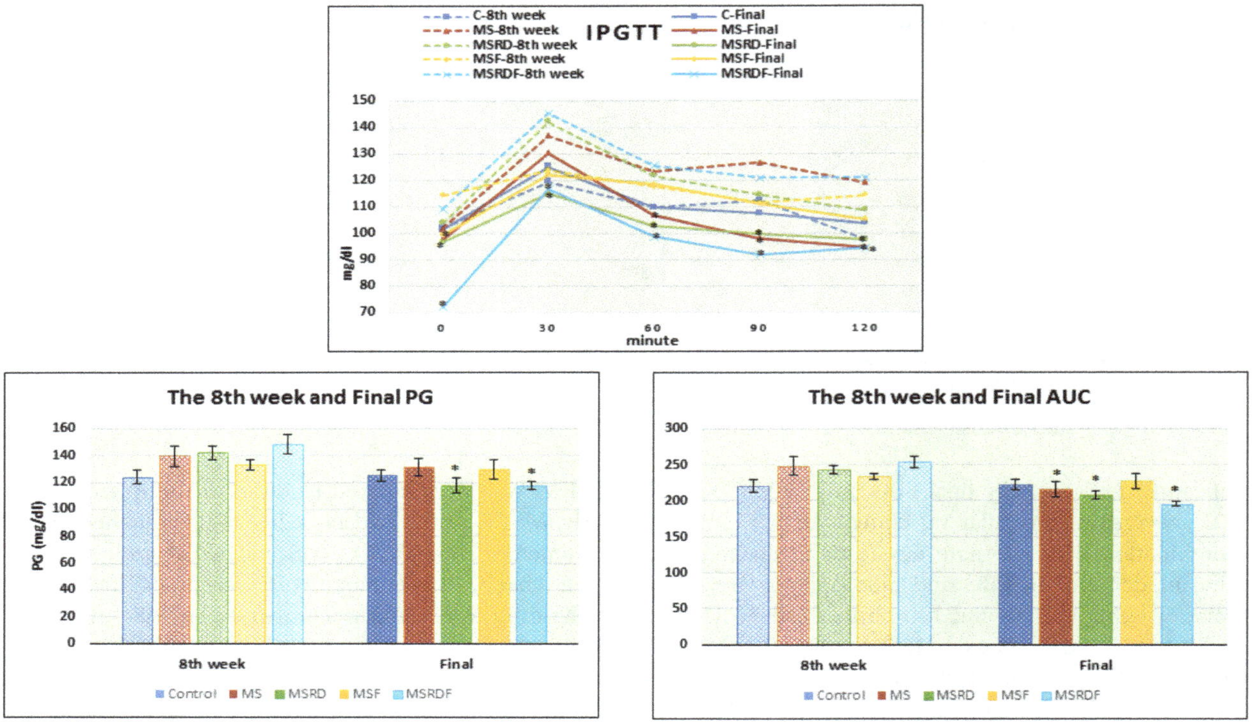

Fig. 3 The 8th week and final glucose homeostasis parameters in the five study groups. *MS* untreated metabolic syndrome group, *MSRD* metabolic syndrome group reverted to regular rat chow, *MSF* metabolic syndrome group on alternate day fasting, *MSRDF* metabolic syndrome group reverted to regular rat chow and on alternate day fasting, *IPGTT* intraperitoneal glucose tolerance test, *PG* peak glycemia, *AUC* area under the curve. Data are expressed as mean ± SEM. * Significance from 8th week value, by Student's "*t*" test for paired data, at $P \leq 0.05$

FBG, IPGTT, PG, AUC, HbA1C, serum fasting insulin, and HOMA-IR

Final values of FBG and blood glucose during IPGTT; PG; and AUC; Hb A1C, all were insignificantly changed in MS group compared to those of the C rats, while the serum fasting insulin level and HOMA-IR were significantly increased in MS group compared to the C group ($P < 0.001$). MSRD group showed non-significant changes in the final values of FBG and blood glucose during IPGTT, PG, and AUC in addition to Hb A1C when compared to those of the MS or C groups. MSRD group showed significant decrease in serum fasting insulin level and HOMA-IR compared to MS group ($P < 0.001$, $P < 0.005$ respectively), and significant increase compared to the C group ($P < 0.001$). MSF group showed significant increase in the levels of blood glucose during IPGTT at 90 min, 120 min ($P < 0.05$), non-significant change in PG and AUC but significant decrease in serum fasting insulin level, HOMA-IR, and Hb A1C compared to MS rats ($P < 0.005$, $P < 0.001$, $P < 0.005$ respectively). Compared to MSRD group, MSF group presented a significantly elevated blood glucose levels during IPGTT at 60 min and 90 min ($P < 0.05$), along with non-significant changes in PG, AUC, serum fasting insulin level, HOMA-IR, and Hb A1C. In comparison to the C group, all the measured glucose homeostasis parameters were not significantly different in MSF rats except for a significantly higher serum fasting insulin and HOMA-IR ($P < 0.001$). MSRDF group exhibited a significant lower level of fasting blood glucose when compared to MSRD, MSF, C, and MS rat groups ($P < 0.005$). The blood glucose levels during IPGTT at 60 min, 90 min, and 120 min were decreased in MSRDF group compared with MSF group ($P < 0.01$, $P < 0.005$, $P < 0.05$ respectively). Compared to the C group, the levels of blood glucose measured during IPGTT in MSRDF group were not significantly different except for a significantly lower value at 90 min ($P < 0.05$). PG was not significantly changed in MSRDF group compared to the other four groups. AUC was significantly decreased in MSRDF group in comparison to MSF and control groups ($P < 0.01$, $P < 0.05$ respectively). Serum fasting insulin and HOMA-IR were significantly decreased in MSRDF group versus MS ($P < 0.001$), MSRD ($P < 0.05$, $P < 0.005$ respectively), and MSF ($P < 0.005$, $P < 0.01$ respectively) groups. HbA1C was decreased in MSRDF group compared with MSRD, MSF, and MS, groups, being significant in MS group only ($P < 0.01$). In comparison to C rats, serum fasting insulin was still significantly higher in MSRDF group ($P < 0.005$),

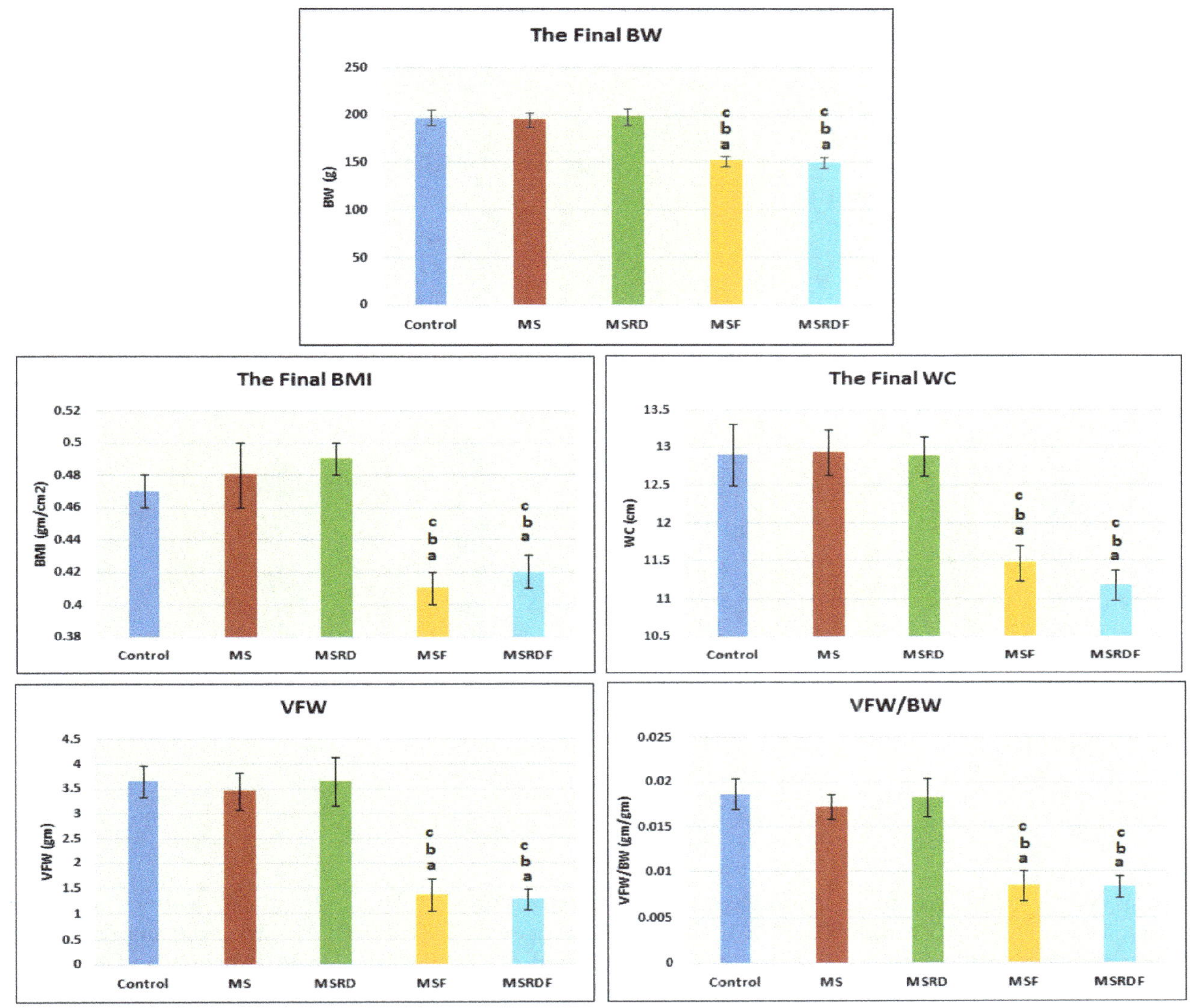

Fig. 4 The final anthropometric and visceral fat parameters in the five study groups. *MS* untreated metabolic syndrome group, *MSRD* metabolic syndrome group reverted to regular rat chow, *MSF* metabolic syndrome group on alternate day fasting, *MSRDF* metabolic syndrome group reverted to regular rat chow and on alternate day fasting, *BW* body weight, *BMI* body mass index, *WC* waist circumference, *VFW* visceral fat weight, *VFW/BW* visceral fat weight/body weight. Data are expressed as mean ± SEM. a: Significance from control group, by LSD test at $P \leq 0.05$. b: Significance from MS group, by LSD test at $P \leq 0.05$. c: Significance from MSRD group, by LSD test at $P \leq 0.05$

while HOMA-IR and HbA1C were not significantly different (Fig. 5 and Table 3).

Lipid profile

MS group showed a significantly higher final serum levels of TGs, TC, and LDL-C associated with a significantly lower HDL-C compared to the C group ($P < 0.001$). MSRD group demonstrated a significantly reduced final serum levels of TGs, TC, and LDL-C ($P < 0.001$, $P < 0.005$, $P < 0.001$ respectively) associated with a significantly elevated HDL-C ($P < 0.001$) compared to the MS group; however, TGs, TC, and LDL-C were still significantly higher ($P < 0.001$, $P < 0.005$, $P < 0.001$ respectively), and HDL-C was significantly lower ($P < 0.001$) compared to the C group. Similarly, MSF group demonstrated a significantly decreased TGs, TC, and LDL-C associated with a significantly elevated HDL-C compared to the MS group ($P < 0.001$); however, TGs, TC, and LDL-C were still significantly higher ($P < 0.005$, $P < 0.05$, $P < 0.05$ respectively), and HDL-C was significantly lower ($P < 0.005$) compared to the C group. On comparing the parameters of lipid profile between the MSRD and MSF groups, non-significant changes were observed. MSRDF group exhibited a significant decrease of the final serum levels of TGs, TC, and LDL-C, along with a rise in HDL-C compared to the MS group ($P <$

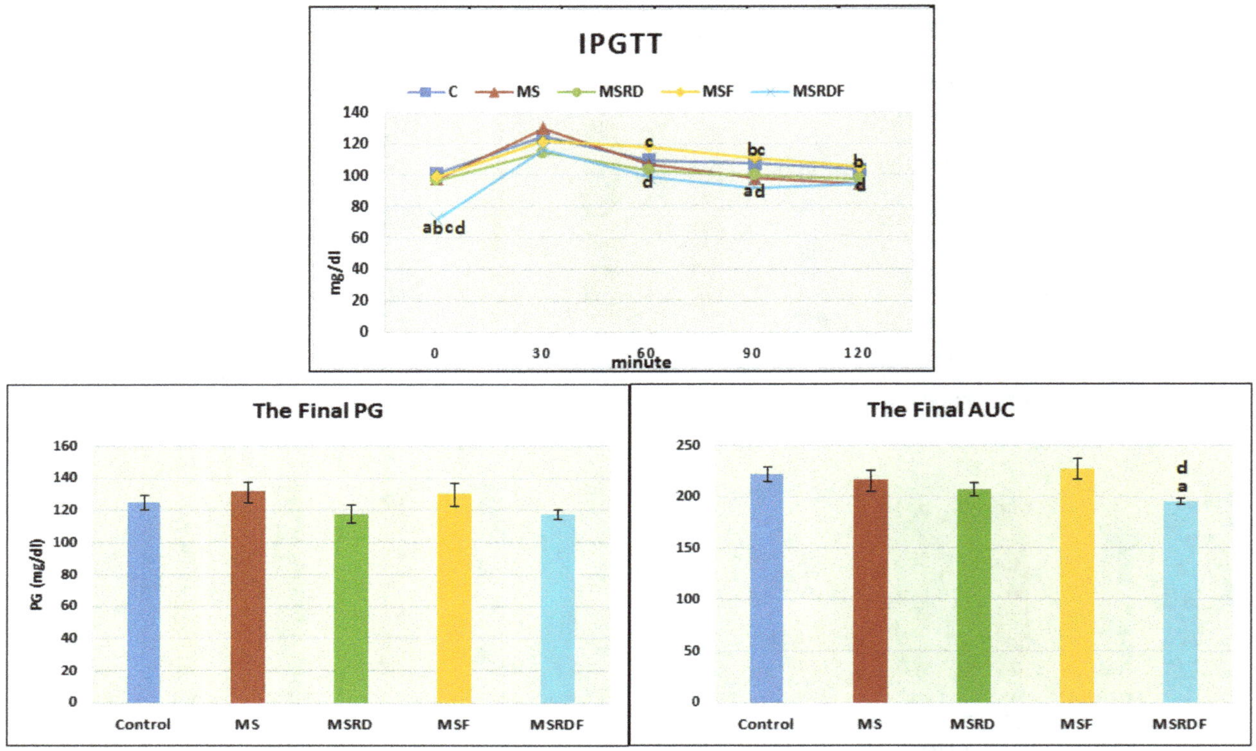

Fig. 5 The final glucose homeostasis parameters in the five study groups. *MS* untreated metabolic syndrome group, *MSRD* metabolic syndrome group reverted to regular rat chow, *MSF* metabolic syndrome group on alternate day fasting, *MSRDF* metabolic syndrome group reverted to regular rat chow and on alternate day fasting, *IPGTT* intraperitoneal glucose tolerance test, *PG* peak glycemia, *AUC* area under the curve. Data are expressed as mean ± SEM. a: Significance from control group, by LSD test at $P \leq 0.05$. b: Significance from MS group, by LSD test at $P \leq 0.05$. c: Significance from MSRD group, by LSD test at $P \leq 0.05$. d: Significance from MSF group by LSD test, at $P \leq 0.05$

0.001) as well as MSRD groups as regards serum levels of TGs, TC, and LDL ($P < 0.05$, $P < 0.005$, and $P < 0.005$, respectively) with insignificant change in HDL-C. Furthermore, in comparison to the MSF group, MSRDF group showed a significant decrease in the final serum levels TC and LDL-C ($P < 0.05$) with no significant changes in TGs or HDL-C. Moreover, the final serum levels of TC and LDL-C in MSRDF group attained those of the controls, yet TGs was still significantly higher ($P < 0.05$) and the HDL-C was significantly lower ($P < 0.005$) than those of the C group (Table 4).

Table 3 The final glucose homeostasis parameters in the five study groups

	Insulin (ng/ml)	HOMA-IR	HbA1C (mg/dl)
C	0.13±0.01 (9)	1.09±0.10 (9)	5.97±0.30 (10)
MS	0.91±0.06^{a} (10)	7.35±0.83^{a} (10)	6.60±0.39 (14)
MSRD	0.61 ±0.07^{a,b} (9)	4.67 ±0.55^{a,b} (9)	6.08±0.52(12)
MSF	0.64±0.07 ^{a,b} (9)	4.46 ±0.52 ^{a,b} (9)	5.25±0.11^{b} (13)
MSRDF	0.39 ±0.05^{a,b,c,d} (9)	2.29±0.35^{b,c,d} (9)	5.23±0.16^{b} (12)

C, control group, MS, untreated metabolic syndrome group, MSRD, metabolic syndrome group reverted to regular rat chow, MSF, metabolic syndrome group on alternate day fasting, MSRDF, metabolic syndrome group reverted to regular rat chow and on alternate day fasting; HOMA-IR, homeostasis model assessment of insulin resistance; HbA1C, glycosylated hemoglobin
Data are expressed as mean ± SEM
In the parenthesis is the number of observations
a: Significance from control group, by LSD test at P ≤0.05
b: Significance from MS group, by LSD test at P ≤0.05
c: Significance from MSRD group, by LSD test at P ≤0.05
d: Significance from MSF group, by LSD test at P ≤0.05

LW, LW/BW, ALT, albumin, bilirubin, MDA, and CRP

MS group showed a significant increase in the final liver weight (LW) and liver weight/body weight ratio (LW/BW) versus the C group ($P < 0.001$). MSRD and MSF groups presented a significant decrease in LW and LW/BW compared to MS group ($P < 0.001$). Also, LW was significantly decreased in MSF group versus MSRD group ($P < 0.05$), while the LW/BW was not significantly changed. In comparison to the control rats, LW/BW was still significantly higher in MSRD and in MSF groups ($P < 0.05$, $P < 0.001$ respectively), but the LW was not significantly different. MRSDF group showed a decrease in LW ($P < 0.001$, $P < 0.001$, $P < 0.05$, respectively) compared to MS, MSRD, and MSF groups as well as LW/BW when compared to the MS and MSF groups only ($P < 0.001$) with the LW in MSRDF group becoming

Table 4 The final lipid profile parameters in the five study groups

	TGs (mg/dl)	TC (mg/dl)	LDL-C (mg/dl)	HDL-C (mg/dl)
C(9)	83.11 ±3.93	144.22 ±4.25	69.16 ±5.09	58.44±1.57
MS (10)	136.30±4.70^{a}	213.00±9.18^{a}	158.34±10.20^{a}	27.40±1.55^{a}
MSRD (9)	107.56±3.22^{a,b}	176.33±5.63 ^{a,b}	109.71±4.96 ^{a,b}	45.11±1.62 ^{a,b}
MSF(9)	103.22±3.67 ^{a,b}	165.67±7.56 ^{a,b}	96.80±8.65 ^{a,b}	48.22±2.60 ^{a,b}
MSRDF (9)	94.89±3.16 ^{a,b,c}	142.89±6.49^{b,c,d}	74.69±6.26 ^{b,c,d}	49.22±2.40^{a,b}

C, control group, MS, untreated metabolic syndrome group, MSRD, metabolic syndrome group reverted to regular rat chow, MSF, metabolic syndrome group on alternate day fasting, MSRDF, metabolic syndrome group reverted to regular rat chow and on alternate day fasting; TGs, triglycerides; TC, total cholesterol; LDL-C, low-density lipoprotein cholesterol; HDL-C, high-density lipoprotein cholesterol
Data are expressed as mean ± SEM
In the parenthesis is the number of observations
a: Significance from control group, by LSD test at P ≤0.05
b: Significance from MS group, by LSD test at P ≤0.05
c: Significance from MSRD group, by LSD test at P ≤0.05
d: Significance from MSF group, by LSD test at P ≤0.05

significantly lower than that of the control rats ($P < 0.05$) and with the LW/BW insignificantly different from control value. MS group demonstrated a significant increase in the serum level of ALT associated with a significantly lower level of serum albumin compared to the C group ($P < 0.001$). Although the levels of serum ALT were significantly decreased associated with a significant increase in serum albumin in MSRD and MSF groups compared to the MS group ($P < 0.001$), yet these parameters were not normalized when compared to control rats. In comparison to the MSRD group, serum level of albumin was not significantly changed in MSF group, but the serum level of ALT was significantly lower ($P < 0.05$). MSRDF rats showed significant decrease of ALT ($P < 0.001$) and non-significant changes of albumin compared to MSRD group, but when compared to MSF group, no significant difference was observed in either ALT or albumin. However, MSRDF group showed a significant decrease in serum ALT together with a significant increase in serum albumin compared to MS group ($P < 0.001$). In comparison to the C group, the serum ALT was not significant, while the serum albumin was significantly lower ($P < 0.05$) in MSRDF group. Concerning the serum bilirubin levels, non-significant changes were recorded among the five study groups (Table 5).

MDA was significantly increased in MS group versus C group ($P < 0.001$), and was significantly decreased in MSRD, MSF, and MSRDF groups in comparison to MS group ($P < 0.001$), though it was still significantly higher than those of the control rats in these three groups ($P < 0.001$, $P < 0.01$, $P < 0.05$ respectively). MSF and MSRDF presented significantly lower liver levels of MDA in comparison to the MSRD rats ($P < 0.05$, $P < 0.01$ respectively). The liver levels of MDA were comparable in MSF and MSRDF groups. Serum level of CRP was

Table 5 The final liver parameters and serum C-reactive protein (CRP) in the five study groups

	LW (gm)	LW/BW (gm/gm)	ALT (U/L)	Albumin (gm/ml)	Bilirubin (mg/dl)	MDA (nmol /gm)	CRP (ng/ml)
C	5.35±0.27 (10)	0.0272 ±0.00096(10)	29.56±1.74 (9)	5.19±0.13 (9)	0.54±0.09 (9)	38.23±2.83 (9)	0.28±0.05 (9)
MS	8.13±0.38^{a} (14)	0.0419± 0.00151^{a}(14)	81.20±1.33^{a} (10)	3.68±0.14^{a} (10)	0.55±0.09 (10)	129.07±4.29^{a} (10)	1.20±0.11^{a} (10)
MSRD	6.21±0.31^{b} (12)	0.0313± 0.00109^{a,b} (12)	44.00±1.56^{a,b} (9)	4.45±0.12^{a,b} (9)	0.48±0.06 (9)	68.90±5.73^{a,b} (9)	0.50±0.07^{b} (9)
MSF	5.21±0.19^{b,c} (13)	0.0345± 0.00063^{a,b} (13)	38.22±1.78^{a,b,c} (9)	4.51±0.14^{a,b} (9)	0.49±0.07 (9)	55.99±4.79^{a,b,c} (9)	0.40±0.07^{b} (9)
MSRDF	4.25±0.31^{a,b,c,d} (12)	0.0283± 0.00141^{b,d} (12)	33.67±1.77^{b,c} (9)	4.77±0.17^{a,b} (9)	0.47±0.06 (9)	51.14±3.61^{a,b,c} (9)	0.33±0.05^{b} (9)

C, control group, MS, untreated metabolic syndrome group, MSRD, metabolic syndrome group reverted to regular rat chow, MSF, metabolic syndrome group on alternate day fasting, MSRDF, metabolic syndrome group reverted to regular rat chow and on alternate day fasting; LW, liver weight; LW/BW, liver weight/body weight; ALT , serum alanine transferase; MDA, malondialdehyde content of liver tissue
Data are expressed as mean ± SEM
In the parenthesis is the number of observations
a: Significance from control group, by LSD test at P ≤0.05
b: Significance from MS group, by LSD test at P ≤0.05
c: Significance from MSRD group, by LSD test at P ≤0.05
d: Significance from MSF group, by LSD test at P ≤0.05

significantly increased in MS group versus C group ($P < 0.001$). MSRD, MSF, and MSRDF groups showed a significant decrease in serum CRP compared to MS group ($P < 0.001$), becoming not significantly different from the level of control rats. The serum level of CRP was not significantly different among MSRD, MSF, and MSRDF groups (Table 5).

Results of correlation study

Serum alanine transferase (ALT) showed significant +ve correlations with VFW, LW, HOMA-IR serum TGs, and LDL-C and significant −ve correlations with serum HDL-C. Serum albumin showed significant -ve correlations with LW. Liver oxidative stress marker [malondialdehyde content of liver tissue (MDA)] showed significant +ve correlations with HOMA-IR and LDL-C and significant −ve correlations with serum HDL-C (Table 6).

Histopathological study

Histopathological examination of livers of the C group stained with H and E stain after 8 weeks, showed branching and anastomosing cords of hepatocytes radiating from the central vein (cv). Livers of the M group showed highly vacuolated hepatocytes at the periphery of the classic hepatic lobule [zone 1] [*]. Mild cellular infiltration is seen (Figs. 6 and 7).

Histopathological examination of livers of the C group stained with H and E stain after 12 weeks showed branching and anastomosing cords of hepatocytes radiating from the central vein (cv). Livers of the MS group showed highly vacuolated hepatocytes at the periphery of the classic hepatic lobule [zone 1]. Livers of the MSRD group showed an apparent moderate decrease in the vacuolated hepatocytes. Livers of the MSF group showed an apparent decrease in the vacuolated hepatocytes. Liver of the MSRDF group showed absence of vacuolated hepatocytes (Fig. 8).

Histopathological examination of livers of the C group stained with periodic acid–Schiff (PAS) stain after 12 weeks showed PAS +ve glycogen granules almost in all hepatocytes. Livers of the MS group showed PAS +ve glycogen granules at the hepatocytes around central vein [zone 3]; vacuolated hepatocytes at the periphery of classic hepatic lobule have no PAS +ve granules. Livers of the MSRD group showed PAS +ve glycogen granules in vacuolated hepatocytes at the periphery of classic hepatic lobule [zone 1], the hepatocytes around central vein have no PAS +ve granules. Livers of the MSF and MSRDF groups did not show PAS +ve glycogen granules (Fig. 9).

Histopathological examination of livers of the C group stained with Maison Trichome stain (MTS) after 12 weeks showed collagen fibers around central vein and in portal area; minimal amount of collagen is seen in between hepatocytes cords. Livers of the MS, MSRD, MSF, and MSRDF groups showed collagen fibers almost comparable to the control group (Fig. 10).

Diagnosis and grading of NAFLD

At the end of 8th week, C group showed 0% steatosis, FC score (1); and M group 69% steatosis, FC score (4).

Four weeks later at the end of the study, C and MSRD F groups showed 0% steatosis, FC score (1); MS group 82% steatosis, FC score (4); and MSRD and MSF groups 42% steatosis, FC score (3).

At the end of 8th week, M group was classified as grade (1) (PF: 0 and AS: 2). Four weeks later at the end of the study, MS, MSRD, and MSF groups were classified as grade (1), MS (PF: 0 and AS: 4), MSRD (PF: 0 and AS: 3), and MSF (PF: 0 and AS: 1) (Table 7).

Table 6 Correlation studies

		VFW	LW	HOMA-IR	TGs	HDL-C	LDL-C
ALT	*r*	**0.419**** (n=46)	**0.759**** (n=46)	**0.687**** (n=46)	**0.818**** (n=46)	**-0.840**** (n=46)	**0.790**** (n=46)
	P	*<0.005*	*<0.001*	*<0.001*	*<0.001*	*<0.001*	*<0.001*
Albumin	*r*	-0.054 (n=46)	**-0.521**** (n=46)	**-0.625**** (n=46)	**-0.765**** (n=46)	**0.655**** (n=46)	**-0.655**** (n=46)
	P	*NS*	*<0.001*	*<0.001*	*<0.001*	*<0.001*	*<0.001*
MDA	*r*	**0.311*** (n=46)	**0.744**** (n=46)	**0.690**** (n=46)	**0.853**** (n=46)	**-0.893**** (n=46)	**0.809**** (n=46)
	P	*<0.05*	*<0.001*	*<0.001*	*<0.001*	*<0.001*	*<0.001*

ALT , serum alanine transferase; MDA, malondialdehyde content of liver tissue; VFW, Visceral Fat Weight; LW, liver weight;HOMA-IR, homeostasis model assessment of insulin resistance; TGs, triglycerides; LDL-C, low-density lipoprotein cholesterol; HDL-C, high-density lipoprotein cholesterol
r: Correlation coefficient
In the parenthesis is the number of observations
**. Correlation is significant at the 0.01 level (2-tailed)
*. Correlation is significant at the 0.05 level (2-tailed)

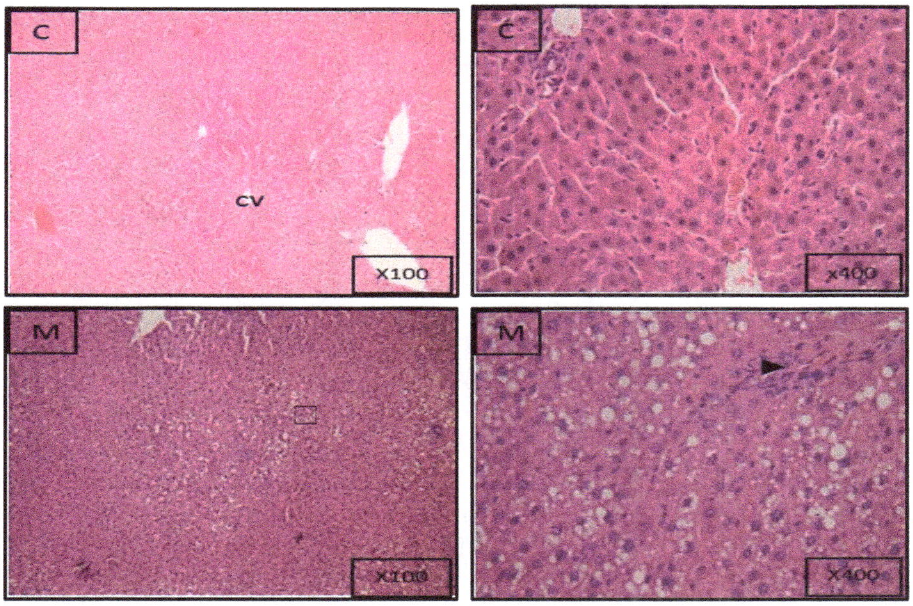

Fig. 6 Liver tissue photomicrograph of control (C) and metabolic syndrome (M) groups after 8 weeks (H&E)

Discussion

Understanding the pathophysiology of MetS is essential, if therapy of MetS-associated NAFLD is to be considered. Pathophysiology of MetS is multifactorial with the unhealthy lifestyle a strongly predisposing factor [42]. Lifestyle aspects include nutrition, physical activity, sleeping hours, smoking, alcohol intake, working hours, hours of watching television, afternoon napping, and social life with friends [42].

Healthy nutrition as described by Mattson et al. [43] includes healthy diet (Mediterranean diet), intake of nutraceuticals, and dietary constriction in the form of caloric restriction or intermittent fasting—defined as periods of unrestricted feeding alternating with periods of caloric restriction.

Unhealthy nutrition is an aspect of unhealthy life style and includes intake of foods with high caloric content, high glycemic index, high content of fructose, high percentage of saturated to polyunsaturated fat, low fruit and vegetable fiber content, as well as irregular eating [44–47].

Garralda-Del-Villar et al. [42] hypothesized that higher adherence to the healthy lifestyle is associated with a lower risk of developing MetS. In the present work, MetS was induced by applying one aspect of unhealthy lifestyle namely unhealthy nutrition in the form of excess fructose intake both in food and drink which mimic the increasing intake of this sweetener in foods and drinks by humans [48]. Fructose content in diet and drink of MS group was equal to starch content in the control rat diet.

The present study was planned to investigate the ability of dietary intervention in the form of reversion to normal diet—with or without adoption of a healthy dietary pattern like zero-calorie intermittent fasting—to cure MetS-associated steatosis which is the hallmark of diagnosis of NAFLD.

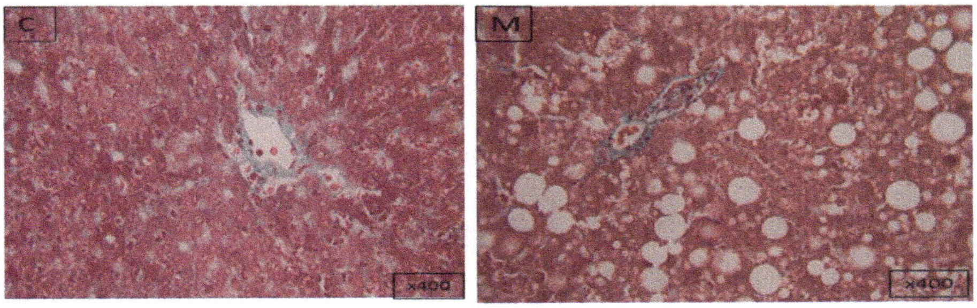

Fig. 7 Liver tissue photomicrograph of control (C) and metabolic syndrome (M) groups after 8 weeks (MT)

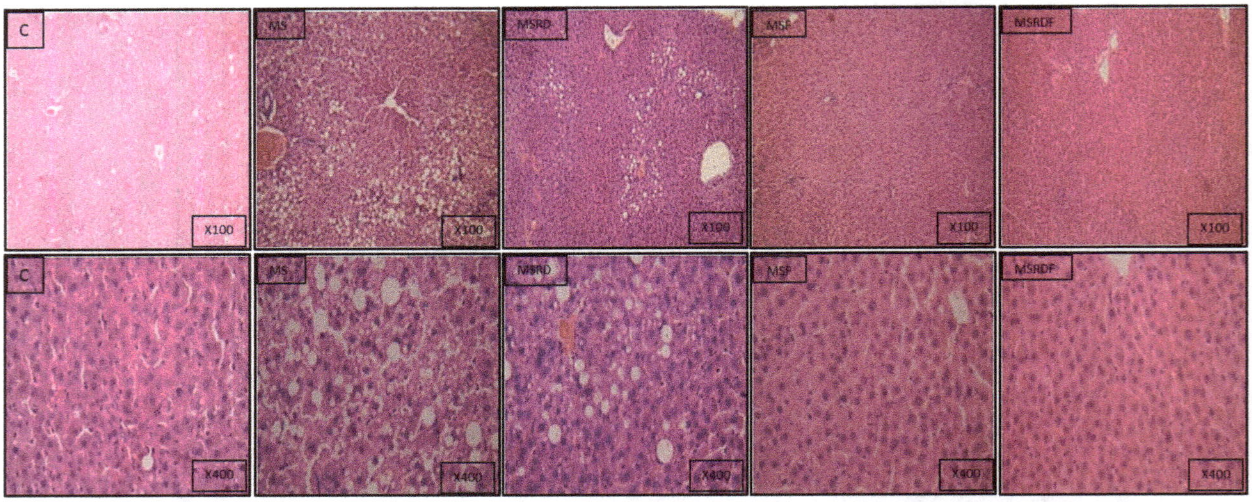

Fig. 8 Liver tissue photomicrograph of the five study groups after 12 weeks (H&E). *C* control group, *MS* untreated metabolic syndrome group, *MSRD* metabolic syndrome group reverted to regular rat chow, *MSF* metabolic syndrome group on alternate day fasting, *MSRDF* metabolic syndrome group reverted to regular rat chow and on alternate day fasting

The results of the present study revealed that 8 weeks of high fructose diet (HFD) was able to induce features of MetS in M rats as evidenced by the significant increase in WC, PG, and AUC as well as the significant decrease of HDL-C compared to control rats. Additionally, in comparison to their initial values, M group presented a significant increase in WC, FBS, PG, AUC, and TG associated with a significant decrease in HDL-C after 8 weeks of HFD.

According to the criteria of harmonizing definition of Alberti et al. [1], M rats, in the present study, showed two criteria of MetS, namely high FBG and low HDL-C, skipping the normal cutoff values of FBG (> 100 mg%), and HDL-C (< 40 mg/dl). Although the cutoff value of WC in the previous definition is not applicable to rats, yet the significant increase in WC in M compared to control rats could be considered the third criterion needed to diagnose MetS in this group. This was consistent with the study of Di Luccia et al. [49], on Sprague-Dawley rats which developed the same MetS criteria, developed in the present study, after 8 weeks of HFD.

Moreover, histopathological study of M rats' livers showed liver steatosis (score-4), hepatocyte ballooning (score-1), and lobular inflammation (score-1), making activity score-2 which both indicate the development of grade-1 NAFLD according to the score of Mendler et al. [40], and highlighting the early emergence of steatohepatitis. Thus, the results of M rats in the present study confirm the close association between unhealthy nutrition in the form of excess fructose intake, MetS, and steatohepatitis and agree with the findings of Mamikutty et al. [50].

At the end of the study, MS rats showed amelioration of two criteria of MetS (VFW, VFW/BW, and FBG) with HDL-C value remaining below the cutoff value of low HDL-C (< 40 mg/dl) according to Alberti et al. [1]. However, liver derangement was evident in the form of significantly increased LW, LW/BW, and serum ALT as well as decreased serum albumin compared to control

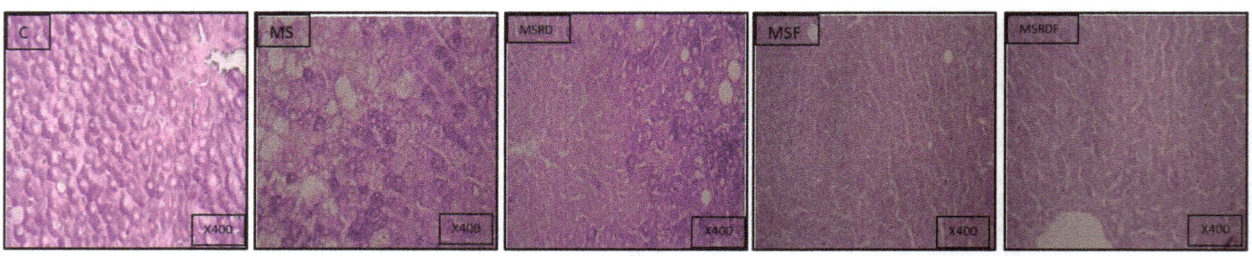

Fig. 9 Liver tissue photomicrograph of the five study groups after 12 weeks (PAS). *C* control group, *MS* untreated metabolic syndrome group, *MSRD* metabolic syndrome group reverted to regular rat chow, *MSF* metabolic syndrome group on alternate day fasting, *MSRDF* metabolic syndrome group reverted to regular rat chow and on alternate day fasting

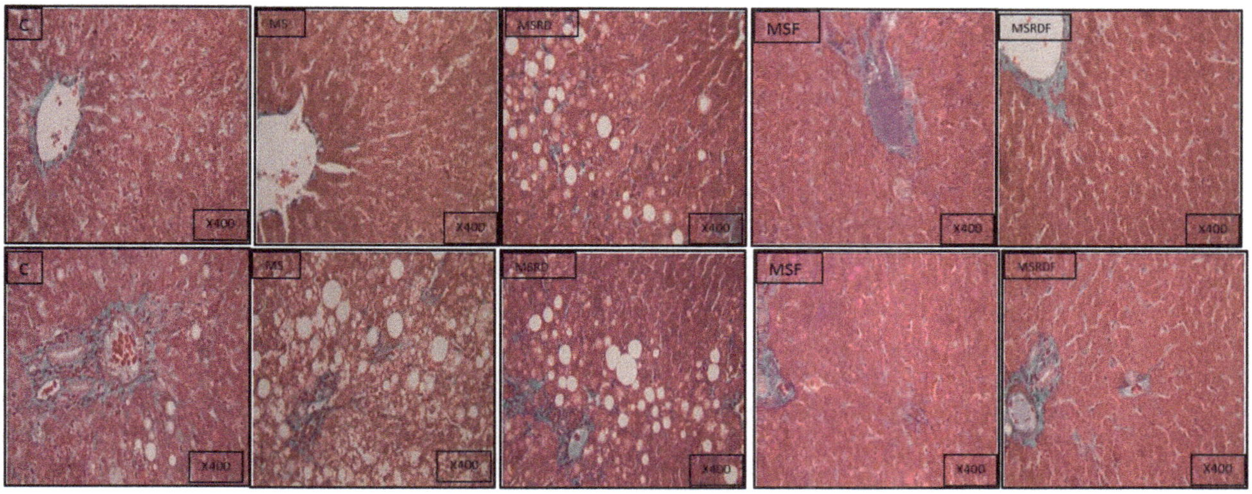

Fig. 10 Liver tissue photomicrograph of the five study groups after 12 weeks (MTS). *C* control group, *MS* untreated metabolic syndrome group, *MSRD* metabolic syndrome group reverted to regular rat chow, *MSF* metabolic syndrome group on alternate day fasting, *MSRDF* metabolic syndrome group reverted to regular rat chow and on alternate day fasting

rats. In support, histological studies revealed progression of their liver fatty changes from 69 to 82% and hepatocyte ballooning score from to 2 with presence of Mallory bodies. Accordingly, the results of MS group at the end of the study indicate that metabolic perturbation induced by high fructose intake is the determinant of NAFLD disease rather than the MetS criteria.

Nutritional intervention, in the present study, namely cessation of fructose intake without caloric restriction in MSRD group, and ADF with continued fructose intake in MSF group resulted in significant amelioration of insulin resistance (serum insulin and HOMA-IR), and dyslipidemia compared to MS rats. The long-term glycemic control parameter (HbA1C) in both groups was declined versus MS rats, approached the control value in both groups and became lower than the normal cutoff value (< 5.7%) according to American diabetes association [51], in MSF group. Such improved glucose homeostasis was further supported by the significant decrease in FBG level at the end of the study versus the 8th week value in

Table 7 Scoring of fatty change (FC score) and grading of NAFLD in the five study groups

FC score 1 < (5%) 2 (5-33%) 3 (34-66%) 4 >(66%		Portal Fibrosis (PF: 0–6)	Activity score (AS: 0–12)				Grade of NAFLD Grade 1 *(PF: 0–2 and AS: 0–4)*, Grade 2 *(PF: 3 or AS: 5–7) and* Grade 3 *(PF: 4–6 or AS: 8–12).*
			Lobular Inflammation and Necrosis (LIN: 0–3)	Mallory Bodies (MB: 0–3)	Hepatocyte Ballooning (HB: 0–3)	Perisinusoidal Fibrosis (PSF: 0–3)	
8th week							
(C)	**1 (0%)**						
(M)	**4 (69%)**	**0**	**1**	**0**	**1**	**0**	Grade 1 (PF: 0 and AS: 2)
Final							
(C)	**1 (0%)**						
(MS)	**4 (82%)**	**0**	**1**	**1**	**2**	**0**	Grade 1(PF: 0 and AS: 4)
(MSRD)	**3 (42%)**	**0**	**1**	**1**	**1**	**0**	Grade 1 (PF: 0 and AS: 3)
(MSF)	**3 (42%)**	**0**	**1**	**0**	**0**	**0**	Grade 1 (PF: 0 and AS: 1)
(MSRDF)	**1 (0%)**						

both MSRD and MSF groups. Alleviation of insulin resistance and dyslipidemia for 4 weeks, herein, contributed to interruption of the pathogenic circuits that lead to oxidative stress and inflammation, as evidenced by the significant decrease in liver MDA, as well as serum CRP, in both groups versus MS rats, resulting in regression of fatty change and abatement of hepatocyte ballooning. Such remarkable effect was able to significantly relive LW, LW/BW, liver injury (decreased ALT), and improve liver function (increased albumin) in both groups versus MS group. Moreover, hepatic steatosis and steatohepatitis were decreased in both groups versus MS rats as demonstrated by the histological studies.

PAS staining of MSRD livers showed increased PAS +ve glycogen granules in zone 1 vacuolated hepatocytes which infer improved insulin resistance in this zone compared to MS group. However, the absence of PAS +ve glycogen granules from zone 3 of MSRD rat livers was in contrast with MS rat livers and might be attributed to either reversal of metabolic zonation of hepatocytes with reversion to regular diet, reversal of insulin resistance with zone 3 hepatocytes becoming more resistant to glycogenic actions of insulin and zone 1 more sensitive to glycogenic actions of insulin with enhanced glucose uptake and glycogenesis in zone 1. The exact changes in oxygen gradient, nutrient flow, and expression of different genes in metabolic syndrome-associated NAFLD should be thoroughly investigated before suggesting a plausible explanation of this alteration in hepatic zonation with reversion to regular diet.

MSF hepatocytes showed no PAS +ve glycogen granules throughout the hepatic lobule which might be attributed to enhanced glycogenolysis and suppressed glycogenesis due to the fasting-associated hormonal changes, an observation that was also seen in the MSRD F rat livers.

Thus, both diet regimens, in the current work, were able to attenuate the metabolic derangement induced by HFD, alleviating liver damage, hepatic steatosis, steatohepatitis, and conserve liver function. It seems likely that both diet regimens used in the current work, equally and positively affected the insulin resistance, long-term glycemic control, dyslipidemia, serum albumin, and CRP as proved by the non-significant changes in these parameters between MSRD and MSF groups. However, ADF was more effective in lowering the liver oxidative stress and mitigating the hepatocellular damage than reversion to regular rat diet, as manifested by the significant decrease in liver MDA and ALT levels along with a lower score of Mallory bodies as well as hepatocyte ballooning in MSF group versus MSRD rats.

Additionally, at the end of the study, the overall obesity parameters (BW) and the visceral obesity parameters (WC) were significantly higher than their matched 8th week values in MSRD group. Also, these parameters together with VFW and VFW/BW were not significantly affected in MSRD group versus controls at the end of the study. These findings indicate that cession of fructose for 4 weeks without caloric restriction neither affected the overall obesity nor the visceral obesity. On the contrary, zero-caloric-intermittent fasting with continued fructose intake, herein, was not only able to significantly decrease the overall and visceral obesity parameters in MSF group at the end of the study period versus their matched values at 8th week, but also, it significantly decreased both in MSF group compared to MS group and MSRD group, becoming even significantly lower than controls. These observations agree with Wan et al. [52], Yang et al. [19], Marinho et al. [53], and Munhoz et al. [54], and denote that caloric restriction by ADF strongly decreased obesity whether overall or visceral, despite the presence of fructose in diet, exceeding the effect of complete cession of fructose in MSRD group. These observations are consistent with Munhoz et al. [54] who found a 35% decrease in total caloric intake and 20.35 % decrease in body weight gain after 12 weeks of ADF in rats.

It is to be noted that reversion to regular rat diet or ADF for 4 weeks did not completely abolish the increase in insulin resistance, dyslipidemia, liver oxidative stress, ALT, and the decrease in albumin induced by HFD during the first 8 weeks of the study period as their levels in both MSRD and MSF groups were still significantly different from those of control rats. Likewise, the hepatic steatosis and steatohepatitis did not normalize in both groups. A longer duration of nutritional intervention might be required for full correction if each diet regimen was applied individually.

Combination of ADF and reversion to regular rat diet resulted in a synergistic impact on glucose homeostasis parameters, leading to a significant decrease in FBG in MSRDF group versus the MS, MSRD, and MSF group, becoming even significantly lower than controls. This was associated with a remarkable enhancement of glucose clearance with improved glucose tolerance as shown by the significant lower AUC in MSRDF group versus both MSF group and control rats. Furthermore, insulin resistance (HOMA-IR) and long-term glycemic control (HbA1C) were normalized in MSRDF group, as both parameters approached the control values.

Furthermore, the parameters of overall obesity and visceral obesity were diminished significantly in MSRDF group compared to MS, MSRD, and control groups. Additionally, combination of the 2 diet regimens significantly improved all lipid profile parameters and attenuated dyslipidemia, liver oxidative stress compared to MS and MSRD rat groups, with CRP and serum albumin still comparable to MSRD group. This was further clarified by the histopathological study of MSRDF rats' livers which revealed resolution of steatosis with FC score-zero and cure of steatohepatitis. Data of these rats indicate that fasting with reversion to normal diet could cure grade-1 NAFLD. Dyslipidemia was also alleviated in MSRDF group versus MSRD and MSF groups, only TC and LDL-C reached the normal control values, while TG was still significantly higher, and HDL-C was significantly lower. The incomplete correction of lipid parameters in MSRDF to control values might explain the failure of the 2 diet regimens in this group to fully ameliorate the liver oxidative stress, hence the serum albumin level was still significantly lower.

Also, of interest was the non-significant changes in obesity parameters, liver MDA, and ALT between MSF and MSRDF group despite their significant decrease in MSRDF versus MSRD group, indicating that caloric restriction by ADF rather than reversion to regular rat diet is responsible for (a) mediating obesity lowering effect and (b) alleviating liver oxidative stress and liver injury in MSRDF group. These observations support our previous assumption that ADF regimen has a dominant effect in alleviating obesity, liver oxidative stress, and liver injury compared to reversion to regular rat diet.

Unpredictably, control rats, in the present study, have developed some features of the MetS on the 8th week, and according to the diagnostic criteria of harmonizing definition of Alberti et al. [1], they were found to have 2 criteria out of 3 needed for MetS diagnosis (low HDL-C 37.7 mg/dl and high FBG glucose100.5 mg/dl). Also, at the end of the study, control rats presented a significantly higher WC versus their matched 8th week value together with high FBG (FBG > 100 mg/dl). These changes might be explained by age progression according to Ghezzi et al. [55] who concluded that the aging process induced metabolic disturbances in Wistar rats and that mature rats (12 months old) showed a significant increase in BW, adiposity, hyperglycemia, as well as dyslipidemia compared to young rats. The absence of liver steatosis in control rats, herein, as demonstrated by the histopathological studies makes the diagnosis of MetS in these rats inappropriate according to Panchal and Brown [56] who included liver dysfunction as a MetS criterion for the animal model of MetS to be validated.

This study has some limitations including lack of caloric intake estimation and lack of fasting control group. Also, it would be of value to determine the local inflammatory response in the liver tissue by estimating TNF-α and/or TGF-β, and that histopathological study was done for 2 rats in each group and not for all rats which made correlation study between NAFLD grading criteria and other parameters inapplicable.

Conclusion

Nutritional interventions by ADF or reversion to regular diet improved glucose homeostasis as well as lipid parameters equally; however, ADF has a greater favorable influence on overall and visceral obesity as well as on liver oxidative stress and hepatocellular damage. Combination of the two regimens is more effective in abating metabolic disturbances, hepatic steatosis, steatohepatitis, and liver injury than each regimen separately. Combination of fructose abstinence and ADF may be used as an effective combination approach for curing grade-1 NAFLD associated with metabolic syndrome.

Abbreviations

ADF: Alternate-day fasting; Alb.: Serum albumin; ALT: Alanine transferase; AUC: Area under the curve; BMI: Body mass index; BW: Body weight; C: Control group; CRP: C-reactive protein; FBG: Fasting blood glucose level; H&E: Hematoxylin and eosin; HbA1C: Glycosylated hemoglobin; HDL-C: High-density lipoprotein cholesterol; HFD: High fructose diet; HFI: High fructose intake; HOMA-IR: Homeostasis model assessment of insulin resistance; IMF: Intermittent fasting; Ins.: Serum insulin; IPGTT: Intraperitoneal glucose tolerance test; LDL-C: Low-density lipoprotein cholesterol; L-MDA: Liver tissue malondialdehyde; LW/BW: Liver weight/body weight ratio; LW: Liver weight; m: Months; M: Metabolic syndrome group; MDA: Malondialdehyde; MetS: Metabolic syndrome; MS: Untreated metabolic syndrome group; MSF: Metabolic syndrome group on alternate-day fasting; MSRD: Metabolic syndrome group reverted to regular rat chow; MSRDF: Metabolic syndrome group reverted to regular rat chow and on alternate-day fasting; NAFL: Nonalcoholic fatty liver; NAFLD: Non-alcoholic fatty liver disease; NASH: Nonalcoholic steatohepatitis; PAS: Periodic acid–Schiff; PG: Peak glycaemia; TC: Serum total cholesterol; TGs: Serum triglycerides; VFW/BW: Visceral fat weight/body weight ratio; VFW: Visceral fat weight; VLDL: Very low-density lipoproteins; WC: Waist circumference

Acknowledgements

Not applicable.

Authors' contributions

NG had performed a fundamental contribution to the design in this study by constructing the experimental protocol. She had followed the experimental plan and involved in the statistical analysis of results. She had included in the writing and final revision of the manuscript. SE had participated in the statistical analysis of results and in the writing of the manuscript. GM had involved in the histological analysis in the study. RM had supervised the experimental work and shared in the writing of the manuscript. MA had carried out the experimental work and assisted in the statistical analysis of results and in the writing of the manuscript. The authors read and approved the final manuscript.

Declarations

Ethics approval and consent to participate

This study was performed according to the guidelines of FMASU, REC, Cairo, Egypt, which conforms to the Guide for the Care and Use of Laboratory Animals published by the US National Institute of Health (NO. FWA 00017585).

Competing interests
The authors declare that they have no competing interests.

References

1. Alberti KG, Eckel RH, Grundy SM, Zimmet PZ, Cleeman JI, Donato KA, Fruchart JC, James WP, Loria CM, Smith SC (2009) Harmonizing the metabolic syndrome: a joint interim statement of the International Diabetes Federation Task Force on Epidemiology and Prevention; National Heart, Lung, and Blood Institute; American Heart Association; World Heart Federation; International Atherosclerosis Society; and International Association for the Study of Obesity. Circulation 120(16):1640–1645
2. Benedict M, Zhang X (2017) Non-alcoholic fatty liver disease: an expanded review. World J Hepatol 9(16):715–732. https://doi.org/10.4254/wjh.v9.i16.715
3. Carr RM, Oranu A, Khungar V (2016) Nonalcoholic fatty liver disease: pathophysiology and management. Gastroenterol Clin N Am 45(4):639–652. https://doi.org/10.1016/j.gtc.2016.07.003
4. Dietrich P, Hellerbrand C (2014) Non-alcoholic fatty liver disease, obesity and the metabolic syndrome. Best Pract Res Clin Gastroenterol 28(4):637–653. https://doi.org/10.1016/j.bpg.2014.07.008
5. Sayiner M, Koenig A, Henry L, Younossi ZM (2016) Epidemiology of nonalcoholic fatty liver disease and nonalcoholic steatohepatitis in the United States and the rest of the world. Clin Liver Dis 20(2):205–214. https://doi.org/10.1016/j.cld.2015.10.001
6. Kanwar P, Kowdley KV (2016) The metabolic syndrome and its influence on nonalcoholic steatohepatitis. Clin Liver Dis 20(2):225–243. https://doi.org/10.1016/j.cld.2015.10.002
7. Hellerbrand C (2010) Pathophysiological similarities and synergisms in alcoholic and non-alcoholic steatohepatitis. Dig Dis 28(6):783–791. https://doi.org/10.1159/000324286
8. Vernon G, Baranova A, Younossi ZM (2011) Systematic review: the epidemiology and natural history of non-alcoholic fatty liver disease and non-alcoholic steatohepatitis in adults. Aliment PharmacolTher 34(3):274–285. https://doi.org/10.1111/j.1365-2036.2011.04724.x
9. Chalasani N, Younossi Z, Lavine JE, Diehl AM, Brunt EM, Cusi K, Charlton M, Sanyal AJ (2012) The diagnosis and management of non-alcoholic fatty liver disease: practice Guideline by the American Association for the Study of Liver Diseases, American College of Gastroenterology, and the American Gastroenterological Association. Hepatology 55(6):2005–2023. https://doi.org/10.1002/hep.25762
10. Calzadilla BL, Adams LA (2016) The natural course of non-alcoholic fatty liver disease. Int J Mol Sci 17
11. Guilherme A, Virbasius JV, Puri V, Czech MP (2008) Adipocyte dysfunctions linking obesity to insulin resistance and type 2 diabetes. Nat Rev Mol Cell Biol 9(5):367–377. https://doi.org/10.1038/nrm2391
12. Cusi K (2009) Role of insulin resistance and lipotoxicity in non-alcoholic steatohepatitis. Clin Liver Dis 13(4):545–563. https://doi.org/10.1016/j.cld.2009.07.009
13. Pappachan JM, Babu S, Krishnan B, Nishal C, Ravindran NC (2017) Non-alcoholic fatty liver disease: a clinical update. Journal of Clinical and Translational Hepatology 5:384–393
14. Marriott BP, Cole N, Lee E (2009) National estimates of dietary fructose intake increased from 1977 to 2004 in the United States. J Nutr 139:1228s–1235s
15. Ter Horst KW, Serlie MJ (2017) Fructose consumption, lipogenesis, and non-alcoholic fatty liver disease. Nutrients 9(9):981. https://doi.org/10.3390/nu9090981
16. Yilmaz Y (2012) Review article: fructose in non-alcoholic fatty liver disease. Aliment PharmacolTher 35(10):1135–1144. https://doi.org/10.1111/j.1365-2036.2012.05080.x
17. Park S, Yoo KM, Hyun JS, Kang S (2017) Intermittent fasting reduces body fat but exacerbates hepatic insulin resistance in young rats regardless of high protein and fat diets. J Nutr Biochem 40:14–22
18. Gotthardt JD, Verpeut JL, Yeomans BL, Yang JA, Yasrebi A, Roepke TA, Bello NT (2016) Intermittent fasting promotes fat loss with lean mass retention, increased hypothalamic norepinephrine content, and increased neuropeptide Y Gene expression in diet-induced obese male mice. Endocrinology 157(2):679–691. https://doi.org/10.1210/en.2015-1622
19. Yang W, Cao M, Mao X, Wei X, Li X, Chen G, Zhang J, Wang Z, Shi J, Huang H, Yao X, Liu C (2016) Alternate-day fasting protects the livers of mice against high-fat diet–induced inflammation associated with the suppression of Toll-like receptor 4/nuclear factor κB signaling. Nutr Res 36:586–593
20. Varady KA, Allister CA, Roohk DJ, Hellerstein MK (2010) Improvements in body fat distribution and circulating adiponectin by alternate-day fasting versus calorie restriction. J Nutr Biochem 21(3):188–195. https://doi.org/10.1016/j.jnutbio.2008.11.001
21. Patel J, Iyer A, Brown L (2009) Evaluation of the chronic complications of diabetes in a high fructose diet in rats. Indian J Biochem Biophys 46(1):66–72
22. Bahgat NM, Abd-El Rahman AM, Ahmed MA, Megahed GK, Abdel Wahed DM, Ali RH (2017) Study of criteria of metabolic syndrome in young female Albino rats on high fructose intake. Ain Shams Medical Journal 68(1):2–3
23. Zhang M, Lv XY, Li J, Xu ZG, Chen L (2008) The characterization of high-fat diet and multiple low-dose streptozotocin induced type 2 diabetes rat model. Exp Diabetes Res 2008 Article ID 704045, 9 pages
24. Matthews JN, Altman DG, Campbell MJ, Royston P (1990) Analysis of serial measurements in medical research. Bmj. 300(6719):230–235. https://doi.org/10.1136/bmj.300.6719.230
25. Bernardis LL (1970) Prediction of carcass fat, water and lean body mass from Lee's nutritive ratio in rats with hypothalamic obesity. Experientia 26(7):789–790. https://doi.org/10.1007/BF02232553
26. Panchal SK, Poudyal H, Iyer A, Nazer R, Alam A, Diwan V, Brown L (2011) High-carbohydrate, high-fat diet–induced metabolic syndrome and cardiovascular remodeling in rats. J Cardiovasc Pharmacol 57(5):611–624. https://doi.org/10.1097/FJC.0b013e31821b1379
27. Fassati p. and prencipe L. (1982) Serum triglycerides determined colorimetrically with an enzyme that produces hydrogen peroxide. clin. Chem 28:2077–2080
28. Tietz N (ed) (1976) Fundamentals of Clinical Chemistry. W.B. Sauders Co, Philadelphia
29. Young D.S. (2001): Effects of diseases on Clinical Lab. Tests 4thadAACC.
30. Doumas B.T. and Biggs H.G. (1976): Standard methods of clinical chemistry, Academic Press, N.Y.7(175).
31. Rand RN, Di Pasqua A (1962) A new diazo method for determination of bilirubin. Clin. Chem 8(6):570–578
32. Golub M (1964) An automated method for determination of serum bilirubin. Clin.Chem 10(5):399–405. https://doi.org/10.1093/clinchem/10.5.399
33. Henry RJ (1964) Clinical chemistry, principles and technics. Harper and Row Publishers, NewYork
34. Satoh K (1978) ClinicaChimica Acta 90:37
35. Ohkawa H, Ohishi W, Yagi K (1979) Anal Biochem 95:351
36. Friedewald WT, Levy RI, Fredrickson DS (1972) Estimation of the concentration of low–density lipoprotein cholesterol in plasma, without use of the preparative ultracentrifuge. Clin Chem 18(6):499–502. https://doi.org/10.1093/clinchem/18.6.499
37. Matthews D, Hosker J, Rudenski A, Naylor B, Treacher D, Turner R (1985) Homeostasis model assessment: insulin resistance and B-cell function from fasting plasma glucose and insulin concentrations in man. Diabetologia 28(7):412–419. https://doi.org/10.1007/BF00280883
38. Burns C, Morris T, Jones B, Koch W, Borer M, Riber U, Bristow A (2010) Proposal to initiate a project to evaluate a candidate International Standard for Human Recombinant Insulin. WHO/BS/10.2143 - Working document QAS/10.381
39. Frishman D, Ardito DM, Graham SM (1992) Performance of glucose monitors. Lab Med 23:3
40. Mendler MH, Kanel G, Govindarajan S (2005) Proposal for a histological scoring and grading system for non-alcoholic fatty liver disease. Liver Int 25: 294–304 r Blackwell Munksgaard 2005
41. Armitage P, Berry G (1987) Statistical methods in medical reserve in left ventricular hypertrophy. Hypertension 5:192–197
42. Garralda-Del-Villar M, Carlos-Chillerón S, Diaz-Gutierrez J, Ruiz-Canela M, Gea A, Martínez-González MA, Bes-Rastrollo M, Ruiz-Estigarribia L, Kales SN, Fernández-Montero A (2018) Healthy lifestyle and incidence of metabolic syndrome in the SUN Cohort. Nutrients. 11(1):65. https://doi.org/10.3390/nu11010065
43. Mattson MP, Allison DB, Fontana L, Harvie M, Longo VD, Malaisse WJ, Mosley M, Notterpek L, Ravussin E, Scheer FA, Seyfried TN, Varady KA, Panda S (2014) Meal frequency and timing in health and disease. Proc Natl Acad Sci U S A 111(47):16647–16653 cited in Rossman MJ, LaRocca TJ, Martens

CR, Seals DR. Healthy lifestyle-based approaches for successful vascular aging. J Appl Physiol (1985). 2018;125(6):1888-1900
44. McKeown NM, Meigs JB, Liu S, Saltzman E, Wilson PW, Jacques PF (2004) Carbohydrate nutrition, insulin resistance, and the prevalence of the metabolic syndrome in the Framingham Offspring Cohort. Diabetes Care 27(2):538–546. https://doi.org/10.2337/diacare.27.2.538
45. Pot G, Hardy R, Stephen A (2014) Irregular consumption of energy intake in meals is associated with a higher cardiometabolic risk in adults of a British birth cohort. Int J Obes 38(12):1518–1524. https://doi.org/10.1038/ijo.2014.51
46. Pot G, Hardy R, Stephen A (2016) Irregularity of energy intake at meals: prospective associations with the metabolic syndrome in adults of the 1946 British birth cohort. Br J Nutr 115(2):315–323. https://doi.org/10.1017/S0007114515004407
47. Ganesan K, Habboush Y, Sultan S (2018) Intermittent fasting: the choice for a healthier lifestyle. Cureus. 10(7):e2947. https://doi.org/10.7759/cureus.2947
48. Taskinen MR, Packard CJ, Borén J (2019) Dietary fructose and the metabolic syndrome. Nutrients. 11(9):1987
49. Di Luccia B, Crescenzo R, Mazzoli A, Cigliano L, Venditti P, Walser JC et al (2015) Rescue of fructose-induced metabolic syndrome by antibiotics or faecal transplantation in a rat model of obesity. PLoS One 10(8):e0134893
50. Mamikutty N, Thent ZC, Haji SF (2015) Fructose-drinking water induced nonalcoholic fatty liver disease and ultrastructural alteration of hepatocyte mitochondria in male Wistar rat. Biomed Res Int 2015:895961
51. American Diabetes Association (2010) Diagnosis and classification of diabetes mellitus. Diabetes care 33(Suppl 1):S62–S69
52. Wan R, Ahmet I, Brown M, Cheng A, Kamimura N, Talan M, Mattson MP (2010) Cardioprotective effect of intermittent fasting is associated with an elevation of adiponectin levels in rats. J Nutr Biochem 21(5):413–417. https://doi.org/10.1016/j.jnutbio.2009.01.020
53. Marinho TDS, Ornellas F, Barbosa-da-Silva S, Mandarim-de-Lacerda CA, Aguila MB (2019) Beneficial effects of intermittent fasting on steatosis and inflammation of the liver in mice fed a high-fat or a high-fructose diet. Nutrition 65:103–112
54. Munhoz AC, Vilas-Boas EA, Panveloski-Costa AC, Leite JSM, Lucena CF, Riva P, Emilio H, Carpinelli AR (2020) Intermittent fasting for twelve weeks leads to increases in fat mass and hyperinsulinemia in young female Wistar rats. Nutrients 12(4):1029. https://doi.org/10.3390/nu12041029
55. Ghezzi AC, Cambri LT, Botezelli JD, Ribeiro C, Dalia RA, de Mello MA (2012) Metabolic syndrome markers in wistar rats of different ages. Diabetol Metab Syndr 4(1):16. https://doi.org/10.1186/1758-5996-4-16
56. Panchal SK, Brown L (2011) Rodent models for metabolic syndrome research. J Biomed Biotechnol 2011:351982

7

SARS-CoV-2-associated gastrointestinal and liver diseases: what is known and what is needed to explore

Dina Sweed[1*], Eman Abdelsameea[2], Esraa A. Khalifa[3], Heba Abdallah[4], Heba Moaz[5], Inas Moaz[6], Shimaa Abdelsattar[7], Nadine Abdel-Rahman[8], Asmaa Mosbeh[1], Hussein A. Elmahdy[9] and Eman Sweed[10]

Abstract

Background: The pandemic of COVID19 which is caused by severe acute respiratory syndrome coronavirus 2 (SARS-CoV-2) was first described in China as an unexplained pneumonia transmitted by respiratory droplets. Gastrointestinal (GI) and liver injury associated with SARS-CoV-2 infection were reported as an early or sole disease manifestation, mainly outside China. The exact mechanism and incidence of GI and liver involvement are not well elucidated.

Main body: We conducted a PubMed search for all articles written in the English language about SARS-CoV-2 affecting the GI and liver. Following data extraction, 590 articles were selected. In addition to respiratory droplets, SARS-CoV-2 may reach the GI system through the fecal-oral route, saliva, and swallowing of nasopharyngeal fluids, while breastmilk and blood transmission were not implicated. Moreover, GI infection may act as a septic focus for viral persistence and transmission to the liver, appendix, and brain. In addition to the direct viral cytopathic effect, the mechanism of injury is multifactorial and is related to genetic and demographic variations. The most frequently reported GI symptoms are diarrhea, nausea, vomiting, abdominal pain, and bleeding. However, liver infection is generally discovered during laboratory testing or a post-mortem. Radiological imaging is the gold standard in diagnosing COVID-19 patients and contributes to understanding the mechanism of extra-thoracic involvement. Medications should be prescribed with caution, especially in chronic GI and liver patients.

Conclusion: GI manifestations are common in COVID-19 patients. Special care should be paid for high-risk patients, older males, and those with background liver disease.

Keywords: COVID-19, Gastrointestinal, Liver, Pathophysiology, SARS-CoV-2

Background

The pandemic of the novel 2019 coronavirus disease (COVID-19) started in December 2019 with an outbreak of unexplained pneumonia in Wuhan, China. Severe acute respiratory syndrome coronavirus 2 (SARS-CoV-2) is primarily transmitted by droplets and aerosols, affecting the respiratory system [1]. In the USA, the first case of SARS-CoV-2-associated gastrointestinal (GI) symptoms had a 2-day history of nausea and vomiting, then progressed to diarrhea upon hospital admission [2]. Subsequently, many studies reported GI and liver infection as the first presentation of COVID-19 with later (or no) respiratory symptoms [3]. This review summarizes the demographic, clinical manifestation, radiological, and pathological findings in COVID-19 patients presenting with GI symptoms to elucidate the route of transmission and mechanism of injury and provide guidance on GI and hepatic treatment in COVID-19 patients.

* Correspondence: dina.sweed@liver.menofia.edu.eg
[1]Pathology Department, National Liver Institute, Menofia University, Shibin El Kom 32511, Egypt
Full list of author information is available at the end of the article

Main text

Material and methods

A thorough PubMed search of all English-language articles published and in-press from December 2019 to December 2020 was done. The search terms were "COVID-19," "SARS-CoV-2," "gastrointestinal," "liver," "diarrhea," "abdominal pain," "nausea," "vomiting," "histopathology," "radiology," "pharmacology," and "liver enzymes." A total of 2160 studies were included in complete data extraction, and a final 590 papers were selected. The papers were reviewed, and data were collected and analyzed by gastroenterology and hepatobiliary specialists.

The mode of transmission of SARS-CoV-2-induced GI and liver diseases

Although inhalation of respiratory droplets is the primary mechanism of SARS-CoV-2 transmission, fecal-oral transmission may be an additional source of GI infection, mainly in children. SARS-CoV-2 viral RNA was detected in the fecal matter for 11.2 to 33 days following viral clearance from the respiratory tract, indicating viral replication in the enterocytes and possible fecal-oral transmission [4]. Saliva and vomit were two additional routes of transmission. SARS-CoV-2 may infect the salivary gland by binding to and secreting from the angiotensin-converting enzyme 2 (ACE2) receptor. Therefore, saliva may play a role in the early stage of viral transmission [5]. The vomit also included viral particles either from nasopharyngeal fluids or the GI tract. The risk of viral transmission is positively correlated with vomiting severity [6]. Portincasa et al. suggest an unconfirmed hypothesis that the virus could translocate from the gut lumen into the liver via portal flow, negatively affecting hepatic cells [7]. SARS-CoV-2 could also reach the appendix via oropharyngeal contamination or appendicolith, resulting in bacterial translocation and appendicitis [8].

One study reported the possibility of SARS-CoV-2 transmission through breastmilk. However, the remaining studies did not find viral transmission in breastmilk, which is supported by the World Health Organization (WHO) that ensured breastfeeding was safe given proper precautions [9]. The low viral load in infected patients' serum makes this transmission route limited or even non-existent [10].

Mechanism of SARS-CoV-2-induced GI and liver diseases (Fig. 1)

Genetic factors

The presence of four primary intestinal transcription factors, caudal type homeobox transcription factor 2 (CDX2), hepatocyte nuclear factor 4 (HNF4), mothers against decapentaplegic homolog 4 (SMAD4), or GATA in the intestine, modulates the function and activity of ACE2 and transmembrane protease serine 2 (TMPR SS2). These results could explain the population's

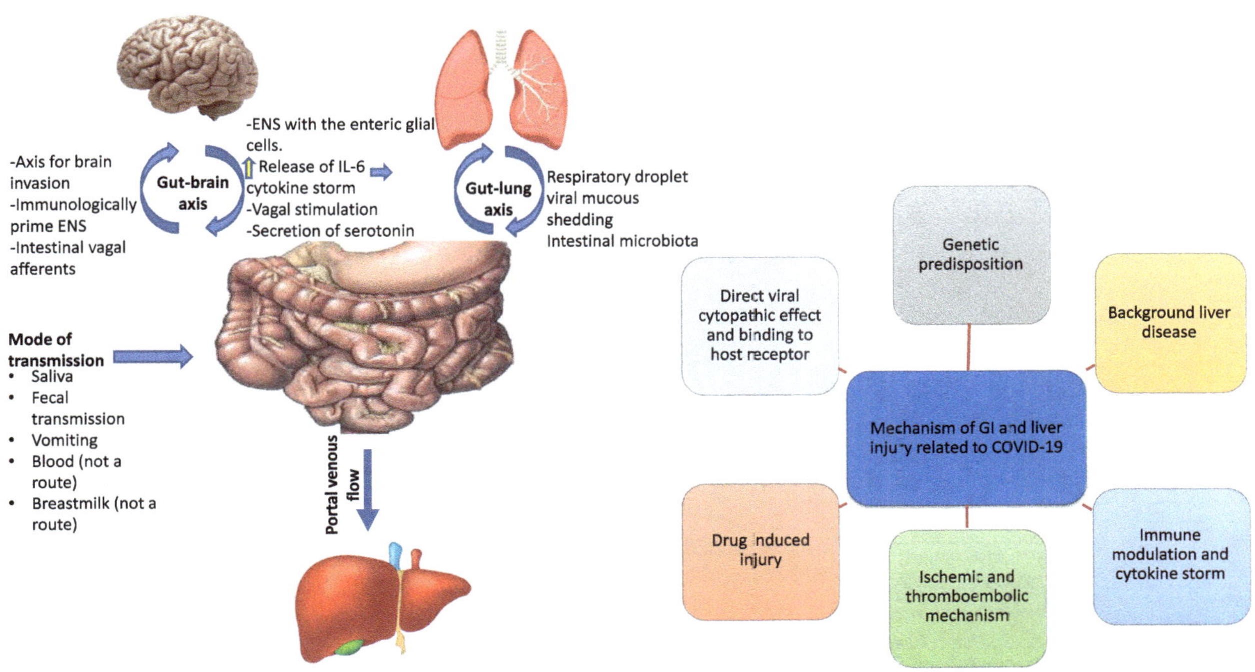

Fig. 1 The route of spread and mechanism of SARS-CoV-2-induced gastrointestinal and liver injury. ENS, enteric nervous system; IL-6, interleukin-6

variable susceptibility to GI symptoms and severity of SARS-CoV-2 infection [11].

Central-neurological mechanism

The gut-brain axis may be a path for SARS-CoV-2 to invade the brain, ascend to the central nervous system (CNS) through intestinal vagal afferents, and immunologically prime the enteric nervous system (ENS). The ENS is strictly interconnected to the enteric glial cells (EGCs), which defend against gut pathogens by activating the Toll-like receptors (TLRs) and other inflammatory mediators. Conversely, SARS-CoV-2 neuroinvasion stimulates serotonin release and provides an alternative central mechanism for GI symptoms [12].

Local mechanisms

Viral-host receptor binding mechanism Coronaviruses are a group of single-stranded enveloped RNA viruses that express four structural proteins: spike glycoprotein, small envelope protein, matrix protein, and nucleocapsid protein, in addition to 16 non-structural proteins [13]. SARS-CoV-2 enters host cells through the interaction between the envelope-anchored viral spike protein and the ACE2 host receptors. ACE2 receptors are widely expressed in various human cells, including the lungs, small intestine, colon, pancreatic islets, kidney, brain, vascular endothelium, and smooth and cardiac muscle [14].

SARS-CoV-2 has a unique structural and functional S protein that facilitates viral entry and replication. The high binding affinity of SARS-CoV-2 for human ACE2, 10–20-fold higher than SARS, increases the viral infectivity [15]. Besides, other host receptors for SARS-CoV-2, specifically CD147, TMPRSS2, endosomal cysteine proteases cathepsin B and L (CatB/L), and furin, are widely distributed in multiple organs, enhancing viral binding and entry. The mechanism of SARS-CoV-2 binding to and entering host cells is illustrated in Fig. 2.

Gut microbiota The gut-lung axis is a bi-directional network in which many respiratory infections often accompany GI symptoms and vice versa. The gut microbiome plays a crucial role in modulating the immune response of SARS-CoV-2 patients to prevent vital organ damage. Alterations to the intestinal microbiota, in conjunction with an impaired immune system, contribute to COVID-19 patients' delayed recovery and mortality [16]. Re-formulating the gut microbiota through nutritional therapy, probiotics, or fecal microbiota transplantation (using standard guidelines) may emerge as a new therapeutic target in disease management [16, 17].

Hypochlorhydria Price suggests that the acidic pH of the normal gastric mucosa inactivates coronaviruses, explaining why the intestinal manifestation is more pronounced than the gastric ones [18]. However, more studies are recommended to evaluate the viral ability to survive and replicate through the extremes of GI pH.

Systemic mechanisms

Immune-related injuries Severe SARS-CoV-2 infection results in a clinical state resembling sepsis due to the massive release of cytokines by the immune system. This cytokine storm involves innate and cellular immunity, including activation of intrahepatic CD4+ and CD8+T-cells, Kupffer cells, activation of B cells, and anti-viral antibodies. These pathways progress toward apoptosis and necrosis of infected cells, resulting in multi-organ failure late in the course of disease [19].

Ischemia-reperfusion injury Severe SARS-CoV-2 cases suffer from ischemia–reperfusion injury through

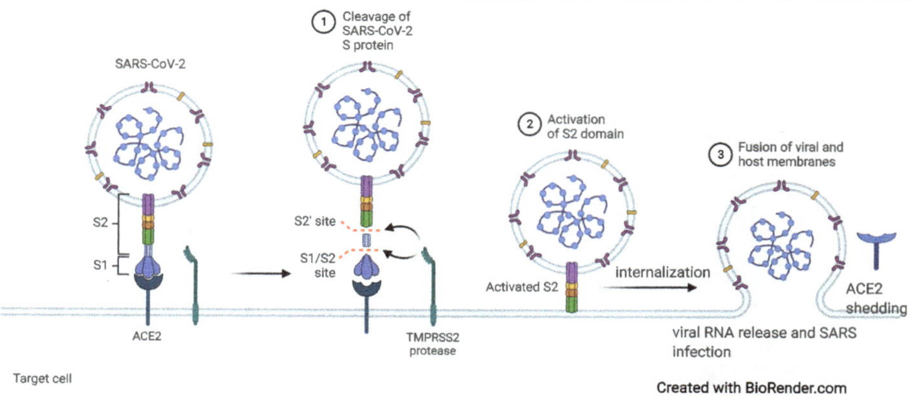

Fig. 2 Coronavirus uses angiotensin-converting enzyme-2 (ACE2) receptor to reach the cells with the binding of the viral spike (S) glycoprotein to cellular receptors via S protein priming by host cell proteases. TMPRSS2, transmembrane protease, serine 2; SARS-CoV-2, severe acute respiratory syndrome coronavirus 2

activation of systemic inflammatory response syndrome (SIRS), SARS, or as a complication of sepsis and hypertension [3].

Drug-induced GI and liver disease Drug therapies for managing SARS-CoV-2 infection are reported to be a direct insult to the GI and liver in variable doses and conditions, discussed in a later section.

Symptoms and signs of GI injury in COVID-19 In a series of > 20,000 hospitalized patients in the UK, the main symptoms of COVID-19 were respiratory (71.6%), followed by enteric symptoms (nausea, abdominal pain, vomiting, and diarrhea) (29%), with 4% of patients complaining of enteric symptoms alone [20]. Patients with GI symptoms experiencing a prolonged period between the onset of symptoms and viral clearance were more likely to have a positive stool test for the virus (73.3% compared to 14.3% with no GI symptoms, $p = 0.033$) [21]. The prevalence of diarrhea was 5–10.3%, nausea and vomiting 5.2–11.7%, abdominal pain 2.7–8.8%, and loss of appetite 15.8%, with few reported cases of GI bleeding [22, 23].

There is no unique esophageal symptom associated with SARS-CoV-2 except for heartburn. Heartburn needs a standard treatment approach with H2 receptor antagonists or proton pump inhibitors (PPIs) [24]. Anorexia is one of the most frequent symptoms reported in COVID-19 patients, mainly associated with malaise and systemic inflammation [25].

Diarrhea may have been the only presentation in 16% of cases [26]. The diarrhea symptoms might last from 1 to 14 days with a mean of 5.4 ± 3.1 days, and the majority of patients experiencing self-limited diarrhea [21]. The possible mechanisms are direct interaction with ACE2 receptors or medications [26].

Epigastric pain, stomachache, and abdominal discomfort have been used to describe abdominal pain [27], and such pain may be a sign of gut nerve inflammation and precede the respiratory symptoms or be the sole manifestation of COVID-19. However, there was no reported data on the quality or nature of the pain characteristic of COVID-19.

Gastrointestinal bleeding in patients with COVID-19 is not as common as other GI symptoms, with a frequency ranging from 4 to 13.7%. A review of 2023 patients with COVID-19 reported only two GI bleeding cases across 15 studies [28]. The cause of bleeding is often not determined, and most patients were treated conservatively. Lower GI bleeding has also been reported in association with COVID-19, necessitating urgent consultation [29]. Ischemia may be the result of thrombotic dysfunction, hypoperfusion, and direct inflammatory effect on GI mucosa.

The prevalence of acute pancreatitis was 0.27% among hospitalized COVID-19 patients with no other identifiable etiology [30].

Laboratory findings on COVID-19-associated GI and liver injury

Figure 3 illustrates the most common laboratory tests specific for GI and liver infection with their possible clinical implications.

General systemic and inflammatory markers (not organ-specific)

COVID-19 patients showed high levels of C-reactive protein (CRP), lactate dehydrogenase (LDH), and α-hydroxybutyrate dehydrogenase (HBDH) as a result of inflammation-inducing GI or liver injury [31]. Interleukin-6 (IL-6) is a crucial cytokine contributing to the host defense by producing acute-phase proteins and proliferation of B-lymphocytes and neutrophils. In the liver, SARS-CoV-2 activates hepatic stellate cells and Kupffer cells to produce many inflammatory factors such as tumor necrosis factor-α (TNF-α), interleukin (IL-6), and chemokines [19]. Moreover, COVID-19 patients with chronic liver disease (CLD) had a higher serum IL-6 level than those without CLD [32].

Laboratory findings specific for GI infection

A high proportion of serum CD19+ B cells, IgA, and low citrulline have been reported in COVID-19 patients presenting with diarrhea, indicating a direct viral cytopathic effect or intestinal ischemia inducing mucosal injury [33]. In contrast, increased serum CCL28 expression was associated with a good mucosal immune response [34]. Fecal calprotectin (FC) has evolved into a reliable biomarker allowing detection of intestinal inflammation in inflammatory bowel disease (IBD) and infectious colitis. High FC in COVID-19 patients indicates an acute GI inflammatory response and/or serves as a potential indicator of the progressive course in IBD patients [35].

Although SARS-CoV-2 induced pancreatic injury, elevated lipase levels exceeding three times the upper limit could be an alarm for GI injury rather than pancreatic injury. However, hyperlipidemia is not considered a marker of severe COVID-19 infection or a poor clinical outcome [36]. Acute hyperglycemia and transient type-2-diabetes also indicate a pancreatic injury and are associated with poor prognosis.

Laboratory findings specific for liver infection

The available liver enzyme data varied widely due to a lack of a standard cut-off point and a consensus definition of severe cases. The prevalence of liver abnormalities has been classified into hepatocyte-type (aspartate aminotransferase [AST]/alanine aminotransferase

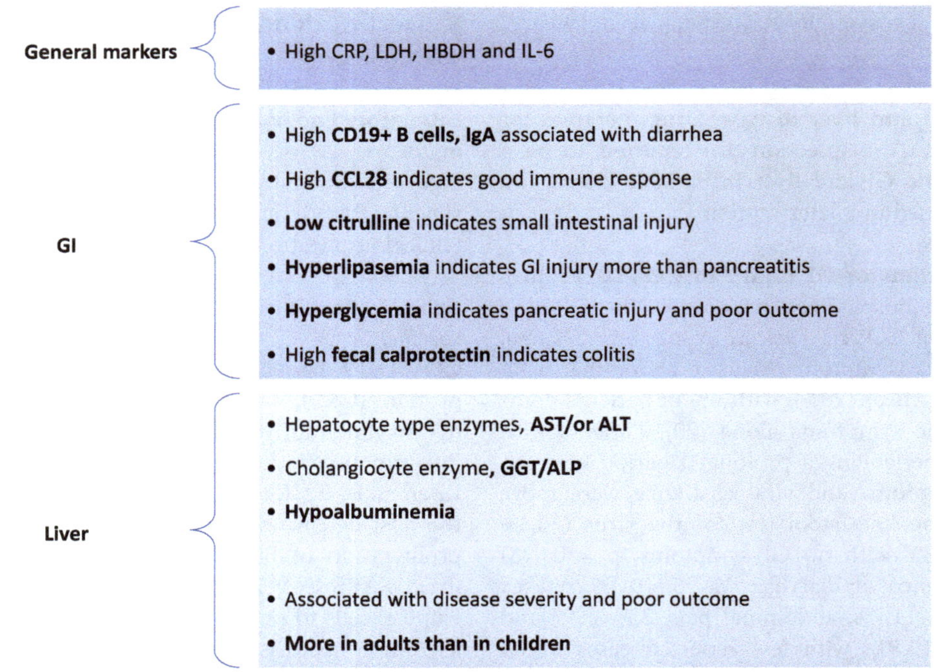

Fig. 3 Laboratory findings in COVID-19 patients presented with GI or liver affection. CRP, C-reactive protein; LDH, lactate dehydrogenase; HBDH, α-hydroxybutyrate dehydrogenase; CCL28, chemokine (C-C motif) ligand 28; GGT, gamma-glutamyl transferase; AST, aspartate aminotransferase; ALT, alanine aminotransferase; ALP, alkaline phosphates; IL-6, interleukin-6

[ALT]) (20.75%), cholangiocyte-type (gamma-glutamyl transferase [GGT]/alkaline phosphatase [ALP]) (29.25%), and mixed types [37]. According to the frequency of elevated hepatocyte-type markers, ALT and AST were found to be elevated in 21.2–25% and 15.2–25% of patients, respectively. AST is typically located in the cytosol and mitochondria of hepatocytes, mainly in zone 3. Therefore, elevated serum AST could reflect direct cytopathic damage of hepatocytes or hypoxic changes. However, AST is not a specific marker for liver injury and has a broader organ distribution, indicating its involvement in multi-organ damage [38].

The prevalence of cholangiocyte-related enzymes showed increased levels of GGT (22.7%) and total bilirubin (9%), though serum ALP is controversial. Since GGT and ALP are expressed in sites other than the bile duct, their level could indicate multi-organ damage and cannot be classified solely as a specific bile duct marker. Furthermore, GGT has been identified as a surrogate marker for increased oxidative stress and chronic inflammation [39]. Therefore, elevated cholangiocyte markers are not specific for bile damage, as shown by rare pathological features of bile damage or cholestasis.

The synthetic liver function is altered by SARS-CoV-2 infection, resulting in hypoalbuminemia, an independent predictor of patient mortality. Albumin deficiency may be related to insufficient protein intake, serum protein exudation due to inflammation, diarrhea, or direct liver injury [40]. Furthermore, hepatic dysfunction badly impacts the coagulative and fibrinolytic pathways, platelet count, neutrophil counts with high neutrophil-to-lymphocyte ratios, and serum ferritin levels [33].

Radiological findings during the SARS-CoV-2 pandemic

Radiology plays a fundamental role in diagnosing COVID-19 patients based on chest findings. rRT-PCR may give initial false-negative results with a sensitivity of 83.3% for early COVID-19. In contrast, typical CT radiological findings demonstrated a sensitivity of nearly 97.2% for diagnosing early COVID-19 and a low rate of missed COVID-19 diagnoses [41, 42]. However, chest CT should not be used exclusively for diagnosing COVID-19 infection, especially in asymptomatic patients [43]. Moreover, abdominal imaging becomes critical in COVID-19 patients who initially or exclusively present with GI symptoms. Abdominal imaging plays a role in determining the mechanism of SARS-CoV-2-induced injury, which may be thromboembolic or non-thromboembolic.

Abdominal imaging findings in patients with SARS-CoV-2 infection

Numerous radiological findings related to COVID-19 have been reported. The findings were separated into four groups to clarify the potential cause of injury (see Fig. 4).

Using contrast-enhanced computed tomography (CECT), enterocolitis of the abdomen was mainly observed in the right-sided colon (ascending colon and transverse colon) but was also involved in any bowel loop [44]. Many bowel ischemia cases in either the small or large bowel were detected by CECT. Occlusive ischemia resulted from thrombosis of the large or small mesenteric arteries, as determined by CT angiography or pathology, respectively. However, non-occlusive bowel ischemia with patent mesenteric arteries was attributed to hypoxia or low cardiac output. In CT angiography, the presence of isolated venous thrombosis in the mesenteric, portal vein, or inferior vena cava was associated with bowel wall edema without evidence of ischemic changes [45]. Pneumatosis intestinalis, a radiological sign suggestive of necrotizing enterocolitis, is another characteristic associated with bowel ischemia in COVID-19 patients. However, pneumatosis intestinalis might be discovered accidentally in the absence of clinical or radiological evidence of bowel ischemia. Epiploic appendagitis and perforation of the small and large bowel have been reported in some cases as direct sequelae of infection or secondary to ischemia [44].

Motility disorders have been identified in few COVID-19 patients, with some exceptions; one case with paralytic ileus resolved after conservative treatment [46]. Another case involved a pediatric patient presenting with abdominal pain and ileocecal intussusception [47]. Motility disorder could be induced by an imbalance of the colon's autonomic innervation, a common feature of coronaviruses. However, further research is recommended to determine if these findings are linked to COVID-19 or concomitant.

Two studies reported the association of appendicitis and mesenteric lymphadenitis with SARS-CoV-2 infections. However, further ancillary studies on the resected specimen were recommended to confirm this hypothesis [8]. Similarly, a COVID-19 case has been identified in which a patient presented with a mild form of pancreatitis, absent of other causes [44].

Hepatic imaging findings in patients with SARS-CoV-2 infection

Hepatic injury was reported frequently in abdominal ultrasound (US) and CT in the form of hepatomegaly, periportal edema, pericholecystic fat stranding, and portal lymphadenopathy. One study showed a significantly lower liver to splenic CT attenuation ratio in COVID-19 patients than in the control group. Assessment of liver stiffness (LS) using combined US and elastography revealed a linear correlation between LS and biochemical markers for acute liver damage, indicating that elastography can be used as a reliable non-invasive indicator of hepatic injury in COVID-19 patients [48].

Hepatic steatosis appearing as a hepatic hypodensity in CT was higher in COVID-19 patients than in the control group. Thus, hepatic steatosis was suggested as a risk factor for SARS-CoV-2 infection [44]. However, it is unknown whether steatosis is a risk factor or a result of COVID-19.

Infectious and direct cytopathic

- **Enterocolitis** (US & CT): CT showed bowel wall thickening (the most common finding in COVID -19 related GI affection), mural hyper-enhancement, mesenteric hypervascularity as wel as mesenteric/peri-colic fat stranding and fluid filled colon in cases with diarrhea.
- **Appendicitis** (US & CT): Thickened appendix with omental stranding and/or fluid.
- **Mesenteric lymphadenitis** (US & CT): Enlarged lymph nodes along the mesenteric axis with/out fluid.
- **Pancreatitis** (US & CT): Edematous pancreas with peri-pancreatic fat stranding.

Ischemic and thrombo-embolic

- **Bowel ischemia** (CT): Dilated bowel caliber, thickened wall with hypo/non-enhancement, mesenteric fat stranding and small amount of ascites. It's either occlusive or non-occlusive.
- **Mesenteric vascular occlusion** (CT angiography): Arterial or venous, absent contrast enhancement of vascular lumen, filling defects or direct visualization of intraluminal hypodense thrombus.

Ischemic or infectious

- **Pneumatosis intestinalis** (X-ray & CT): Gas foci within the bowel wall. It's either ischemic (life threatening) or benign (spontaneous resolution).
- **Small and large bowel perforation** (X-ray or CT): Primarily suspected by pneumoperitoneum. More specific findings were found in CT of some patients such as frank discontinuity of a thickened loop, pericecal hematoma with active bleeding, large bowel dilatation with contrast leakage and fluid contrast layering at the recto-vesical pouch.
- **Epiploic appendigitis** (CT): Stranding of the omentum around a well-defined pericolic ovoid shaped fatty area.

Motility disorder

- **Paralytic ileus** (X-ray& CT): Distended bowel loops from the anus to the duodenum, filled with fluid and air–fluid levels.
- **Ileocecal intussusception** (US &CT): Target sign of alternating bowel wall layers.

Fig. 4 Abdominal radiological findings of COVID-19-associated GI symptoms. CT, computed tomography; US, ultrasound; GI, gastrointestinal

Biliary system manifestations were reported in COVID-19 patients in the form of bile stasis with subsequent gall bladder distention and sludge formation [44]. Furthermore, edema of the gall bladder wall, hepatic bed, and pericholecystic fat stranding were observed independently or as part of hepatic injury.

Finally, solid organ acute infarction was reported in two COVID-19 patients, involving the kidney, spleen, or liver [44].

Histopathological findings of COVID-19-associated GI and liver injury

The role of histopathology in the diagnosis of COVID-19 aims to detect viral host receptors, assess pathological features, visualize viral particles, and understand disease mechanisms. Moreover, virus detection by immunohistochemistry (IHC) can be recognized directly by the pathologist, saving time and money to confirm a potential suspected case of COVID-19.

Pathological findings of GI-related COVID-19

The small intestine, primarily absorptive and crypt enterocytes but not goblet, Paneth, or enteroendocrine cells, expressed more ACE2 receptors than other GI sites [49]. Furthermore, histopathological analysis of 14 GI specimens obtained either post-mortem or by resection revealed ischemic changes in the form of mucosal necrosis or transmural hemorrhagic infarction [50]. The possible etiology of ischemia was thrombi in mucosal or mesenteric blood vessels in six cases, vasculitis and endothelial inflammation in four cases, and mixed thrombi and endotheliitis in two cases. Hobnail modifications of the endothelial cells with bizarre nuclear shapes have been also reported [51]. Inflammation was evident in seven cases: two of lymphoplasmacytic nature, two of acute nature, and three of undefined nature. Three cases of microscopic colitis were reported; however, there is insufficient evidence to determine whether these cases are SARS-CoV-2 related or incidental findings. There were seven attempts to detect SARS-CoV-2 viral particles in GI specimens. Positive viral particles were observed in the mucosa and the endothelial cells in five and two cases, respectively [51]. Moreover, Stah et al. detected intact viral particles in the bowel endothelium 8 weeks after initial infection and viral clearing in respiratory and blood specimens [52]. However, negative results were reported in six cases: two for the esophagus, two for the colon, one for the stomach, and one for the duodenum. The two reported appendicitis cases showed mucosal necrosis, non-caseating granulomas, and a foreign body reaction associated with severe mesenteric necrotizing lymphadenitis or ulcerophelgmonous [8].

Pathological findings of liver-related COVID-19

There has been a limited pathology role in diagnosing liver-associated COVID-19 abnormalities, with the majority of specimens obtained post-mortem [32, 53–55]. Histopathological characteristics varied, with most cases exhibiting a mixed pattern of injury. Histopathological changes included steatosis, either microvesicular and/or macrovesicular (61/95), inflammation with variable distribution including portal, sinusoidal, lobular, or panacinar (64/101), vascular abnormalities (54 cases), endotheliitis (3 cases), and lobular necrosis/apoptosis (15 cases). Other pathological findings reported in low frequency included Kupffer cell hyperplasia, giant cells transformation, lobular cholestasis, granuloma, and type II fibrinogen deposition. Moreover, bile duct damage was reported in only two cases. Numerous experiments used various techniques to visualize the viral particles, including electron microscopy (EM), polymerase chain reaction (PCR), or even IHC, with positive findings encountered in 15/22 cases [54, 55]. Rather than viral particles, some authors interpreted the EM findings as clathrin-coated vesicles, which are involved in synaptic vesicle reconstitution, or multi-vesicular bodies, which are routinely discovered post-mortem. Several studies have conducted a C4d IHC test to assess immunological background, and only one case was positive (1/50) [54–56].

The histopathological findings of steatosis, acute hepatitis, and positive viral tissue detection indicate a poor patient outcome. Histopathological observations were interpreted to gain a better understanding of the potential mechanism of injury (see Fig. 5).

Management therapies in SARS-CoV-2-associated GI and liver diseases

Treatment of COVID-19 associated GI or liver infection aims to clear the viral infection, relieve symptoms, and stabilize patients with previous GI or liver diseases. All therapies are critical for their anti-inflammatory properties and reduce viral entry, host receptor binding, and replication.

In addition to viral target therapies, symptomatic treatment is discussed, including oral or intravenous hydration and antiemetic medications. The anti-diarrheal agent loperamide can be used in patients without fever or bloody stools and after ruling out other infectious causes. Patients with non-variceal upper GI bleeding can be conservatively treated with PPIs and coagulation optimization without endoscopic intervention. However, PPIs are associated with hypochlorhydria, which increases the risk of SARS-CoV-2 entering the gut from the stomach, causing viral infection. Therefore, PPIs should be used at the lowest effective dose (once daily) [57]. Similarly, endoscopic evaluation for lower GI

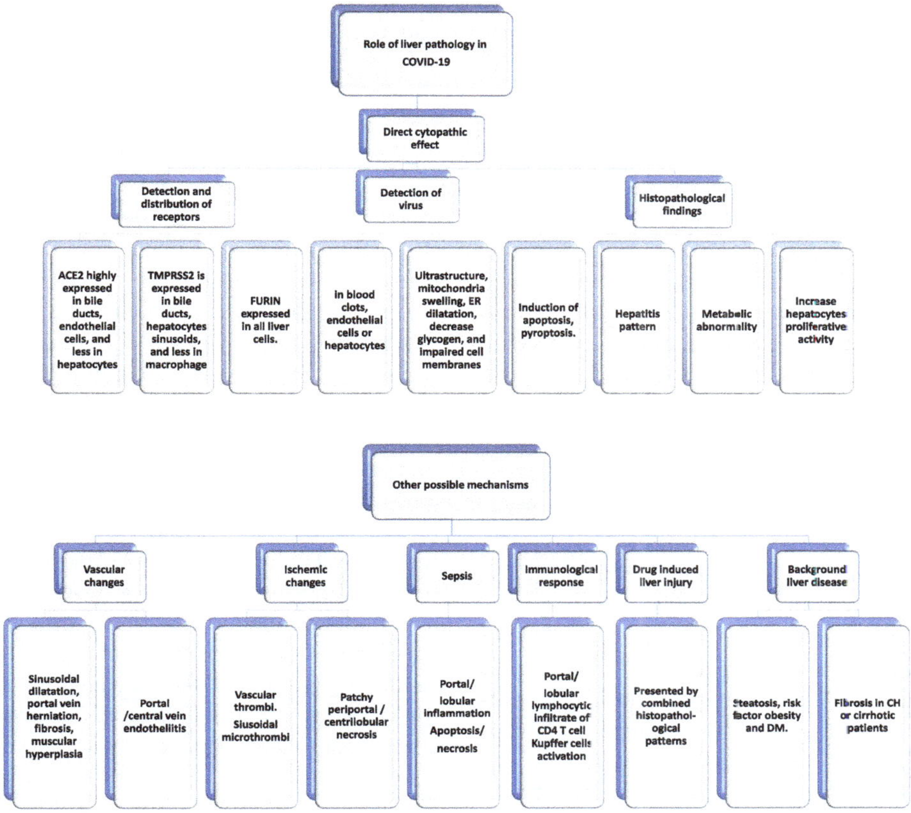

Fig. 5 The role of pathology in understanding SARS-CoV-2-induced liver injury mechanism. ACE2, angiotensin-converting enzyme-2; TMPRSS2, transmembrane protease, serine 2

bleeding might be initially postponed until acute disease resolution. For patients with severe COVID-19-associated liver damage, hepatoprotective, anti-inflammatory, and jaundice-reducing agents, as well as vitamin E, are recommended [58].

Management of background GI and liver diseases during the SARS-CoV-2 pandemic

Many studies discussed the strategies for managing IBD patients during the SARS-CoV-2 pandemic in connection with several factors, mainly proper interpretation of the complaint, whether related to COVID-19 or acute flaring of the primary disease. For active IBD patients without SARS-CoV-2 infection, adding or escalating anti-inflammatory or biologic therapy for symptomatic improvement and remission induction may be involved. However, systemic glucocorticoids should be used at the lowest effective therapeutic dose [59]. On the other hand, the aim of therapy in patients with inflammatory bowel disease (IBD) infected with SARS-CoV-2 is to minimize immunosuppression during active viral infection to avoid viral complications (e.g., pneumonia). Two strategies are proposed for COVID-19 patients with IBD in remission: continue therapy indefinitely with budesonide, aminosalicylates, sulfasalazine, topical glucocorticoids, and antibiotics [59], or temporarily adjust medication until symptoms resolve, including systemic glucocorticoids and immunomodulators [60].

Immunosuppressive therapy reduction or discontinuation is not recommended for asymptomatic patients who have undergone liver transplantation and post-transplant treatment unless they are SARS-CoV-2 positive. Similarly, HCC-related treatments should be administered without any delay.

Drug-induced GI and liver injury (DILI)

Certain drugs are alleged to play a role in GI and liver injury. The possible mechanisms include reactive metabolites and oxidative stress, idiosyncratic through drug-cytochrome P-450 interaction, or synergistic inflammatory response [61–63]. Table 1 summarizes the potential therapeutic agents, their mechanism of action, common side effects relating to the GI and liver, and possible drug-drug interactions (DDIs).

Hepatic patients with non-alcoholic fatty liver disease (NAFLD) infected with SARS-CoV-2 might be more susceptible to DILI [64]. Dexamethasone was found to decrease mortality rates among COVID-19 patients; however, it may lead to chronic hepatitis B virus (HBV) reactivation. Similarly, tocilizumab, an IL-6 blocker, increases HBV reactivation risk. Therefore, hepatitis B surface antigen (HBsAg)-positive patients should also be treated with anti-viral medication for the duration of steroid therapy.

For patients with severe alcoholic or autoimmune hepatitis, caution must be taken when suggesting the initiation of steroids or other immunosuppressive therapy [65]. Regimens containing chloroquine or remdesivir were generally considered safe. Hydroxychloroquine should be treated for cardiac arrhythmias in patients receiving hepatitis C treatment [66].

Demographic data of SARS-CoV-2-associated GI and liver infection

Geographical distribution of GI symptoms

The SARS-CoV-2 associated with GI manifestations was reported later in the COVID-19 pandemic. A potential reason is that the prevalence of GI symptoms is 2–3 times lower in China, the epicenter of the outbreak, than in western countries, primarily Europe and the USA; however, there was no statistically significant difference between the country-based studies [23]. Furthermore, an analysis of Chinese studies showed a constant low prevalence of diarrhea and vomiting before, during, and after April [67]. These observed differences could result from variability in SARS-CoV-2 host receptor gene expression, coagulation activity, and health care access amongst different socio-economic groups and ethnicities, all of which affect COVID-19 pathogenesis. Chinese populations have a lower risk of thrombo-embolic complications than other ethnic groups, which reduces the severity of COVID-19 [68]. However, geographic differences between countries remain unexplored.

Age-related GI and liver symptoms

COVID-19 patients with GI symptoms ranged in age from 1 day to 92 years, with a pooled mean age of 48.7 ± 16.5 years [39]. The frequency of patients presenting with COVID-19-related GI symptoms did not show much variance, remaining at nearly 10% for all age groups [69]. Age was positively correlated with the severity of GI symptoms and mortality. Possible factors include low expression of ACE receptors, lower intensity of viral exposure, the protective effects of live vaccines, increased susceptibility to recurrent infections, and the difference in the adaptive, cellular immunity, and microbiota in children. In contrast to the age-related vascular and endothelial damage, prior coronavirus exposure and associated comorbidities negatively impact the disease course in the elderly [70].

Gender differences of SARS-CoV-2-associated GI and liver symptoms

According to a recent meta-analysis by Kaur et al., which included 6635 COVID-19 patients, COVID-19-infected individuals were predominantly male. However, the manifestation of GI symptoms was significantly different between males and females. Self-reported GI symptom frequency during the COVID-19 course was significantly higher among women than men ($P < 0.001$). Zouh et al. found a significantly higher proportion of female COVID-19 patients with GI symptoms associated with COVID-19 [71]. The exact mechanism is not elucidated; however, it could be hormonal modulation of the gustatory system. Notably, global data suggested male gender is a negative indicator of disease severity and mortality. Factors responsible for higher male mortality could include higher rates of smoking, respiratory tract infection, proinflammatory cytokines, and the immunosuppressive effect of testosterone. However, Agrawal et al. suggested that the estrogen-enhancing effect and the localization of immune response genes on X-chromosome may protect females [72].

The prognosis of SARS-CoV-2-induced GI and liver infection

There was no consensus regarding the impact of GI symptoms on the COVID-19 course. Studies reported no significant difference in the prevalence of diarrhea, nausea, or vomiting between severe and non-severe patients [22]. Another study reported patients presenting with COVID-19-related GI symptoms to have a low mortality rate compared to those without GI symptoms [73]. In contrast, other studies reported a poor outcome for COVID-19 patients who presented with GI symptoms, especially abdominal pain [69, 74]. The low prognostic impact of GI symptoms could be related to the marked electrolyte imbalance, gut dysbiosis, ischemic-reperfusion injury, and associated neurological manifestations.

Notably, there was a consensus of the poor prognostic impact of elevated liver enzymes on COVID-19 patients [69]. In extreme COVID-19 patients, hypoalbuminemia, high GGT, aminotransferase (AST > ALT), and bilirubin rather than serum ALP levels were observed [39].

The impact of background GI and liver diseases on the outcome of SARS-CoV-2 infection

There was no correlation between autoimmune GI diseases and the increased risk of SARS-CoV-2 infection. Patients with IBD are not at greater risk and can maintain remission with maintenance therapy [59]. Similarly, celiac disease patients showed no increased risk for

Table 1 Potential GI and liver adverse effects and drug interaction profile of COVID-19 investigational drugs

	Mechanism of action	GI affection	Liver affection	Major drug-drug interactions
Chloroquine/ hydroxychloroquine [80]	Interferences with terminal glycosylation of ACE2 receptor Blocks viral entry by increasing endosomal pH and inhibiting viral fusion to the cell membrane	Nausea, vomiting, weight loss, abdominal pain	Rare elevations in aminotransferases. Most reactions are Idiosyncrasy or oxidative stress.	A moderate inhibitor of CYP2D6 and P-gp Significant particularly with anti-rejection immunosuppressants. Weak interaction with tenofovir/ entecavir Hydroxychloroquine given to a patient taking hepatitis c treatment should monitor for cardiac arrhythmia
Ivermectin [81]	Inhibition of viral IMPα/β1-mediated nuclear import, which reduces the replication of the virus and so the viral load	Nausea, vomiting, diarrhea	Very few reports on elevated liver enzymes or jaundice	Avoid concomitant use of ivermectin with other drugs that enhance GABA activity
Nitazoxanide [82]	Antiparasitic drug has broad-spectrum anti-viral activity	Abdominal pain (8%), diarrhea (2%), nausea (3%), vomiting (1%)	Increased ALT: <1%	Rapidly hydrolyzed to tizoxanide. which is highly protein-bound (>99%), so caution when giving with other highly protein-bound drugs with narrow therapeutic indices.
Atazanavir [83]	Protease inhibitors	Diarrhea, nausea, vomiting, abdominal pain	Indirect hyperbilirubinemia with overt jaundice Elevation of hepatic enzymes especially in patients with underlying HBV or HCV co-infection	Inhibitor of CYP3A4 and CYP2C9 PPI decreases its concentrations. Tenofovir and efavirenz should not be co-administered with atazanavir
Favipiravir [84]	RNA-dependent RNA polymerase inhibitor	Nausea/vomiting (5–15%), diarrhea (5%)	Liver enzyme abnormalities	Inhibitor for: CYP2C8 and aldehyde oxidase
Interferon beta [85]	Cytokines with anti-viral and immunomodulatory effects.	Nausea, vomiting	Elevated liver enzymes	DDI potential not fully evaluated. Possible inhibitor of CYP enzymes
Lopinavir/ritonavir [86]	HIV protease inhibitor/ CYP450inhibitor	Nausea/vomiting (5–10%), abdominal pain (1–10%), diarrhea (10–30%), dysgeusia (< 2%), increased serum amylase/lipase.	Hepatotoxicity ranges from mild elevations in aminotransferases to acute liver failure. Recovery takes 1–2 mo. Might include drug-cytochrome P-450 interaction	Substrate for: CYP3A4, CYP2D6, P-gp Inducer for: CYP1A2, CYP2B6, CYP2C8, CYP2C9, CYP2C19, UGT1A1 Inhibitor for: CYP3A4 Increased levels of Immunosuppressive drugs (calcineurin and mTOR inhibitors). Moderate interaction risk with tenofovir with renal functions monitoring. Lopinavir/ ritonavir increase concentrations of hepatitis C treatment.
Remdesivir [87]	RNA-dependent RNA polymerase inhibitor	Nausea, vomiting	Deranged liver enzymes Hepatotoxicity reported; frequency is not yet known.	NA
Ribavirin [88]	Inhibit capping of viral messenger RNA, and the viral RNA-dependent polymerase	Nausea	Hepatotoxicity	NA
Anakinra [89]	IL-1R inhibitor	Rare abdominal pain, nausea, diarrhea	Hepatobiliary disorders: Elevated transaminases, noninfectious hepatitis	No effect on CYP450.
Baricitinib [90]	JAK1 and JAK2 inhibitor Inhibit viral endocytosis	Bowel perforation, nausea, vomiting	Hepatitis B reactivation	Partially metabolized by CYP3A4 and a substrate for OAT3 and P-gp OAT3 inhibitors cause a significant effect on baricitinib exposure
Dexamethasone/ Hydrocortisone [59]	Reduction of IL-8, monocyte chemo-attractant protein-1,	Nausea, peptic ulcers	NA	Aspirin can increase the risk of bleeding when used with it

Table 1 Potential GI and liver adverse effects and drug interaction profile of COVID-19 investigational drugs *(Continued)*

	Mechanism of action	GI affection	Liver affection	Major drug-drug interactions
	and Th1 chemokine IFN-γ-inducible protein-10			
Ruxolitinib [91]	Selective JAK inhibitors	NA	Increased ALT Increased AST	Metabolized by CYP3A4 and CYP2C9. So, it is liable to DDIs with inhibitors or inducers of these enzymes. Ruxolitinib may inhibit BCRP and P-gp, and caution is indicated with co-administering with substrates of these transporters with narrow therapeutic indices.
Sarilumab [92]	IL-6R inhibitor	Few cases of gastrointestinal perforation	Increased ALT	No effect on CYP450
Tocilizumab [93]	IL-6R inhibitor (Curbs cytokine release syndrome)	Bowel perforation, pancreatitis, abdominal pain	Elevated liver enzymes, Reactivation of chronic hepatitis B	No effect on CYP450

ACE angiotensin-converting enzyme, *ALT* alanine aminotransferase, *AST* aspartate aminotransferase, *BCRP* breast cancer resistance protein, *COVID-19* coronavirus disease-19, *CYP* cytochrome P450, *DDI* drug-drug interaction, *GABA* γ-aminobutyric acid, *GI* gastrointestinal, *HIV* human immunodeficiency virus, *IFN* interferon, *IL* interleukin, *IMP* α/β-mediated nuclear import, *JAK* Janus kinase, *OAT* organic anion transporter, *P-gp* P-glycoprotein, *PPI* proton pump inhibitor, *Th* t-helper, *TOR* target of rapamycin

SARS-CoV-2 infection or primary disease complications [75].

In CLD patients, SARS-CoV-2 infection stimulates inflammatory mediators and decreases ACE2 expression, aggravating liver cirrhosis [76]. Furthermore, NAFLD patients infected with SARS-CoV-2 might be more vulnerable to DILI, a cytokine storm, and ischemic damage to the liver [77]. Similarly, HBV patients coinfected with SARS-CoV-2 could experience HBV reactivation following therapy [78]. Therefore, the liver function in patients with CLD should be monitored regularly throughout the SARS-CoV-2 infection.

Discussion

The digestive tract may serve as a possible route of SARS-CoV-2 transmission to the liver, appendix, and brain. The virus reaches the gut through fecal transmission, saliva, or vomiting. The persistence of viral indicators in the stool may be used as a surrogate monitor for recurrent infection [27]. A GI and liver injury mechanism is a multi-hit hypothesis requiring interaction between genetics, multiple organ cross-talk, and vascular and inflammatory response [4]. Demographic studies have proposed a low prevalence of COVID-19-associated GI symptoms in China compared to other countries; however, there is no consensus on gender or age as predicting factors [27]. The high-risk factors include the male gender, old age, anorexia, abdominal pain, liver enzyme abnormalities, and the histopathological findings of steatosis, acute hepatitis, and positive viral tissue detection. Surprisingly, SARS-CoV-2 infection may worsen the background liver disease, with low or no impact on pre-existing GI diseases [76].

Typical GI symptoms experienced by some COVID-19 patients included diarrhea, nausea, vomiting, and abdominal pain, which may even necessitate surgical interventions [20, 29]. Therefore, all patients with GI symptoms should be eligible for SARS-CoV-2 testing as these symptoms may precede the respiratory symptoms or be the only symptoms [23]. In contrast, liver injury is observed during laboratory investigation or post-mortem pathological studies. Liver function tests should be monitored even in the absence of hepatic symptoms. Abnormalities in liver enzymes are reported in similar frequencies despite the presence of pre-existing liver disease [79], and unexplained elevation of ALT/AST, an increase of bilirubin, and reduced albumin levels in a clinically suspect patient may indicate COVID-19 infection. The mechanism of GI injury is multifactorial, with infection and ischemic-thromboembolic alteration playing a significant role. A subsequent intestinal malabsorption, imbalance in intestinal secretions, intestinal dysbiosis, and activation of the enteric nervous system exacerbate the GI infection. Even more, the mucosal injury could mediate viral spread throughout the bowel wall [26].

Similarly, the mechanism of liver injury is multifactorial, confirmed by mixed histopathological findings, laboratory results, and radiological investigations. The direct viral cytopathic effect has been explained by broad hepatic SARS-CoV-2 host receptor distributions [15]. Vascular alterations result from increased blood flow, endothelial injury, endotheliitis, thrombosis, and concomitant thrombotic changes in the pulmonary vessels [54]. However, Lagana et al. reported that liver vascular abnormalities do not correlate with pulmonary dysfunction [55]. The lack of pathological features of ischemia did not explain the elevated serum aminotransferase levels in COVID-19 patients but rather raises the possibility of another mechanism other than hypoxic-ischemic injury. Similarly, the pathological findings of sepsis are reported only in four cases [55]. The immunological and cytokine storm mechanism contributes significantly to liver damage by releasing inflammatory mediators and activating different immune cells [19]. The expression of C4d was focally positive in only one case [54, 55]. Therefore, the immunological response is more cellular than humoral. DILI is a possible mechanism, though it is still a diagnosis of exclusion. The presence of steatosis and mixed histopathological findings supports drug-induced damage [55]. However, Wang et al. found no significant differences in drug adherence between patients with normal and abnormal liver enzymes [22]. Moreover, hepatotoxicity usually occurs after long-term antiviral therapy. Finally, most histopathological changes in the liver were limited or related to underlying liver diseases [53].

Suggestions for future research

COVID-19 associated with GI and liver injury is an emerging research era with many questions with no definite answers. The mechanism by which some individuals experience GI symptoms rather than respiratory symptoms is not well elucidated. The route of GI transmission and the virus's ability to survive the extremes of GI pH require further studies. The reliable role of elevated liver enzymes during SARS-CoV-2 infection must also be investigated because liver damage is usually an incidental finding in the routine laboratory or pathological investigation. Improving the histopathological tools in detecting viral particles could aid in elucidating disease mechanisms. More studies are recommended to identify the essential structural proteins of SARS-CoV-2 that promote tissue invasion and replication. Accordingly, improved selective and targeted therapeutic agents could be developed.

Conclusions

SARS-CoV-2 infection resulted in GI and liver disease through multi-hit complex mechanisms. GI manifestations are normal in COVID-19 patients, and particular attention should be given to high-risk patients, including those who are older, male, and have abdominal pain, elevated liver enzymes, or background liver disease.

Abbreviations

SARS-CoV-2: Severe acute respiratory syndrome coronavirus 2; GI: Gastrointestinal; COVID-19: Novel 2019 coronavirus disease; ACE2: Angiotensin-converting enzyme 2; TMPRSS2: Transmembrane protease serine 2; ENS: Enteric nervous system; EGCs: Enteric glial cells; TLRs: Toll-like receptors; CatB/L: Cathepsin B and L; SIRS: Systemic inflammatory response syndrome; PPIs: Proton pump inhibitors; CRP: C-reactive protein; LDH: Lactate dehydrogenase; HBDH: α-hydroxybutyrate dehydrogenase; IL-6: Interleukin-6; TNF-α: Tumor necrosis factor-α; CLD: Chronic liver disease; FC: Fecal calprotectin; IBD: Inflammatory bowel disease; AST: Aspartate aminotransferase; ALT: Alanine aminotransferase; GGT: Gamma-glutamyl transferase; ALP: Alkaline phosphatase; CECT: Contrast-enhanced computed tomography; US: Ultrasound; LS: Liver stiffness; EM: Electron microscopy; PCR: Polymerase chain reaction; HC: Immunohistochemistry; DDI: Drug-drug interactions; DLI: Drug induced liver injury; HBV: Hepatitis B virus; HBsAg: Hepatitis B surface antigen; NAFLD: Non-alcoholic fatty liver disease

Acknowledgements

Not applicable.

Authors' contributions

All authors of this paper have participated in its drafting and approved the final version submitted. DS wrote the pathological part, EA wrote the GI and hepatology part, EK wrote the radiological part, HA and SA wrote the biochemical and mechanism of disease, HM wrote the mode of spread and mechanism of disease, IM made the online search and wrote the epidemiological part, NA contributed to paper editing, and ES wrote the pharmacological part. All authors acquired and interpreted the collected data. DS, AM, HE, and ES revised and edited the final version.

Declarations

Ethics approval and consent to participate

Not applicable.

Competing interests

The authors have no conflicts of interest to declare.

Author details

[1]Pathology Department, National Liver Institute, Menofia University, Shibin El Kom 32511, Egypt. [2]Hepatology and Gastroenterology Department, National Liver Institute, Menofia University, Shibin El Kom, Egypt. [3]Radiology Department, Faculty of Medicine, Menofia University, Shibin El Kom, Egypt. [4]Clinical Pathology Department, National Liver Institute, Menofia University, Shibin El Kom, Egypt. [5]Microbiology Department, Faculty of Medicine, Menofia University, Shibin El Kom, Egypt. [6]Epidemiology and Preventive Medicine Department, Menofia University, Shibin El Kom, Egypt. [7]Clinical Biochemistry, and Molecular Diagnostics Department, National Liver Institute, Menofia University, Shibin El Kom, Egypt. [8]Ohio State College of Medicine, Columbus, OH, USA. [9]Biochemistry Department, Faculty of Science, Cairo University, Giza, Egypt. [10]Clinical Pharmacology Department, Faculty of Medicine, Menofia University, Shibin El Kom, Egypt.

References

1. Li Q, Guan X, Wu P, Wang X, Zhou L, Tong Y, Ren R, Leung KSM, Lau EHY, Wong JY, Xing X, Xiang N, Wu Y, Li C, Chen Q, Li D, Liu T, Zhao J, Liu M, Tu W, Chen C, Jin L, Yang R, Wang Q, Zhou S, Wang R, Liu H, Luo Y, Liu Y, Shao G, Li H, Tao Z, Yang Y, Deng Z, Liu B, Ma Z, Zhang Y, Shi G, Lam TTY, Wu JT, Gao GF, Cowling BJ, Yang B, Leung GM, Feng Z (2020) Early transmission din Wuhan, China, of novel coronavirus-infected pneumonia. N Engl J Med 382(13):1199–1207. https://doi.org/10.1056/NEJMoa2001316
2. Holshue ML, DeBolt C, Lindquist S, Lofy KH, Wiesman J, Bruce H, Spitters C, Ericson K, Wilkerson S, Tural A, Diaz G, Cohn A, Fox L, Patel A, Gerber SI, Kim L, Tong S, Lu X, Lindstrom S, Pallansch MA, Weldon WC, Biggs HM, Uyeki TM, Pillai SK, Washington State -nCo VCIT (2020) First case of 2019 novel coronavirus in the United States. N Engl J Med 382(10):929–936. https://doi.org/10.1056/NEJMoa2001191
3. Zhong P, Xu J, Yang D, Shen Y, Wang L, Feng Y, Du C, Song Y, Wu C, Hu X, Sun Y (2020) COVID-19-associated gastrointestinal and liver injury: clinical features and potential mechanisms. Signal Transduction and Targeted Therapy 5(1):256. https://doi.org/10.1038/s41392-020-00373-7

4. Pamplona J, Solano R, Soler C, Sabat M (2020) Epidemiological approximation of the enteric manifestation and possible fecal–oral transmission in COVID-19: a preliminary systematic review. Eur J Gastroenterol Hepatol Publish Ahead of Print. https://doi.org/10.1097/MEG.0000000000001934
5. Li Y, Ren B, Peng X, Hu T, Li J, Gong T, Tang B, Xu X, Zhou X (2020) Saliva is a non-negligible factor in the spread of COVID-19. Mol Oral Microbiol 35(4): 141–145. https://doi.org/10.1111/omi.12289
6. Jones DL, Baluja MQ, Graham DW, Corbishley A, McDonald JE, Malham SK, Hillary LS, Connor TR, Gaze WH, Moura IB, Wilcox MH, Farkas K (2020) Shedding of SARS-CoV-2 in feces and urine and its potential role in person-to-person transmission and the environment-based spread of COVID-19. Sci Total Environ 749:141364 https://doi.org/10.1016/j.scitotenv.2020.141364
7. Portincasa P, Krawczyk M, Machill A, Lammert F, Di Ciaula A (2020) Hepatic consequences of COVID-19 infection. Lapping or biting? Eur J Intern Med 77:18–24. https://doi.org/10.1016/j.ejim.2020.05.035
8. Ahmad S, Ahmed RN, Jani P, Ullah M, Aboulgheit H (2020) SARS-CoV-2 isolation from an appendix. J Surg Case Rep 2020(8):rjaa245. https://doi.org/10.1093/jscr/rjaa245
9. Groß R, Conzelmann C, Müller JA, Stenger S, Steinhart K, Kirchhoff F, Münch J (2020) Detection of SARS-CoV-2 in human breastmilk. Lancet 395(10239): 1757–1758. https://doi.org/10.1016/S0140-6736(20)31181-8
10. Cho HJ, Koo JW, Roh SK, Kim YK, Suh JS, Moon JH, Sohn SK, Baek DW (2020) COVID-19 transmission and blood transfusion: a case report. Journal of Infection and Public Health 13(11):1678–1679 https://doi.org/10.1016/j.jiph.2020.05.001
11. Chen L, Marishta A, Ellison CE, Verzi MP (2021) Identification of transcription factors regulating SARS-CoV-2 entry genes in the intestine. Cell Mol Gastroenterol Hepatol 11(1):181–184. https://doi.org/10.1016/j.jcmgh.2020.08.005
12. DosSantos MF, Devalle S, Aran V, Capra D, Roque NR, Coelho-Aguiar JM, TCLdSe S, Subilhaga JG, Pereira CM, D'Andrea Meira I, Niemeyer Soares Filho P, Moura-Neto V (2020) Neuromechanisms of SARS-CoV-2: a review. Front Neuroanat 14:37. https://doi.org/10.3389/fnana.2020.00037
13. Fändriks L (2009) The angiotensin II type 2 receptor and the gastrointestinal tract. J Renin-Angiotensin-Aldosterone Syst 11(1):43–48. https://doi.org/10.1177/1470320309347788
14. Garg M, Angus PW, Burrell LM, Herath C, Gibson PR, Lubel JS (2012) Review article: the pathophysiological roles of the renin-angiotensin system in the gastrointestinal tract. Aliment Pharmacol Ther 35(4):414–428. https://doi.org/10.1111/j.1365-2036.2011.04971.x
15. Davidson Anne M, Wysocki J, Batlle D (2020) Interaction of SARS-CoV-2 and other coronavirus with ACE (angiotensin-converting enzyme)-2 as their main receptor. Hypertension 76(5):1339–1349. https://doi.org/10.1161/HYPERTENSIONAHA.120.15256
16. Ahlawat S, Asha SKK (2020) Immunological co-ordination between gut and lungs in SARS-CoV-2 infection. Virus Res 286:198103–198103. https://doi.org/10.1016/j.virusres.2020.198103
17. Panchal P, Budree S, Scheeler A, Medina G, Seng M, Wong WF, Eliott R, Mitchell T, Kassam Z, Allegretti JR, Osman M (2018) Scaling safe access to fecal microbiota transplantation: past, present, and future. Current Gastroenterology Reports 20(4):14. https://doi.org/10.1007/s11894-018-0619-8
18. Price E (2020) Could the severity of COVID-19 be increased by low gastric acidity? Crit Care 24(1):456. https://doi.org/10.1186/s13054-020-03182-0
19. Castelli V, Cimini A, Ferri C (2020) Cytokine storm in COVID-19: "when you come out of the storm, you won't be the same person who walked in". Front Immunol 11:2132–2132. https://doi.org/10.3389/fimmu.2020.02132
20. Docherty AB, Harrison EM, Green CA, Hardwick HE, Pius R, Norman L, Holden KA, Read JM, Dondelinger F, Carson G, Merson L, Lee J, Plotkin D, Sigfrid L, Halpin S, Jackson C, Gamble C, Horby PW, Nguyen-Van-Tam JS, Ho A, Russell CD, Dunning J, Openshaw PJ, Baillie JK, Semple MG, investigators IC (2020) Features of 20 133 UK patients in hospital with covid-19 using the ISARIC WHO Clinical Characterisation Protocol: prospective observational cohort study. BMJ 369:m1985-m1985. doi:https://doi.org/10.1136/bmj.m1985
21. Han C, Duan C, Zhang S, Spiegel B, Shi H, Wang W, Zhang L, Lin R, Liu J, Ding Z, Hou X (2020) Digestive symptoms in COVID-19 patients with mild disease severity: clinical presentation, stool viral RNA testing, and outcomes. Am J Gastroenterol 115(6):916–923. https://doi.org/10.14309/ajg.0000000000000664
22. Wang H, Qiu P, Liu J, Wang F, Zhao Q (2020) The liver injury and gastrointestinal symptoms in patients with coronavirus disease 19: a systematic review and meta-analysis. Clin Res Hepatol Gastroenterol 44(5): 653–661. https://doi.org/10.1016/j.clinre.2020.04.012
23. Sultan S, Altayar O, Siddique SM, Davitkov P, Feuerstein JD, Lim JK, Falck-Ytter Y, El-Serag HB, AGAIEa (2020) AGA Institute rapid review of the gastrointestinal and liver manifestations of COVID-19, meta-analysis of international data, and recommendations for the consultative management of patients with COVID-19. Gastroenterology 159(1):320–334.e327. https://doi.org/10.1053/j.gastro.2020.05.001
24. Freedberg DE, Conigliaro J, Wang TC, Tracey KJ, Callahan MV, Abrams JA, Famotidine Research G (2020) Famotidine use is associated with improved clinical outcomes in hospitalized COVID-19 patients: a propensity score matched retrospective cohort study. Gastroenterology 159(3):1129–1131.e1123. https://doi.org/10.1053/j.gastro.2020.05.053
25. Hunt RH, East JE, Lanas A, Malfertheiner P, Satsangi J, Scarpignato C, Webb GJ (2020) COVID-19 and gastrointestinal disease: implications for the gastroenterologist. Dig Dis. https://doi.org/10.1159/000512152
26. Luo S, Zhang X, Xu H (2020) Don't overlook digestive symptoms in patients with 2019 novel coronavirus disease (COVID-19). Clin Gastroenterol Hepatol 18(7):1636–1637. https://doi.org/10.1016/j.cgh.2020.03.043
27. Cheung KS, Hung IFN, Chan PPY, Lung KC, Tso E, Liu R, Ng YY, Chu MY, Chung TWH, Tam AR, Yip CCY, Leung K-H, Fung AY-F, Zhang RR, Lin Y, Cheng HM, Zhang AJX, To KKW, Chan K-H, Yuen K-Y, Leung WK (2020) Gastrointestinal manifestations of SARS-CoV-2 infection and virus load in fecal samples from a Hong Kong cohort: systematic review and meta-analysis. Gastroenterology 159(1):81–95. https://doi.org/10.1053/j.gastro.2020.03.065
28. Tian Y, Rong L, Nian W, He Y (2020) Review article: gastrointestinal features in COVID-19 and the possibility of faecal transmission. Aliment Pharmacol Ther 51(9):843–851. https://doi.org/10.1111/apt.15731
29. Chan KH, Lim SL, Damati A, Maruboyina SP, Bondili L, Abu Hanoud A, Slim J (2020) Coronavirus disease 2019 (COVID-19) and ischemic colitis: an under-recognized complication. Am J Emerg Med 38(12):2758.e2751–2758.e2754. https://doi.org/10.1016/j.ajem.2020.05.072
30. Inamdar S, Benias PC, Liu Y, Sejpal DV, Satapathy SK, Trindade AJ (2020) Prevalence, risk factors, and outcomes of hospitalized patients with coronavirus disease 2019 presenting as acute pancreatitis. Gastroenterology 159(6):2226–2228.e2222 https://doi.org/10.1053/j.gastro.2020.08.044
31. Zhang H, Liao Y-S, Gong J, Liu J, Xia X, Zhang H (2020) Clinical characteristics of coronavirus disease (COVID-19) patients with gastrointestinal symptoms: a report of 164 cases. Dig Liver Dis 52(10):1076–1079. https://doi.org/10.1016/j.dld.2020.04.034
32. Xu Z, Shi L, Wang Y, Zhang J, Huang L, Zhang C, Liu S, Zhao P, Liu H, Zhu L, Tai Y, Bai C, Gao T, Song J, Xia P, Dong J, Zhao J, Wang F-S (2020) Pathological findings of COVID-19 associated with acute respiratory distress syndrome. Lancet Respir Med 8(4):420–422. https://doi.org/10.1016/S2213-2600(20)30076-X
33. Zhang L, Han C, Zhang S, Duan C, Shang H, Bai T, Hou X (2020) Diarrhea and altered inflammatory cytokine pattern in severe coronavirus disease 2019: impact on disease course and in-hospital mortality. Journal of Gastroenterology and Hepatology n/a (n/a) 36(2):421–429. https://doi.org/10.1111/jgh.15166
34. Yan Y, Jiang X, Wang X, Liu B, Ding H, Jiang M, Yang Z, Dai Y, Ding D, Yu H, Zhang S, Liu J, Sha M, Lui C, Qiu Y, Lu H, Hu Q (2021) CCL28 mucosal expression in SARS-CoV-2-infected patients with diarrhea in relation to disease severity. J Infect 82(1):e19–e21. https://doi.org/10.1016/j.jinf.2020.08.042
35. Effenberger M, Grabherr F, Mayr L, Schwaerzler J, Nairz M, Seifert M, Hilbe R, Seiwald S, Scholl-Buergi S, Fritsche G, Bellmann-Weiler R, Weiss G, Müller T, Adolph TE, Tilg H (2020) Faecal calprotectin indicates intestinal inflammation in COVID-19. Gut 69(8):1543–1544. https://doi.org/10.1136/gutjnl-2020-321388
36. Aghemo A, Piovani D, Parigi TL, Brunetta E, Pugliese N, Vespa E, Omodei PD, Preatoni P, Lleo A, Repici A, Voza A, Cecconi M, Malesci A, Bonovas S, Danese S, Humanitas C-TF (2020) COVID-19 digestive system involvement and clinical outcomes in a large academic hospital in Milan, Italy. Clin Gastroenterol Hepatol 18 (10):2366-2368.e2363. 18(10):2366–2368.e3. https://doi.org/10.1016/j.cgh.2020.05.011
37. Cai Q, Huang D, Yu H, Zhu Z, Xia Z, Su Y, Li Z, Zhou G, Gou J, Qu J, Sun Y, Liu Y, He Q, Chen J, Liu L, Xu L (2020) COVID-19: abnormal liver function tests. J Hepatol 73(3):566–574. https://doi.org/10.1016/j.jhep.2020.04.006
38. Ferm S, Fisher C, Pakala T, Tong M, Shah D, Schwarzbaum D, Cooley V, Hussain S, Kim SH (2020) Analysis of gastrointestinal and hepatic

manifestations of SARS-CoV-2 infection in 892 patients in Queens, NY. Clin Gastroenterol Hepatol 18(10):2378–2379.e2371. https://doi.org/10.1016/j.cgh.2020.05.049
39. Kumar-M P, Mishra S, Jha DK, Shukla J, Choudhury A, Mohindra R, Mandavdhare HS, Dutta U, Sharma V (2020) Coronavirus disease (COVID-19) and the liver: a comprehensive systematic review and meta-analysis. Hepatol Int 14(5):711–722. https://doi.org/10.1007/s12072-020-10071-9
40. Huang W, Li C, Wang Z, Wang H, Zhou N, Jiang J, Ni L, Zhang XA, Wang D-W (2020) Decreased serum albumin level indicates poor prognosis of COVID-19 patients: hepatic injury analysis from 2,623 hospitalized cases. Sci China Life Sci 63(11):1678–1687. https://doi.org/10.1007/s11427-020-1733-4
41. Li Y, Xia L (2020) Coronavirus disease 2019 (COVID-19): role of chest CT in diagnosis and management. Am J Roentgenol 214(6):1280–1286. https://doi.org/10.2214/AJR.20.22954
42. Long C, Xu H, Shen Q, Zhang X, Fan B, Wang C, Zeng B, Li Z, Li X, Li H (2020) Diagnosis of the coronavirus disease (COVID-19): rRT-PCR or CT? Eur J Radiol 126:108961–108961. https://doi.org/10.1016/j.ejrad.2020.108961
43. Kovács A, Palásti P, Veréb D, Bozsik B, Palkó A, Kincses ZT (2021) The sensitivity and specificity of chest CT in the diagnosis of COVID-19. Eur Radiol 31(5):2819–2824. https://doi.org/10.1007/s00330-020-07347-x
44. Bhayana R, Som A, Li MD, Carey DE, Anderson MA, Blake MA, Catalano O, Gee MS, Hahn PF, Harisinghani M, Kilcoyne A, Lee SI, Mojtahed A, Pandharipande PV, Pierce TT, Rosman DA, Saini S, Samir AE, Simeone JF, Gervais DA, Velmahos G, Misdraji J, Kambadakone A (2020) Abdominal imaging findings in COVID-19: preliminary observations. Radiology 297(1): E207–E215. https://doi.org/10.1148/radiol.2020201908
45. Thuluva SK, Zhu H, Tan MML, Gupta S, Yeong KY, Cheong Wah ST, Lin L, Yap ES (2020) A 29-year-old male construction worker from India who presented with left-sided abdominal pain due to isolated superior mesenteric vein thrombosis associated with SARS-CoV-2 infection. Am J Case Rep 21:e926785. https://doi.org/10.12659/AJCR.926785
46. Ibrahim YS, Karuppasamy G, Parambil JV, Alsoub H, Al-Shokri SD (2020) Case Report: Paralytic ileus: a potential extrapulmonary manifestation of severe COVID-19. Am J Trop Med Hyg 103(4):1600–1603. https://doi.org/10.4269/ajtmh.20-0894
47. Martínez-Castaño I, Calabuig-Barbero E, González-Piñera J, López-Ayala JM (2020) COVID-19 infection is a diagnostic challenge in infants with ileocecal intussusception. Pediatr Emerg Care 36(6):e368. https://doi.org/10.1097/PEC.0000000000002155
48. Effenberger M, Grander C, Fritsche G, Bellmann-Weiler R, Hartig F, Wildner S, Seiwald S, Adolph TE, Zoller H, Weiss G, Tilg H (2020) Liver stiffness by transient elastography accompanies illness severity in COVID-19. BMJ Open Gastroenterology 7(1):e000445. https://doi.org/10.1136/bmjgast-2020-000445
49. Zhang H, Li HB, Lyu JR, Lei XM, Li W, Wu G, Lyu J, Dai ZM (2020) Specific ACE2 expression in small intestinal enterocytes may cause gastrointestinal symptoms and injury after 2019-nCoV infection. International journal of infectious diseases : IJID : official publication of the International Society for Infectious Diseases 96:19–24. https://doi.org/10.1016/j.ijid.2020.04.027
50. Ignat M, Philouze G, Aussenac-Belle L, Faucher V, Collange O, Mutter D, Pessaux P (2020) Small bowel ischemia and SARS-CoV-2 infection: an underdiagnosed distinct clinical entity. Surgery 168(1):14–16. https://doi.org/10.1016/j.surg.2020.04.035
51. Carnevale S, Beretta P, Morbini P (2020) Direct endothelial damage and vasculitis due to SARS-CoV-2 in small bowel submucosa of COVID-19 patient with diarrhea. J Med Virol 93(1):61–63. https://doi.org/10.1002/jmv.26119
52. Stahl K, Bräsen JH, Hoeper MM, David S (2020) Direct evidence of SARS-CoV-2 in gut endothelium. Intensive Care Med 46(11):2081–2082. https://doi.org/10.1007/s00134-020-06237-6
53. Tian S, Xiong Y, Liu H, Niu L, Guo J, Liao M, Xiao S-Y (2020) Pathological study of the 2019 novel coronavirus disease (COVID-19) through postmortem core biopsies. Mod Pathol 33(6):1007–1014. https://doi.org/10.1038/s41379-020-0536-x
54. Sonzogni A, Previtali G, Seghezzi M, Grazia Alessio M, Gianatti A, Licini L, Morotti D, Zerbi P, Carsana L, Rossi R, Lauri E, Pellegrinelli A, Nebuloni M (2020) Liver histopathology in severe COVID 19 respiratory failure is suggestive of vascular alterations. Liver Int 40(9):2110–2116 https://doi.org/10.1111/liv.14601
55. Lagana SM, Kudose S, Iuga AC, Lee MJ, Fazlollahi L, Remotti HE, Del Portillo A, De Michele S, de Gonzalez AK, Saqi A, Khairallah P, Chong AM, Park H, Uhlemann A-C, Lefkowitch JH, Verna EC (2020) Hepatic pathology in patients dying of COVID-19: a series of 40 cases including clinical, histologic, and virologic data. Mod Pathol 33(11):2147–2155. https://doi.org/10.1038/s41379-020-00649-x
56. Fiel MI, El Jamal SM, Paniz-Mondolfi A, Gordon RE, Reidy J, Bandovic J, Advani R, Kilaru S, Pourmand K, Ward S, Thung SN, Schiano T (2020) Findings of severe hepatic severe acute respiratory syndrome coronavirus-2 infection. Cell Mol Gastroenterol Hepatol 11(3):763–770. https://doi.org/10.1016/j.jcmgh.2020.09.015
57. Almario CV, Chey WD, Spiegel BMR (2020) Increased risk of COVID-19 among users of proton pump inhibitors. Am J Gastroenterol 115(10):1707–1715. https://doi.org/10.14309/ajg.0000000000000798
58. Wu J, Song S, Cao H-C, Li L-J (2020) Liver diseases in COVID-19: etiology, treatment and prognosis. World J Gastroenterol 26(19):2286–2293. https://doi.org/10.3748/wjg.v26.i19.2286
59. Rubin DT, Feuerstein JD, Wang AY, Cohen RD (2020) AGA Clinical Practice Update on Management of Inflammatory Bowel Disease During the COVID-19 Pandemic: Expert Commentary. Gastroenterology 159(1):350–357. https://doi.org/10.1053/j.gastro.2020.04.012
60. Brenner EJ, Ungaro RC, Gearry RB, Kaplan GG, Kissous-Hunt M, Lewis JD, Ng SC, Rahier J-F, Reinisch W, Ruemmele FM, Steinwurz F, Underwood FE, Zhang X, Colombel J-F, Kappelman MD (2020) Corticosteroids, but not TNF antagonists, are associated with adverse COVID-19 outcomes in patients with inflammatory bowel diseases: results from an international registry. Gastroenterology 159(2): 481–491.e3. https://doi.org/10.1053/j.gastro.2020.05.032
61. Ellison CA, Blackwell SB (2020) Acute hepatocellular injury associated with azithromycin. J Pharm Pract 34(3):493–496. https://doi.org/10.1177/089719001989428
62. Makin AJ, Wendon J, Fitt S, Portmann BC, Williams R (1994) Fulminant hepatic failure secondary to hydroxychloroquine. Gut 35(4):569–570. https://doi.org/10.1136/gut.35.4.569
63. Liu J, Cao R, Xu M, Wang X, Zhang H, Hu H, Li Y, Hu Z, Zhong W, Wang M (2020) Hydroxychloroquine, a less toxic derivative of chloroquine, is effective in inhibiting SARS-CoV-2 infection in vitro. Cell Discovery 6(1):16. https://doi.org/10.1038/s41421-020-0156-0
64. Huang C, Wang Y, Li X, Ren L, Zhao J, Hu Y, Zhang L, Fan G, Xu J, Gu X, Cheng Z, Yu T, Xia J, Wei Y, Wu W, Xie X, Yin W, Li H, Liu M, Xiao Y, Gao H, Guo L, Xie J, Wang G, Jiang R, Gao Z, Jin Q, Wang J, Cao B (2020) Clinical features of patients infected with 2019 novel coronavirus in Wuhan, China. Lancet 395(10223):497–506. https://doi.org/10.1016/S0140-6736(20)30183-5
65. Wong GL-H, Wong VW-S, Thompson A, Jia J, Hou J, Lesmana CRA, Susilo A, Tanaka Y, Chan W-K, Gane E, Ong-Go AK, Lim S-G, Ahn SH, Yu M-L, Piratvisuth T, Chan HL-Y (2020) Management of patients with liver derangement during the COVID-19 pandemic: an Asia-Pacific position statement. The Lancet Gastroenterology & Hepatology 5(8):776–787. https://doi.org/10.1016/S2468-1253(20)30190-4
66. Ganne-Carrié N, Fontaine H, Dumortier J, Boursier J, Bureau C, Leroy V, Bourlière M, Afef FAftSotL (2020) Suggestions for the care of patients with liver disease during the Coronavirus 2019 pandemic. Clin Res Hepatol Gastroenterol 44(3):275–281. https://doi.org/10.1016/j.clinre.2020.04.001
67. Dorrell RD, Dougherty MK, Barash EL, Lichtig AE, Clayton SB, Jensen ET (2020) Gastrointestinal and hepatic manifestations of COVID-19: a systematic review and meta-analysis. JGH Open 5(1):107–115. https://doi.org/10.1002/jgh3.12456
68. Abdelzaher H, Saleh BM, Ismail HA, Hafiz M, Gabal MA, Mahmoud M, Hashish S, Gawad RMA, Gharieb RY, Abdelnaser A (2020) COVID-19 genetic and environmental risk factors: a look at the evidence. Front Pharmacol 11: 579415–579415. https://doi.org/10.3389/fphar.2020.579415
69. Mao R, Qiu Y, He J-S, Tan J-Y, Li X-H, Liang J, Shen J, Zhu L-R, Chen Y, Iacucci M, Ng SC, Ghosh S, Chen M-H (2020) Manifestations and prognosis of gastrointestinal and liver involvement in patients with COVID-19: a systematic review and meta-analysis. The Lancet Gastroenterology & Hepatology 5(7):667–678. https://doi.org/10.1016/S2468-1253(20)30126-6
70. Zimmermann P, Curtis N (2020) Why is COVID-19 less severe in children? A review of the proposed mechanisms underlying the age-related difference in severity of SARS-CoV-2 infections. Arch Dis Child 106(5):429–439. https://doi.org/10.1136/archdischild-2020-320338
71. Zhou Z, Zhao N, Shu Y, Han S, Chen B, Shu X (2020) Effect of gastrointestinal symptoms in patients with COVID-19. Gastroenterology 158(8):2294–2297. https://doi.org/10.1053/j.gastro.2020.03.020
72. Agrawal H, Das N, Nathani S, Saha S, Saini S, Kakar SS, Roy P (2020) An assessment on impact of COVID-19 infection in a gender specific manner. Stem Cell Rev Rep 17(1):94–112. https://doi.org/10.1007/s12015-020-10048-z

73. Hajifathalian K, Krisko T, Mehta A, Kumar S, Schwartz R, Fortune B, Sharaiha RZ, group* W-Gr (2020) Gastrointestinal and hepatic manifestations of 2019 novel coronavirus disease in a large cohort of infected patients from New York: clinical implications. Gastroenterology 159(3):1137–1140.e1132. https://doi.org/10.1053/j.gastro.2020.05.010
74. Chen R, Yu Y-L, Li W, Liu Y, Lu J-X, Chen F, Zhou Q, Xia Z-Y, Gao L, Meng Q-T, Ma D (2020) Gastrointestinal symptoms associated with unfavorable prognosis of COVID-19 patients: a retrospective study. Front Med (Lausanne) 7:608259–608259. https://doi.org/10.3389/fmed.2020.608259
75. Zingone F, D'Odorico A, Lorenzon G, Marsilio I, Farinati F, Savarino EV (2020) Risk of COVID-19 in celiac disease patients. Autoimmun Rev 19(10):102639–102639. https://doi.org/10.1016/j.autrev.2020.102639
76. Iavarone M, D'Ambrosio R, Soria A, Triolo M, Pugliese N, Del Poggio P, Perricone G, Massironi S, Spinetti A, Buscarini E, Viganò M, Carriero C, Fagiuoli S, Aghemo A, Belli LS, Lucà M, Pedaci M, Rimondi A, Rumi MG, Invernizzi P, Bonfanti P, Lampertico P (2020) High rates of 30-day mortality in patients with cirrhosis and COVID-19. J Hepatol 73(5):1063–1071. https://doi.org/10.1016/j.jhep.2020.06.001
77. Ji D, Qin E, Xu J, Zhang D, Cheng G, Wang Y, Lau G (2020) Non-alcoholic fatty liver diseases in patients with COVID-19: a retrospective study. J Hepatol 73(2):451–453. https://doi.org/10.1016/j.jhep.2020.03.044
78. Liu J, Wang T, Cai Q, Sun L, Huang D, Zhou G, He Q, Wang F-S, Liu L, Chen J (2020) Longitudinal changes of liver function and hepatitis B reactivation in COVID-19 patients with pre-existing chronic hepatitis B virus infection. Hepatol Res 50(11):1211–1221. https://doi.org/10.1111/hepr.13553
79. Singh S, Khan A (2020) Clinical characteristics and outcomes of coronavirus disease 2019 among patients with preexisting liver disease in the United States: a multicenter research network study. Gastroenterology 159(2):768–771.e3. https://doi.org/10.1053/j.gastro.2020.04.064
80. Hashimoto T, Perlot T, Rehman A, Trichereau J, Ishiguro H, Paolino M, Sigl V, Hanada T, Hanada R, Lipinski S, Wild B, Camargo SMR, Singer D, Richter A, Kuba K, Fukamizu A, Schreiber S, Clevers H, Verrey F, Rosenstiel P, Penninger JM (2012) ACE2 links amino acid malnutrition to microbial ecology and intestinal inflammation. Nature 487(7408):477–481. https://doi.org/10.1038/nature11228
81. Kaur H, Shekhar N, Sharma S, Sarma P, Prakash A, Medhi B (2021) Ivermectin as a potential drug for treatment of COVID-19: an in-sync review with clinical and computational attributes. Pharmacol Rep 73(3):1–14. https://doi.org/10.1007/s43440-020-00195-y
82. Fox LM, Saravolatz LD (2005) Nitazoxanide: a new thiazolide antiparasitic agent. Clin Infect Dis 40(8):1173–1180. https://doi.org/10.1086/428839
83. Aygün İ, Kaya M, Alhajj R (2020) Identifying side effects of commonly used drugs in the treatment of Covid 19. Sci Rep 10(1):21508. https://doi.org/10.1038/s41598-020-78697-1
84. Du Y-X, Chen X-P (2020) Favipiravir: pharmacokinetics and concerns about clinical trials for 2019-nCoV infection. Clinical Pharmacology & Therapeutics 108(2):242–247 https://doi.org/10.1002/cpt.1844
85. Okuno H, Takasu M, Kano H, Seki T, Shiozaki Y, Inoue K (1993) Depression of drug-metabolizing activity in the human liver by interferon-β. Hepatology (Baltimore, Md) 17(1):65–69 https://doi.org/10.1002/hep.1840170113
86. Horby PW, Mafham M, Bell JL, Linsell L, Staplin N, Emberson J, Palfreeman A, Raw J, Elmahi E, Prudon B, Green C, Carley S, Chadwick D, Davies M, Wise MP, Baillie JK, Chappell LC, Faust SN, Jaki T, Jefferey K, Lim WS, Montgomery A, Rowan K, Juszczak E, Haynes R, Landray MJ (2020) Lopinavir–ritonavir in patients admitted to hospital with COVID-19 (RECOVERY): a randomised, controlled, open-label, platform trial. Lancet 396(10259):1345–1352. https://doi.org/10.1016/S0140-6736(20)32013-4
87. Wang M, Cao R, Zhang L, Yang X, Liu J, Xu M, Shi Z, Hu Z, Zhong W, Xiao G (2020) Remdesivir and chloroquine effectively inhibit the recently emerged novel coronavirus (2019-nCoV) in vitro. Cell Res 30(3):269–271. https://doi.org/10.1038/s41422-020-0282-0
88. Tong S, Su Y, Yu Y, Wu C, Chen J, Wang S, Jiang J (2020) Ribavirin therapy for severe COVID-19: a retrospective cohort study. Int J Antimicrob Agents 56(3):106114–106114. https://doi.org/10.1016/j.ijantimicag.2020.106114
89. Khan NA (2020) Anakinra for severe forms of COVID-19. The Lancet Rheumatology 2(10):e586–e587. https://doi.org/10.1016/S2665-9913(20)30273-3
90. Richardson P, Griffin I, Tucker C, Smith D, Oechsle O, Phelan A, Rawling M, Savory E, Stebbing J (2020) Baricitinib as potential treatment for 2019-nCoV acute respiratory disease. Lancet 395(10223):e30–e31. https://doi.org/10.1016/S0140-6736(20)30304-4
91. La Rosée F, La Rosée P (2020) Ruxolitinib in COVID-19 hyperinflammation and haematologic malignancies. Acta Haematol 144(3):246–249. https://doi.org/10.1159/000510770
92. Khiali S, Rezagholizadeh A, Entezari-Maleki T (2020) A comprehensive review on sarilumab in COVID-19. Expert Opin Biol Ther 21(5):1–12. https://doi.org/10.1080/14712598.2021.1847269
93. Chen L-F, Mo Y-Q, Jing J, Ma J-D, Zheng D-H, Dai L (2017) Short-course tocilizumab increases risk of hepatitis B virus reactivation in patients with rheumatoid arthritis: a prospective clinical observation. Int J Rheum Dis 20(7):859–869 https://doi.org/10.1111/1756-185X.13010

8

Study of hepatitis B virus infection, reactivation among patients with chronic hepatitis C infection treated by direct antiviral agents (DAAs)

Haitham A. Azeem[1*], Ashraf M. Alkabeer[2], Ali Sobhy Mohammed[3] and Amira Ahmed Hussein[4]

Abstract

Background: Hepatitis B virus (HBV) may reactivate when treating chronic hepatitis C (CHC) with direct-acting antivirals (DAA). We aimed to investigate the risk of HBV infection and reactivation during DAA therapy by performing a prospective observational study carried on 200 patients positive for chronic HCV who were candidates for treatment by DAA therapy according to the Egyptian guidelines from February 2019 to December 2019; the patients identified to carry HBsAg at baseline or with positive HBc Abs were further assessed for other HBV markers: hepatitis B e antigen at baseline, and serum HBV DNA quantitative measurement at baseline, week 4 of treatment, end of treatment. On the other hand, recent infection by HBV among those patients was observed.

Results: Of all participants, 49% were males and 51% were females, aged above 18 years. There is a highly statistically significant difference (p-value < 0.05) between HCV RNA PCR (at the beginning, at the end of 4 weeks, and at the end of 12 weeks) in studied patients. There was a highly statistically significant difference found between the liver function tests at the beginning, at the end of 4 weeks, and at the end of 12 weeks of treatment where it shows improvement except for serum albumin. At beginning of the study, there were 34 patients who are co-infected with HCV and HBV with quantitative PCR test for HBV DNA ≥ 20 IU/ml. After 1 month of DAA therapy, reactivation was detected in 6 cases (4 occult cases show reverse seroconversion (became HBs Ag positive), and 2 co-infected cases show increased HBV DNA > 1000 IU/L above the baseline level). In addition, 3 new cases acquired recent infection with the positivity of HBc IgM and detectable levels of HBV DNA. After 3 months of study, reactivation was detected in one patient with co-infection (where increased HBV DNA > 1000 IU/L above the baseline level), and 5 new cases acquired recent infection late in the study.

Conclusion: Screening for HBV infection prior to DAA therapy is required to detect recent infection of reactivation of previous infection during or after DAA therapy.

Keywords: HBV reactivation, DAA therapy, Chronic HCV infection

* Correspondence: Haithamaly.44@Azhar.edu.eg
[1]Department of Internal Medicine, Assiut College of Medicine, Al-Azhar University, Assiut, Egypt
Full list of author information is available at the end of the article

Background

Hepatitis C virus (HCV) infection is the leading cause of cirrhosis, hepatic decompensation, hepatocellular carcinoma, and liver transplantation [1–3]. Globally, due to the shared modes of transmission, co-infection with both hepatitis B virus (HBV) and hepatitis C virus (HCV) is not uncommon. This is especially so in high-risk populations such as intravenous drug abusers, patients on hemodialysis, patients who have received an organ transplant, human immunodeficiency virus-positive patients, and b-thalassemia patients [4]. Hepatitis B is a potentially life-threatening liver infection caused by the hepatitis B virus (HBV). It is a major global health problem and can cause chronic infection and puts people at high risk of death from cirrhosis and liver cancer [5–7]. The landscape of HCV management was dramatically changed by the recent advent of direct-acting antivirals (DAAs) for chronic hepatitis C virus (HCV) infection, where DAA regimens are associated with a sustained virological response (SVR) rate of > 90–95% and are considered safe; nevertheless, a few complications have been reported including reactivation of hepatitis B virus (HBV) [8–10]. Recommendations have been made by the American Association for the Study of Liver Diseases (AASLD)/Infectious Diseases Society of America (IDSA) and European Association for the Study of the Liver (EASL) to screen all CHC patients before DAA therapy for hepatitis B surface antigen (HBsAg), hepatitis B surface antibody, and hepatitis B core antibody. However, whether serum or plasma HBV DNA measurement is necessary [4]. So, we assessed the potential risk of hepatitis B virus (HBV) reactivation in patients receiving direct-acting antiviral agent (DAA)-based therapy for patients with chronic HCV.

Methods

Study design

This prospective observational study was carried on 200 patients positive for chronic HCV (positive antibody to HCV and positive HCV RNA), from February 2019 to December 2019, who were candidates for treatment by DAA therapy according to the Egyptian guidelines and systematically assessed for their eligibility for DAA therapy through a standardized clinical and virological assessment, including complete blood count, liver profile included, alanine aminotransferase (ALT), aspartate aminotransferase (AST), bilirubin, albumin, creatinine, prothrombin time, (MINI VIDAS®, Biomerieux, France), HBsAg, and HBc antibodies (Stat Fax 4200, Dia Sorin, USA), done for all patients, and abdominal ultrasonography (US) in addition to hepatic transient elastography by fibroscan for all participants. Some patients underwent liver biopsy. Patients with the following characteristics were ineligible for DAAs according to the national guidelines: Child-Pugh class C cirrhosis, hepatocellular carcinoma (HCC) or liver metastases, platelet counts < 50 10^9 cells/L, current pregnancy, or breast-feeding. Also, patients under immunosuppressive drugs or with hepatorenal syndrome were excluded. Written consent was obtained from all participants; the patients identified to carry HBsAg at baseline or with positive HBc Abs were further assessed for other HBV markers: hepatitis B e antigen (HBeAg, Stat Fax 4200, Dia Sorin, USA) at baseline and serum HBV DNA quantitative measurement (DT Lite Real Time PCR, DNA-Technology, Russia, limit of detection: 25 IU/ml) at baseline, week 4 of treatment, end of treatment, and 12 weeks post-treatment. All patients received HCV antiviral therapy according to the Egyptian guidelines. SVR was assessed at 12 weeks after the end of treatment using HCV RNA. *The following definitions were considered:*

➢ Chronic hepatitis B (CHB) according to [11]

- HBsAg present for ≥ 6 months.
- Serum HBV DNA varies from undetectable to several billion IU/ml.
- Subdivided into HBeAg positive and negative. HBV DNA levels are typically > 20,000 IU/mL in HBeAg-positive CHB, and lower values (2000–20,000 IU/mL) are often seen in HBeAg-negative CHB.
- Normal or elevated ALT and/or AST levels.
- Liver biopsy results showing chronic hepatitis with variable necroinflammation and/or fibrosis.

➢ *Virological response* to HCV antiviral therapy defined by undetectable HCV-RNA during treatment and sustained virological response (SVR) at week 12 of post-treatment follow-up.

➢ *HBV reactivation according to AASLD-IDSA* recommendations [11]; loss of HBV immune control in HBsAg-positive, anti-HBc-positive, HBsAg-negative, or anti-HBc-positive patients receiving immunosuppressive therapy for a concomitant medical condition; a rise in HBV DNA compared to baseline (or an absolute level of HBV DNA when a baseline is unavailable); and reverse seroconversion (seroreversion) from HBsAg-negative to HBsAg-positive for HBsAg-negative, anti-HBc-positive patients.

Statistical analysis

Data were verified, coded by the researcher, and analyzed using IBM-SPSS 21.0 (IBM-SPSS Inc., Chicago, IL, USA). Descriptive statistics such as means, standard deviations, medians, and ranges were calculated. Test of significances: chi-square test was calculated to compare the frequencies among the groups. For continuous variables, independent t-test analysis was carried out to compare the means of normally distributed data.

Table 1 Comparison between HCV RNA PCR results in the studied patients

N = 200		At the start of treatment		After 1 month of treatment		At the end of treatment		P-value
HCV RNA PCR	**Negative**	0	0%	190	95%	196	98%	**P1 < 0.001 HS**
	Positive	200	100%	10	5%	4	2%	**P2 = 0.04 S** **P3 < 0.001 HS**

X^2: chi-square test
S: *p*-value < 0.05 is considered significant
HS: *p*-value < 0.001 is considered highly significant
P1: refers to the statistical difference between the start of DAA and 1 month after DAA
P2: refers to the statistical difference between the start of DAA and at the end of DAA
P3: refers to the statistical difference between 1 month after DAA and at the end of DAA

➢ Probability (*P*-value)
- *P*-value < 0.05 was considered significant.
- *P*-value < 0.001 was considered highly significant.
- *P*-value > 0.05 was considered insignificant.
- P1 refers to the statistical difference between the start of DAA and 1 month after DAA.
- P2 refers to the statistical difference between the start of DAA and the end of DAA.
- P3 refers to the statistical difference between 1 month after DAA and the end of DAA.

Results

In the current study, 200 patients were enrolled, 15% of them were aged < 40 years, 29.5% aged from 40 to 50 years, and 55.5% aged > 50 years. Of all participants, 49% were males and 51% were females. All patients were positive for HCV Abs and HCV RNA PCR quantitative test, and all were candidates for DAA therapy. There is a highly statistically significant difference (*p*-value < 0.05) between HCV RNA PCR (at the beginning, at the end of 4 weeks, and at the end of 12 weeks) in the studied patients (Table 1). There is no statistically significant difference (*p*-value > 0.05) between HBV DNA PCR quantitative test results (at the beginning, at the end of 4 weeks, and at the end of 12 weeks) (Table 2). The means of liver function prior to DAA therapy were ALT (60), AST (55.6), ALP (285.3), GGT (60), bilirubin (2.3), Alb (2.2), and, lasty, INR (1.2) (Table 4).

No statistically significant differences were found between liver ultrasound findings and fibroscan at the beginning, at the end of 4 weeks, and at the end of 12 weeks of treatment by DAAs (*p*-value > 0.05) (Table 3). A highly statistically significant difference was found between liver function tests at the beginning, at the end of 4 weeks, and at the end of 12 weeks of treatment (*p*-value < 0.001) (Table 4), where it shows improvements except for albumin; there was no statistically significant difference observed in the studied patients (Table 4). At beginning of the study, there were 34 patients who are co-infected with HCV and HBV with quantitative PCR test for HBV DNA ≥ 20 IU/ml, 30 patients with positive HBsAg, and 4 patients with positive HBc Ab (IgM). In addition to 5 cases with occult HBV infection with negative HBs Ag and positivity of anti-HBc IgG, 6 patients were immunized against HBV with positive anti-HBs Ab (Table 5). Fourteen patients were with HBV PCR < 2000 IU/ml with normal enzymes and not received antiviral therapy, and 20 patients were on antiviral drugs for HBV; their fibroscan range from f0 to f1 in 15 patients and from f1 to f2 in 5 patients. Abdominal ultrasound shows fatty liver in 17 patients and liver cirrhosis in 3 patients.

After 1 month of starting (DAAs), laboratory and serological investigations for all patients show that PCR for HCV RNA was still positive in 10 (5%) patients and became negative in all other patients. At the end of DAA therapy, only 4 (2%) patients were still positive for HCV PCR (Table 6).

Associated improvement in liver functions was observed (Table 4). Abdominal ultrasound throughout the study was normal in 115 patients, fatty infiltration in 57 patients, and cirrhotic changes in 28 patients (Table 4). Also, the fibroscan ranged between f3 and f4 in 32 patients, f1 and f2 in 55 patients, and f0 and f1 in 113 patients throughout the study without changes (Table 6).

As regards other hepatitis B virology markers, no statistically significant difference was found at the beginning, at the end of 4 weeks, and at the end of 12 weeks

Table 2 Comparison between HBV DNA PCR results in the studied patients

N = 200		At the start of treatment	After 1 month of treatment	At the end of treatment	P-value
HBV DNA PCR	**Negative**	166 (83%)	159 (79.5%)	154 (77%)	P1 = 0.253 NS
	Positive	34 (17%)	41 (20.5%)	46 (23%)	P2 = 0.064 NS P3 = 0.475 NS

X^2: chi-square test
S: *p*-value < 0.05 is considered significant
HS: *p*-value < 0.001 is considered highly significant
P1: refers to the statistical difference between the start of DAA and 1 month after DAA
P2: refers to the statistical difference between the start of DAA and the end of DAA
P3: refers to the statistical difference between 1 month after DAA and the end of DAA

Table 3 Comparison between liver function results in the studied patients

N = 200		At the start of treatment	After 1 month of treatment	At the end of treatment	*P*-value
ALT	**Mean**	60.5	51.3	37.2	**P1 = < 0.001 HS**
	± SD	12.3	11.8	7.9	**P2 = < 0.001 HS** **P3 = < 0.001 HS**
AST	**Mean**	55.6	42.3	35.7	**P1 = < 0.001 HS**
	± SD	13.2	12.7	10.2	**P2 = < 0.001 HS** **P3 = < 0.001 HS**
ALP	**Mean**	285.3	120.6	90.2	**P1 = < 0.001 HS**
	± SD	36.4	24.3	19.5	**P2 = < 0.001 HS** **P3 = < 0.001 HS**
GGT	**Mean**	60.7	55.2	25.8	**P1 = < 0.001 HS**
	± SD	17.8	15.5	13.2	**P2 = < 0.001 HS** **P3 = < 0.001 HS**
Total bilirubin	**Mean**	2.3	1.5	1.01	**P1 = < 0.001 HS**
	±SD	0.9	0.8	0.5	**P2 = < 0.001 HS** **P3 = < 0.001 HS**
Direct bilirubin	**Mean**	0.9	0.5	0.1	**P1 = < 0.001 HS**
	± SD	0.3	0.1	0.02	**P2 = < 0.001 HS** **P3 = < 0.001 HS**
Albumin	**Mean**	2.2	2.3	2.4	P1 = 0.151 NS
	± SD	0.9	0.4	1.2	P2 = 0.06 NS P3 = 264 NS
INR	**Mean**	1.2	1.09	1.1	**P1 = < 0.001 HS**
	± SD	0.2	0.3	0.2	**P2 = < 0.001 HS** **P3 = < 0.001 HS**

X^2: Chi-square test
S: *p*-value < 0.05 is considered significant
HS: *p*-value < 0.001 is considered highly significant
P1: refers to the statistical difference between the start of DAA and 1 month after DAA
P2: refers to the statistical difference between the start of DAA and the end of DAA
P3: refers to the statistical difference between 1 month after DAA and the end of DAA

of treatment by DAAs (*p*-value > 0.05), except for HBc Ab (IgM), where it increased with statistically significant difference between the studied patients (during and after treatment) (Table 5). As regards laboratory finding at the start of the study, there was a positivity of HBsAg in 34 cases co-infected with HBV (with positive HBs Ag and detectable HBV DNA > 20 IU/ml) in addition to 5 occult HBV (with negative HBs Ag and positivity of HBc IgG and detectable levels of HBV DNA) (Table 7).

After 1 month of DAA therapy, reactivation was detected in 6 cases (4 occult cases show reverse seroconversion (became HBs Ag positive), and 2 co-infected cases show increased HBV DNA > 1000 IU/L above the baseline level). In addition, 3 new cases acquired recent infection with the positivity of HBc IgM and detectable levels of HBV DNA (Table 7).

After 3 months of study, reactivation was detected in one patient with co-infection (where increased HBV DNA > 1000 IU/L above the baseline level), and 5 new cases acquired recent infection late in the study (Table 7).

Discussion

HCV is a worldwide infection affecting about 180 million persons with the highest prevalence in Egypt. ASAL D (2015) demonstrated that the American Association Study of Liver Disease suggests that all HCV patients

Table 4 Comparison between U/S results in the studied patients

N = 200	At the start of treatment	After 1 month of treatment	At the end of treatment	p-value
Abdominal ultrasounds				
Normal	**115 (57.5%)**	**115 (57.5%)**	**114 (57%)**	p1 = 1.0 NS
Fatty	**57 (28.5%)**	**57 (28.5%)**	**58 (29%)**	p2 = 0.993NS
Cirrhotic	**28 (14%)**	**28 (14%)**	**28 (14%)**	p3 = 0.993 NS

X^2: chi-square test
S: *p*-value < 0.05 is considered significant
HS: *p*-value < 0.001 is considered highly significant
P1: refers to the statistical difference between the start of DAA and 1 month after DAA
P2: refers to the statistical difference between the start of DAA and the end of DAA
P3: refers to the statistical difference between 1 month after DAA and the end of DAA

Table 5 Comparison between hepatitis virology markers in the studied patients

N = 200	At the start of treatment		After 1 month of treatment		At the end of treatment		*P*-value
HCV Ab							
Negative	0	0%	0	0%	0	0%	–
Positive	200	100%	200	100%	200	100%	
HBs Ag							
Negative	166	83%	159	79.5%	154	77%	P1 = 0.439 NS P2 = 0.064 NS P3 = 0.279 NS
Positive	34	17%	41	20.5%	46	23%	
HBs Ab							
Negative	194	97%	194	97%	194	97%	P1 = 1.0 NS P2 = 1.0 NS P3 = 1.0 NS
Positive	6	3%	6	3%	6	3%	
HBc Ab							
IgG							
Negative	165	82.5%	165	82.5%	164	82%	P1 = 0.585 NS P2 = 0.585 NS P3 = 1.0 NS
Positive	35	17.5%	35	17.5%	36	18%	
IgM							
Negative	196	98%	193	%	189	94.5%	P1 = 0.521 NS **P2 = 0.009 S** **P3 = 0.043 S**
Positive	4	2%	7	3%	11	5.5%	
HB e Ag							
Negative	194	97%	194	97%	193	96.5%	P1 = 0.759 NS P2 = 0.778 NS P3 = 0.557 NS
Positive	6	3%	6	3%	7	3.5%	
HB e Ab							
Negative	180	90%	178	89%	178	89%	P1 = 0.744 NS P2 = 0.744 NS P3 = 1.0 NS
Positive	20	10%	22	11%	22	11%	

X^2: chi-square test
S: *p*-value < 0.05 is considered significant
HS: *p*-value < 0.001 is considered highly significant
P1: refers to the statistical difference between the start of DAA and 1 month after DAA
P2: refers to the statistical difference between the start of DAA and the end of DAA
P3: refers to the statistical difference between 1 month after DAA and the end of DAA

who are about to initiate DAA therapy should be assessed for HBV co-infection by checking for the presence of HBsAg, anti-HBs, and anti-HBc. In addition, patients with positive HBsAg should be tested for HBV DNA viral load before the initiation of DAA therapy. The patients who meet the criteria for HBV treatment due to active HBV infection should initiate the HBV treatment before or during the HCV treatment. The patients with low or undetectable HBV DNA levels should be monitored at regular intervals (usually no more than once every 4 weeks) for HBV reactivation, and the patients with HBV DNA levels that meet treatment criteria should initiate HBV therapy. For those patients with positive anti-HBc or anti-HBs and anti-HBc, there are no sufficient recommendations; however, there is a risk of HBV reactivation in the case of elevated liver

Table 6 Comparison between fibroscan results in the studied patients

		At the start of treatment		1 month of treatment		At the end of treatment		*P*-value
Fibroscan	**F0–F1**	113	56.5%	113	56.5%	111	55.5%	P1 = 1.0 NS P2 = 0.973 NS P3 = 0.973 NS
	F1–F2	55	27.5%	55	27.5%	57	28.5%	
	F3–F4	32	16.5%	32	16.5%	32	16.5%	

X^2: chi-square test
S: *p*-value < 0.05 is considered significant
HS: *p*-value < 0.001 is considered highly significant
P1: refers to the statistical difference between the start of DAA and 1 month after DAA
P2: refers to the statistical difference between the start of DAA and the end of DAA
P3: refers to the statistical difference between 1 month after DAA and the end of DAA

Table 7 Comparison between HBV DNA PCR results in the studied patients

N = 15	At the start of treatment	1 month of treatment	At the end of treatment	*P*-value
HBV DNA PCR				
Negative	12 (80%)	5 (33.3%)	0 (0%)	**P1 = 0.009 HS**
Positive	3 (20%)	10 (66.7%)	15 (10%)	**P2 < 0.001 HS** **P3 = 0.014 S**

X^2: chi-square test
S: *p*-value < 0.05 is considered significant
HS: *p*-value < 0.001 is considered highly significant
P1: refers to the statistical difference between the start of DAA and 1 month after DAA
P2: refers to the statistical difference between the start of DAA and the end of DAA
P3: refers to the statistical difference between 1 month after DAA and the end of DAA

enzymes during or after DAA therapy. This prospective study was carried on 200 patients with chronic HCV infection who visited our outpatient clinic in Al-Azhar University Hospital and Aswan antiviral unit who started DAA-based therapy, and the patients were evaluated for HBV reactivation during and after DAA therapy; 34 of them had chronic HBV.

In the current study, 15% of cases aged < 40 years, 29.5% aged between 40 and 50 years, and 55.5% aged > 50 years, and 49% were males and 51% were females; this agreed with the Egyptian Demographic Health Survey (EDHS) that estimated the prevalence of HCV antibodies and HCV RNA in HCV patients, commonest among the 15–59 years age group [12, 13], which may be as a result of continuing exposure and increased risk of infection in this age group [14], and this was nearly in agreement with Kawagishi and Suda's study that included 191 patients with HCV infection who received IFN-free DAA therapies where the mean age was 69 years and 86% of cases were males; also, our documented age was agreed with Lin et al.'s study [15] where the mean age of studied cases was 59.9 years and males represented 58% of cases. In the current study, no statistically significant differences were found between ultrasonographic and fibroscan findings in the enrolled cases at the start of the study, 1 month after, and after treatment (*p*-value > 0.05), while in Lin et al.'s study [15], they used APRI score (this is an AST to Platelet Ratio Index) that was the main tool used to determine liver cirrhosis status. In a meta-analysis of 40 studies, investigators concluded that an APRI score > 1.0 had a sensitivity of 76% and a specificity of 72% for predicting cirrhosis. In addition, APRI score > 0.7 had a sensitivity of 77% and a specificity of 72% for predicting significant hepatic fibrosis [16]. Our findings were agreeing with Yeh et al.'s study [17], where they did not observe any HBV-related ALT flare (abrupt rise of ALT level to > 5 times the upper limit of normal during chronic (HBV) infection or hepatic decompensation, but were antagonistic as regards to ALT, where there was no ALT elevation before or at the peak of HBV DNA levels in HBsAg-positive patients with HBV reactivation, indicating that on-treatment ALT monitoring may not be sensitive enough to detect HBV reactivation) [17]. Most patients in Belperio et al.'s study [18] appeared to have "silent" or "mild" HBV reactivation characterized by normal ALT or less than a 2-fold change in ALT. The occurrence of HBV reactivation without hepatitis in the setting of DAA treatment has also been observed as the most common presentation by others. The observed incidence of HBV reactivation among HBsAg-positive patients of 8.3% (7/84) and the incidence of HBV reactivation with evidence of biochemical hepatitis of 2.4% (2/84) warrant use of HBV prophylaxis in this setting. Notably, there was an apparent lack of association with baseline HBV DNA levels as 3 of the 8 with reactivation had undetectable pre-DAA HBV DNA levels. HBV reactivation was detected in 6 patients (12.8%) during treatment and reach to 7 patients (17.9%) after treatment, and this was higher than Belperio et al.'s study [18]; 62,290 patients infected with HCV were retrospectively assessed having completed oral DAA treatment. Among the 377 patients (0.6%) who were known to be HBsAg-positive prior to DAA initiation, 96 (25.5%) were on HBV treatment at the start of DAA therapy. HBV reactivation was defined by a > 1000 IU/mL increase in HBV DNA occurring while on DAA treatment. Eight of the cases occurred in patients known to be HBsAg positive, and 1 case occurred in a patient known only to be isolated anti-HBc-positive whereas HBV reactivation occurred in HCV infected patients with and without detectable HBV DNA prior to DAA initiation. HBV reactivation did not appear to be impacted by baseline HCV RNA level, presence of cirrhosis, or HCV DAA regimen. The rate of reactivation of HBV infection in the current study is higher than the reported HBV reactivation rate of 1–2% per year in persons with inactive disease. Thus, providers should recognize that patients with isolated anti-HBc are at some risk, albeit less, and that identifying these patients prior to DAA treatment and assessing HBV DNA status can heighten recognition of reactivation [19]. Our study was in line with Cheng et al.'s study [20], which reported 327 patients receiving pan oral DAA agents for HCV infections in areas endemic for HBV in China. Ten patients were positive for hepatitis B surface antigen (HBsAg), and 124 patients had occult HBV infection. HBV reactivation was determined by measuring HBV DNA and HBsAg status in serial serum samples collected every 2 weeks during DAA treatment and then every 4 weeks after treatment until week 12. In the total study population, 10 patients (3.1%) had hepatitis; 3 cases were associated with HBV reactivation (1 case not in the icteric phase, 1 case in the icteric phase, and 1 case with liver failure) and 7 from other causes. Testing positive for HBsAg before DAA treatment was a strong risk factor for developing hepatitis during treatment (hazard ratio, 15.0; $P < .001$). The study had some limitations; were we are unable to identify some detailed information that might have had an effect on HBV reactivation such as HBsAg level, anti-HBs titer, and HBV genotype. In addition, the type of DAAs is not included in the study which may play a role in reactivation of previous HBV infection.

Conclusion

Screening for HBV infection prior to DAA therapy is required to detect recent infection and reactivation of previous infection during or after DAA therapy which may affect the outcome of DAA therapy.

Abbreviation

DAAs: Direct antiviral agents

Acknowledgements

None

Authors' contributions

HA is the corresponding author for the submission and revised the manuscript. AM was responsible for the analysis of the data. Laboratory investigations were performed by AS. AH was responsible for the data collection. All authors have read and approved the final manuscript.

Declarations

Ethics approval and consent to participate

The local ethical committee (Al-Azhar University Hospitals, Assiut) approved the study, but the reference number is not applicable, and a written consent for participation was taken from all patients.

Competing interests

The authors declare that they have no competing interests.

Author details

[1]Department of Internal Medicine, Assiut College of Medicine, Al-Azhar University, Assiut, Egypt. [2]Department of Internal Medicine, Assiut College of Medicine, Al-Azhar University, Assiut, Egypt. [3]Department of Clinical Pathology, Assiut College of Medicine, Al-Azhar University, Assiut, Egypt. [4]Department of Internal Medicine, Al-Sebaia Central Hospital, Aswan, Egypt.

References

1. Kao JH et al (2016) Hepatitis C virus infection in Taiwan: past, present, and future. J Formos Med Assoc 115(2):65–66. https://doi.org/10.1016/j.jfma.2015.06.012
2. Abo-Amer YE et al (2018) Declining prevalence of hepatitis C virus among university students in one of the main governorates in Egypt. Infect Drug Resist 11:2435–2441. https://doi.org/10.2147/IDR.S183462 eCollection 2018. PMID: 30538509
3. Abd-elsalam S et al (2019) Sofosbuvir, pegylated interferon and ribavirin in the treatment of an Egyptian cohort with hepatitis C virus infection in real-life clinical practice. Infect Disord Drug Targets 19(2):179–184. https://doi.org/10.2174/1871526518666180912121835 PMID: 30207250
4. Liu C-H, Liu C-J, Su T-H, Fang Y-J, Chen et al (2017) Hepatitis B virus reactivation in patients receiving interferon-free direct-acting antiviral agents for chronic hepatitis C virus infection. Infect Dis Soc Am. 2017;4(1): ofx028.
5. World Health Organization (2019) Progress report on HIV, viral hepatitis, and sexually transmitted infections 2019. Accountability for the global health sector strategies, 2016–2021. Geneva: World Health Organization; 2019 (WHO/CDS/HIV/19.7). License: CC BY-NC-SA 3.0 IGO.
6. Soliman H, Ziada D, Salama M, Hamisa M, Badawi R, Hawash N, Selim A, Abd-Elsalam S (2020) Predictors for fibrosis regression in chronic HCV patients after the treatment with DAAS: results of a real-world cohort study. Endocr Metab Immune Disord Drug Targets 20(1):104–111. https://doi.org/10.2174/1871530319666190826150344 PMID: 31448717
7. Hanafy AS, Soliman S, Abd-Elsalam S (2019) Rescue therapy for chronic hepatitis C virus infection after repeated treatment failures: impact on disease progression and risk of hepatocellular carcinoma. Hepatol Res 49(4): 377–384. https://doi.org/10.1111/hepr.13303 Epub 2019 Jan 28. PMID: 30570817
8. European Association for the Study of the Liver (2017) EASL Recommendations on treatment of hepatitis C 2016. J Hepatol 66(1):153–194. https://doi.org/10.1016/j.jhep.2016.09.001
9. Elfert A et al (2020) Treatment of hepatitis C cirrhotic patients with directly acting antivirals: a multicenter study. Infect Disord Drug Targets. https://doi.org/10.2174/1871526520666201019122205 Online ahead of print. PMID: 33076813
10. Abdel-Noor R, Watany M, Abd-Elsalam S, ElKhalawany W, Soliman S, Badawi R (2020) Is hepatitis B surface antigen (HB s Ag) enough alone as a screening test for HBV infection in rheumatic disease patients before starting immunosuppressive therapies? A cross-sectional study. Infect Disord Drug Targets 20(6):878–883. https://doi.org/10.2174/1871526519666191212094141 PMID: 31830889
11. AASLD-IDSA (2016) recommendations for testing, managing and treating adults infected with hepatitis C virus. Hepatology 62:932–954
12. Kandeel A, Genedy M, El-Refai S, Funk A, Fontanet A, Talaat M (2016) The prevalence of hepatitis C virus infection in Egypt 2015: implications for future policy on prevention and treatment. Liver Int 37(1):45–53
13. Mohamed AA, el-Toukhy NETR, Said EM, Gabal HMR, AbdelAziz H, Doss W, el-Hanafi H, el Deeb HH, Mahmoud S, Elkadeem M, Shalby HS, Abd-Elsalam S (2020) Hepatitis C virus: efficacy of new DAAs regimens. Infect Disord Drug Targets 20(2):143–149. https://doi.org/10.2174/1871526519666190121114003 PMID: 30663575
14. Matheï C, Buntinx F, Van Damme P (2001) Is the prevalence of hepatitis c virus (HCV) RNA in anti-HCV–positive injection drug users positively correlated with age? J Infect Dis 184(5):659–660. https://doi.org/10.1086/322795
15. Lin ZH, Xin YN, Dong QJ et al (2015) Evaluation of aspartate aminotransferase-to-platelet ratio index as a non-invasive marker for liver cirrhosis. Clin Diagn Res 9(11):OC22–OC24
16. Lin ZH, Xin YN, Dong QJ, Wang Q, Jiang XJ, Zhan SH, Sun Y, Xuan SY (2011) Performance of the aspartate aminotransferase-to-platelet ratio index for the staging of hepatitis C-related fibrosis: an updated meta-analysis. Hepatology 53(3):726–736. https://doi.org/10.1002/hep.24105

17. Yeh ML, Huang CF, Hsieh MH, Ko YM, Chen KY, Liu TW, Lin YH, Liang PC, Hsieh MY, Lin ZY, Chen SC, Huang CI, Huang JF, Kuo PL, Dai CY, Yu ML, Chuang WL (2017) Reactivation of hepatitis B in patients of chronic hepatitis C with hepatitis B virus infection treated with direct acting antivirals. J Gastroenterol Hepatol 32(10):1754–1762. https://doi.org/10.1111/jgh.13771
18. Belperio PS, Shahoumian TA, Mole LA, Backus LI (2017) Evaluation of hepatitis B reactivation among 62,920 veterans treated with oral hepatitis C antivirals. Hepatology 66:27–36
19. Terrault NA, Bzowej NH, Chang KM, Hwang JP, Jonas MM, Murad MH (2016) American Association for the Study of Liver Diseases. AASLD guidelines for treatment of chronic hepatitis B. Hepatology 63(1):261–283. https://doi.org/10.1002/hep.28156
20. Wang C, Ji D, Chen J, Shao Q, Li B, Clin JL (2016) Hepatitis due to reactivation of hepatitis B virus in endemic areas among patients with hepatitis C treated with direct-acting antiviral agents. Gastroenterol Hepatol 15(1):132–136

9

Egyptian protocol for living donor liver transplantation (LDLT) during SARS-CoV-2 pandemic

Hany Said Abd Elbaset[1], Ahmad Mohammad Sultan[2], Iman Fawzy Montasser[3], Hossam E. M. Soliman[4], Mohamed Elayashy[5], Nahed A. Makhlouf[6*] and Scientific Committee of Ministry of Health (MOH) National Project of Waiting Lists, Egypt

Abstract

Background: The current SARS-CoV-2 pandemic may negatively impact the care of liver transplant candidates and recipients.

Main body of the abstract: Accordingly, each country must have its national guidelines based on the current situation and according to available tools. Liver Transplantation Scientific Committee of Waiting List Project in Egypt was established in 13 April 2020. One of the major objectives of this Scientific Committee is the preparation of national protocol for Transplant Centers in Egypt to deal with living donor liver transplantation (LDLT) during SARS-CoV-2 pandemic.

Conclusions: The protocol highlights basic hospital requirements for LDLT during SARS-CoV-2 pandemic, the patient selection from the waiting list, management of patients on the waiting list, and post-transplant management.

Keywords: SARS-CoV-2, LDLT, Egyptian national protocol, Waiting list project

Background

COVID-19 is the disease caused by an emerging coronavirus named severe acute respiratory syndrome coronavirus-2 (SARS-CoV-2) that was initially detected in Wuhan City, Hubei Province of China in December 2019. This virus spread across China and then spread worldwide and finally has been declared a pandemic [1, 2].

SARS-CoV-2 infection is acquired from anyone who is shedding the virus. Person-to-person transmission was detected through close exposure (< 6 feet) to an infected person with COVID-19, mainly via respiratory droplets produced when the infected case coughs or sneezes. The transmission frequently occurred from symptomatic persons with COVID-19 through droplet spread. Less frequently infection acquired from asymptomatic person has occurred, and the transmission is presumed to be possible from close contact with contaminated objects [1].

Older patients and those with pre-existing medical health problems are at risk of having severe course of disease. It is unclear to what degree chronic liver diseases should be considered as risk factors, due to insufficient clinical studies [3]. However, patients with end-stage liver disease are at increased risk of infection due to cirrhosis-associated immune dysfunction [4].

Between 1990 and August 2013, 3804 liver transplants were performed in Arab Countries, with Living Donor Liver Transplantation (LDLT) represented 80%. A lot of Egyptian patients were suffering from end-stage liver disease (ESLD), and necessitating liver transplantation (LT). More than 50% of transplanted cases in Arab

* Correspondence: nahedmak@yahoo.com; nahed.mak@aun.edu.eg
Hany Said Abd Elbaset is the Head of the Scientific Committee.
[6]Tropical Medicine and Gastroenterology, Medical Team of Liver Transplantation at Al-Rajhi Liver Hospital, Faculty of Medicine, Assiut University, Assiut, Egypt
Full list of author information is available at the end of the article

countries were reported from Egypt. The regulations for LDLT were made by the Egyptian medical syndicate [5], whereas deceased donor (cadaveric) liver transplant (DDLT) has not yet been authorized. Between July 2018 and January 2020, 380 LDLT operations were performed in Egypt [Data were obtained from Ministry of Health (MOH)] registery database for National Project of Waiting Lists, Egypt).

Information on transplant recipients with COVID-19 are still few and based on published case reports or case series but accumulating experience is going on. However, based on previous data from other viruses including SARS, serious infection in the immunocompromised persons such as organ transplant recipients has happened. Mild affection has also been observed. The risk factors for severe infection have not been completely known. The American Society of Transplantation anticipated a greater viral load and shedding in transplant recipients that could result in more infectivity and spread to other persons [1]. The current pandemic requires unusual allocation of healthcare resources which may negatively impact the care of patients with chronic liver disease [3].

Main text

Rational

Each country with limited resources must have its national guidelines for LDLT during SARS-CoV-2 pandemic based on the current situation and according to the local resources and available tools.

Aims of this protocol

1- Basic hospital requirements for LDLT during SARS-CoV-2 pandemic.
2 Patient selection from the waiting list.
3 Management of patients on the waiting list for LDLT.
4 Post-transplant management.

Hospital requirements for LDLT during SARS-CoV-2 pandemic

Basic hospital staff, facilities, and equipment required to restart LDLT program during the pandemic:

a) Presence of sufficient staff for initial evaluation of cases based on symptoms, background, and exposure history (e.g., fever, respiratory symptoms, loss of taste or smell, contact with proven case of SARS-CoV-2 infection) by using rapid questionnaire survey.
b) Nasopharyngeal swab for SARS-CoV-2 PCR laboratory facilities: Nasopharyngeal swab must be done for both recipient and donor 48 h before hospital admission and 24 h before the operation.
c) High-resolution CT chest for both recipient and donor on hospital admission.
d) Laboratory facilities and infection control team facilities for screening, early detection of suspected cases including hospital staff, potential donors, and recipients.
e) Provide safe pathway for both recipient and donor including operative rooms, ICU, ward, necessary equipment such as ventilators, ultrasound, and duplex equipment.

Medical staff precautions and protection:

a) Personal Protective Equipments (PPE) must be provided to all operative team, ICU staff, ward staff, radiology and laboratory staff i.e. (All medical persons and workers who are in contact with donor and recipient in perioperative care) (detailed infection prevention and control procedures during SARS-COV-2 pandemic, Additional file 1: Annex 1)
b) Any medical staff with a history of contact with confirmed cases of COVID-19 without wearing full PPE must be temporary excluded from the team for home isolation for 14 days +/− nasopharyngeal swab if needed (i.e., if any suggestive symptoms appear like fever, cough) [6].

Patient selection from the waiting list

Basic precautions needed for potential recipients for LDLT:

Recipients of LDLT and donor candidates must have home isolation and personal distancing for a minimum of 10 days, counting back from the planned date of transplantation. Reporting any fever or respiratory symptoms to the transplant team by phone [7].

Initial evaluation before admission:

Evaluation is based on symptoms, background, and exposure history (e.g., fever, respiratory symptoms, loss of taste or smell, contact with proven case of SARS-COV-2 infection) and by the latest updated rapid survey questionnaire provided and updated by MOH.

Nasopharyngeal swab for SARS-CoV-2 PCR:

Nasopharyngeal swab must be done for both recipient and donor 48 h before hospital admission and 24 h before the operation [3, 7].

High-resolution CT chest for both recipient and donor on hospital admission.

As negative nasopharyngeal swab results do not completely exclude SARS-CoV-2 infection [8], so CT chest is mandatory during the pandemic.

The transplant team must explain to potential recipients and their relatives the risk of SARS-CoV-2

infection aggravation under post-transplant immunosuppression [7].

Recipient selection, Table 1.

***High priority for liver transplantation** denotes mortality risk on the waiting list overweighs the risk of SARS-CoV-2 infection.

Moderate risk: Case by case discussion with Liver Transplantation Team, but the Scientific Committee of MOH national project of waiting lists does not recommend transplantation in the current situation.

Transplant candidate with a history of confirmed COVID-19 disease:

- Non-urgent transplantation should be avoided.
- If urgent transplantation is indicated:
- Nasopharyngeal/oropharyngeal PCR should be negative twice (at least 48 h apart).
- Complete resolution of clinical, laboratory, or radiological findings.
- Ideal disease-free interval is unknown but not less than 20 days from disease onset, and better to be more than 37 days [1, 9].

Recommendations for the donors (pre-operative test and management) [1, 3, 10]:

a) Only the donor with low risk is accepted.

No direct contact with a positive or suspected patient. No suspicious symptoms as follows:

- Fever (> 38 °C).
- Malaise or flu-like symptoms, +/− myalgias.
- New cough.
- Shortness of breath.
- Unexplained abdominal pain, nausea, and/or diarrhea.
- Loss of sense of taste and/or smell.

b) Recommendation for home isolation 14 days before hospital admission.
c) Complete blood count (CBC) shows no leucopenia and C-reactive protein (CRP) is negative
d) Radiological chest X-ray and high-resolution CT should be negative for any suspected lesion.
e) Nasopharyngeal/oropharyngeal PCR should be done twice in the week before transplantation with 48-72 h apart.
f) High-risk donors who have direct contact with positive or suspected patient with any suspicious symptom should be advised to postpone donation for 28 days after symptom resolution and have a negative PCR test.
g) Detailed informed SARS-CoV-2 infection risk consent should be taken from the donor [11]

Management of potential recipients on the waiting list for LDLT

a) All potential recipients on the waiting list should be regularly followed up either by phone contact or transplant clinic visits whenever needed.
b) Monthly update of Child-Pugh and MELD scores (weekly update if MELD> 25).
c) Abdominal ultrasound/duplex and alpha-fetoprotein every 3 months.
d) Triphasic CT portography if the results of ultrasound/duplex is suspicious.
e) Weekly arrangement of waiting list by liver transplant team in each center according to Child-Pugh, MELD score, HCC characteristics of potential recipients.
f) Mortality/dropout on the waiting list must be recorded including date, time on waiting list, and cause of death/dropout.

Table 1 Recipient selection for LDLT during SARS-CoV-2 pandemic

	High priority risk group*	Moderate risk group
Criteria	• Fulminant liver failure • MELD equal or greater than 20 • Child-Pugh class C (score 10). • Previous history of HRS. • Previous history SBP. • Benign (PVT) grade II. • HCC within Milan unfit for bridge (Child-Pugh late B or C). • HCC beyond Milan within UCSF with a good response of downstaging after 3 months.	• MELD 15—19 • HCC within Milan fit for bridge therapy.
Decision	Proceed for transplantation with precautions	Complete donor preparation, close follow up on the waiting list

MELD model for end stage liver disease; *HRS* hepato-renal syndrome; *SBP* spontaneous bacterial peritonitis; *PVT* portal vein thrombosis; *HCC* hepatocellular carcinoma; *UCSF* University of California San Francisco;* high priority for liver transplantation denotes mortality risk on the waiting list overweighs the risk of SARS-CoV-2 infection

g) We recommend that specialized centers for liver transplantation provide easily accessible contact information to facilitate immediate hepatology consultations to the local health care providers if needed.
h) Include nasopharyngeal swab PCR testing for COVID-19 disease for patients with acute on chronic liver failure [3].
i) Counseling of liver transplant candidates for vaccination against *Streptococcus pneumoniae* and influenza [3].
j) Detailed informed Covid-19 disease risk consent for recipient before the operation [11]

Post-transplant management

Immunosuppressant protocol:

Maintain the usual protocol of immunosuppressants which is based on calcineurin inhibitors (CNIs), mycophenolate mofetil (MMF) and steroid, and at the usually recommended target levels.

For a recipient with proven post-transplant Covid-19 disease:

a) Data from different liver transplant centers are scarce and there is no consensus on how to deal with immunosuppressant drugs in such situation. So far there have been no specific recommendations in terms of course or management of liver transplanted patients from major Societies. Some reports suggest decreasing immunosuppression for infected recipients, if no recent rejection episodes. Paradoxically, others suggest that a reactive immune response might be the cause for severe tissue damage and that immunosuppression might be protective from the postulated cytokine storm [12, 13].
b) The national recommendations include reduction/hold of CNI dose, according to disease severity and radiological finding in CT chest. This must be done as case by case discussion in a multidisciplinary team with a senior chest consultant, transplant hepatology consultant, and ICU consultant in severe cases.
c) **MMF/Azathioprine (AZA)** hold should be discussed on a case by case basis. It is essential to consider reducing azathioprine or mycophenolate dosages, especially in the setting of lymphopenia, fever, or worsening pneumonia attributed to COVID-19 [14].
d) Patients who develop adult respiratory distress syndrome (ARDS), use steroid dose as recommended by Covid protocol prepared by MOH [15]. Methylprednisolone 1 mg/kg/day for 3-5 days then oral steroids in tapering dose over 4-6 weeks.
e) Drug-drug interactions with immunosuppressant medications need to be evaluated and managed [15].
f) We recommend regular telephone communication between the liver transplant team (or Central Transplant Committee) and health care physicians caring for liver transplant recipient with proven COVID-19 positive at isolation hospital.

Post-transplant clinic and follow up visits:

a) For recipients who transplanted more than 3 months, the follow-up can be made through telemedicine with the transplant team according to scheduled visits as usual or exceptional telemedicine if any new developed symptoms or whenever needed. Hospital visit and/or admission whenever needed according to clinical judgment by the transplant physician in charge with the case [12, 16]. All recipients discharged from the hospital with educational booklet information that includes the alarm symptoms (e.g., fever, cough, vomiting, or diarrhea) and contact details for the transplant team members.
b) Early postoperative period: less than 3 months from the operation, regular post-operative follow-up visits as per center protocol. Limit the number of patients who visit the transplant clinic, and limit the number of family members/friends who accompany patients in their visits. Special precautions on hand hygiene, wearing face mask throughout the visit, well-aerated rooms for waiting, keep distance 2 m between patients at waiting area, and decontamination of the waiting area should be practiced, etc. [12].
c) Transplant recipients should be educated about the importance of performing frequent hand hygiene, cleaning frequently touched surfaces, avoidance of crowded public places, and applying social distancing, staying away from individuals who are ill [17].

Vaccination:

The usual vaccination of liver transplant recipients against *Streptococcus pneumoniae* and influenza is strongly recommended [3].

Travel restriction for transplant recipients:

It is essential to postpone all non-essential travel for transplant recipients. We also recommend that transplant patients' immediate household contacts should not travel to high-risk areas [1]. Recipients transplanted from rural areas are instructed to stay nearby to their transplant centers at least for the first 3 months.

Conclusion

The preparation of a national protocol for Transplant Centers in Egypt to deal with LDLT during SARS-CoV-2 pandemic is essential. This protocol highlighted basic hospital requirements, the patient selection from the waiting list, management of patients on the waiting list, and post-transplant management during SARS-CoV-2 pandemic. Regular and frequent updates are essentially needed according to any emerging data.

Abbreviations

LDLT: Living donor liver transplantation; SARS-CoV-2: Severe acute respiratory syndrome coronavirus-2; COVID-19: Coronavirus disease 2019; ESLD: End-stage liver disease; DDLT: Deceased donor (cadaveric) liver transplant; PPE: Personal protective equipments; MOH: Ministry of health; MELD: Model for end-stage liver disease; HRS: Hepato-renal syndrome; SBP: Spontaneous bacterial peritonitis; PVT: Portal vein thrombosis; HCC: Hepatocellular carcinoma; UCSF: University of California San Francisco; CNIs: Calcineurin inhibitors; MMF: Mycophenolate Mofetil; AZA: Azathioprine; ARDS: Adult respiratory distress syndrome

Acknowledgements

The authors would like to thank all members of the national project of management of patients on waiting lists, MOH, Egypt.

Authors' contributions

H S A and A M S were responsible for the concept, the plan of the work, and final revision. I F M shared in the literature review, design, writing of the manuscript, and initial revision. H E M S and M E shared in writing Additional file 1: Annex 1 and final revision, NA M shared in the literature review, writing of the manuscript, and she is the corresponding author. All Authors have read and approved the final manuscript.

Ethics approval and consent to participate

Not applicable.

Competing interests

The authors declare that they have no competing interests.

Author details

[1]HPB Surgery and Liver Transplantation, Ain Shams University, Cairo, Egypt. [2]GI Surgery, Liver Transplantation Unit, Gastrointestinal Surgical Center, Mansoura University, Mansoura, Egypt. [3]Tropical Medicine and Gastroenterology, Ain Shams University, Cairo, Egypt. [4]Professor of HPB Surgery and Liver Transplantation, National Liver Institute, Menoufia University, Menuofia, Egypt. [5]Anesthesia, Intensive Care and Pain Management, Cairo University, Cairo, Egypt. [6]Tropical Medicine and Gastroenterology, Medical Team of Liver Transplantation at Al-Rajhi Liver Hospital, Faculty of Medicine, Assiut University, Assiut, Egypt.

References

1. American Society of Transplantation (2020) 2019-nCoV (coronavirus): FAQs for organ donation and transplantation https://www.myast.org/sites/default/files/COVID19%20FAQ%20Tx%20Centers%2003.20.2020-FINAL.pdf
2. Wang C, Horby Peter W, Hayden Frederick G, Gao George F (2020) A novel coronavirus outbreak of global health concern. Lancet. 395(10223):470–473
3. Boettler T, Newsome PN, Mondelli MU, Maticic M, Cordero E, Cornberg M, Berg T (2020) Care of patients with liver disease during the COVID-19 pandemic: EASL-ESCMID position paper. JHEP Reports 2(3):100113. https://doi.org/10.1016/j.jhepr.2020.100113
4. Albillos A, Lario M, Álvarez-Mon M (2014) Cirrhosis-associated immune dysfunction: distinctive features and clinical relevance. J Hepatol 61: 1385–1396
5. Amer, Marwan (2016) Living donor liver transplantation in Egypt. Hepato Biliary Surg Nutr 5(2):98–106
6. Egyptian Ministry of Health and Population (2020) Coronavirus disease 2019 (COVID-19) SARS COV2. Management Guide.Vesion 1. Egypt, pp 1–24
7. Japan Society of Transplantation (2020) Basic guidelines in transplantation medicine for new coronavirus infection (COVID-19), 2nd edn
8. Winichakoon P, Chaiwarith R, Liwsrisakun C et al (2020) Negative nasopharyngeal and oropharyngeal swab does not rule out COVID-19. J Clin Microbiol 58:e00297–e00220
9. Zhou F, Yu T, Du R, Fan G, Liu Y, Liu Z et al (2020) Clinical course and risk factors for mortality of adult inpatients with COVID-19 in Wuhan, China: a retrospective cohort study. Lancet 395:1054–1062
10. Fix OK, Hameed B, Fontana RJ, Kwok RM, McGuire BM, Mulligan DC et al (2020) Clinical best practice advice for hepatology and liver transplant providers during the COVID-19 pandemic: AASLD expert panel consensus statement. Hepatology 72(1):287First published: 16 April 2020. https://doi.org/10.1002/hep.31281
11. American Society of Transplantation (2020) COVID-19 organ donation and transplantation town hall (donor issues and candidate concerns): American Society of Transplantation Available from: https://www.youtube.com/watch?reload=9&v=0xaFpTba0T8&t=accessed April 13, 2020
12. AASLD. American Association for the Study of Liver Diseases (2020) Clinical insights for hepatology and liver transplant providers during the COVID-19 pandemic. Released: April 7
13. D'Antiga L (2020) Coronaviruses and immunosuppressed patients. The facts during the third epidemic. Liver Transp 26(6):832–834
14. Zhu L, Xu X, Ma K, Yang J, Guan H, Chen S et al (2020) Successful recovery of COVID-19 pneumonia in a renal transplant recipient with long-term immunosuppression. Am J Transplant 20(3) 1859–1963
15. Egyptian Ministry of Health and Population (2020) Management guidelines for COVID-19. Patients with special medical conditions. Egypt, April
16. Terry K (2020) Telehealth seen as a key tool to fight COVID-19. The hospitalist https://www.thehospitalist.org/hospitalist/article/218574/coronavirus-updates/telehealth-seen-key-tool-help-fight-covid-19
17. Center for Disease Control and Prevention (CDC) (2019) Coronavirus disease 2019 (COVID-19). Cleaning and disinfection for community facilities https://www.cdc.gov/coronavirus/2019ncov/community/organizations/cleaning-disinfection.html

10

Performance of albumin-bilirubin score in prediction of hepatic encephalopathy in cirrhotic patients with acute variceal bleeding

Rehab Elsayed Elsafty, Abdallah Ahmed Elsawy*, Ahmed Fawzy Selim and Atef Mohamed Taha

Abstract

Background: Hepatic encephalopathy exacerbates the morbidity, delays hospital discharge, and increases the rate of readmissions of cirrhotic patients, particularly those are admitted by acute variceal bleeding. We evaluated the performance of albumin-bilirubin score in prediction of hepatic encephalopathy in cirrhotic patients with acute variceal bleeding, in comparison to Child-Pugh and MELD scores. This prospective cohort study was conducted on 250 cirrhotic patients who were consecutively presented by acute variceal bleeding in the period from January to December 2020 at Tanta university emergency hospital. Albumin-bilirubin, Child-Pugh, and MELD scores were measured at admission, and then all patients were followed up for 4 weeks after endoscopic bleeding control for possible occurrence of hepatic encephalopathy

Results: Albumin-bilirubin, Child-Pugh, and MELD scores had significant performances in prediction of hepatic encephalopathy in cirrhotic patients with acute variceal bleeding; in this regard, albumin-bilirubin score had the highest accuracy (AUC 0.858, CI 0.802-0.914, sig 0.000) followed by Child-Pugh score (AUC 0.654, CI 0.574–0.735, sig 0.001) and then MELD score (AUC 0.602, CI 0.519–0.686, sig 0.031). The cumulative incidence of hepatic encephalopathy in cirrhotic patients with albumin-bilirubin grade 3 was found to be significantly more than that present in albumin-bilirubin grade 2; most of these hepatic encephalopathy cases occurred in the first 2 weeks of follow-up period.

Conclusions: Albumin-bilirubin score has a significant performance in risk prediction of hepatic encephalopathy in cirrhotic patients with acute variceal bleeding better than Child-Pugh and MELD scores. Albumin-bilirubin grades could be used as a risk stratifying tool to triage cirrhotic patients who will benefit from early discharge after bleeding control and those patients who will benefit from prophylactic measures for hepatic encephalopathy.

Keywords: Albumin-bilirubin score, Prediction, Hepatic encephalopathy, Variceal bleeding, Cirrhosis

Background

Hepatic encephalopathy (HE) exacerbates the morbidity and delays hospital discharge as well as increases the rate of hospital readmissions of cirrhotic patients, particularly those are admitted by acute variceal bleeding (AVB) [1–5]. The varying severity of liver decompensation is related to both the incidence and prevalence of hepatic encephalopathy in cirrhotic patients [1, 6]; the underlying residual liver functions are commonly and widely evaluated by Child-Pugh score [7]; however, this score has some limitations due to the interrelation between albumin and ascites and the subjective assessment of encephalopathy and ascites [8]. The new albumin-bilirubin (ALBI) score was developed previously by Johnson et al.; this

* Correspondence: abdallahelsawy@hotmail.com
Department of Internal Medicine, Faculty of Medicine, Tanta University, Tanta, Egypt

model depends on two objectively evaluated parameters (serum albumin and serum bilirubin); it assesses the degree of underlying hepatic reserve function in cirrhotic patients and has a high degree of performance in prediction of mortality due to liver failure [9]. This score was widely validated in many reports [10–13]. In this study, we assessed the performance of albumin-bilirubin score in prediction of hepatic encephalopathy in cirrhotic patients with acute variceal bleeding, in comparison to Child-Pugh and MELD scores.

Methods

Study design

This is a prospective cohort study that was conducted in accordance to strengthening the reporting of observational studies in epidemiology (STROBE) guidelines [14].

Source of data and potential eligible population

This study was conducted at adult gastroenterology unit of internal medicine department at Tanta university hospitals, in the period from January 2020 to December 2020 on a total of 319 patients who were admitted consecutively by acute upper gastro-intestinal bleeding (hematemesis and/or melena); all patients were resuscitated and then they were evaluated by upper gastrointestinal (GIT) endoscopy for assessment and control of bleeding source. Our eligible participants were recruited in accordance to our inclusion and exclusion criteria that were assessed within the first 24 h after admission.

Exclusion and inclusion criteria

Fifty-four patients were excluded as they did not fulfill study inclusion criteria (31 patients were excluded due to non-variceal upper GIT bleeding, 9 patients excluded as they were clinically unfit for upper GIT endoscopy, 10 patients were excluded due to failure of endoscopic control of variceal bleeding, 4 patients were excluded because cirrhosis was not confirmed), five patients were excluded as they were presented by hepatic encephalopathy before upper GIT endoscopy, three patients were excluded as they died shortly after admission during preoperative resuscitation, and seven patients were excluded as they refused follow-up in our unit. Therefore, the eligibility criteria were fulfilled in only 250 cirrhotic patients who were presented consecutively by acute variceal bleeding and were controlled successfully by upper GIT endoscopy.

Data collection

Each patient was meticulously evaluated after admission and resuscitation with or without blood transfusion, and then upper GIT endoscopy was done within 12 h from the occurrence of hematemesis and/or melena for fit patients to diagnose and control of bleeding source; all the operators were highly experienced physicians at our endoscopy unit. The following first admission criteria were evaluated for all patients who fulfilled our inclusion criteria: demographic criteria (age and sex), clinical criteria (presence of hematemesis and/or melena, ascites, spleen diameter, variceal grading, endoscopic modality of variceal bleeding control and their need for blood transfusion), and laboratory criteria (AST, ALT, s.albumin. s.bilirubin, INR, s.creatinine, platelet count, hemoglobin). The collected patients' laboratory data were used to calculate Child-Pugh, MELD, and albumin-bilirubin (ALBI) scores. Albumin-bilirubin score was calculated using the following formula [(log10 bilirubin in μmol/L × 0.66) + (albumin in g/L × − 0.085)]. Levels ≤ − 2.6 was considered as ALBI grade 1, levels > − 1.39 was considered as ALBI grade 3, and other levels were considered as ALBI grade 2 [9]. All patients were followed up for 4 weeks for possible occurrence of hepatic encephalopathy; we considered the day of hematemesis or the day of first appearance of melena as the initiation time point of follow-up period; all patients were followed up firstly at our emergency unit for few days and then completed the follow-up period at internal wards of our gastroenterology unit or at our outpatient clinic through scheduled examinations every week, as illustrated in study participants' flow diagram (Fig. 1). All patients received broad spectrum antibiotics routinely for at least 1 week after endoscopy as a prophylactic measure for post-endoscopic bacterial infection.

Statistical analysis methods

We used IBM SPSS, version 23 statistic software (IBM, NY, USA), for both summarization and statistical analysis of our collected data. The mean and standard deviation (SD) was used for normally distributed quantitative data while the median and interquartile range (IQR) was calculated for abnormally distributed quantitative data; however, all qualitative data were tabulated as frequency and relative frequency tables. Receiver operating characteristic (ROC) curves were calculated for our ALBI, Child-Pugh, and MELD scores, and their areas under the ROC curve (AUC) were computed. The cumulative incidence functions for hepatic encephalopathy in-between ALBI grades were illustrated using Kaplan-Meier curve and analyzed using the Log Rank test. *P* values less than 0.05 were considered statistically significant.

Results

Table 1 of our results shows the main demographic, clinical, and laboratory baseline criteria for study eligible

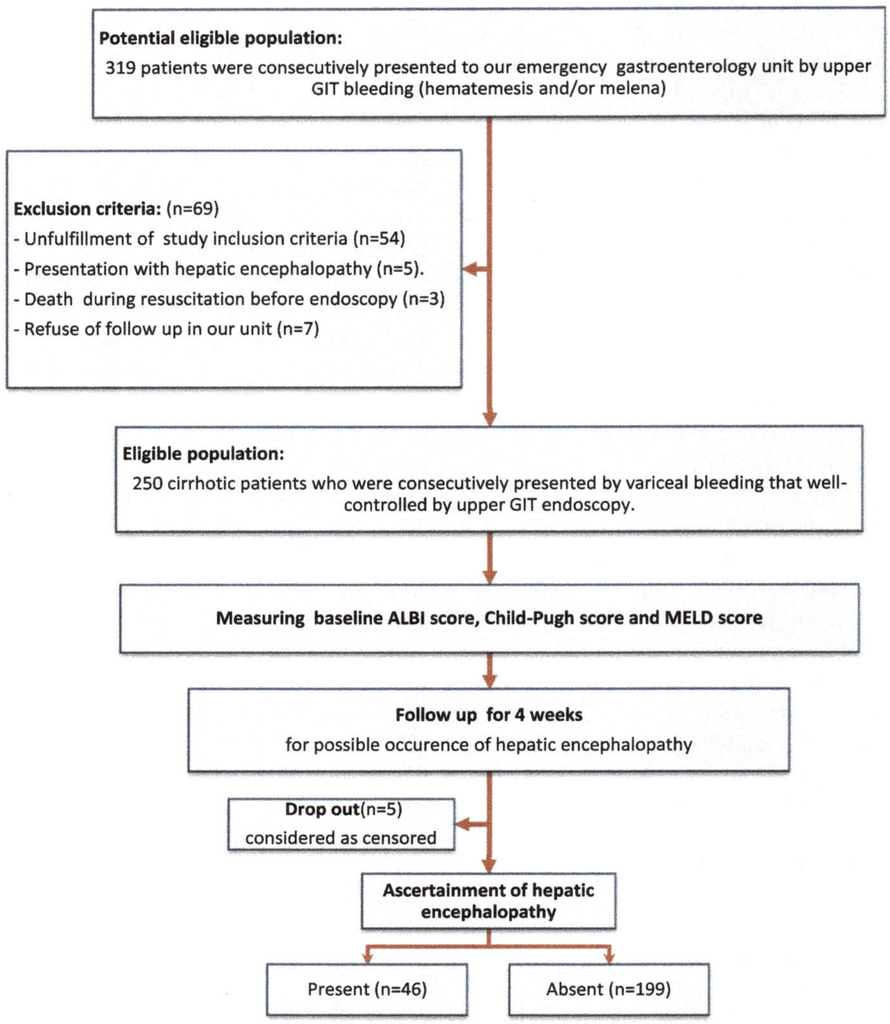

Fig. 1 Participants' flow diagram

population as well as their baseline scores of liver functions (Child-Pugh, MELD, and ALBI scores).

Table 2 of our results shows cross-tabulation of hepatic encephalopathy versus deferent grades of ALBI score along the follow-up period; the cumulative incidence of HE in our study was found to be 18.3% (46 HE cases) after 4 weeks follow-up time; 39 of these HE cases (84.8%) occurred in patients with ALBI grade 3 while the remaining 7 HE cases (15.2%) occurred in patients with ALBI grade 2.

Figure 2 of our results illustrates the receiver operating criteria curve for baseline ALBI, Child-Pugh, and MELD scores in prediction of hepatic encephalopathy with AUC and their respective confidence intervals and significance values (AUC 0.858, 0.654, and 0.602; CI 0.802–0.914, 0.574–0.735, and 0.519–0.686 with sig 0.000, 0.001, and 0.031 for ALBI, Child-Pugh, and MELD scores respectively.

Figure 3 of our results illustrates cumulative incidence function for different ALBI grades as a risk factor predicting hepatic encephalopathy, in which there was a significant difference between ALBI grade 2 and ALBI grade 3 (sig = 0.000).

Discussion

Acute variceal bleeding is a known predisposing risk factor for hepatic encephalopathy in cirrhotic patients [1, 3]; this may exacerbate the morbidity and delay hospital discharge as well as increase the rate of hospital readmissions and mortality in those patients [1–6]; consequently, early administration of appropriate prophylactic measures for HE in risky patients with AVB may mitigate both morbidity and mortality burden as well as alleviate the possible shortage of hospital places especially in emergency situations.

Table 1 Main baseline participants' criteria:

Baseline criteria for eligible population		Value		
Demographic criteria				
• **Age** (years)		Mean (SD)	58	(9.1)
• **Sex**	• **Male**	Count (%)	160	(64%)
	• **Female**	Count (%)	90	(36%)
	• **Total**	Count (%)	250	(100%)
Patients clinical criteria				
• **Presentation**	• **Hematemesis**	Count (%)	52	21%
	• **Melena**	Count (%)	37	15%
	• **Combined hematemesis and melena**	Count (%)	161	64%
• **Previous variceal bleeding**		Count (%)	105	42%
• **Variceal grading**	• **Grade 1**	Count (%)	10	4%
	• **Grade 2**	Count (%)	102	41%
	• **Grade 3**	Count (%)	138	55%
• **Variceal bleeding control**	• **EBL**	Count (%)	42	17%
	• **EIT**	Count (%)	208	83%
• **Need for blood transfusion**		Count (%)	163	65%
• **Ascites**	• **No ascites**	Count (%)	33	(13.2%)
	• **Mild to moderate**	Count (%)	141	(56.4%)
	• **Massive**	Count (%)	76	(30.4%)
• **Spleen diameter** (cm)		Median (IQR)	15	(3)
• **HCC**		Count (%)	22	(9%)
• **Etiology of cirrhosis**	• **CHC**	Count (%)	196	(78.4%)
	• **CHB**	Count (%)	21	(8.4%)
	• **CHC and CHB**	Count (%)	9	(3.6%)
	• **Other**	Count (%)	24	(9.6%)
Laboratory parameters				
• **ALT** (IU/L)		Mean (SD)	43.3	(11.66)
• **AST** (IU/L)		Mean (SD)	47.6	(10.73)
• **S. albumin** (gm/l)		Mean (SD)	28.9	(3.42)
• **S. bilirubin** (mg/dl)		Median (IQR)	2.5	(1.4)
• **INR**		Median (IQR)	2.1	(0.30)
• **S. creatinine** (mg/dl)		Median (IQR)	1.2	(0.2)
• **Platelets** ($\times 10^3/mm^3$)		Median (IQR)	145	(54)
• **Hemoglobin** (g/dl)		Median (IQR)	9.6	(0.9)
Evaluated scores for liver functions				
• **Child-Pugh score**		Median (IQR)	10	(3)
• **MELD score**		Median (IQR)	19.8	(4.4)
• **ALBI score**		Median (IQR)	-1.4	(0.6)
• **ALBI grade**	• **ALBI grade 1**	Count (%)	0	(0%)
	• **ALBI grade 2**	Count (%)	118	(47.2%)
	• **ALBI grade 3**	Count (%)	132	(52.8%)

EBL endoscopic band ligation, *EIT* endoscopic injection therapy, *HCC* hepatocellular carcinoma, *CHC* chronic hepatitis C, *CHB* chronic hepatitis B, *ALT* alanine aminotransferase, *AST* aspartate aminotransferase, *INR* international normalized ratio, *MELD* modified end-\stage liver disease, *ALBI* albumin-bilirubin, *SD* standard deviation, *IQR* interquartile range

Table 2 ALBI grades versus hepatic encephalopathy cross-tabulation

		Hepatic encephalopathy						Sig.	Risk estimate (95% CI)
		Present (n = 46)					Absent (n = 204)		
		1st week	2nd week	3rd week	4th week	Total			
ALBI grade 2 (n = 118)	Count (%)	2 (28.6%)	4 (57.1%)	1 (14.3%)	0 (0.0%)	7 (5.9%)	111 (94.1%)	< 0.0005	4.98 (2.31–10.75)
ALBI grade 3 (n = 132)	Count (%)	14 (35.9%)	18 (46.2%)	5 (12.8%)	2 (5.1%)	39 (29.5%)	93 (70.5%)		

ALBI grade albumin-bilirubin grade

In this respect, the risk stratification of those cirrhotic patients with AVB at hospital admissions could be helpful for early prediction of possible occurrence of HE even after bleeding control; these predictors were evaluated in many reports [15, 16]. One of these risk stratifying factors is the underlying liver function which is commonly assessed by Child-Pugh score [7]; however, this score may be limited by the interrelation between albumin and ascites and the subjective assessment of encephalopathy and ascites [8]. In our study, we used the new ALBI score for the underlying liver functions as a risk stratifying factor for prediction of HE in cirrhotic patients with AVB; we hypothesized that this score has a better performance in comparison to Child-Pugh and MELD scores as it depends on only two objectively assessed parameters (serum albumin and serum bilirubin).

First of all, we found that the cumulative incidence of HE in our patients were about 18.3% within 4 weeks follow-up period, and the reported cumulative incidences of HE after AVB have great variability; it was reported as 16.9% by Win J et al. [17], 31.4% by Fouad TR et al. [18], 40% by Sharma P et al. [19], and 54.5% by Higuera-de-la-Tijera F et al. [20]; this wide discrepancy may be due to the wide variability of the underlying reserve liver functions, variability in follow-up periods, and variability in modalities of variceal bleeding control. Various prophylactic measures of HE in cirrhotic patients after acute upper GIT bleeding were studied in many reports and were found to significantly improve the incidence rates of HE in those patients; these measures aim to eliminate the blood from GIT to decrease the absorption of its toxic products which is the main mechanism of HE after AVB [17–20].

As regards the accuracy of ALBI score in prediction of HE in cirrhotic patients with AVB in comparison to both Child-Pugh and MELD scores, we found that all of these scores had a significant performance; however, we found that ALBI score had the highest performance followed by Child-Pugh score then MELD score. Fouad TR et al. [18] reported a similar conclusion to ours as they identified the possible risk prediction of HE for ALBI score in comparable to Child-Pugh and MELD scores.

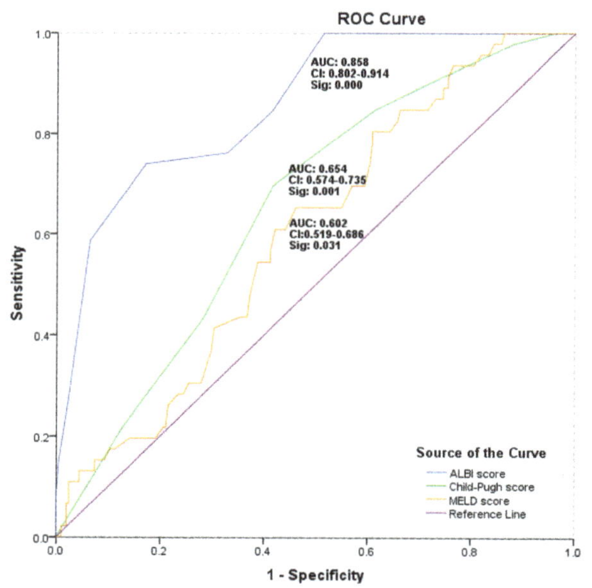

Fig. 2 ROC curve for ALBI, Child-Pugh, and MELD scores in prediction of hepatic encephalopathy

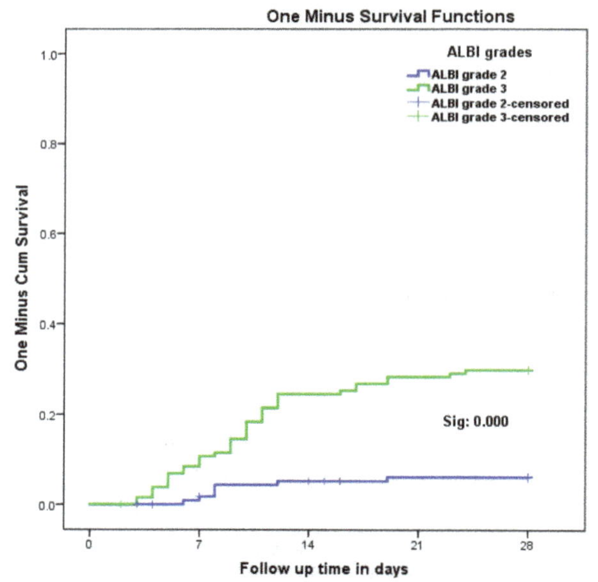

Fig. 3 Cumulative incidence function for different ALBI grades in prediction of hepatic encephalopathy

In our study, we used ALBI grades for risk stratifying of our patients, and we found that the cumulative incidence function of HE in cirrhotic patients with ALBI grade 3 was significantly more than that present in ALBI grade 2; most of these HE cases occurred in the first 2 weeks of follow-up period, so we could suggest that early hospital discharge for those cirrhotic patients after good control of AVB could be possible in absence of ALBI grade 3; this is the same concept that was reported by Fouad TR et al. [18]. At the same time, we could encourage the administration of prophylactic measures for those cirrhotic patients with ALBI grade 3 who are admitted with AVB.

Our study has some limitations; the first limitation is the uni-centericity of this study, and the second is that the methods of follow-up were not the same for all patients; however, we tried to select the most appropriate method for each patient; the third limitation is that we did not assess the possible hazard of rebleeding; however, we found only 11 cases (4.4%) of mild rebleeding episodes that were appropriately controlled. Lastly, we did not correlate between ALBI score and different stages of HE; however, we focused in our study on the possible predictive performance of ALBI score for possible occurrence of HE.

Conclusion

We could conclude that albumin-bilirubin score has a significant performance in risk prediction of hepatic encephalopathy in cirrhotic patients with acute variceal bleeding better than both Child-Pugh and MELD scores. Albumin-bilirubin grades could be used as a risk stratifying tool to triage cirrhotic patients who will benefit from early discharge after bleeding control and those patients who will benefit from prophylactic measures for hepatic encephalopathy.

Abbreviations

ALBI: Albumin-bilirubin; ALT: Alanine aminotransferase; AST: Aspartate aminotransferase; AUC: Area under the curve; AVB: Acute variceal bleeding; CHB: Chronic hepatitis B; CHC: Chronic hepatitis C; CI: Confidence interval; EBL: Endoscopic band ligation; EIT: Endoscopic injection therapy; GIT: Gastrointestinal; HCC: Hepatocellular carcinoma; HE: Hepatic encephalopathy; INR: International normalized ratio; IQR: Interquartile range; MELD: Modified end-stage liver disease; ROC: Receiver operating characteristics; SD: Standard deviation; Sig: Significance

Acknowledgements

We would like to thank all staff members in Gastroenterology Unit of Internal Medicine department at Tanta University Hospital that assisted us in this study.

Authors' contributions

All authors read and approved the final manuscript, according to the following respective roles of each author: REE shared in the study conception and design, data collection, and data interpretation. AAE shared in the study conception and design, data collection, data analysis, and data interpretation and is the corresponding author. AFS shared in the study conception and design, data collection, and data interpretation. AMT shared in the study conception and design, data collection, and data interpretation.

Declarations

Ethics approval and consent to participate

The present study was conducted in accordance with the Declaration of Helsinki. The study protocol was approved by the ethics committee of Tanta Faculty of Medicine (No: 19/12/33594). All patients provided written informed consent. The results of the research were used only in scientific purposes and not in any other aims.

Competing interests

The authors declare that they have no competing interests.

References

1. American Association for the Study of Liver Diseases; European Association for the Study of the Liver (2014) Hepatic encephalopathy in chronic liver disease: 2014 practice guideline by the European Association for the Study of the Liver and the American Association for the Study of Liver Diseases. J Hepatol 61(3):642–659
2. Bleibel W, Al-Osaimi AM (2012) Hepatic encephalopathy. Saudi J Gastroenterol 18(5):301–309. https://doi.org/10.4103/1319-3767.101123
3. Patidar KR, Bajaj JS (2015) Covert and overt hepatic encephalopathy: diagnosis and management. Clin Gastroenterol Hepatol 13(12):2048–2061. https://doi.org/10.1016/j.cgh.2015.06.039
4. Volk ML, Tocco RS, Bazick J, Rakoski MO, Lok AS (2012) Hospital readmissions among patients with decompensated cirrhosis. Am J Gastroenterol 107(2):247–252. https://doi.org/10.1038/ajg.2011.314
5. Seraj SM, Campbell EJ, Argyropoulos SK, Wegermann K, Chung RT, Richter JM (2017) Hospital readmissions in decompensated cirrhotics: factors pointing toward a prevention strategy. World J Gastroenterol 23(37):6868–6876. https://doi.org/10.3748/wjg.v23.i37.6868
6. Del Piccolo F, Sacerdoti D, Amodio P, Bombonato G, Bolognesi M, Mapelli D et al (2003) Central nervous system alterations in liver cirrhosis: the role of portal-systemic shunt and portal hypoperfusion. Metab Brain Dis 18(1):51–62. https://doi.org/10.1023/A:1021930702815
7. Pugh R, Murray-lyon I, Dawson J (1973) Transection of the oesophagus for bleeding oesophageal varices. Br J Surg 60(8):646–649. https://doi.org/10.1002/bjs.1800600817
8. Wang YY, Zhao XH, Ma L, Ye JZ, Wu FX, Tang J, You XM, Xiang BD, Li LQ (2018) Comparison of the ability of Child-Pugh score, MELD score, and ICG-R15 to assess preoperative hepatic functional reserve in patients with hepatocellular carcinoma. J Surg Oncol 118(3):440–445. https://doi.org/10.1002/jso.25184
9. Johnson PJ, Berhane S, Kagebayashi C, Satomura S, Teng M, Reeves HL, O'Beirne J, Fox R, Skowronska A, Palmer D, Yeo W, Mo F, Lai P, Iñarrairaegui M, Chan SL, Sangro B, Miksad R, Tada T, Kumada T, Toyoda H (2015) Assessment of liver function in patients with hepatocellular carcinoma: a new evidence-based approach-the ALBI grade. J Clin Oncol 33(6):550–558. https://doi.org/10.1200/JCO.2014.57.9151
10. Hiraoka A, Kumada T, Michitaka K, Kudo M (2019) Newly proposed ALBI grade and ALBI-T score as tools for assessment of hepatic function and prognosis in hepatocellular carcinoma patients. Liver Cancer 8(5):312–325. https://doi.org/10.1159/000494844
11. Wang YY, Zhong JH, Su ZY, Huang JF, Lu SD, Xiang BD, Ma L, Qi LN, Ou BN, Li LQ (2016) Albumin-bilirubin versus Child-Pugh score as a predictor of outcome after liver resection for hepatocellular carcinoma. Br J Surg 103(6):725–734. https://doi.org/10.1002/bjs.10095
12. Toyoda H, Lai PB, O'Beirne J, Chong CC, Berhane S, Reeves H et al (2016) Long-term impact of liver function on curative therapy for hepatocellular carcinoma: application of the ALBI grade. Br J Cancer 114(7):744–750. https://doi.org/10.1038/bjc.2016.33
13. Hiraoka A, Kumada T, Nouso K, Tsuji K, Itobayashi E, Hirooka M, Kariyama K, Ishikawa T, Tada T, Toyoda H, Kawasaki H, Hiasa Y, Michitaka K (2016) Proposed new sub-grouping for intermediate-stage hepatocellular carcinoma using albumin-bilirubin grade. Oncology. 91(3):153–161. https://doi.org/10.1159/000447061
14. Vandenbroucke JP, von Elm E, Altman DG, Gøtzsche PC, Mulrow CD, Pocock SJ, Poole C, Schlesselman JJ, Egger M, STROBE Initiative (2014) Strengthening the Reporting of Observational Studies in Epidemiology (STROBE): explanation and elaboration. Int J Surg 12(12):1500–1524. https://doi.org/10.1016/j.ijsu.2014.07.014

15. Rattanasupar A, Tiawijit N, Rachatapantanakorn B (2014) Predictive factor for hepatic encephalopathy in cirrhotic patients who presented with acute variceal bleeding. J Med Assoc Thail 97(6):567–573
16. Kumar AS, Sibia RS (2015) Predictors of in-hospital mortality among patients presenting with variceal gastrointestinal bleeding. Saudi J Gastroenterol 21(1):43–46. https://doi.org/10.4103/1319-3767.151226
17. Wen J, Liu Q, Song J, Tong M, Peng L, Liang H (2013) Lactulose is highly potential in prophylaxis of hepatic encephalopathy in patients with cirrhosis and upper gastrointestinal bleeding: results of a controlled randomized trial. Digestion. 87(2):132–138. https://doi.org/10.1159/000346083
18. Fouad TR, Abdelsameea E, Abdel-Razek W, Attia A, Mohamed A, Metwally K, Naguib M, Waked I (2019) Upper gastrointestinal bleeding in Egyptian patients with cirrhosis: post-therapeutic outcome and prognostic indicators. J Gastroenterol Hepatol 34(9):1604–1610. https://doi.org/10.1111/jgh.14659
19. Sharma P, Agrawal A, Sharma BC, Sarin SK (2011) Prophylaxis of hepatic encephalopathy in acute variceal bleed: a randomized controlled trial of lactulose versus no lactulose. J Gastroenterol Hepatol 26(6):996–1003. https://doi.org/10.1111/j.1440-1746.2010.06596.x
20. Higuera-de-la-Tijera F, Servín-Caamaño AI, Salas-Gordillo F, Pérez-Hernández JL, Abdo-Francis JM, Camacho-Aguilera J et al (2018) Primary prophylaxis to prevent the development of hepatic encephalopathy in cirrhotic patients with acute variceal bleeding. Can J Gastroenterol Hepatol 2018:3015891

11

Validity of routine biochemical and ultrasound scores for prediction of hepatic fibrosis and steatosis in NAFLD

Rasha Eletreby[1*], Zeinab Abdellatif[1], Yasmine Gaber[1], Ahmed Ramadan[1], Naglaa Ahmad[2], Hany Khattab[3], Mohamed Said[1] and Yasmin Saad[1]

Abstract

Background: We evaluated the validity of some non-invasive scores and ultrasound findings to predict fibrosis and steatosis in a cohort of NAFLD patients who underwent liver biopsy. Ninety-seven NAFLD patients were enrolled and classified into NASH (66) and simple steatosis groups (31) based on liver biopsy. ROC curves were constructed for Fibrosis-4 index (FIB4), aspartate aminotransferase to platelet ratio index (APRI), and NAFLD fibrosis score (NFS) in fibrosis prediction, also for (hepatic steatosis index; HSI, fatty liver index; FLI) and ultrasonographic subcutaneous and visceral adipose tissue measurements (SAT and VAT) for steatosis prediction.

Results: FIB4 had AUC of 0.6, APRI and NFS at cutoffs of 0.3 and -2.4 had AUC of 0.64 and 0.63 in detecting the presence of any grade of fibrosis, and of (0.52, 0.55, and 0.58) for significant fibrosis. FIB4 at a cut-off of (0.76) had the highest AUC in detecting any grade of fibrosis in the simple steatosis group (0.81). SAT (at cutoff of 2.1 and 2.5) was superior to VAT. HSI (at cutoff 45.35 and 45.7) was superior to FLI in detecting moderate or marked steatosis.

Conclusion: FIB4 and NFS can be used in screening for silent liver disease with ongoing fibrosis in simple steatosis. They are unsatisfactory predictors for significant fibrosis in NAFLD. SAT is better than VAT in predicting moderate steatosis and is slightly better than biochemical HSI.

Keywords: NAFLD, Fibrosis progression, Steatosis, Non-invasive assessment

Background

NAFLD represents the most common liver disorder in Western countries, with 17–46% prevalence among adults [1]. In Egypt, the prevalence of NAFLD is rising owing to rising prevalence of obesity. NAFLD was found in 57.65% of a cohort of obese Egyptian adolescents in one study [2].

NAFLD is tightly associated with several risk factors; the presence of which impacts the severity and progression of the disease. The most important risk factors are known to be insulin resistance (IR) and metabolic syndrome (MetS) [3].

* Correspondence: r_m_tawfik@yahoo.com
[1]Endemic Medicine and Hepatology Department, Cairo University, Cairo, Egypt
Full list of author information is available at the end of the article

The diagnosis of NASH provides important prognostic information and indicates an increased risk of fibrosis progression, cirrhosis, and possibly HCC. It also prompts closer follow-up and possibly a greater need for more intensive therapy [4]. Similarly, steatosis should be documented whenever NAFLD is suspected as the primary disease or as a coexisting condition as it predicts future diabetes mellitus, cardiovascular events, and arterial hypertension [4].

Unfortunately, the standard diagnostic tool for NASH, namely, liver biopsy, has significant limitations such as sampling variability [5], being prohibitively expensive and relatively invasive with some morbidity and very rare mortality risk [6]. Also, quantification of fat content is not of interest in clinical practice, except as a surrogate of treatment efficacy, and is therefore not generally recommended. Imaging, especially ultrasound is the preferred tool for diagnosis of NAFLD being cheaper and more available than MRI; the gold standard. However, imaging has the limitation of low sensitivity in the detection of mild degrees of steatosis; hence, it is not suitable for screening purposes [4].

Recent guidelines started to support the use of non-invasive biomarkers and scores of fibrosis and steatosis, as well as transient elastography ± controlled attenuation parameter (CAP), as acceptable non-invasive procedures for fibrosis/steatosis assessment in NAFLD cases [4].

Among non-invasive markers for fibrosis assessment, the FIB4 index has been independently validated in subjects with HCV infection. It is a simple and relatively inexpensive method that correlates with the stage of fibrosis [7]. Another simple fibrosis scoring system is the NAFLD fibrosis score (NFS) which was found to independently identify patients with and without advanced fibrosis at initial NAFLD diagnosis [8].

Fatty liver index (FLI) and hepatic steatosis index (HSI), on the other side; are steatosis scores that were found to reliably predict the presence, rather than the severity, of steatosis [9].

In the current study, we aim to evaluate the validity of three non-invasive fibrosis markers, namely, FIB-4, APRI, and NFS, in detecting both significant fibrosis in patients with NAFLD, and any stage of fibrosis in the subgroup of patients with simple steatosis. As well as to compare the diagnostic performance of two other non-invasive hepatic steatosis indices (HSI and FLI) to US findings (grading of liver brightness and subcutaneous and visceral fat measurements) versus liver biopsy as a gold standard, being cheap, simple, readily available indices for steatosis detection in NAFLD patients in the setting of low socioeconomic status and high prevalence, and morbidity of NAFLD.

Methods

The current study included 97 NAFLD patients who sought medical advice at NASH multi-disciplinary clinic, Kasr Alainy Hospital, Cairo University, Cairo, Egypt. The clinic involves a multidisciplinary team including hepatologists, nutritionists, pathologists, endocrinologists, endoscopists, and bariatric surgeons.

Among 250 patients presented to the NAFLD clinic, 97 patients enrolled after exclusion of those with positive viral hepatitis markers and those who did not consent for liver biopsy. The study was conducted in the period from July 2014 to July 2016.

Patients who fulfilled the following inclusion criteria were recruited.

- Age ≥ 18 years.
- Bright liver by ultrasound.
- Negative hepatitis markers (negative HBsAg, HBcAb, HCVAb).
- Negative history of other chronic liver diseases as autoimmune hepatitis, primary biliary cirrhosis, etc.

Enrolled patients were subjected to the following:

- Informed consent: All patients enrolled had signed an informed consent form. The study was carried out per the Helsinki Declaration [10] and was approved by the ethical committee of the endemic medicine department, Kasr Alainy Hospital, Cairo University.

- Clinical evaluation including sex, age, body-mass index (BMI), history of DM, HTN, or any comorbidities, detailed dietary questionnaire, and anthropometric measurements.

- Laboratory investigations in the form of liver biochemical profile (BIL, AST, ALT, ALP, GGT, INR), lipid profile (cholesterol, triglycerides, HDL, LDL), and fasting blood glucose.

- Calculation of fibrosis indices:

- *Calculation of APRI by the formula* [(AST/upper limit of normal × 100)/platelet count] [11]. Where, non- significant fibrosis (< F2): < 0.7, significant fibrosis (≥ F2-< F4): 0.7-<1 and cirrhosis (F4): ≥ 1.
- *Calculation of FIB-4 by the formula* (Age × AST/platelet count × sqr ALT) [12]. Non-significant fibrosis (< F2) was identified as FIB4 < 1.45, significant fibrosis (≥ F2-<F4): 1.45-<3.25 and cirrhosis (F4): ≥ 3.25.
- Calculation of NAFLD fibrosis score:

The NFS is composed of 6 variables, including age, hyperglycemia, BMI, platelet count, albumin, and AST/ALT ratio.

NAFLD fibrosis score = −1.675 + 0.037 × age (year) + 0.094 × BMI (kg/m2) + 1.13 × IFG/diabetes (yes = 1, no = 0) + 0.99 × AST/ALT ratio − 0.013 × platelet count (× 109/L) − 0.66 × albumin(g/dL) [8]. NAFLD patients with a score less than −1.5 were classified as "low probability of advanced liver fibrosis," and those patients with a score of at least −1.5 were classified as "intermediate or high probability of advanced liver fibrosis" [8].

- Calculation of steatosis indices:

- Hepatic steatosis index (HSI) [13]

HSI = 8 × ALT/AST + BMI + 2, if DM; +2, if female with values < 30 ruling out and values > 36 ruling in steatosis.

- Fatty liver index (FLI) [14]

FLI = logistic (0.953 × ln (TG)+0.139 × BMI+0.718 × ln(γGT) +0.053 × waist−15.745) × 100; where logistic(x)

= 1/(1+e $^{-x}$) denotes the logistic function and ln the natural logarithm.

Values < 30 rule out and values > 60 rules in steatosis.

- Abdominal ultrasonography: Real-time abdominal US was done using a transabdominal 4C-AH46701AA machine with a 1-5MHZ convex linear transducer, with a built-in color flow mapping (CFM) and Doppler functions. US evaluation included subcutaneous adipose tissue (SAT) measurement and visceral adipose tissue (VAT) measurement. The appearance of the liver concerning size, echo pattern, presence of hepatic focal lesion/s and portal vein patency, scanning for spleen, examination for ascites, abdominal lymphadenopathy, and abdominal masses, together with scanning for other abdominal and pelvic organ.

- Liver biopsy: All enrolled patients had undergone liver biopsy to differentiate NAFL from NASH, with the calculation of NAFLD activity score (NAS). The NAS is the sum of the biopsy scores for steatosis (0 to 3), lobular inflammation (0 to 3), and hepatocellular ballooning (0 to 2), in addition to the calculation of the fibrosis stage (0 to 4). A NAS < 3 corresponds to NAFL, 3 to 4 corresponds to borderline NASH, and a score ≥ 5 corresponds to NASH [15]. Steatosis grades were also determined (mild, moderate, severe) [16].

Statistical methods

- Numerical variables are presented as mean (standard deviation); while categorical variables are presented as numbers and percentages.
- Logistic regression analysis was done to identify predictors of the presence of NASH, NAS score ≥ 5, and to identify predictors of NAS score > 4. Logistic regression analysis was done to identify factors associated with higher grades of fibrosis.
- ROC curves were constructed to analyze the discriminatory power of non-invasive fibrosis markers, Fib4, APRI, and NFS, for the prediction of the presence of fibrosis, and another time for predicting significant fibrosis, with liver biopsy being the gold standard.
- (ROC) curve analysis was used to identify the best cut-off value of various liver fat indices for detecting moderate/marked steatosis
- Data analysis was done using Statistics/Data Analysis (STATA) version 13.1 software.

Results

Baseline characters of the study population

Mean age was 42 years, 74.2% were females, mean BMI was 34.3, 20.6% were diabetic, 59% had macro- and microvesicular steatosis in liver biopsy. 17/80 (21.3%) patients had severe steatosis. In total, 20.6% (20/97) had significant fibrosis (≥ F2). Two patients (2.1%) had severe inflammation. Two subgroups have been then identified: the NASH group (66 patients) and the simple steatosis group (31 patients). DM, female waist circumference, fasting blood sugar, and fibrosis stage were statistically different between both groups (Table 1). Patients with marked steatosis had statistically significant higher ALT (*p* 0.04), as well as a higher number of patients with grade III liver brightness by ultrasound (*p* <0.0001).

Risk factors for significant and higher grades of fibrosis

Albumin, bilirubin, and NFS were significantly associated with significant fibrosis on performing univariate logistic regression (Table 2).

Risk factors for the presence of fibrosis in simple steatosis subgroup

Higher age, lower serum albumin, NFS, and FIB4 were significantly associated with the presence of fibrosis despite the absence of inflammation in studied biopsies (Table 3).

Sensitivity and specificity of different indices for fibrosis prediction

At a cutoff of 0.76, FIB4 was 83.3% sensitive, 69.2% specific, with an accuracy of 77.4%, positive likelihood ratio (LR+) of 2.7, and negative likelihood ratio (LR–) of 0.2 for detection of fibrosis in patients with simple steatosis. APRI had sensitivity, specificity, and accuracy rates of 66.1%, 61.3%, and 65.6% at the cutoff of 0.30 in the detection of any grade of fibrosis. A cutoff value of –2.44 NFS had sensitivity, specificity, LR+, and LR– of 73.44%, 51.6%, +1.52, and –0.51 in detecting the presence of any grade of fibrosis (Fig. 1).

AUC of different markers in fibrosis prediction

FIB4, APRI, and NFS had acceptable and comparable AUC of 0.60, 0.64, 0.63 in detecting the presence of any grade of fibrosis, however, all markers were poor predictors of significant fibrosis ≥ F2 (AUC: 0.52, 0.55, 0.58) (Fig. 1, Table 4).

In the subgroup of patients with simple steatosis (NAS score of ≤ 4); FIB4 had the highest AUC curve compared to NFS and APRI in the detection of any grade of fibrosis (0.81 versus 0.74 and 0.78) (Fig. 1, Table 4).

AUC for HSI and FLI in the prediction of different grades of steatosis

HSI was superior to FLI in detecting either moderate or marked steatosis. At the cutoff of 45.35, HSI had the sensitivity of 73.17%, specificity of 58.06%, LR+ of 1.74, LR– of 0.5, and accuracy of 66.67% in predicting moderate steatosis with AUC of 0.64, and nearly the same percentages with less accuracy in detecting marked steatosis

Table 1 Baseline characteristics of the study population

		The whole group	NAS < 4 (*n* = 31)	NAS ≥ 4 (*n* = 66)	*P* value
Age		42.02 (8.99)	42 (10.44)	42.03 (8.30)	0.9
Gender Male/female		25 (25.8%)/72 (74.2%)	10 (32.2%)/21(67.7%)	15 (22.72%)/51 (77.27%)	0.3
Residence Rural/urban		18 (27.3%)/48 (72.7%)	4 (12.9%)/16 (51.61%)	14 (21.21%)/32 (48.48%)	0.4
Diabetes mellitus		20 (20.6%)	2 (6.45%)	18 (27.27%)	0.01
Hypertension		13 (13.40%)	2 (6.45%)	11 (16.67%)	0.1
BMI median (IQR)		32.9 (29.15-38.14)	32 (28-35.99)	33.05 (30-38.86)	0.2
Waist circumference	Males Median (IQR)	55 (16.84%)	44 (40-50)	52 (49-62)	0.07
	Females Median (IQR)	81 (38.41%)	48.5 (45-56)	68 (55-127)	0.01
Laboratory parameters					
Hemoglobin		12.91 (1.70)	12.61 (2.08)	13.05 (1.49)	0.2
Platelets		272.12 (69.69)	272.97 (62.003)	271.72 (73.52)	0.9
AST median (IQR)		30 (22-41.5)	27 (22-34)	30 (23-44)	0.06
ALT median (IQR)		32.5 (21-57)	26 (18-38)	40 (23-60)	0.01
Bilirubin median (IQR)		0.56 (0.4-0.9)	0.5 (0.4-0.84)	0.6 (0.4-0.9)	0.8
Albumin		4.27 (0.43)	4.21 (0.48)	4.30 (0.41)	0.4
INR		1.001 (0.09)	1.01 (0.05)	0.99 (0.10)	0.7
Cholesterol median (IQR)		202 (177-229)	202 (166-225)	202 (180-234)	0.4
Triglycerides median (IQR)		140 (100-180)	141 (96-200)	135.5 (100-179.5)	0.9
FBG median (IQR)		99.5 (90-110)	92 (86-101)	100 (90-116)	0.04
Liver biopsy					
Type of steatosis	Macro and microvesicular	29 (59.2%)	10	19	0.3
	Macrovesicular	12 (24.5%)	4	8	
	Microvesicular	8 (16.3%)	5	3	
Fibrosis stage	F0	31 (31.96%)	13	18	0.04
	F1	46 (47.42%)	17	29	
	F2	17 (17.5%)	1	16	
	F3	2 (2.1%)	0	2	
	F4	1 (1.03%)	0	1	

Unless otherwise stated, numerical variables presented as mean (SD)

at a cutoff value of 45.7 (sensitivity was 73.33%, specificity was 50.88%, LR+ was 1.49, LR− was 0.52, while accuracy was 55.6%) with AUC of 0.66. On the other hand, FLI had AUCs of 0.52 and 0.56 for predicting the presence of moderate and marked steatosis (Fig. 2).

AUC for ultrasound parameters (SAT and VAT) in the prediction of different grades of steatosis

SAT shows a higher AUC for predicting moderate steatosis (AUC 0.66 vs 0.56) and nearly equal AUC as VAT for detecting marked steatosis (AUC 0.57 vs 0.60). A cutoff value of 2.1, SAT had a sensitivity of 81.25%, specificity of 60%, LR+ of 2.03, LR− of 0.3, and accuracy of 73.08% in detecting moderate steatosis. For predicting marked steatosis, SAT had a sensitivity of 62.5%, specificity of 66.7%, LR+ of 1.9, LR− of 0.6, and accuracy of 65.4% at cutoff value of 2.5. On the other hand, at a cutoff value of 1.8, VAT showed a sensitivity of 66.67%, specificity of 52.63%, LR+ of 1.41, LR− of 0.63, and accuracy of 58.06% in predicting marked steatosis (Fig. 3).

Discussion

In this cross-sectional observational study, we aimed to evaluate the role of some non-invasive, simple, readily

Table 2 Univariate logistic regression analysis for factors associated with significant fibrosis ≥ F2 in NAFLD patients

	Odds ratio (95% conf. interval)	*P* value
Age	1.01 (0.96-1.06)	0.7
Gender (female)	1.62 (0.62-4.18)	0.3
DM	3.24 (0.9-12.03)	0.07
BMI > 35	1.18 (0.49-2.87)	0.7
AST	1.02 (0.99-1.05)	0.1
ALT	1.004 (0.99-1.02)	0.5
ALP	1.01 (0.99-1.02)	0.3
GGT	0.99 (0.98-1.004)	0.2
Triglycerides	0.99 (0.99-1.001)	0.1
Cholesterol	0.99 (0.98-1.01)	0.4
Albumin	0.31 (0.11-0.89)	**0.03**
Bilirubin	7.19 (1.59-32.50)	**0.01**
APRI	3.18 (0.52-19.51)	0.2
FIB4	2.17 (0.80-5.87)	0.1
NFS	1.41 (1.1-1.89)	**0.02**

available, and cheap indices, namely, FIB-4, APRI, and NFS in the detection of significant fibrosis (≥ F2) in patients with NAFLD, as well as their role in detecting any stage of fibrosis in a subgroup of patients with simple steatosis. Similarly, we could evaluate the predictability of other non-invasive steatosis indices (HSI and FLI) and compare them to US findings (grading of liver brightness and subcutaneous and visceral fat measurements) taking liver biopsy results as a standard in diagnosis and grading of hepatic steatosis/fibrosis.

Significant fibrosis (≥ F2) was observed in 20.6%, while advanced fibrosis (F3-4) was seen in 3.1% of patients.

Table 3 Predictors of higher grades of fibrosis in simple steatosis group (NAS score ≤ 4) (n = 31)

	Odds ratio (95% conf. interval)	*P* value
Age	1.1 (1.04-1.18)	0.04
Gender (female)	3 (0.63-14.23)	0.1
BMI > 35	1.12 (0.24-5.21)	0.9
AST	1.06 (0.98-1.14)	0.1
ALT	1.01 (0.97-1.05)	0.6
ALP	0.99 (0.98-1.02)	0.9
GGT	0.99 (0.98-1.01)	0.7
Triglycerides	0.99 (0.98-1.003)	0.2
Cholesterol	0.99 (0.98-1.01)	0.6
Albumin	0.1 (0.01-0.67)	0.02
FIB4	10.73 (1.41-81.54)	0.02
NFS	1.94 (1.11-3.40)	0.02

According to the National Health and Nutrition Examination Survey conducted in 1988-1994, advanced fibrosis (NFS > 0.676) was only observed in 3.2% of patients with NAFLD [17].

In this study, the prevalence of T2DM was significantly higher in the NASH group compared to the simple steatosis one. It is well known that diabetes risk and type 2 DM (T2DM) are closely associated with the severity of NAFLD, progression to NASH, advanced fibrosis, and HCC development [18].

Regression analysis for predictors of significant fibrosis revealed that lower serum albumin, higher bilirubin, and NFS were significantly associated with higher grades of fibrosis (≥ F1). Several studies revealed that NFS is an important predictor of advanced fibrosis in NAFLD patients [19].

Although patients with simple steatosis without inflammation were considered for a long time to have a benign course with little progression [1], this view has been modified by results of different studies demonstrating that steatosis alone may progress to NASH with fibrosis, however, at a slower rate [20].

In the subgroup of patients with simple steatosis, predictors of fibrosis were older age, lower serum albumin, FIB4, and NFS. The importance of identifying patients who had fibrosis is that this could carry the risk of progressing to NASH. In one study by Pais et al., 64% of 25 patients with simple steatosis developed NASH after an average of 3.7 years. They showed that severe ballooning, presence of bridging fibrosis, older age, and deterioration of metabolic risk factors were associated with a more rapid progression [21].

In the current study, FIB4, APRI, and NFS had comparable AUC for detecting the presence of any grade of fibrosis. Detecting the early stages of fibrosis is of great importance in preventing disease progression to minimize complications [22]. On the other hand, all markers were poor predictors of significant fibrosis ≥ F2. Contrarily, Castera in 2018 reported AUC for transient elastography, FIB-4, and the NAFLD fibrosis scores in diagnosing severe fibrosis-cirrhosis of 0.88, 0.84, and 0.84 respectively [23]. Mohamed et al. studied the diagnostic performance of FIB4, NFS, and APRI in NAFLD. They found AUC for advanced fibrosis of 0.936, 0.916, and 0.907 [24]. Also, in a meta-analysis of 13 studies consisting of 3064 patients, NFS had an AUROC of 0.85 for predicting advanced fibrosis [25]. This difference may be related to the small number of patients with advanced fibrosis (≥ F3) in our study (3%).On the other hand, Nones et al. evaluated results of FIB4, APRI, and NFS in 67 patients with NAFLD, the best diagnostic accuracy was achieved with FIB 4 model (AUROC = 0.83) versus APRI and NFS. Again, the difference may be attributed to the higher number of patients with advanced

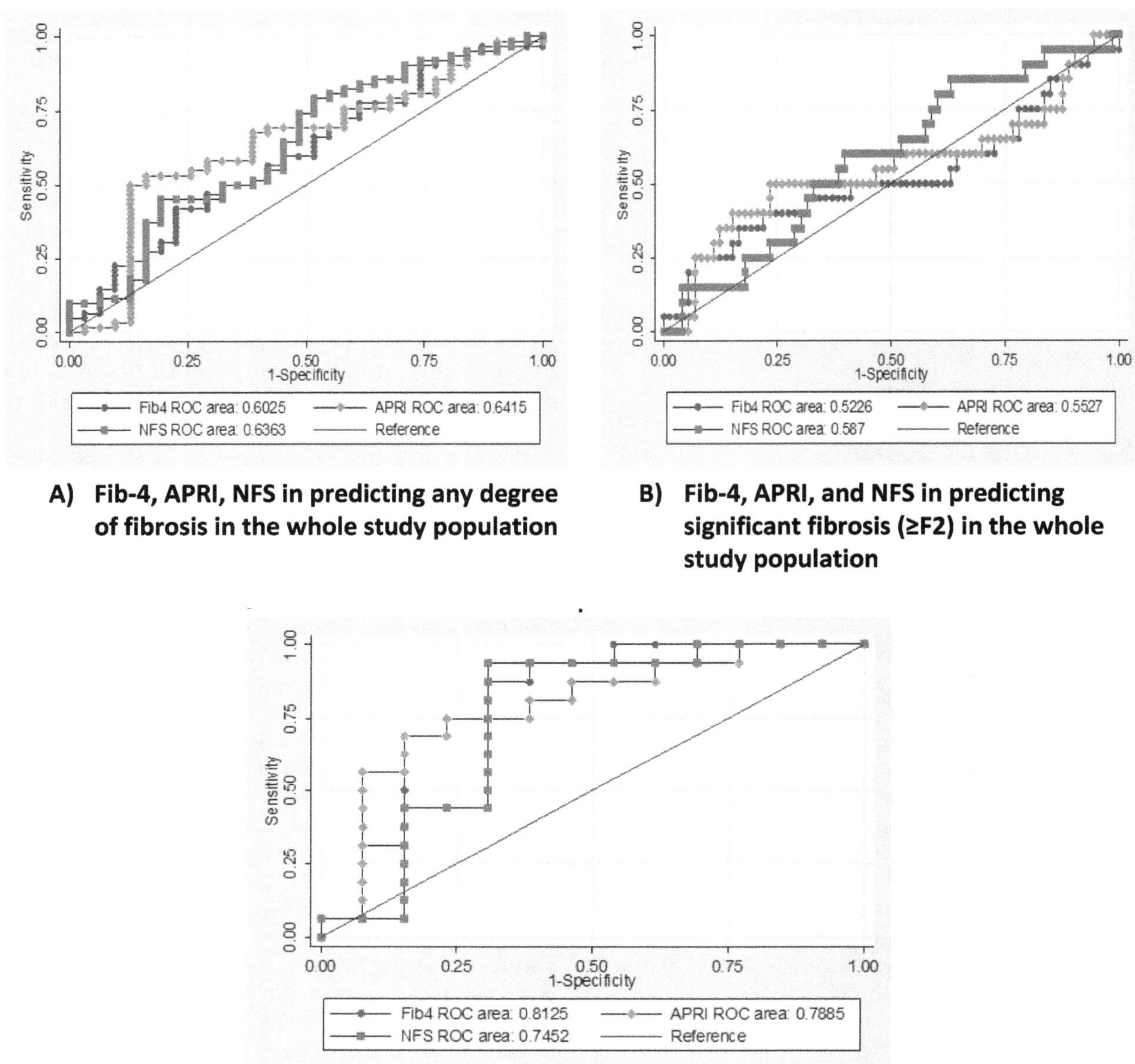

A) Fib-4, APRI, NFS in predicting any degree of fibrosis in the whole study population

B) Fib-4, APRI, and NFS in predicting significant fibrosis (≥F2) in the whole study population

C) Fib-4, APRI, NFS in predicting any degree of fibrosis in the subset of patients with simple steatosis (NAS≤4)

Fig. 1 ROC curves for predictivity of FIB4, APRI, NFS of different degrees of fibrosis. (**A**) Fib-4, APRI, NFS in predicting any degree of fibrosis in the whole study population. (**B**) Fib-4, APRI, and NFS in predicting significant fibrosis (≥ F2) in the whole study population. (**C**) Fib-4, APRI, NFS in predicting any degree of fibrosis in the subset of patients with simple steatosis (NAS ≤ 4)

fibrosis (≥ F3) in his study 18 (26.86%) compared to the current one (3%) [26].

Among non-invasive scores of hepatic steatosis, the hepatic steatosis index (HSI) has been derived from data of a Korean cross-sectional study that involved more than 10,000 patients and has been validated against ultrasound [13]. It is a promising score that seems to predict incident metabolic syndrome [27]. In the current study, HSI has been validated against liver biopsy results and showed acceptable AUC in the prediction of moderate and marked steatosis. Our results go hand in hand with those of Fedchuk et al., where HSI had an AUC of 0.65 in the prediction of the presence of hepatic steatosis [9].

The fatty liver index (FLI) was mentioned as one of the best-validated steatosis scores, as it has been externally validated in the general population or grade 3

Table 4 AUROC of tested markers in detection of presence of fibrosis as well as significant fibrosis in the whole cohort and in simple steatosis subgroup

	AUROC (95% conf. interval) for detection of		
	Presence of fibrosis	**Significant fibrosis**	**Presence of fibrosis in simple steatosis subgroup**
APRI	0.64 (0.52-0.76) (Cutoff: 0.30)	0.55 (0.4-0.72)	0.788 (0.61-0.97)
FIB4	0.60 (0.48-0.73)	0.52 (0.4-0.69)	0.81 (0.64-0.98)
NFS	0.64 (0.51-0.76)	0.58 (0.45-0.73)	0.74 (0.53-0.95)

obese persons and can variably predict metabolic, hepatic, and cardiovascular outcomes/mortality [4]. However, in the current study, FLI had unsatisfactory AUC for predicting the presence of moderate and marked steatosis and was inferior to HSI. The discrepancy maybe since the fatty liver index (FLI) has only been validated against liver ultrasonography in published studies [28] rather than liver biopsy that has been taken in our study.

Despite its limitations, ultrasound is still recommended by EASL 2016 guidelines to be the preferred first-line diagnostic procedure for imaging of NAFLD, as it provides additional diagnostic hepatobiliary information [4]. In the current study, subcutaneous adipose tissue (SAT) showed better AUC than visceral adipose tissue (VAT) in predicting moderate steatosis and similar AUC in predicting marked hepatic steatosis. Lower AUC for detection of marked steatosis in the current

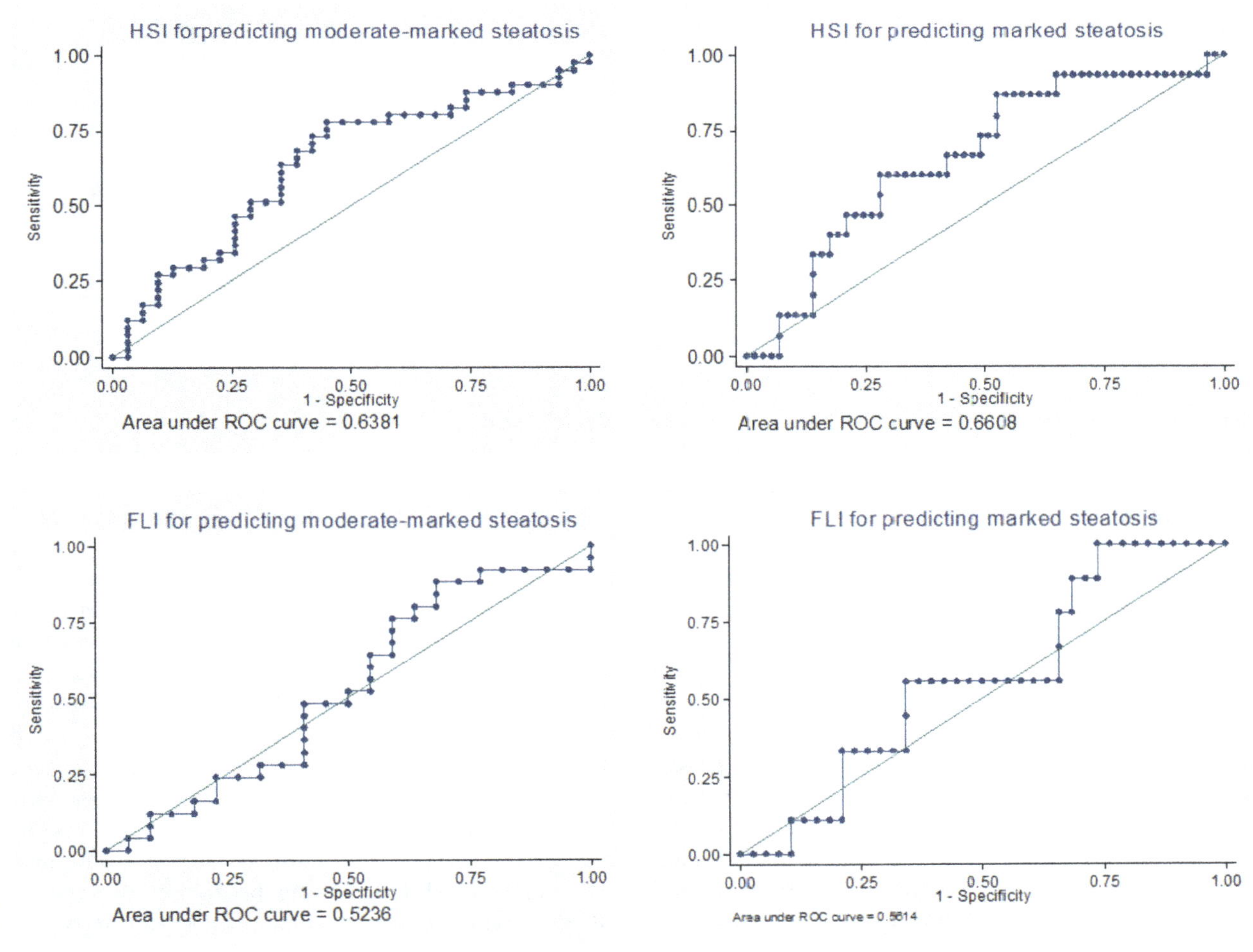

Fig. 2 ROC curve for HSI and FLI in the prediction of moderate/marked steatosis

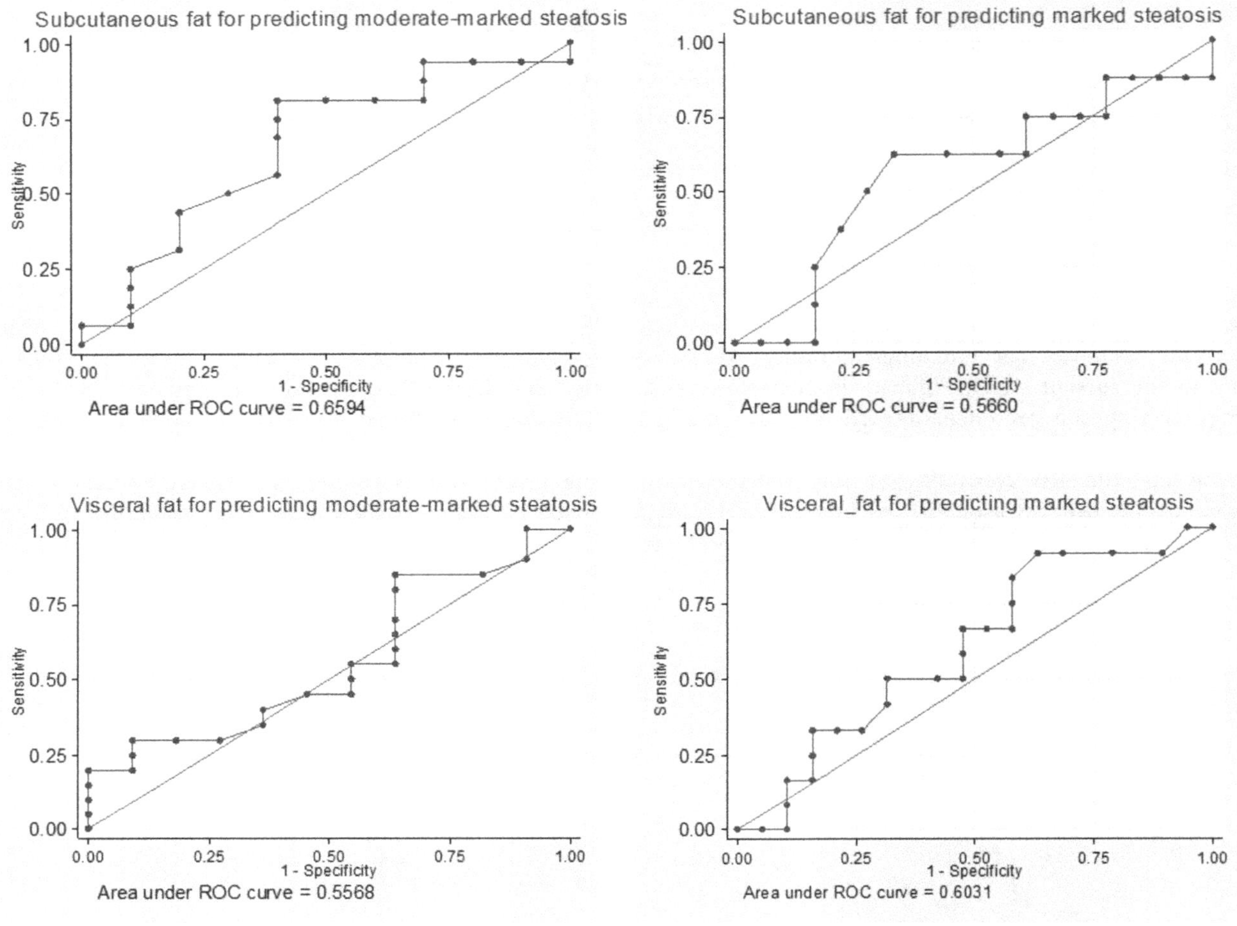

Fig. 3 ROC curve for SAT and VAT in the prediction of moderate/marked steatosis

study may be due to the technical limitation of higher waist circumference and obesity of this cohort.

In the current study, subcutaneous adipose tissue (SAT) showed the best results among all tested non-invasive measures, namely, serum biomarkers (HSI and FLI) as well as visceral adipose tissue (VAT) by ultrasound in detecting moderate steatosis.

The main point of strength of the current study is the presence of liver biopsy results as a gold standard for comparison with non-invasive markers. Note that many other published studies lack the results of liver biopsy and compare the accuracy of non-invasive biochemical markers with imaging or controlled attenuation parameter (CAP) measures which are still not considered the gold standard for fibrosis/steatosis diagnosis. The main limitation of our study is that the main cohort of patients has no or mild degree fibrosis (F0-F1) by liver biopsy (79%), while significant and advanced fibrosis was present in 21% which may have affected the results.

Conclusion

Based on the results of the current study, we can conclude that FIB4 could be used as a screening tool for silent liver disease with ongoing fibrosis in NAFL D patients with simple steatosis, which warrants closer follow-up and more intensive therapies. However, FIB4, APRI, and NFS are still unsatisfactory non-invasive markers for the detection of significant fibrosis in NASH patients and further studies are needed to reach optimal markers. We can also conclude that ultrasound assessment of subcutaneous adipose tissue (SAT) rather than visceral adipose tissue (VAT) performs well in the prediction of moderate steatosis and slightly better than hepatic steatosis index (HSI) which proves also to be a good noninvasive biochemical tool in the prediction of moderate steatosis and performs better than the fatty liver index.

Abbreviations
APRI: AST to platelet ratio index; FIB 4: Fibrosis score 4; NAFLD: Non-alcoholic fatty liver disease; NAS: NAFLD activity score; NASH: Non-alcoholic steatohepatitis; NFS: NAFLD fibrosis score

Acknowledgements
No agency to be acknowledged

Authors' contributions
The authors read and approved the final manuscript; all authors contributed to the work. MS: Idea of the study. Revision of the manuscript. YS: Idea of the study, revision of the manuscript, and mastering the clinical work and connections with other specialists. RE: Drafting the manuscript and the corresponding author. ZA: Doing the statistical tests for the study. AR: Patient follow-up in the clinic and collecting data. YG: Patient follow-up in the clinic and collecting data. NA: Clinical follow-up of patients from the endocrinological point of view. HK: Doing the histopathological examination for liver biopsies. Taken from patients for the staging of steatosis and fibrosis.

Declarations

Ethics approval and consent to participate
All patients signed informed consent. The study was carried out following the Helsinki Declaration [10] and was approved by the local ethical committee of the Endemic Medicine Department, Kasr Alainy Hospital, Cairo University; hence, it did not have an ethics committee's reference number.

Competing interests
No competing interests

Author details
[1]Endemic Medicine and Hepatology Department, Cairo University, Cairo, Egypt. [2]Internal Medicine Department, Endocrine Section, Faculty of Medicine, Cairo University, Cairo, Egypt. [3]Pathology Department, Faculty of Medicine, Cairo University, Cairo, Egypt.

References
1. Vernon G, Baranova A, Younossi ZM (2011) Systematic review: the epidemiology and natural history of non-alcoholic fatty liver disease and non-alcoholic steatohepatitis in adults. Aliment Pharmacol Ther 34(3):274–285. https://doi.org/10.1111/j.1365-2036.2011.04724.x
2. Zaki ME, Ezzat W, Elhosary YA, Saleh OM (2013) Factors associated with nonalcoholic fatty liver disease in obese adolescents Macedonian. J Med Sci 6:273–277
3. Gaggini M, Morelli M, Buzzigoli E, DeFronzo RA, Bugianesi E, Gastaldelli A (2013) Non-alcoholic fatty liver disease (NAFLD) and its connection with insulin resistance, dyslipidemia, atherosclerosis, and coronary heart disease. Nutrients 5(5):1544–1560. https://doi.org/10.3390/nu5051544
4. (2016) EASL–EASD–EASO Clinical Practice Guidelines for the management of non-alcoholic fatty liver disease. *J Hepatol* 64(6):1388–1402. https://doi.org/10.1016/j.jhep.2015.11.004
5. Ratziu V, Charlotte F, Heurtier A, Gombert S, Giral P, Bruckert E, Grimaldi A, Capron F, Poynard T, LIDO Study Group (2005) Sampling variability of liver biopsy in nonalcoholic fatty liver disease. Gastroenterology 128(7):1898–1906. https://doi.org/10.1053/j.gastro.2005.03.084
6. Chalasani N, Younossi Z, Lavine JE, Charlton M, Cusi K, Rinella M et al (2018) The diagnosis and management of nonalcoholic fatty liver disease practice guidance from the American Association for the Study of Liver Diseases. Hepatology 67(1)
7. Shah AG, Lydecker A, Murray K, Tetri BN, Contos MJ, Sanyal AJ, NASH Clinical Research Network (2009) Use of the FIB4 index for non-invasive evaluation of fibrosis in non-alcoholic fatty liver disease. Clin Gastroenterol Hepatol 7(10):1104–1112. https://doi.org/10.1016/j.cgh.2009.05.033
8. Angulo P, Hui JM, Marchesini G, Bugianesi E, George J, Farrell GC, Enders F, Saksena S, Burt AD, Bida JP, Lindor K, Sanderson SO, Lenzi M, Adams LA, Kench J, Therneau TM, Day CP (2007) The NAFLD fibrosis score: a noninvasive system that identifies liver fibrosis in patients with NAFLD. Hepatology 45(4):846–854. https://doi.org/10.1002/hep.21496
9. Fedchuk L, Nascimbeni F, Pais R, Charlotte F, Housset C, Ratziu V, the LIDO Study Group (2014) Performance and limitations of steatosis biomarkers in patients with nonalcoholic fatty liver disease. Aliment Pharmacol Ther 40(10):1209–1222. https://doi.org/10.1111/apt.12963
10. World Medical Association (2013) Declaration of Helsinki: ethical principles for medical research involving human subjects. JAMA 310:2191–2194
11. Shaheen AA, Myers RP (2007) Diagnostic accuracy of the aspartate aminotransferase-to-platelet ratio index for the prediction of hepatitis C-related fibrosis: a systematic review. Hepatology 46(3):912–921. https://doi.org/10.1002/hep.21835
12. Sterling RK, Lissen E, Clumeck N, Sola F, Correa MC, Montaner J (2006) et. al: Development of a simple noninvasive index to predict significant fibrosis patients with HIV/HCV co-infection. Hepatology 43(6):1317–1325. https://doi.org/10.1002/hep.21178
13. Lee JH, Kim D, Kim HJ, Lee CH, Yang JI Kim W, Kim YJ, Yoon JH, Cho SH, Sung MW, Lee HS (2010) Hepatic steatosis index: a simple screening tool reflecting nonalcoholic fatty liver disease. Dig Liver Dis 42(7):503–508. https://doi.org/10.1016/j.dld.2009.08.002
14. Bedogni G, Bellentani S, Miglioli L, Masutti F, Passalacqua M, Castiglione A, Tiribelli C (2006) The fatty liver index: a simple and accurate predictor of hepatic steatosis in the general population. BMC Gastroenterol 6(1):33. https://doi.org/10.1186/1471-230X-6-33
15. Kleiner DE, Brunt EM, Van Natta M, Behling C, Contos MJ, Cummings OW et al (2005) Design and validation of a histological scoring system for nonalcoholic fatty liver disease. Hepatology. 41(6):1313–1321. https://doi.org/10.1002/hep.20701
16. Brunt EM, Janney CG, Di Bisceglie AM, Neuschwander-Tetri BA, Bacon BR (1999) Nonalcoholic steatohepatitis: a proposal for grading and staging the histological lesions. Am J Gastroenterol 94(9):2467–2474. https://doi.org/10.1111/j.1572-0241.1999.01377.x
17. Kim D, Kim WR, Kim HJ, Therneau TM (2013) Association between noninvasive fibrosis markers and mortality among adults with nonalcoholic fatty liver disease in the United States. Hepatology. 57(4):1357–1365. https://doi.org/10.1002/hep.26156
18. Loomba R, Abraham M, Unal A, Wilson L, Lavine J, Doo E et al (2012) Association between diabetes, family history of diabetes, and risk of nonalcoholic steatohepatitis and fibrosis. Hepatology 56(3):943–951. https://doi.org/10.1002/hep.25772
19. Pérez-Gutiérrez OZ, Hernández-Rocha C, Candia-Balboa RA, , Arrese MA, Benítez C, Brizuela-Alcántara DC, Méndez-Sánchez N, Uribe M, Chávez-Tapia NC Validation study of systems for noninvasive diagnosis of fibrosis in nonalcoholic fatty liver disease in Latin population. Ann Hepatol 2013; 12: 416–424, 3, DOI: https://doi.org/10.1016/S1665-2681(19)31004-X.
20. Harrison SA, Torgerson S, Hayashi PH (2003) The natural history of nonalcoholic fatty liver disease: a clinical histopathological study. Am J Gastroenterol 98(9):2042–2047. https://doi.org/10.1111/j.1572-0241.2003.07659.x
21. Pais R, Charlotte F, Fedchuk L, Bedossa P, Lebray P, Poynard T, Ratziu V, LIDO Study Group (2013) A systematic review of follow-up biopsies reveals disease progression in patients with non-alcoholic fatty liver. J Hepatol 59(3):550–556. https://doi.org/10.1016/j.jhep.2013.04.027
22. Cleveland E, Bandy A, Van-Wagner LB (2018) Diagnostic challenges of nonalcoholic fatty liver disease/nonalcoholic steatohepatitis. Clin Liver Dis 11(4)
23. Castera (2018) Diagnosis of non-alcoholic fatty liver disease/non-alcoholic steatohepatitis: non-invasive tests are enough. Liver Int 38:67–70
24. Mohamed RA, Nabiha MI, ElShobakya MB, Khattab HM (2014) The value of noninvasive scoring systems for the diagnosis of advanced fibrosis in Egyptian patients with nonalcoholic fatty liver disease. Egypt Soc Intern Med 26(4):162–169. https://doi.org/10.4103/1110-7782.148151
25. Musso G, Gambino R, Cassader M, Pagano G (2011) Meta-analysis: Natural history of non-alcoholic fatty liver disease (NAFLD) and diagnostic accuracy

of non-invasive tests for liver disease severity. Ann Med 43(8):617–649. https://doi.org/10.3109/07853890.2010.518623
26. Nones RB, Ivantes CP, Pedroso MLA (2017) Can FIB4 and NAFLD fibrosis scores help endocrinologists refer patients with non-alcoholic fatty liver disease to a hepatologist? Arch Endocrinol Metab 61(3):276–281. https://doi.org/10.1590/2359-3997000000233
27. Cicero AF, D'Addato S, Reggi A, Reggiani GM, Borghi C (2013) Hepatic steatosis index and lipid accumulation product as middle-term predictors of incident metabolic syndrome in a large population sample: data from the Brisighella Heart Study. Intern Emerg Med 8(3):265–267. https://doi.org/10.1007/s11739-012-0875-9
28. Kim JH, Kwon SY, Lee SW, Lee CH (2011) Validation of fatty liver index and lipid accumulation product for predicting fatty liver in Korean population. Liver Int 31(10):1600–1601. https://doi.org/10.1111/j.1478-3231.2011.02580.x

12

Intrathoracic rupture of hydatid cyst of the liver in children: a report of two cases

Rachida Laamiri[1*], Sahla Sellami[1], Nahla Kechiche[1], Mabrouk Abdelaali[2], Mongi Mekki[1] and Mohsen Belghith[1]

Abstract

Background: Intrathoracic rupture of hepatic hydatid cyst is a rare but dangerous complication. Its occurrence in children is exceptional as diagnosis and management constitute real challenges. We report two cases of intrathoracic rupture of hepatic hydatid cyst in children.

Case presentation: Our patients were respectively 12-year-old boy and 9-year-old girl, known cases of respiratory symptoms, diagnosed initially for pleuropneumonia. The CT scan established the diagnosis of intrathoracic rupture of hepatic hydatid cyst in the pleural cavity for the first patient and in the bronchial tree for the second. An emergency surgery was performed for both. The second patient developed broncho-biliary fistulas during the post-operative course which necessitated a re-intervention. A recurrence was noted at follow-up for the second patient.

Conclusion: Intrathoracic rupture of hepatic hydatid cyst is a serious complication which can occur even in children. Its diagnosis needs a high index of suspicion. The surgical approach remains controversial and there is a lack of consensus about the best way of management. Recurrence may occur despite appropriate treatment.

Keywords: Intrathoracic rupture, Hepatic hydatid cyst, Children, Diagnosis, Management

Background

The hydatid disease is an endemic parasitic pathology in the Mediterranean countries including Tunisia that can be observed at any age [1]. The most commonly affected organ in children is the lung at first followed by liver [1, 2]. Some complicated forms can cause morbidity and mortality. Intrathoracic rupture is a rare but dangerous complication that may occur even in children with challenges in terms of diagnosis and treatment [3].

We are presenting two cases of intrathoracic rupture in children and discussing the diagnosis and management of this complication.

Case presentation

Case 1

A 12-year-old boy presented to the Paediatrics Emergency Care for dyspnea, right side chest pain, and fever of around 7 days of evolution. The physical examination revealed fever, bronchial rales, and no breath sounds on the right lung base. The chest X-ray showed moderate right-sided pleural effusion. The diagnosis of a right pleuropneumonia was initially retained and treated with antibiotics: vancomycin and cefotaxime initially for 4 days with no improvement. A thoracoabdominal CT scan was then performed showing a collapsed hydatid cyst of the hepatic dome, a detached laminated membrane in the pleural cavity (Fig. 1) with a collapse of the inferior side of the right lung, and a 3-cm breach in the right diaphragm. An emergency laparotomy via right subcostal approach was performed revealing (Fig. 2) a hydatid cyst with a tear of the superior surface on the hepatic dome without biliary fistula, a 3-cm large diaphragmatic breach through which seropurulent fluid, daughter vesicles, and germinative membrane disseminated to pleural cavity. Phreno-pulmonary and hepato-diaphragmatic disconnection were performed. The pleural cavity was irrigated with hypertonic saline through the breach with the evacuation of the membrane. Diaphragmatic closure was achieved and a

* Correspondence: lamiri.rachida@yahoo.fr
[1]Pediatric Surgery Department, University Hospital, University of Monastir, Monastir, Tunisia
Full list of author information is available at the end of the article

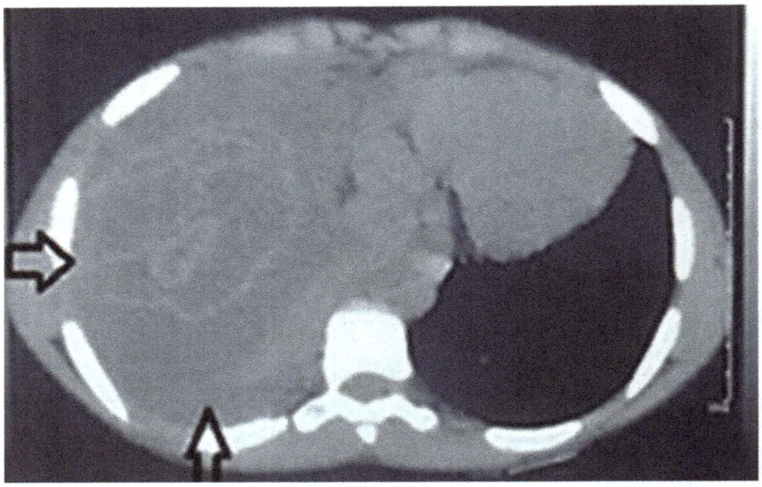

Fig. 1 CT scan showing a detached laminated membrane in the pleural cavity

chest tube was inserted. Albendazole therapy was administered for 6 months after an uneventful post-operative course. No recurrence or other hydatid localizations were detected after 2 years of follow-up.

Case 2

A 9-year-old girl presented to Pediatric Emergency Care for cough, hemoptysis, and chest pain of around 10 days of evolution. On examination, her temperature was 38.6 °C, auscultation found bronchial rales and decreased breath sound on the right lung base, and abdominal examination revealed right abdominal tenderness. Chest X-ray showed right-sided pleural effusion suggesting pleuropneumonia treated with antibiotics: penicillin and gentamicin initially with no improvement of clinical and paraclinical features after 5 days. Therefore, a thoracoabdominal CT scan was performed revealing a hydatid cyst of the hepatic dome complicated by intrathoracic rupture into the bronchial tree (Fig. 3). The patient underwent an emergency surgery via right subcostal approach. After performing diaphragmatic disconnection, exploration revealed a collapsed liver hydatid cyst and a

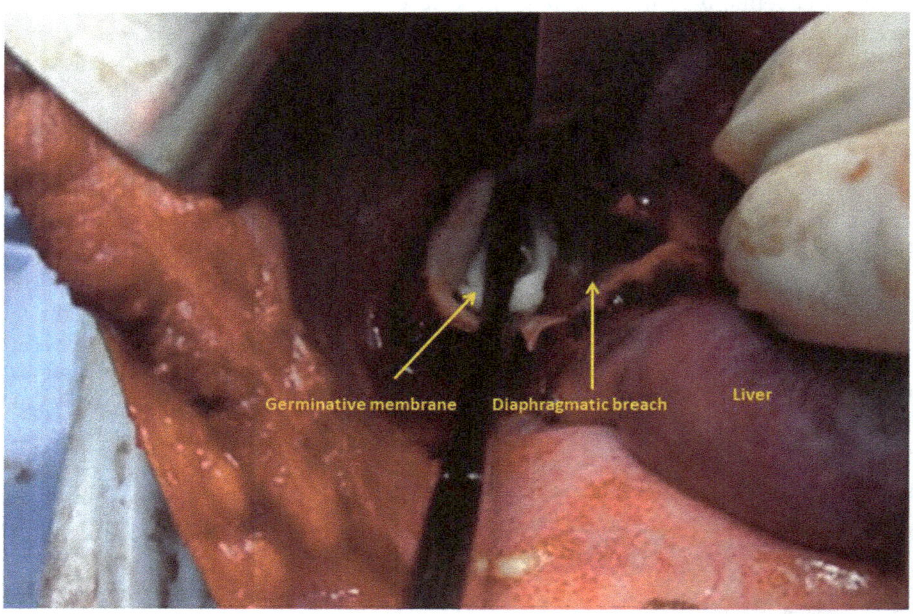

Fig. 2 Surgical specimen revealing an hydatid cyst on the hepatic dome and a 3-cm large diaphragmatic breach through which germinative membrane disseminated to pleural cavity

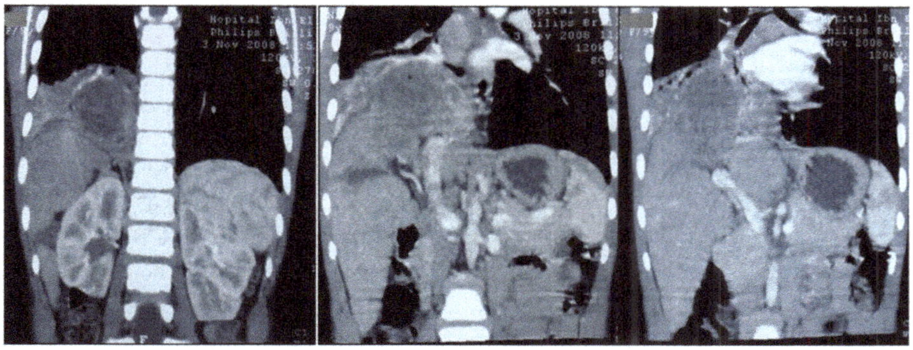

Fig. 3 CT scan revealing a hydatid cyst of the hepatic dome complicated by intrathoracic rupture into the bronchial tree

diaphragmatic breach of 5 cm through which the germinative membrane disseminated to the lung, an excision of the membrane was performed through the breach. The treatment of pulmonary lesions was impossible via abdominal approach; therefore, posterolateral thoracotomy in the sixth intercostal space was performed allowing closure of bronchial fistulas and the diaphragmatic breach; a chest tube and abdominal drain were inserted. Postoperative day (POD) 3, our patient presented biliptysis. A thoraco-abdominal CT scan was realized the next day and revealed a diaphragmatic breach with bronchobilary fistula; the patient was then re-operated via subcostal approach. A minimally biliary fistula was found, diaphragmatic closure was achieved before insertion of the drainage tube into the cystic duct. No complication appeared in evolution, and our patient was discharged 19 days after second surgery. Albendazole therapy was administered for 6 months. After 2 years of follow-up, she presented pleural hydatid cyst recurrence of 2.4 cm treated successfully with albendazole.

Discussion

Intrathoracic rupture of hepatic hydatid cyst is a rare clinical pathology with a reported frequency of 0.6 to 1.6% in adult population [4]. The rupture into the pleural cavity is less common than in the bronchial tree [5]. Several factors explain this complication: the negative intrathoracic pressure which tends to aspirate the hepatic hydatid cyst, the mechanical compression exerted by the cyst on the diaphragm leading to muscles erosion, the infection of the cyst leading to muscle necrosis, and in the case of biliary fistulas, the caustic feature of the bile caused a chemical erosion of the diaphragm, lung, and pleura [6]. This complication results from the long evolution of a hydatid cyst of the hepatic dome and generally reported in young adults [3, 7]. Caustic action on the lung or bronchial tree caused by the bile will damage the pulmonary parenchyma with lesions ranging from simple hydatid pneumonia to the constitution of a cave. Once the cyst gets through the diaphragm, different lesional aspects may result, classified according to Mestiri et al. into 4 types and 9 subtypes [8]. Referring to this classification, our patients are classified respectively as type IVb and Ib.

Intrathoracic rupture is usually revealed through respiratory and thoracic symptoms. Hydatic vomica and pathognomonic hydaticoptysis of hydatid disease are less commonly reported [3].

Chest X-ray is not very helpful. It shows a right lower lobe opacity or pleural effusion. An ultrasound exam is essential for some authors as it shows the hepatic hydatid cyst and its close connection with thoracic lesions, visualizes the diaphragmatic discontinuity, highlights thoracic lesions, and explores the biliary tract [3]. However, CT scan is more effective than ultrasound in assessing pulmonary pleural and parenchymal lesions [3]. In our patients, the chest X-ray showed right sided pleural effusion. The lack of clinical improvement leads us to suspect lung hydatid cyst rupture in the pleural cavity as our patients come from an endemic echinococcosis area. We completed this by CT scan to establish our diagnosis.

The surgical approach to treat hepatic hydatid cyst with thoracic involvement is controversial [3, 4, 9]. Surgery can be performed by thoracotomy only, thoracophrenolaparotomy, laparotomy only, or associated with thoracotomy [7]. The abdominal approach enables to treat the liver cyst, to evacuate the pleural cavity through the diaphragmatic breccia and to restore the diaphragm [9]. The treatment of pleuropulmonary lesions have been reported to represent the limitation of this approach in adult because the important lesions of the pulmonary parenchyma required a regulated resection such as lobectomy or segmentectomy [3, 7]. The thoracic approach offering adequate access to treat both thoracic and abdominal lesions is defended by some authors [4, 5, 10, 11].

In pediatrics population, surgery must be conservative and most of pulmonary lesions caused by hepatic hydatid rupture are minimal and located on the lower or middle pulmonary lobe [5, 7]. That is why we prefer abdominal approach only to treat hepatic hydatid cyst with thoracic involvement. For our first patient, given the absence of significant pleuro-pulmonary lesions, the abdominal approach proved to be effective and safe. For the second patient bronchial fistulas treatment was impossible by the laparotomy which required additional thoracic approach.

Medical adjuvant treatment is indicated when hydatid disease dissemination and total cysts resection is not possible. Albendazole (10 mg/kg/day given b.i.d) for 6 months is the current recommended therapy when indicated. Prophylactic measures should always be taken in endemic areas [11].

Despite diagnosis and therapeutic progress, this complication has high mortality and recurrence rate (7.5%; 16%) [3–5].

Conclusion

Intrathoracic rupture of hepatic hydatid cyst is a rare but a serious complication which can occur even in children. The treatment is essentially surgical; the approach is controversial and depends on the anatomic type of lesion. The prevention from this complication involves early diagnosis and primary prevention of hydatid disease.

Acknowledgements
Not applicable

Authors' contributions
RL: has drafted the work, SS: traduction (English), NK: traduction (English), AM: analyzes radiologic exams, MM: has substantively revised the work, MB: has substantively revised the work. All the authors have read and approved the manuscript.

Declarations

Ethics approval and consent to participate
We had the agreement of the ethics committee of our medical school of Monastir.

Competing interests
The authors declare that they have no competing interests.

Author details
[1]Pediatric Surgery Department, University Hospital, University of Monastir, Monastir, Tunisia. [2]Imagery Department, University Hospital, University of Monastir, Monastir, Tunisia.

References

1. M'rad S, Oudni-M'rad M, Boubaker G, Bouazzi L, Gorcii M, Nouri A et al (2012) Étude rétrospective de la distribution et de la fertilité des kystes hydatiques chez l'enfant en Tunisie. Pathol Biol (Paris) Jun 60(3):166–169. https://doi.org/10.1016/j.patbio.2011.03.002
2. Eyüboğlu TŞ, Gürsoy TR, Aslan AT, Pekcan S, Budakoğlu İİ (2019) Ten-year follow-up of children with hydatid cysts. Turk Pediatri Ars 54(3):173–178. https://doi.org/10.14744/TurkPediatriArs.2019.24119
3. Kilani T, El Hammami S, Horchani H, Ben Miled-Mrad K, Hantous S, Mestiri I et al (2001) Hydatid disease of the liver with thoracic involvement. World J Surg 1:40–45
4. Belliraj L, Alzouma II, Ammor FZ, Harmouchi H, Rabiou S, Lakrambi M et al (2017) La prise en charge des kystes hydatiques du foie (KHF) rompus dans le thorax à propos de 31 cas. Rev Mal Respir 34(Suppl):A99
5. Msougar Y, Lakranbi M, Bouchikh M, Ouadnouni Y, Maidi M, Fenan H et al (2010) La place de la thoracotomie dans le traitement des kystes hydatiques abdominaux rompus dans le thorax. Rev Mal Respir 5:417–420
6. Kilani T, Daoues A, Horchani H, Sellami M (1991) Place de la thoracotomie dans les complications thoraciques des kystes hydatiques du foie. Ann. Chir Thorac Cardiovasc 45:705
7. Rabiou S, Harmouchi H, Belliraj L, Ammor FZ, Issoufou I, Sidibé K et al (2017) Management for ruptured liver hydatid cysts in the chest: experience of a Moroccan center. Clin Surg 2:1757
8. Mestiri S, Kilani T, Thameur H, Sassi S (1987) Thoracic migrations of hydatid cysts of the liver : proposal for a classification. Lyon Chir 1:12–16
9. Sakhri J, Benali A, Letaief R, Derbel F, Dahmen Y, Ben Hadj Hmida R (1996) Les kystes hydatiques du foie rompus dans le thorax : aspects diagnostiques et thérapeutiques. J Chir 133(9-10):437–441
10. Rabiou S, Lakranbi M, Ouadnouni Y, Panaro F, Smahi M (2017) Surgical management of hydatid Bilio-bronchial fistula by exclusive thoracotomy. Int J Surg 41:112–118. https://doi.org/10.1016/j.ijsu.2017.03.074
11. Kabiri H, El Maslout A, Benosman A (2001) Thoracic rupture of hepatic hydatidosis (123 cases). Ann Thorac Surg 72(6):1883–1886. https://doi.org/10.1016/S0003-4975(01)03204-0

13

Clinical utility of ABCB1 single nucleotide polymorphism on tacrolimus dose requirements in Egyptian liver transplant patients

Azza Abd El-rahman Saab[1], Eman Saleh El-hadidi[1], Maha Mohsen Hussein[2], Maram Saeed Abd El-baki Shararah[1] and Heba Hassan Aly[1*]

Abstract

Background: Liver transplantation (LT) is the only effective radical cure for all types of end-stage liver diseases. Major advances have been made in the field of liver transplantation due to improvements in surgical techniques and organ conservation as well as optimization of intensive care and immunosuppressive management. We aimed to assess the influence of ABCB1 gene polymorphism of liver transplant recipients on blood level and dose requirements of oral tacrolimus, in an attempt to help in designing an individualized tacrolimus regimen for Egyptian liver transplant recipient. The study included 25 liver transplant recipients and their respective 25 donors. All subjects of this study were subjected to full medical history, clinical evaluation, laboratory investigations, and ABCB1 gene polymorphism evaluation by RT-PCR. Tacrolimus concentration was evaluated for all the recipients during the first 3 months post transplantation.

Results: The present study revealed that the presence of CC genotype was significantly correlated to the effect on tacrolimus C/D ratio and weight-adjusted tacrolimus dose during the first week of the first and 2nd months ($Z = -2.108$, $P < 0.05$) but not the 3rd month post transplantation (p-value >0.05). Subjects carrying CC genotype required higher doses of tacrolimus to achieve the desired trough levels compared to subjects carrying CT and TT genotypes. The same effect was observed over the whole period of the study but the results were statistically non-significant (p-value>0.05). Recipients who received liver tissue from donors carrying CC genotype also required higher doses of tacrolimus and reached lower levels of blood tacrolimus trough levels.

Conclusion: The present study revealed that ABCB1 CC genotype of both recipients and donors of liver transplantation was significantly associated with increased required tacrolimus dose early after liver transplantation reaching statistically significant level in the first week of the first and second months.

Keywords: ABCB1 single nucleotide, Polymorphism tacrolimus dose, Liver transplant

* Correspondence: hebahassan@med.asu.edu.eg
[1]Clinical Pathology Department, Faculty of Medicine, Ain Shams University, Cairo, Egypt
Full list of author information is available at the end of the article

Background

Liver transplantation (LT) is the only effective radical cure for all types of end stage liver diseases providing new hope for these patients. Immunosuppressant is the main preventive and treatment measure for organ transplant rejections. The appropriate use of immunosuppressant is directly related to the survival of the liver transplant recipients [1].

Tacrolimus is an immunosuppressant widely used in liver transplant patients. Tacrolimus is a calcineurin inhibitor, which is an enzyme that activates T-cells of the immune system. Due to its narrow therapeutic index and high inter- and intra-individual pharmacokinetic variability, the administration regimens of this drug need to be closely monitored [2]. The optimal trough levels were expected to be between 5 and 10 ng/ml for a better survival rate after liver transplantation [3].

Tacrolimus is a metabolic substrate for (CYP450) 3A enzymes in particular CYP3A5. The efflux of tacrolimus is through P-glycoprotein (P-gp) transporter, which together with CYP3A determines tacrolimus oral clearance [4].

Physiologically, P-gp is present on the surface of biliary canalicular hepatocytes, luminal surface of columnar epithelial cells of the lower gastrointestinal tract (GIT), liver, pancreas, small and large intestines, jejunum, and colon. P-gp alters the pharmacokinetics of some drugs including tacrolimus by reducing their intestinal absorption while enhancing their biliary excretion through the liver and tubular excretion in the kidney [5].

P-gp is encoded by the ABCB1 gene. Numerous single nucleotide polymorphisms occur in coding and non-coding regions which might influence mRNA expression and protein translation and folding, and finally affect drug pharmacokinetic characteristics [6].

Many studies revealed that substitution of cytosine (C) by thymine (T) in the ABCB1 gene in exon 27 was connected with the change of expression and activity of P-gp [7].

Aim of the work

The aim of the present work was to assess the influence of ABCB1 gene polymorphism of liver transplant recipients and their respective donors on blood level and dose requirements of oral tacrolimus, in an attempt to help in designing an individualized tacrolimus regimen for Egyptian liver transplant recipient.

Methods

This study is a cross-sectional study which was conducted from February 2020 to October 2020 on twenty-five (25) liver transplant recipients and their respective donors. They were recruited from Ain Shams Center of Organ Transplantation (ASCOT). An informed verbal consent was taken from all participants. The study protocol was approved by the Research Ethics Committee at Ain Shams University Faculty of Medicine.

Liver transplantation recipients (*n*=25)

This group included twenty-five (25) patients who had liver transplantation. They were 20 males and 5 females with age ranged from 36 to 67 years.

Liver transplantation donors (*n*=25)

This group included respective donors of liver transplant recipients; they were 18 males and 7 females with age ranged from 18 to 41 years. Subjects who had acute rejection or graft failure, less than 18 years old, and those who developed tacrolimus-related complications early in the post transplantation period necessitating change of immunosuppressant regimen were excluded from our study.

All individuals in this study were subjected to the following

Full medical history, clinical evaluation, and laboratory investigations in the form of total and direct bilirubin, urea, and creatinine. ALT, AST, total protein and albumin, CBC, INR, determination of ABCB1 gene polymorphism using real time-polymerase chain reaction technique (RT-PCR), tacrolimus concentration/dose ratio (C/D ratio) calculated with trough concentration, and weight-standardized 24-h tacrolimus dose (mg/kg/d).

Sampling

Seven milliliters of venous blood were collected 2 h before the next tacrolimus dose under complete aseptic precautions divided into three types of tubes as follows:

Citrate vacutainer for assay of coagulation profile, plain tube containing gel for serum separation to perform AST, ALT, total protein, total and direct bilirubin, tri-potassium ethylene diamine tetra acetate "k3 EDTA" vacutainer for complete blood count (CBC), TAC concentration, and RT-PCR.

Blood collected in plain tubes was left for 20 min to clot then centrifuged at 2000–3000 RPM for 10 min. The sera were separated for assay of liver profile and serum creatinine. EDTA vacutainer collected for assay of ABCB1 polymorphism were stored at –70 °C as whole blood till the time of analysis. Repeated freezing/thawing of samples was avoided.

Methods

a. Analytical methods

1. Assay of tacrolimus trough level

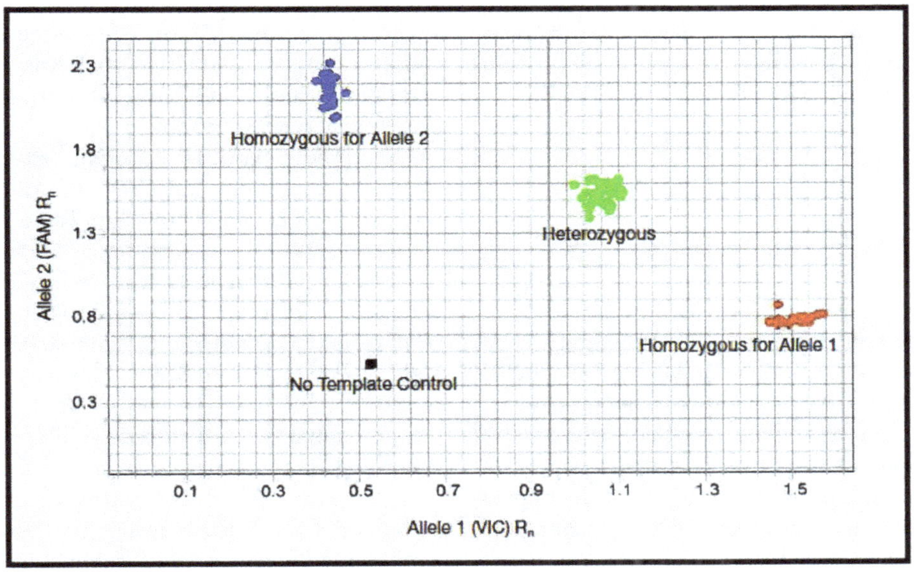

Fig. 1 Allelic discrimination plot

Done by Abbott ARCHITECT tacrolimus competitive immunoassay method with chemiluminescent microparticle immunoassay (CMIA) technology. According to the manufacturer's instructions, blood specimens were pretreated by rapidly vortex mixing of 200 μL of EDTA whole blood with 200 μL of precipitation reagent, followed by centrifugation to obtain clear supernatant for analysis. Tacrolimus in the specimen competes with tacrolimus acridinium-labeled conjugate for the available binding sites on the anti-tacrolimus antibody-coated paramagnetic microparticles. The resulting chemiluminescent signal is indirectly related to the amount of tacrolimus in the specimen.

2. Assay of ABCB1polymorphism by real-time PCR

Detection of ABCB1 polymorphism (rs1045642) was performed by TaqMan real-time PCR kit supplied by Thermo Scientific[1]. The technique was done in three main steps: extraction of genomic DNA from peripheral blood leucocytes in an EDTA whole blood sample, amplification of the extracted DNA, and allelic discrimination by real-time PCR.

Principle

TaqMan genotyping assays genotype SNPs using the 5′ nuclease assay for amplifying and detecting specific SNP alleles in purified genomic DNA samples. Each TaqMan genotyping assay contains two primers for amplifying the sequence of interest and two TaqMan probes for detecting alleles. The presence of two probe pairs in each reaction allows genotyping of the two possible variant alleles at the SNP site in a DNA target sequence. The genotyping assay determines the presence or absence of a SNP based on the change in fluorescence of the dyes associated with the probes.

Result interpretation

A substantial increase in FAM dye florescence only indicates homozygosity for allele 1 (Wild allele), substantial increase in VIC dye florescence only indicates homozygosity for allele 2 (Mutant allele), and substantial increase in both VIC and FAM dye fluorescence indicates allele 1 allele 2 heterozygosity (Fig. 1).

b. Statistical methods

Data were collected, revised, coded, and entered to the Statistical Package for Social Science (IBM SPSS) version 23 for data analysis.

The Friedman test used is a non-parametric statistical test used to detect differences in treatments across multiple test attempts. The chi-square test (χ^2) is applied to study the association between each 2 variables (Pearson chi-square) or comparison between 2 independent groups as regards the categorical data. Mann–Whitney U test is a test to compare nonparametric data.

Results

The results obtained in the present study are shown in Tables 1, 2, 3, 4, 5, 6, 7, and 8.

[1]** Thermo Scientific: 168 Third Avenue, Waltham, MA, USA 02451.

Table 1 Comparison between recipient and donors regarding ABCB1 genotype and its allele distribution (by chi-square test)

		Recipient		Donor		χ^2	P-value	Sig.
		No.	%	No.	%			
ABCB1	**CC**	11	44.0%	15	60.0%	1.377	0.502	NS
	CT	12	48.0%	9	36.0%			
	TT	2	8.0%	1	4.0%			
Allele	**C**	34	68.0%	39	78.0%	1.268	0.260	NS
	T	16	32.0%	11	22.0%			

Table 1 demonstrates descriptive and comparative statistics of the genotype and allele frequencies of ABCB1 gene polymorphism (rs1045642) between donors and recipients. The CC genotype (wild type) constituted 60% and 44% for the donors and recipients respectively, while TT genotype (Mutant type) constituted 4% of the donors and 8% of the recipients. Thirty-six (36%) of donors and 48% of recipients had CT genotype.

Follow-up for concentration/dose ratio (C/D), tacrolimus dose, and tacrolimus concentration among the recipients during the first 4 weeks post transplantation are shown in Table 2. The results of follow-up for C/D ratio and required tacrolimus dose in relation to genotype of the recipient was significant in the first week of the first month post transplantation (p-value <0.05). During the 1st week, C/D ratio median value was significantly lower in subjects with CC genotype (median (IQR) = 48) compared to subjects with TT and CT genotypes (median (IQR) = 134.9). The dose requirements needed to reach the trough level was significantly higher in subjects with CC genotype compared to subjects with TT and CT genotypes ranging (0.01–0.7mg/kg/day) and (0.01–0.09mg/kg/day) respectively (p-value <0.05). Follow-up of C/D ratio, dose, and concentration of tacrolimus in the next 3 weeks was statistically non-significant (p-value>0.05) (Table 3).

Recipients group were followed up in time intervals of 2 months and 3 months post transplantation; C/D ratio was significantly lower and required dose was significantly higher in recipients carrying CC genotype median = 63.5 compared to C/D ratio of median = 126.5 for the recipients carrying CT or TT genotype during the 2nd month post transplantation, while the effect of genotype was statistically non-significant during the 3rd month post transplantation (Table 4).

The donors' group's genotype effect on tacrolimus dose, concentration, and C/D ratio during the 1st, 2nd, and 3rd months is illustrated in Tables 5 and 6. C/D ratio during the 1st week post-transplantation was significantly higher in subjects who received liver tissue from TT and CT genotype compared to subjects who received liver tissue CC genotype (p-value <0.05), whereas the results were non-significant during the following 3 months.

Study subjects were further subdivided into 4 groups according to genotype of donor and recipient. Groups 1 and 2 are compared as regards C/D ratio, tacrolimus dose, and trough level during the first 3 months post transplantation as shown in Table 7. In these groups, the recipient genotype is CC while donor genotype is either CC or CT/TT for groups 1 and 2 respectively. C/D ratio of group 1 (median (IQR) = 44.1) compared to C/D ratio of group 2 (median (IQR) = 113) was statistically significant during the 1st week post transplantation. There was no statistical significance during the next 3 months between the 2 groups.

In groups 3 and 4, the recipient genotype is CT/TT while donor genotype is either CC or CT/TT respectively. C/D ratio, tacrolimus dose, and trough level during the 1st 3 months post transplantation in Table 8 show no statistical significance between the 2 groups.

P-value >0.05, non-significant (NS); P-value <0.05, significant (S); P-value< 0.01, highly significant (HS)

P-value >0.05, non-significant (NS); P-value <0.05, significant (S); P-value< 0.01, highly significant (HS)

P-value >0.05, non-significant (NS); P-value <0.05, significant (S); P-value< 0.01, highly significant (HS)

Discussion

Tacrolimus (also known as FK506), a calcineurin inhibitor (CNI), is the cornerstone in the immunosuppressive

Table 2 Follow-up for C/D, tacrolimus dose, and tacrolimus concentration among recipients during the first 4 weeks post transplantation (Friedman test)

		1st week No. = 25	2nd week No. = 25	3rd week No. = 25	4th week No. = 25	Test value	P-value	Sig.
C/D	**Median (IQR)**	98.8 (46–140)	95.2 (66.3–122.4)	105 (66–131.4)	117.3 (91.2–134.7)	1.289	0.732	NS
	Range	22.5–350	33.75–740	38.16–310	62.1–326.0			
Dose (mg/kg/day)	**Median (IQR)**	0.05 (0.03–0.07)	0.06 (0.04–0.08)	0.06 (0.04–0.08)	0.05 (0.04–0.07)	4.915	0.178	NS
	Range	0.01–0.7	0.01–4	0.02–5.2	0.02–4.5			
Trough level (ng/dl)	**Median (IQR)**	4.25 (2.40–5.30)	5.1 (3.9–6.8)	5.7 (4.5–6.9)	5.7 (5–6.5)	5.331	0.004	HS
	Range	0.9–7.9	2.7–9.6	2.9–15	1.4–14.5			

Table 3 Relation of ABCB1 genotype and C/D ratio and tacrolimus dose and concentration among the recipient group during the first month post transplantation (Mann–Whitney test)

		ABCB1		Z	*P*-value	Sig.
		CC	CT+TT			
C/D 1st wk	**Median (IQR)**	48 (39–100)	134.95 (76.6–158)	−2.108	0.035	S
	Range	32–221	22.5–350			
Tac dose (mg/kg/day)	**Median (IQR)**	0.07 (0.05–0.1)	0.04 (0.03–0.06)	−2.095	0.036	S
	Range	0.01–0.7	0.01–0.09			
Trough level (ng/dl)	**Median (IQR)**	4.14 (1.8–4.9)	4.43 (2.6–5.8)	−0.904	0.366	NS
	Range	1–6.8	0.9–7.9			
C/D 2nd wk	**Median (IQR)**	75.5 (66–113.75)	100.25 (75–147.2)	−1.123	0.262	NS
	Range	54.5–170	33.75–740			
Tac dose (mg/kg/day)	**Median (IQR)**	0.06 (0.05–0.08)	0.06 (0.04–0.08)	−0.359	0.719	NS
	Range	0.03–4	0.01–1.5			
Trough level (ng/dl)	**Median (IQR)**	4.45 (3.7–6.8)	5.6 (3.9–7.4)	−0.411	0.681	NS
	Range	2.8–8.5	2.7–9.6			
C/D 3rd wk	**Median (IQR)**	105 (60–116)	106.3 (66.24–137.5)	−0.876	0.381	NS
	Range	38.16–169	57.3–310			
Tac dose (mg/kg/day)	**Median (IQR)**	0.05 (0.04–0.09)	0.06 (0.03–0.07)	−0.358	0.720	NS
	Range	0.02–4.5	0.02–0.09			
Trough level (ng/dl)	**Median (IQR)**	5.2 (3.6–6.5)	5.8 (4.8–7.8)	−0.849	0.396	NS
	Range	3.16–10.4	2.9–15			
C/D 4th wk	**Median (IQR)**	91.2 (70.0–123.5)	122.25 (110–162)	2.1325	0.063	NS
	Range	62.1–167	72.32–326.0			
Tac dose (mg/kg/day)	**Median (IQR)**	0.06 (0.04–0.09)	0.06 (0.04–0.07)	−0.111	0.912	NS
	Range	0.02–5.2	0.03–0.1			
Trough level (ng/dl)	**Median (IQR)**	5.7 (3–6.1)	5.85 (5–8.4)	−1.233	0.217	NS
	Range	1.4–7.75	2.2–14.5			

Table 4 Relation of ABCB1 genotype and C/D ratio, tacrolimus dose, and trough levels among the recipient group 2 months and 3 months post transplantation (Mann–Whitney test)

ABCB1		CC	CT+TT	Z	*P*-value	Sig.
2nd month						
Dose	**Median (IQR)**	0.1 (0.07–0.1)	0.05(0.03–0.08)	−1.902	0.050	S
	Range	0.04–0.1	0.02–0.1			
Trough level	**Median (IQR)**	5.3(3.8–10.6)	6.65(6.05–7.8)	−0.797	0.426	NS
	Range	2.9–12.9	2.2–14.6			
C/D	**Median (IQR)**	63.5(49–106)	126.5(88.25–207.5)	−2.154	0.031	S
	Range	47–143	55–486			
3rd month						
Dose	**Median (IQR)**	0.08(0.05–0.09)	0.05(0.03–0.07)	−1.508	0.132	NS
	Range	0.02–0.1	0.01–0.1			
Trough level	**Median (IQR)**	4.95(4.5–7.4)	5.8(3.3–7)	−0.188	0.851	NS
	Range	3.2–8.8	1.4–9.1			
C/D	**Median (IQR)**	76.5(61–176)	122(84.5–147.5)	−0.469	0.639	NS
	Range	32–225	47–205			

P-value >0.05, non-significant (NS); *P*-value <0.05, significant (S); *P*-value< 0.01, highly significant (HS)

Table 5 Relation of ABCB1 genotype and C/D ratio and tacrolimus dose and concentration among the donors' group in relation to ABCB1 genotype (Mann–Whitney test)

		ABCB1		U test	P-value	Sig.
		CC	CT+TT			
C/D 1st wk	Median (IQR)	70 (34.5–132.5)	131.7 (100–160.3)	−2.164	0.030	S
	Range	22.5–350	48–294.4			
Tac dose (mg/kg/day)	Median (IQR)	0.06 (0.04–0.07)	0.04 (0.03–0.09)	−0.950	0.342	NS
	Range	0.01–0.1	0.01–0.7			
Trough level (ng/dl)	Median (IQR)	4.14 (2.10–4.60)	5.10 (2.60–6.70)	−1.526	0.127	NS
	Range	0.9–5.8	1–7.9			
C/D 2nd wk	Median (IQR)	95.2 (66.3–122.4)	93.85 (56–147.2)	−0.055	0.956	NS
	Range	33.75–187.5	54.5–740			
Tac dose (mg/kg/day)	Median (IQR)	0.06 (0.04–0.08)	0.07 (0.05–0.1)	−1.092	0.275	NS
	Range	0.03–0.1	0.01–4			
Trough level (ng/dl)	Median (IQR)	4.60 (3.70–8.00)	5.10 (4.45–6.20)	−0.361	0.718	NS
	Range	2.7–9.6	2.7–7.4			
C/D 3rd wk	Median (IQR)	78 (61.6–116)	125.75 (98.6–169)	−1.609	0.108	NS
	Range	38.16–310	57.3–200.3			
Tac dose (mg/kg/day)	Median (IQR)	0.06 (0.04–0.08)	0.06 (0.04–0.08)	−0.168	0.867	NS
	Range	0.02–0.1	0.02–5.2			
Trough level (ng/dl)	Median (IQR)	5.20 (3.60–6.50)	5.75 (5.20–7.80)	−0.971	0.331	NS
	Range	2.9–9.3	3.16–15			
C/D4th wk	Median (IQR)	122 (99.5–162)	99.45 (79.0–123.5)	0.998	0.318	NS
	Range	62.1–250	70.0–326.0			
Tac dose (mg/kg/day)	Median (IQR)	0.04 (0.03–0.06)	0.06 (0.04–0.07)	−0.926	0.355	NS
	Range	0.02–0.2	0.02–4.5			
Trough level (ng/dl)	Median (IQR)	5.60 (5.00–6.50)	6.10 (4.17–8.50)	−0.694	0.487	NS
	Range	2.2–8.4	1.4–14.5			

P-value >0.05, non-significant (NS); *P*-value <0.05, significant (S); *P*-value< 0.01, highly significant (HS)

Table 6 Relation of ABCB1 genotype and C/D ratio, tacrolimus dose, and trough levels among the donor group 2 months and 3 months post transplantation (Mann–Whitney test)

ABCB1		CC	CT+TT	U test	*P*-value	Sig.
2nd month						
Dose	Median (IQR)	0.05(0.04–0.08)	0.08(0.04–0.1)	−0.812	0.417	NS
	Range	0.02–0.1	0.03–0.1			
Trough level	Median (IQR)	6.65(5.9–8.1)	6.05(5.1–9.85)	−0.222	0.824	NS
	Range	2.2–10.6	3.8–14.6			
C/D	Median (IQR)	108(82.5–167)	86(54.5–184.5)	−0.355	0.722	NS
	Range	49–213	47–486			
3rd month						
Dose	Median (IQR)	0.05(0.03–0.06)	0.08(0.05–0.1)	−1.878	0.060	NS
	Range	0.01–0.07	0.02–0.1			
Trough level	Median (IQR)	5.4(2.1–8.2)	5.35(4.5–6.95)	−0.089	0.929	NS
	Range	1.4–9.1	3.2–7.4			
C/D	Median (IQR)	142.5(71–150)	90.5(59.5–119.75)	−1.422	0.155	NS
	Range	47–225	32–205			

P-value >0.05, non-significant (NS); *P*-value <0.05, significant (S); *P*-value< 0.01, highly significant (HS)

Table 7 C/D ratio in correlation with different genotype of donor when recipient genotype is CC (Mann–Whitney test)

		Group 1 (CC/CC) No. = 7	Group 2 (CC/CT or TT) No. = 4	U test	*P*-value	Sig.
1st wk						
C/D ratio	**Median (IQR)**	44.1(34.5–70)	113(74–173.5)	−2.268	0.023	S
	Range	32–75.2	48–221			
Dose	**Median (IQR)**	0.07(0.05–0.09)	0.07(0.02–0.4)	0.000	1.000	NS
	Range	0.05–0.1	0.01–0.7			
Trough level	**Median (IQR)**	4.14(2.4–4.4)	3.55(1.4–6.05)	−0.189	0.850	NS
	Range	1.6–4.9	1–6.8			
2nd wk						
C/D	**Median (IQR)**	92.5(66.3–122.4)	65.45(55.25–94.33)	−1.323	0.186	NS
	Range	66–170	54.5–113.75			
Dose	**Median (IQR)**	0.06(0.04–0.08)	0.08(0.06–2.05)	−1.245	0.213	NS
	Range	0.03–0.08	0.05–4			
Trough level	**Median (IQR)**	4.2(3.7–8.4)	4.78(3.63–5.3)	−0.379	0.705	NS
	Range	3.7–8.5	2.8–5.5			
3rd wk						
C/D	**Median (IQR)**	78(53.6–112)	125.3(82.5–157.3)	−1.136	0.256	NS
	Range	38.16–116	60–169			
Dose	**Median (IQR)**	0.06(0.04–0.09)	0.07(0.04–2.64)	−0.190	0.849	NS
	Range	0.02–0.1	0.02–5.2			
Trough level	**Median (IQR)**	5.2(3.6–6.5)	5.2(3.88–8.1)	0.000	1.000	NS
	Range	3.3–9	3.16–10.4			
4th wk						
C/D	**Median (IQR)**	99.5(63–141)	107.35(85.1–285.75)	−0.756	0.450	NS
	Range	62.1–167	79–448			
Dose	**Median (IQR)**	0.05(0.04–0.09)	0.04(0.02–2.28)	−0.579	0.563	NS
	Range	0.04–0.2	0.02–4.5			
Trough level	**Median (IQR)**	5.85(5.2–6.5)	3.51(2.13–5.14)	−1.492	0.136	NS
	Range	3–7.75	1.4–6.1			
2 months						
Dose	**Median (IQR)**	0.1(0.04–0.1)	0.09(0.07–0.1)	−0.232	0.817	NS
	Range	0.04–0.1	0.07–0.1			
Trough level	**Median (IQR)**	5.9(2.9–10.6)	4.7(3.8–12.9)	−0.218	0.827	NS
	Range	2.9–10.6	3.8–12.9			
C/D	**Median (IQR)**	73(49–106)	54(47–143)	−0.218	0.827	NS
	Range	49–106	47–143			
3 months						
Dose	**Median (IQR)**	0.05(0.02–0.07)	0.09(0.08–0.1)	−1.964	0.050	NS
	Range	0.02–0.07	0.08–0.1			
Trough level	**Median (IQR)**	5(4.5–8.8)	4.9(3.2–7.4)	−0.655	0.513	NS
	Range	4.5–8.8	3.2–7.4			
C/D	**Median (IQR)**	176(71–225)	61(32–82)	−1.528	0.127	NS
	Range	71–225	32–82			

P > 0.05, non-significant; *P* < 0.05, significant; *P* < 0.01, highly significant

Table 8 C/D ratio in correlation with different genotype of donor when recipient genotype is CT or TT (Mann–Whitney test)

		Group 3 (CT or TT/CC) No. = 8	Group 4 (CT or TT/CT or TT) No. = 6	U test	P-value	Sig.
1st wk						
C/D ratio	**Median (IQR)**	115.65(55.55–150.75)	138.7(113.5–160.3)	−0.775	0.439	NS
	Range	22.5–350	72–294.4			
Dose	**Median (IQR)**	0.05(0.04–0.06)	0.04(0.03–0.05)	−0.589	0.556	NS
	Range	0.01–0.06	0.02–0.09			
Trough level	**Median (IQR)**	4.18(1.95–4.95)	5.6(4.2–6.7)	−1.678	0.093	NS
	Range	0.9–5.8	2.6–7.9			
2nd wk						
C/D	**Median (IQR)**	100.25(65.1–126)	121.2(92.5–176.4)	−0.711	0.477	NS
	Range	33.75–187.5	54.7–740			
Dose	**Median (IQR)**	0.06(0.04–0.08)	0.07(0.04–0.1)	−0.393	0.694	NS
	Range	0.04–0.1	0.01–1.5			
Trough level	**Median (IQR)**	5.35(3.5–7.75)	5.65(5–6.3)	−0.065	0.948	NS
	Range	2.7–9.6	2.7–7.4			
3rd wk						
C/D	**Median (IQR)**	76.35(63.92–124)	125.75(98.6–196)	−0.904	0.366	NS
	Range	58–310	57.3–200.3			
Dose	**Median (IQR)**	0.07(0.05–0.07)	0.05(0.04–0.08)	−0.327	0.744	NS
	Range	0.03–0.1	0.03–0.1			
Trough level	**Median (IQR)**	5.35(4–7.7)	6.3(5.5–7.8)	−1.033	0.302	NS
	Range	2.9–9.3	5.2–15			
4th wk						
C/D	**Median (IQR)**	128.6(119.65–191)	114.45(91.4–133)	−1.291	0.197	NS
	Range	110–250	72.32–326.4			
Dose	**Median (IQR)**	0.04(0.02–0.06)	0.07(0.05–0.07)	−1.899	0.058	NS
	Range	0.02–0.07	0.04–0.09			
Trough level	**Median (IQR)**	5.15(4.75–6.55)	7.5(6.1–8.5)	−2.200	0.028	S
	Range	2.2–8.4	5.46–14.5			
2 months						
Dose	**Median (IQR)**	0.04(0.03–0.08)	0.05(0.03–0.1)	−0.575	0.565	NS
	Range	0.02–0.08	0.03–0.1			
Trough level	**Median (IQR)**	6.7(6.4–8.1)	6.2(5.9–6.8)	−0.568	0.570	NS
	Range	2.2–8.4	5.5–14.6			
C/D	**Median (IQR)**	140(94–202)	113(59–226)	−0.081	0.935	NS
	Range	82.5–213	55–486			
3 months						
Dose	**Median (IQR)**	0.04(0.03–0.06)	0.05(0.04–0.07)	−0.818	0.414	NS
	Range	0.01–0.07	0.02–0.1			
Trough level	**Median (IQR)**	5.8(1.5–8.2)	5.8(4.5–6.9)	−0.082	0.935	NS
	Range	1.4–9.1	4.5–7			
C/D	**Median (IQR)**	140(70–150)	112.5(99–127)	−0.407	0.684	NS
	Range	47–150	58–205			

$P > 0.05$, non-significant; $P < 0.05$, significant; $P < 0.01$, highly significant
Group 1 (CC/CC), group 2 (CC/CT or TT), group 3 (CT or TT/CC), and group 4 (CT or TT/CT or TT)

regimen post liver transplantation. By suppressing calcineurin activity, interleukin-2 (IL-2) production by T-cells is also reduced which affects proliferation and maturation of T-cells exerting immunosuppression effect. Therapeutic use of tacrolimus is complicated by its narrow therapeutic index, interpatient pharmacokinetics' variability, and the risk of drug interactions with co-administrated medications [8].

Passage of the drug across biological membranes is mostly regulated by membrane transporters. These membrane proteins determine the distribution of different drugs throughout the body, and they are hence major determinants of drug pharmacokinetic/pharmacodynamics profile [9]. The oral bioavailability of tacrolimus varies greatly between individuals and largely depends on the activity of cytochrome P4503A (CYP3A) subfamily and P-glycoprotein (P-gp) which is an efflux transporter encoded by the MDR1/ABCB1 [adenosine triphosphate (ATP)-binding cassette subfamily B, member 1] gene.

The ABCB1 gene has been extensively studied for characteristic polymorphisms and it has been shown that many of these polymorphisms may be linked with the function of P-glycoprotein. About 50 SNPs for ABCB1 have been identified. The most frequently studied polymorphisms for ABCB1 gene are C1236T (rs1128503), G2677T/A (rs2032582), and C3435T (rs1045642) [10]. The possible influence of genetic polymorphisms of P-gp in transplant recipients have been indicated as one of the most important variables affecting the pharmacokinetics of immunosuppressive drugs [11].

The aim of the present work was to assess the influence of ABCB1 gene polymorphism (rs1045642) of liver transplant recipients and donors on blood level and dose requirements of oral tacrolimus, in an attempt to help in designing an individualized tacrolimus regimen for Egyptian liver transplant recipient. The study was conducted on 25 patients who received liver transplantation in liver transplantation unit at Ain Shams University Specialized hospitals and their 25 respective donors.

Liver transplant recipients in the present study were given the same drug formulation through the same route of administration; they all received oral tacrolimus in the form of immediate release Prograf®.

Pediatric and elderly individuals over 65 years were excluded. This exclusion was to avoid variability in tacrolimus pharmacokinetics that might be introduced by age differences [12].

All individuals in this study were subjected to full medical history, clinical evaluation, and laboratory investigations in the form of total and direct bilirubin, urea, and creatinine. ALT, AST, total protein and albumin, CBC, INR, determination of ABCB1 gene polymorphism using real-time-polymerase chain reaction technique (RT-PCR), tacrolimus blood concentration using chemiluminescent microparticle immunoassay (CMIA) tacrolimus assay on the Abbott Architect® analyzer. Concentration/dose ratio (C/D ratio) calculated with trough concentration and weight-standardized 24-h tacrolimus dose (mg/kg/d).

In the present study, ABCB1 CC genotype was detected in 11 (44%) recipients and 14 (56%) were CT and TT genotype, while the donors with CC genotype were 15 (60%) and those with CT/TT genotype were 10 (40%), respectively.

The genotype distribution of our study was similar to a study by Abd El-Hakim et al. [13] who reported the presence of CT and TT genotypes in 26 recipients (54%) while CC genotype was detected in 22 subjects (45.8%) of the enrolled 48 subjects. On the other hand, Venuto et al. [14] reported that of 149 American patients, 57 (38.3%) were CC genotype while 92 patients (61.7%) were CT/TT genotype. Moreover, Denga et al. [15] who genotyped 136 Chinese liver transplant recipients for ABCB1 polymorphism also found that 52 subjects (38.2%) were CC genotype while 84 subjects (61.7%) were CT/TT genotypes.

Similarly, Bonate et al. [16] showed that genotype distribution differs between races (African, American and Caucasians) affecting required doses in order to attain comparable tacrolimus levels. Ethnic variations would explain the different genotype distribution reported by different studies.

In our study, tacrolimus daily dose was significantly increased to achieve adequate levels among recipients carrying ABCB1 CC genotype compared to recipients carrying CT and TT genotypes during the 1st week. Thus, C/D ratio was significantly lower in recipients carrying CC genotype compared to those carrying CT or TT genotypes.

Our study subjects were followed up for 3 months. Tacrolimus dose was significantly higher in recipients with CC genotype with concomitant decrease in C/D ratio during the first week of the 2nd month. These changes were also observed during 2nd, 3rd, and 4th weeks of the first month and also during the rest of the study period although not reaching statistical significance.

It is noteworthy that during the follow-up, seven recipients experienced tacrolimus side effects as hallucinations and tacrolimus resistance by the end of 1st month requiring change of the immunosuppressant. Out of these 7 recipients, 5 were CC genotype (71.4%) and the remaining were CT genotype. These patients required high doses of tacrolimus but failed to reach the sufficient trough level for the optimum immunosuppression.

These findings were similar to the results reported by Helal et al. [7] who also observed an increase in required tacrolimus dose among recipients with CC genotype compared to CT and TT genotypes.

Staatz et al. [17] studied the effect of different genotype on tacrolimus pharmacokinetics in renal transplant patients and demonstrated a higher tacrolimus concentration and a lower dose requirement in patients with TT variant genotype than in those with the CC wild-type genotype denoting lower functional activity of P-glycoprotein in the variant genotype. This was also observed by Vafadari et al. [18] who reported that TT homozygous patients' T-cells have a less active efflux pump, hence more inhibition of the production of IL-2 resulting in a better graft survival and less graft rejection.

Moreover, in a study by Gérard et al. [19], 66 adult liver recipients receiving oral tacrolimus were included in this study. Data were collected from day 1 to day 25 post-transplantation showing an approximately 1.5-fold difference in tacrolimus estimated clearance between TT and CC recipients being higher in CC genotype.

On the other hand, Kurzawski et al. [20] found no significant difference reported for tacrolimus dose or C/D between the different ABCB1 (rs1045642) genotypes in a study held on 241 kidney transplant patients through the 1st year post transplantation.

These results were also reported by Suzuki et al. [21] who investigated a total of 80 consecutive living-donor liver transplant (LDLT) recipients on tacrolimus. Sixty (60) patients were completely followed for 7 days early after liver transplantation in order to evaluate the pharmacokinetics. No effect of ABCB1 polymorphism on the required dose was observed.

A similar non-significant result by [22] was also reported in meta-analysis carried out to evaluate how recipient ABCB1 (n = 318) genotypes influence tacrolimus pharmacokinetics till 1 month of transplantation. It was reported that the recipient ABCB1 3435 C > T polymorphism has no significant influence on tacrolimus pharmacokinetics till 1 month of transplant.

A follow-up study of 51 Caucasian patients by Provenzani et al. [23] at 1, 3, and 6 months after transplantation as regards the ABCB1 SNPs did not show any appreciable influence on tacrolimus dosing requirements.

In the previous mentioned studies, the difference in follow-up period could possibly be an explanation as prolonged follow-up is subjected to factors such as introduction of other immunosuppressant with subsequent reduction of tacrolimus while short period of follow-up could be affected by patients loss as a result of death from complications. Also, inter-individual variability is high as regards dose modifications to reach sufficient trough levels of about (8–10 ng/dl).

To evaluate the effect of the donor genotype on the recipient response, study subjects were further subdivided into 4 groups. Recipient is CC and donor is CC in group 1. Recipient genotype is CC and donor genotype is CT/TT in group 2. Recipient is CT/TT and donor is CC in group 3, recipient genotype is CT/TT, and donor genotype is CT/TT in group 4.

Our study shows statistical significance between group 1 and 2 during the first week post transplantation as regards C/D ratio. Decreased C/D ratio in group 1 intensifies the effect of combined effect of CC genotype of recipient and donor. Sixty (60%) of donors carried CC genotype. Their corresponding recipients required higher tacrolimus dose than those who received from CT or TT genotypes. Their drug concentration was also lower which was associated with a significantly lower levels of C/D compared to 40% who received liver transplantation from CT and TT genotypes. Otherwise, the genotype had no statistical significance during the follow-up at 2 and 3 months.

Both groups 3 and 4 show no statistical significance when compared as regards C/D ratio, tacrolimus dose, or trough levels during the 1st, 2nd, and 3rd months.

A study done by Gómez-Bravo et al. [24] evaluated the impact of ABCB1 genotypes of graft and patient on tacrolimus dosage requirement and on the incidence of acute rejection among adult Caucasian Spanish liver transplant recipients. In the 98 subjects of this study, no consistent evidence has been found that the ABCB1 genotype of either recipient or the graft has a significant influence on the distribution of tacrolimus or the incidence of acute rejection or other adverse events.

The clinical outcome at 2-year follow-up study by Glowacki et al. [25] on 209 French renal transplant recipients who received tacrolimus as the main immunosuppressant did not appear to be related to the donor or recipient ABCB1 3435C>T polymorphism and no difference was reported regarding the required dose between the subjects of the study.

The effect of recipient genotype was more prominent than that of the donor's because recipients with CC genotype showed an expression of P-gp not only in the liver but also in the duodenum endothelium, kidney, adrenal gland, and pancreas two times higher compared to individuals with TT and CT genotypes while the donor effect is only related to the transplanted liver; therefore, CC-genotyped recipients experience reduced intestinal absorption of orally administered drugs including tacrolimus and enhanced biliary excretion through the liver and tubular excretion in the kidney [26].

Conclusion

The present study revealed that ABCB1 CC genotype of both recipients and donors of liver transplantation was significantly associated with increased required tacrolimus dose early after liver transplantation reaching statistically significant level in the first week of the first and second months. Further studies are recommended using a larger sample size and longer duration of follow-up.

Abbreviations

C/D ratio: Concentration dose ratio,; CYP450: Cytochrome P450; CMIA: Chemiluminescent microparticle immunoassay; CNI: Calcinurin inhibitor; IQR: Interquartile range; LT: Liver transplantation; P-gp: Permeability glycoprotein; RT-PCR: Real-time polymerase chain reaction

Acknowledgements

Not applicable

Authors' contributions

AS drafted the manuscript; HA carried out the molecular genetic studies, participated in the sequence alignment, and participated in study design. MS carried out the molecular genetic studies, participated in the sequence alignment and performed statistical analysis. MM participated in the study design. The late EE made the study design. All authors read and approved the final manuscript.

Declarations

Ethics approval and consent to participate

Research of Ethics committee, Faculty of Medicine, Ain Shams University FWA 00017585.

Competing interests

The authors declare that they have no competing interests.

Author details

[1]Clinical Pathology Department, Faculty of Medicine, Ain Shams University, Cairo, Egypt. [2]Internal Medicine, Hepatology and Gastroenterology Department, Faculty of Medicine, Ain Shams University, Cairo, Egypt.

References

1. Lu YX, Su QH, Wu KH, Ren YP, Li L, Zhou TY, Lu W (2015) A population pharmacokinetic study of tacrolimus in healthy Chinese volunteers and liver transplant patients. Acta Pharmacologica Sinica 36(2):281–288
2. Penninga L, Moller CH, Gustafsson F, Steinbruchel DA and Cluud C (2010) Tacrolimus versus cyclosporine as primary immunosuppession after heart transplantation: Systemic review with meta analysis and trial sequential analysis of randomised trials. Eur J clin pharmacol 66:1177–1187
3. Jia JJ, Lin BY, He JJ, Geng L, Kadel D, Wang L, Yu DD, Shen T, Yang Z, Ye YF, Zhou L (2014) "Minimizing tacrolimus"strategy and long-term survival after liver transplantation. World Journal of Gastroenterology: WJG 20(32):11363
4. Beckebaum S, Cicinnati VR, Radtke A, Kabar I (2013) Calcineurin inhibitors in liver transplantation–still champions or threatened by serious competitors. Liver International 33(5):656–665
5. Gameiro M, Silva R, Rocha-Pereira C, Carmo H, Carvalho F, Bastos MD, Remião F (2017) Cellular models and in vitro assays for the screening of modulators of P-gp, MRP1 and BCRP. Molecules 22(4):–600
6. Coller JK, Ramachandran J, John L, Tuke J, Wigg A, Doogue M (2019) The impact of liver transplant recipient and donor genetic variability on tacrolimus exposure and transplant outcome. British Journal of Clinical Pharmacology 85(9):2170–2175
7. Helal M, Obada M, Abd Elrazek W, Safar M, Abd El-Hakim T, El-Said H (2017) Effect of ABCB1 (3435C> T) and CYP3A5 (6986A> G) genes polymorphism on tacrolimus concentrations and dosage requirements in liver transplant patients. Egyptian Journal of Medical Human Genetics 18(3):261–268
8. Wang N, Zhang Y, Yang JW, Zhu LQ (2016) Effects on Pharmacokinetics of Tacrolimus in Liver Transplant Patients. SM J Pharmac. Ther 2(1):1012
9. Abel B, Sajid A, Lusvarghi S, Murakami M, Chufan EE, Gottesman MM, Durell SR, Ambudkar SV (2020) Reversing the direction of drug transport mediated by the human multidrug transporter P-glycoprotein. Proc Natl Acad Sci 117(47):29609–17
10. Jeleń A, Zawadzka I, Pietrzak J (2020) The impact of ABCB1 gene polymorphism and its expression on non-small-cell lung cancer development, progression and therapy – preliminary report. Sci Rep 10:6188
11. Guang L, LiQin Z, Jian WY, Yuan Z, YaQing J, Yan WZ (2015) Effects of CYP3A5 genotypes, ABCB1 C3435T and G2677T/A polymorphism on pharmacokinetics of Tacrolimus in Chinese adult liver transplant patients. Xenobiotica 45(9):840–6
12. Ebid AH, Mohamed S, Mira A, Saleh A (2019) Pharmacokinetics of tacrolimus in Egyptian liver transplant recipients: role of the classic co-variables. Journal of Advanced Pharmacy Research 3(4):182–193
13. Abd El-Hakim T, Helal M, Obada M, Abd Elrazek W, Safan M, El-Said H (2017) Effect of ABCB1 (3435C> T) and CYP3A5 (6986A> G) genes polymorphism on tacrolimus concentrations and dosage requirements in liver transplant patients. Egyptian J Med Human Genet 18(3):261–8
14. Venuto RC, Meaney CJ, Chang S, Leca N, Consiglio JD, Wilding GE, Brazeau D, Gundroo A, Nainani N, Morse SE, Cooper LM (2015) Association of extrarenal adverse effects of posttransplant immunosuppression with sex and ABCB1 haplotypes. Medicine 94(37):–1315
15. Deng, R.; Liao, Y.; Li, Y.; Tang, J (2018). Association of CYP3A5, CYP2C8, and ABCB1 polymorphisms with early renal injury in Chinese liver transplant recipients receiving tacrolimus. InTransplantation proceedings; 50(10): 3258-3265. Elsevier.
16. Bonate P, Lu Z, Keirns J (2019) Population pharmacokinetics of immediate- and prolonged-release tacrolimus formulations in liver, kidney and heart transplant recipients. Br J Clin Pharmacol 85(8):1692–703
17. Staatz CE, Goodman LK, Tett SE (2010) Effect of CYP3A and ABCB1 single nucleotide polymorphisms on the pharmacokinetics and pharmacodynamics of calcineurin inhibitors: Part I. Clinical Pharmacokinetics 49(3):141–175
18. Vafadari R, Bouamar R, Hesselink DA, Kraaijeveld R, van Schaik RH, Weimar W, Baan CC, van Gelder T (2013) Genetic polymorphisms in ABCB1 influence the pharmacodynamics of tacrolimus. Therapeutic Drug Monitoring 35(4): 459–465
19. Gérard C, Stocco J, Hulin A, Blanchet B, Verstuyft C, Durand F, Conti F, Duvoux C, Tod M (2014) Determination of the most influential sources of variability in tacrolimus trough blood concentrations in adult liver transplant recipients: a bottom-up approach. The AAPS Journal 16(3):379–391
20. Kurzawski M, Dąbrowska J, Dziewanowski K, Domański L, Perużyńska M, Droździk M (2014) CYP3A5 and CYP3A4, but not ABCB1 polymorphisms affect tacrolimus dose-adjusted trough concentrations in kidney transplant recipients. Pharmacogenomics 15(2):179–188
21. Suzuki H, Miyata Y, Akamatsu N, Sugawara Y, Kaneko J, Yamamoto T, Arita J, Sakamoto Y, Hasegawa K, Tamura S, Kokudo N (2016) Pharmacokinetics of a Once-Daily Dose of Tacrolimus Early After Liver Transplantation: With Special Reference to CYP3A5 and ABCB1 Single Nucleotide Polymorphisms. Ann Transplant 21:491–499
22. Naushad SM, Pavani A, Rupasree Y, Hussain T, Alrokayan SA, Kutala VK (2019) Recipient ABCB1, donor and recipient CYP3A5 genotypes influence tacrolimus pharmacokinetics in liver transplant cases. Pharmacological Reports 71(3):385–392
23. Provenzani A, Notarbartolo M, Labbozzetta M, Poma P, Vizzini G, Salis P, Caccamo C, Bertani T, Palazzo U, Polidori P, Gridelli B (2011) Influence of CYP3A5 and ABCB1 gene polymorphisms and other factors on tacrolimus dosing in Caucasian liver and kidney transplant patients. International Journal of Molecular Medicine 28(6):1093–1102
24. Gómez-Bravo MA, Salcedo M, Fondevila C, Suarez F, Castellote J, Rufian S, Pons JA, Alamo JM, Millán O, Brunet M (2013) Impact of donor and recipient CYP3A5 and ABCB1 genetic polymorphisms on tacrolimus dosage requirements and rejection in Caucasian Spanish liver transplant patients. The Journal of Clinical Pharmacology 53(11):1146–1154

25. Glowacki F, Lionet A, Buob D, Labalette M, Allorge D, Provôt F, Hazzan M, Noël C, Broly F, Cauffiez C (2011) CYP3A5 and ABCB1 polymorphisms in donor and recipient: impact on tacrolimus dose requirements and clinical outcome after renal transplantation. Nephrology Dialysis Transplantation 26(9):3046–3050
26. Brodin B and Saaby L (2017) A Critical View on In Vitro Analysis of P-glycoprotein (P-gp) Transport Kinetics. J Pharm Sci 106(9):2257–2264

Sofosbuvir/ledipasvir safety and efficacy for HCV patients with haemodialysis and liver cirrhosis: a small retrospective study

Ebtisam Boushi[1], Khaled Cheha[1], Noha Hedar[1], Rasha Almokdad[1], Mohammed Waleed Alassi[1] and Ameer Kakaje[2,3*]

Abstract

Background: Hepatitis C virus (HCV) infection is a high prevalent disease. Sofosbuvir/ledipasvir (SOF/LDV) can successfully treat HCV and it was until recently that SOF/LDV was approved by the FDA in haemodialysis patients, but not in patients with liver cirrhosis. This study reports patients on haemodialysis and compensated liver cirrhosis who used this regiment. This is a retrospective study on patients who were on haemodialysis and used SOF/LDV for HCV treatment in one secondary health care facility (a hospital). Treatment consisted of 400g SOF and of 90g LDV once daily. Patients were assessed for HCV RNA at the end of treatment after 12 weeks and after 24 weeks for patients. New symptoms were also assessed.

Results: Our sample contained 16 males and 5 females with a mean age of 40.9 years. Nineteen patients had no cirrhosis of the liver, and the other two had clinical and radiological cirrhosis and had Child–Turcotte–Pugh (CTP) type B. Full follow-up was for only 20 patients and they all had HCV resolved as one patient had died from a stroke. Other factors were assessed such as HCV genotypes, but treatment had the same results with no difference in symptoms development ($p>0.05$). Twelve patients had HCV genotype 1, eight patients had HCV genotype 4, and one patient had HCV genotype 5.

Conclusion: Despite the small sample size, SOF/LDV combination is suggested to be effective in patients on haemodialysis and who had compensated cirrhosis and CTP type B without the need of dose adjustment or increase duration of treatment, and there were no major complications overall.

Keywords: Cirrhosis, End-stage kidney disease, Haemodialysis, Sofosbuvir/ledipasvir, HCV

Background

Hepatitis C virus (HCV) infection has a prevalence of 3% worldwide, it is more frequent in long-term haemodialysis patients and it reached 7.5% in developed countries. Nevertheless, it was demonstrated that having a positive anti-HCV serologic was associated with a higher incidence of chronic kidney disease (CKD) in the population [1, 2]. Furthermore, there was an increase of extrahepatic manifestation in CKD patients with chronic HCV such as an increased risk of 51% of proteinuria [2]. Moreover, haemodialysis itself is a major risk for HCV despite blood testing which is one of major causes of chronic liver disease in such patients [3], and it substantially increases mortality [4].

Antiviral therapy has a positive outcome on patients on haemodialysis as it increased survival [5]. Sofosbuvir/ledipasvir (SOF/LDV) combination is considered one of the treatment combinations for HCV as they have 100% eradication rate in acutely affected HCV genotype 1. Sofosbuvir is also approved for genotypes 1 through 6

*Correspondence: ameer.kakaje@hotmail.com
[2] Faculty of medicine, Damascus University, Damascus, Syria
Full list of author information is available at the end of the article

[6]. Food and Drug Administration (FDA) has recently approved for regiments containing sofosbuvir/ledipasvir (SOF/LDV) for HCV treatment in renal disease with estimated glomerular filtration rate (eGFR) <30 and haemodialysis [7, 8]. However, not much data about using this regime in decompensating liver disease is available. And therefore it is still not recommended [9]. SOF/LDV treatment can go for 12 weeks, and the recommended doses were at 400 mg for sofosbuvir, and 90 mg for ledipasvir daily [6].

Prevalence for HCV varies across the world with developing countries having the highest rates [10]. Syria has been suffering from war since 2011, and its medical sector and economy have taken a huge hit as only 1.5 hospital beds with only 1.22 physicians were dedicated for each 1000 of population [11]. SOF/LDV combination is commonly used in Syria despite the global restrictions and high prices on drugs. These restrictions made it hard to obtain other alternatives in Syria for patients such as in cases with CKD and cirrhosis. This study contains 21 patients who used SOF/LDV regiment at Damascus Hospital although they had end-stage renal disease (ESRD) and were on haemodialysis with two patients having cirrhosis.

Methods

This study included 21 patients who presented at Damascus Hospital in the period between February 2018 and August 2019. All patients used SOF/LDV for HCV and were on haemodialysis from ESKD.

Patient and ethical consent

This study was ethically and scientifically approved by Damascus Hospital ethical committee, and gastroenterology department number 113297ب. Patient written consent was taken before administration of drugs. Risks and benefits were explained, and patients agreed on taking the drugs. Patients' oral consent was later taken for collecting and publishing their data for research purposes.

Inclusion/exclusion criteria

Our sample included patients who had HCV diagnosed by polymerase chain reaction (PCR), had ESRD (GFR <15 mL/min), and were on haemodialysis when initiating HCV treatment. PCR is the best diagnostic method in haemodialysis patients [12]. We did not enrol patients who had other severe uncontrolled comorbidities that were not directly related to HCV, cirrhosis, or renal failure, such as uncontrolled diabetes with persistent high HbA1c and severe uncontrolled hypertension. We enrolled patients who used SOF/LDV for the treatment of HCV. No patient received other treatment for HCV before initiating SOF/LDV (naïve).

Child–Turcotte–Pugh (CTP) was used to determine the severity of cirrhosis. CTP is based on multiple factors, encephalopathy, ascites, bilirubin, albumin, and prothrombin time. CTP was used as it is an easy method to use in the daily practice with a high prognostic accuracy in 6-month period [13]. Cirrhosis was diagnosed based on radiological, and clinical features, not by using invasive procedures.

Dosing

Standard doses for SOF/LDV were indicated as it was found that no adjustment is needed for ESRD patients who are on haemodialysis. Doses were 90 mg for ledipasvir, and 400 mg for sofosbuvir for once daily for 12 week [7, 8].

Progress

Only reported symptoms that newly developed or exacerbated after treatment initiation were reported. Assessment for new symptoms and routine blood tests (full blood count, urea, electrolytes, creatinine, and liver function tests) were conducted at the beginning, middle (6-week period), and at the end of treatment period which was after 12 weeks to determine if any changes in labs were transient or not and to check for new symptoms. These tests and examination were conducted 1 day before haemodialysis.

HCV PCR testing was conducted at the beginning, after 12 weeks (end treatment response or ETR), and after ETR by 12 weeks to assess sustained virological response (SVR12) as no longer follow-ups were possible (SVR24). Any patient who had haemoglobin below 11 was considered as anaemic.

Statistical analysis

Data was processed using IBM SPSS software version 25 for Windows (SPSS Inc, IL, USA). Chi-square, Fisher's exact, independent *T*, and one-way ANNOVA tests were performed to determine the statistical significance between the groups of cases and controls. Values of less than 0.05 for the two-tailed *P* values were considered statistically significant. However, multivariate tests were avoided due to large amounts of variables and small sample size.

Results

Our sample included 16 males (76.2%) and five females (23.8%) with a mean age of 40.90 ± 11.05 years. Two male patients were single (12.5%), one was engaged (6.25%), and 13 were married (81.25%). In contrast, one female patient was single (20%), and four were married (80%). While ten male patients lived in the suburbs (62.5%), and six male patients lived in an urban area (37.5%), all female patients lived in suburbs. Three males and one female patient had a history of smoking with an average of 22.5 pack/year history. None of the patients drank alcohol regularly. One patient had a haemorrhagic stroke in week 5 of treatment and died. The remaining 20 patients continued treatment until the end, and one of them had successful renal transplant after SVR12.

There were no significant differences in routine blood between before and after the treatment for all types in our research.

All patients who were followed up until SVR12 had 0 copies of HCV RNA when using PCR when finishing 12 weeks of treatment. No patient declared medication ceasing due to adverse effect or deteriorating of the symptoms. No major changes were found in liver and renal function during the study period. No major complications or deaths were declared except for one patient who had the stroke.

HCV genotypes

Ten patients (47.6%) had HCV genotype 1a, two (9.5%) genotype 1b, eight (38.1%) genotype 4, and one (4.8%) genotype 5. All females had no cirrhosis whereas two males (17.6%) had clinical and radiological findings of cirrhosis with CTP B (Fig. 1). HCV genotype 1b was associated with having a headache (p=0.047). Having a headache was also associated with female gender (p=0.026). However, having a headache overall was only in one patient. No statistically significant differences were found when comparing HCV genotype with any of the other symptoms, or smoking (p<0.05). HCV genotypes were also not associated with gender, and CTP scores (p<0.05).

CTP score and symptoms

At the end of follow-up, newly developed symptoms were recorded for 17 patients containing the two patients with CTP B. The other 3 patients' follow-ups were not valid, and the final fourth patient had a stroke at week 5.

Out of the 17 patients, four (23.5%) developed lethargy or "an increased in tiredness", one (5.9%) developed sustained headache, seven (41.2%) declared an increase of nausea, five (29.4%) declared an increased frequency of passing stools, four (23.5%) an increased dizziness, one (5.9%) an increased shortness of breath, five (29.4%) an increased insomnia, eight (47.1%) an increased arthralgia, and six (35.3%) an increased mood swings or more negative mood (Table 1).

Developing new symptoms were not statistically significantly associated with gender, or smoking (p<0.05). Developing arthralgia was insignificantly associated with smoking (p=0.072). However, CTP scores were associated with developing dizziness (p=0.007) as all patients with CTP B (2 patients) had dizziness. Moreover, CTP B was associated with a shortness of breath (p=0.005) and nausea (p=0.072) as only one patient had shortness of breath, and he had CTP type B. There were no patients

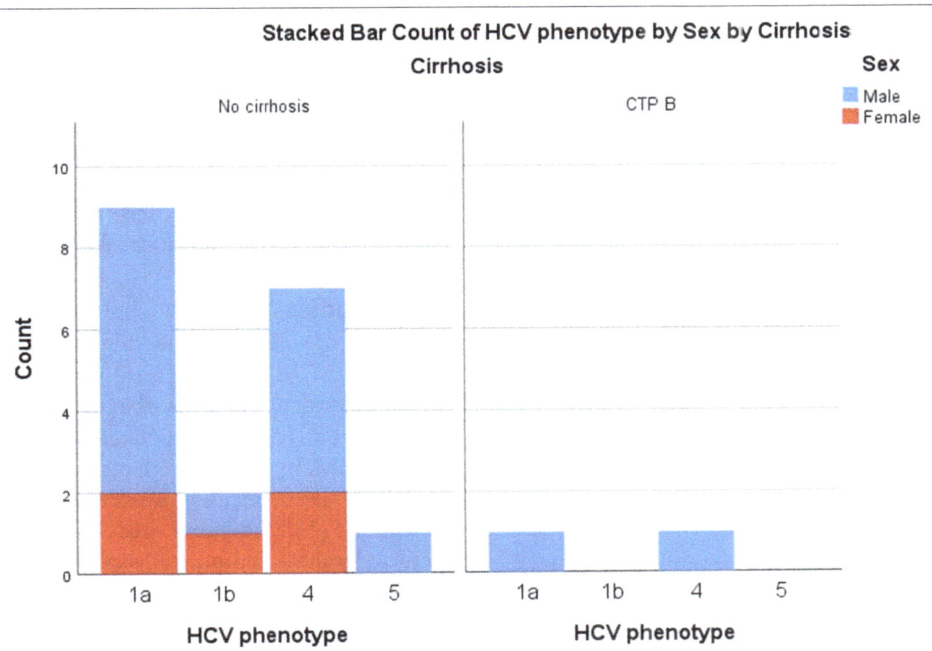

Fig. 1 HCV phenotypes and CTP of the participants

Table 1 Symptoms developed in patients after 12 weeks of treatment

Characteristic	Negative	Positive
HCV 1a (*n*=10)		
Lethargy	6	2
Headache	8	0
Nausea	4	4
Diarrhoea	6	2
Dizziness	6	2
Shortness of breath	7	1
Insomnia	5	3
Arthralgia	4	4
Mood disturbances	4	4
HCV 1b (*n*=2)		
Lethargy	1	1
Headache	1	1
Nausea	1	1
Diarrhoea	0	2
Dizziness	2	0
Shortness of breath	2	0
Insomnia	2	0
Arthralgia	1	1
Mood disturbances	2	0
HCV 4 (*n*=8)		
Lethargy	5	1
Headache	6	0
Nausea	4	2
Diarrhoea	5	1
Dizziness	4	2
Shortness of breath	6	0
Insomnia	4	2
Arthralgia	3	3
Mood disturbances	4	2
HCV 5 (*n*=1)		
Lethargy	1	0
Headache	1	0
Nausea	1	0
Diarrhoea	1	0
Dizziness	1	0
Shortness of breath	1	0
Insomnia	1	0
Arthralgia	1	0
Mood disturbances	1	0

who developed any new pulmonary, or dermatology symptoms, or coughing.

CBC and symptoms

Mean haemoglobin level and platelet count for patients who achieved SVR12 were respectively 9.04 g/dl and 201,712 $\times$ 10^9 per litter when medications were initiated, and 9.95 g/dl and 205,750 $\times$ 10^9 per litter after 12 weeks. Moreover, 16 patients had an anaemia (Hb<11 g/dl) when initiating drugs with levels ranging from 6.3 to 12.40 g/dl. No statistically significant difference was found when comparing HCV RNA copies when diagnosed, age, haemoglobin level, and platelet counts at the beginning or the end, with developing lethargy, nausea, diarrhoea, dizziness, shortness of breath, insomnia, arthralgia, and mood disturbances ($p<0.05$). There were no statistically significant differences when comparing age, haemoglobin level at the beginning or the end, HCV RNA copies when diagnosed with developing headache ($p<0.05$). However, it was found that having lower platelets when diagnosed or after 12 weeks of treatment was correlated with having a headache ($p=0.040$ and $p=0.086$ respectively).

Other variables

No statistically significant differences were found when comparing HCV RNA copies with smoking cigarettes, amount smoked, haemoglobin levels, and platelet counts ($p<0.05$).

Discussion

Our study

All patients had no evidence of HCV on PCR when followed up despite having ESRD and regardless of having CTP type B at SVR12. No significant side effects were developed regardless of having the clinical and radiological cirrhosis and CTP type B or not. No dose adjustment was required in the two patients of CTP B, and SOF/LDV was effective in patients with HCV genotypes of 1a, 1b, 4, and 5.

Interestingly, a slight improvement in anaemia and low platelets was noticed after HCV treatment for some patients. No associations were found between any of the variables of HCV genotypes, symptoms developed, HCV RNA copies when diagnosed, HCV genotypes, gender, cigarette smoking, amount smoked, and having CTP B.

Other studies

A decline of eGFR and anaemia were observed in a large study of SOF/LDV in ESRD [8]. However, using the alternative older drugs such as ribavirin, interferon (IFN) alfa, or pegylated IFN was associated with more severe anaemia [14]. Many adverse effects were noticed for LDV/SOF treatment, but they were mild to moderate in 93% of patients [15]. Fatigue, headache, insomnia, and nausea were the most common adverse effects [15], and anaemia has occurred in some patients [16]. Sofosbuvir is the first peg-interferon-free combination regimen with high SVR rates. It has fewer side effects and requires shorter treatment compared to old drugs [10, 17]. We speculated that anaemia was alleviated as the chronic infection (HCV) was resolved and thus slightly improving the anaemia, or it was just coincidental.

In decompensated liver failure, more adverse effects were found, mainly in CTP B and C. However, many studies found that most of these effects were from ribavirin [9]. Other studies also found that SVR was lower in high CTP scores with higher relapse. These studies used the same fixed dose of SOF/LDV despite the cirrhosis. However, these drugs are still not recommended in hepatic decompensation until more studies are conducted [9]. SOF/LDV is indicated in patients with HCV who did not benefit from peginterferon alfa plus ribavirin and who is treatment naïve without cirrhosis or with compensated cirrhosis [17]. In our study, regular doses were used for SOF/LDV for 12 weeks with no major side effects.

Limitations

No data was available on eGFR or ECG changes after giving the medications; data only contained full-blood count, electrolytes, liver function creatinine, and urea levels which were not substantially changed throughout the study and we could not include more tests or take more frequent test which means that there was a possibility to miss point changes in values. Some patients' follow-ups for symptoms were missing, and new symptoms could not be accurately determined if they were from medications, or other causes. No weekly visits were scheduled which could have left a gab in new or transient symptoms detection as visits and blood testing were only scheduled on the first day, 6 weeks, and 12 weeks after initiating the medication. Drugs were not administered before the haemodialysis so we could not observe the direct effect of haemodialysis on the drug. Moreover, the effect of other medications, and medical conditions, and the aetiology of ESRD and HCV were not studied. Our sample study was small, particularly for patients with cirrhosis with CTP B as they were only two patients and for patients with particular HCV genotypes. Finally, longer follow-ups were not feasible due to limited resources of the hospital and most patients not being compliant for longer follow-ups.

Conclusions

The results suggest that sofosbuvir/ledipasvir can be used in renal failure patients on haemodialysis to treat HCV genotypes 1a, 1b, 4 and 5, and when having clinical and radiological cirrhosis with CTP B. No dose adjustment or an increase of duration was required. Also, no additional severe symptoms were developed in patients with CTP B in comparison to the other patients. Treatment was administered after the haemodialysis. Further studies on larger study groups should be conducted to confirm these findings. Our sample size was small and contained only two patients with cirrhosis which was diagnosed on radiological and clinical basis.

Abbreviations

CTP: Child–Turcotte–Pugh; CKD: Chronic kidney disease; ESRD: End-stage renal disease; ETR: End treatment response; eGFR: Estimated glomerular filtration rate; Hb: Haemoglobin; HCV: Hepatitis C virus; IFN: Interferon; PCR: Polymerase chain reaction; RNA: Ribonucleic acid; SOF/LDV: Sofosbuvir/ledipasvir; SVR: Sustained virological response.

Acknowledgements

This study has a preprint on https://doi.org/10.21203/rs.3.rs-21371/v2 and on https://www.researchsquare.com/article/rs-21371/v1.

Authors' contributions

All authors adhere to the ICMJE definition of authorship and they have complete access to the study data that support the publication. EB: conceptualisation, supervision, validation, reviewing and editing the draft, project administration, and resources. KC: supervision, validation, project administration, and resources. NH: data curation, investigation, reviewing and editing the draft, supervision, visualization, resources, and software. RA: investigation, methodology, project administration, resources, and visualization. MWA: reviewing the draft and software. All authors read and approved the final manuscript. AK: visualization, writing original draft, revewing and editing, software, data curation, methodology, and formal analysis.

Declarations

Ethics approval and consent to participate

This study was ethically and scientifically approved by Damascus Hospital ethical committee, and gastroenterology department number 113297ب. Patient's written consent was taken before administration of drugs as this drug regime was not approved at the time of treatment for haemodialysis patients. Risks and benefits were explained and patients agreed on taken the drugs

Competing interests

No competing interests to declare.

Author details

[1]Gastroenterology department, Damascus Hospital, Damascus, Syria. [2]Faculty of medicine, Damascus University, Damascus, Syria. [3]University Hospital Geelong, Barwon Health, Victoria, Australia.

References

1. Goodkin DA, Bieber B, Jadoul M, Martin P, Kanda E, Pisoni RL (2017) Mortality, hospitalization, and quality of life among patients with hepatitis C infection on hemodialysis. Clin J Am Soc Nephrol 12(2):287–297
2. Fabrizi F, Verdesca S, Messa P, Martin P (2015) Hepatitis C virus infection increases the risk of developing chronic kidney disease: a systematic review and meta-analysis. Digest Dis Sci 60(12):3801–3813
3. Marinaki S (2015) Hepatitis C in hemodialysis patients. World J Hepatol 7(3):548 https://doi.org/10.4254/wjh.v7.i3.548. ISSN: 1948-5182

4. Kalantar-Zadeh K, Kilpatrick RD, McAllister CJ, Miller LG, Daar ES, Gjertson DW et al (2007) Hepatitis C virus and death risk in hemodialysis patients. J Am Soc Nephrol. 18(5):1584–1593
5. Söderholm J, Millbourn C, Büsch K (2018) et a. Higher risk of renal disease in chronic hepatitis C patients: Antiviral therapy survival benefit in patients on hemodialysis. J Hepatol. 68(5):904–911
6. Zeuzem S (2017) Treatment options in hepatitis C: the current state of the art. Deutsches Aerzteblatt Online. https://doi.org/10.3238/arztebl.2017.0011. ISSN: 1866-0452
7. AASLD-IDSA. HCV guidance: recommendations for testing, managing, and treating hepatitis C; patients with renal impairment [updated December 10, 2019; cited 2020 February 14]. Available from: https://www.hcvguidelines.org/unique-populations/renal-impairment.
8. Butt AA, Ren Y, Puenpatom A, Arduino JM, Kumar R, Abou-Samra AB (2018) Effectiveness, treatment completion and safety of sofosbuvir/ledipasvir and paritaprevir/ritonavir/ombitasvir + dasabuvir in patients with chronic kidney disease: an ERCHIVES study. Alimentary Pharmacol Ther 48(1):35–43
9. AASLD-IDSA. HCV guidance: recommendations for testing, managing, and treating hepatitis C; patients with decompensated cirrhosis [updated November 6, 2019; cited 2020 March 9]. Available from: https://www.hcvguidelines.org/unique-populations/decompensated-cirrhosis.
10. Mohamed AA, Hepatitis C (2015) Virus: a global view. World J Hepatol. 7(26):2676. https://doi.org/10.4254/wjh.v7.i26.2676. ISSN: 1948-5182
11. Agency. CgCI. Middle East :: Syria [updated FEBRUARY 20, 2020. Available from: https://www.cia.gov/library/publications/resources/the-world-factbook/geos/sy.html.
12. Firdaus R, Saha K, Biswas A, Sadhukhan PC (2015) Current molecular methods for the detection of hepatitis C virus in high risk group population: a systematic review. World J Virol. 4(1):25–32
13. Wu S-L, Zheng Y-X, Tian Z-W, Chen M-S, Tan H-Z (2018) Scoring systems for prediction of mortality in decompensated liver cirrhosis: a meta-analysis of test accuracy. World Journal of Clinical Cases. 6(15):995–1006
14. Sulkowski MS (2003) Anemia in the treatment of hepatitis C virus infection. Clinical Infectious Diseases. 37(s4):S315–SS22
15. Afdhal N, Zeuzem S, Kwo P, Chojkier M, Gitlin N, Puoti M et al (2014) Ledipasvir and sofosbuvir for untreated HCV genotype 1 infection. New England Journal of Medicine. 370(20):1889–1898
16. Ferreira VL, Assis Jarek NA, Tonin FS, Borba HHL, Wiens A, Muzzillo DA et al (2017) Ledipasvir/sofosbuvir with or without ribavirin for the treatment of chronic hepatitis C genotype 1: a pairwise meta-analysis. Journal of Gastroenterology and Hepatology. 32(4):749–755
17. Ledipasvir/sofosbuvir (Harvoni): for the treatment of cronic hepatitis C virus (CHC) G1 infection in adults [Internet]. Ottawa (ON): Canadian Agency for Drugs and Technologies in Health; 2015. https://www.ncbi.nlm.nih.gov/books/NBK362646/

15

Resuming post living donor liver transplantation in the COVID-19 pandemic: real-life experience, single-center experience

Abeer Awad Abdellatif[1*], Mohamad Sherif Mogawer[1], Mostafa El- Shazli[2], Hanaa El-Karaksy[3], Ayman Salah[2], Amany Abdel-Maqsod[1], Mona El-Amir[1], Mohamed Said[4], Naglaa Zayed[5], Karim Hosny[3], Hadeel Gamal Eldeen[6], Ayman M. A. Osman[7], Doaa A. Mansour[2], Ahmed Nabil[2], Ahmed Abdel-Ghani[1], Engy A. Mogahed[3] and Noha A. Yasin[3]

Abstract

Background: Solid organ transplantation (SOT) service has been disrupted during the current coronavirus disease 2019 (COVID-19) pandemic, which deferred the service in most centers worldwide. As the pandemic persists, there will be an urgency to identify the best and safest practices for resuming activities as areas re-open. Resuming activity is a difficult issue, in particular, the decision of reopening after a period of slowing down or complete cessation of activities.

Objectives: To share our experience in resuming living donor liver transplantation (LDLT) in the context of the COVID-19 pandemic in the Liver Transplantation Unit of El-Manial Specialized Hospital, Cairo University, Egypt, and to review the obstacles that we have faced.

Material and methods: This study is a single-center study. We resumed LDLT by the 26th of August 2020 after a period of closure from the 1st of March 2020. We have taken a lot of steps in order to prevent COVID-19 transmission among transplant patients and healthcare workers (HCWs).

Results: In our study, we reported three LDLT recipients, once resuming the transplantation till now. All our recipients and donors tested negative for SARS-CoV-2 by nasopharyngeal RT-PCR a day before the transplantation. Unfortunately, one of them developed COVID-19 infection. We managed rapidly to isolate him in a single room, restricting one team of HCWs to deal with him with strict personal protective measures. Finally, the patient improved and was discharged in a good condition. The second patient ran a smooth course apart from FK neurotoxicity which improved with proper management. The third patient experienced a sharp rise in bilirubin and transaminases on day 14 that was attributed to drug toxicity vs. rejection and managed by discontinuing the offending drugs and pulse steroids. In addition, one of our head nurses tested positive for SARS-CoV-2 that was manageable with self-isolation.

Conclusion: Careful patient, donor, personnel screening is mandatory. Adequate supply of personal protective equipments, effective infection control policies, and appropriate administrative modifications are needed for a safe return of LDLT practice.

*Correspondence: beero4a@yahoo.com
[1] Hepatogastroenterology, Liver Transplantation Unit, Internal Medicine Department, Kasr Al-Aini Hospitals, Cairo University, Kasr Al-Aini Street, Cairo PO: 11451, Egypt
Full list of author information is available at the end of the article

Keywords: COVID-19, Egypt, Liver transplantation, Single-center experience

Introduction

Since December 2019, the whole world suffers from a novel coronavirus named severe acute respiratory syndrome coronavirus-2 (SARS-CoV-2) that was declared by the World Health Organization (WHO) as a global pandemic on March 11, 2020; since then, the entire health care environment, especially liver transplant (LT) services, has been affected worldwide [1].

Solid organ transplantation (SOT) is facing many challenges that have been created during the COVID-19 pandemic. Therefore, service provision, restructuring outpatient care, careful screening, donor and recipient selection, and performing LT with limited resources should be redesigned in the post-COVID era [2].

As the pandemic persists, there will be an urgency to identify the best and safest practices for resuming activities as areas re-open. In particular, the decision about resuming SOT remains the most challenging [3].

Indeed, the limitation of data and the highly dynamic COVID-19 pandemic makes a high challenge to weigh the risks and benefits of resuming the SOT amidst fluctuating SARS-CoV-2 community transmission [3].

Owing to the long-term immunosuppressive drugs that LT recipients are exposed to, they may be more susceptible to severe COVID-19 infection with a worse prognosis when compared with the general population. The decision to defer the SOT or not, during this pandemic, is still debatable among many countries especially with the continuing increase in the number of COVID patients in those countries [4].

Many centers suggested that transplantation should be deferred, while others recommended performing transplantation under strict infection precautions and after careful risk assessments. Moreover, the decision should rely upon certain considerations, as center capability regarding the availability of beds in the intensive care unit (ICU), ventilators, and available donated blood [5].

There are still limited published data on the experience with SOT during the COVID-19 era.

Aim of the work

To share our experience in resuming living donor liver transplantation (LDLT) in the context of the COVID-19 pandemic in the Liver Transplantation Unit of El-Manial Specialized Hospital, Cairo University, Egypt, and to report the obstacles we faced.

Methodology

This study is a single-center study. Oral and written informed consents were obtained from the patients or from their eligible relatives.

We resumed the LDLT program in our unit at El-Manial Specialized Hospital, Cairo University, by the 26th of August 2020 after a period of closure from the 1st of March 2020. We planned to transplant one case every 21 days to ensure the best quality of service as well as patients' safety.

We have taken a lot of steps in order to prevent COVID-19 transmission among transplant patients and healthcare workers (HCWs) as working in small subgroups and segregating the teams taking care of immediate post-LT patients from pre-LT patients and from other patients. All organ donor teams, transplant providers, and support staff were aware of this risk and have taken appropriate respiratory contact precautions. Our transplant team members were divided into 4 teams which allowed the continuation of services if any team member became exposed to, or infected with COVID-19. We emphasized to our post-transplant patients about preventive measures that should be followed such as frequent hand washing, cleaning frequently touched surfaces, staying away from large crowds, staying away from individuals who are ill, and refraining from travel during this pandemic. Periodical training and auditing were held by the infection control team to ensure the continuous awareness with the strict infection precautions, proper donning and doffing of personal protective equipment (PPE), and also to observe that these measures were followed strictly by all the HCWs.

Measures to minimize infection risk included maintaining physical distance (1–2 m), washing hands frequently (at least 20 s with soap), minimum hospital visits after transplant and regularly disinfecting surfaces, avoiding hand-face contact as much as possible, and avoiding close contact with patients and if contact is unavoidable, the use of an N95 mask and full PPE was emphasized. All HCWs had to wear (at a minimum) a surgical mask in all clinical settings even in regular staff meetings.

All the patients (recipient and donor) were subjected to thorough history taking for the presence of fever or respiratory symptoms, as well as contact and travel history. Lastly, a COVID-19 test was performed as a final step to exclude asymptomatic COVID-19 infection before proceeding to surgery.

During the transplantation surgery and because the donor and recipient were negative for COVID-19, the surgeons did not require additional use of protective wear. However, during aerosol-generating procedures like intubation and extubation, the anesthesiologists were wearing full PPE.

Recipients were nursed strictly in a single room with only one team of nurses till discharge while applying strict standard and droplets precautions. They were monitored closely for the development of infective symptoms and tested for COVID-19 promptly if any symptoms were reported.

Furthermore, we tried to minimize the number of staff contact with the transplanted patient as possible and all non-essential contact was minimized. Periodic testing of HCWs was performed regularly (twice per month) by nasopharyngeal RT-PCR. Active surveillance was ensured in order to prevent viral spread among HCWs.

Results

First of all, before starting the transplantation process, a key point was to consider the availability of operating theater, medical staff members, and ICU beds, as these resources may be diverted to the care of patients with COVID-19.

All patients, donors, and personnel were provided with surgical masks and supplies to perform hand hygiene at the entrance of the transplant unit. Before transplantation, both living donors and recipients underwent nasopharyngeal swabs for SARS-CoV-2 by RT-PCR, as well as chest computed tomography (CT) scans the day before the transplantation. Only donors and recipients who tested negative were eligible for transplantation. Suspected or confirmed COVID-19 patients were eliminated from the donation/transplantation process.

High-performance PPE, i.e., an N95 or FFP2/FFP3 respirator, a hairnet, a double pair of gloves, a disposable waterproof surgical gown, a face shield or goggles, and work safety clogs all are supplied to all medical staff and HCWs who get in direct contact with the transplanted patient.

From the 26th of August, we transplanted three patients. All our recipients and donors tested negative for SARS-CoV-2 by nasopharyngeal RT-PCR a day before the transplantation. The first one was a 2.5-year-old child who underwent LDLT for Crigler–Najjar syndrome type I on 26/8/2020. His donor was his 35-year-old father who was medically free. On day 8 post-transplant the patient started to develop fever reaching 38.5°C. Abdominal ultrasound revealed 300 cc of clear appearing subphrenic collection secondary to a minimal biliary leak, for which a pigtail was inserted guided by ultrasonography. Culture and sensitivity of the drained fluid revealed no bacterial growth. Few days later the collection totally resolved while a low-grade fever persisted. On day 11, the patient developed high-grade fever (40°C), tachycardia (130 b/min), and tachypnea (RR=30) for which he was readmitted to the ICU, a nasopharyngeal swab for SARS-CoV-2 was done by RT-PCR and proved positive; CT chest was normal. We managed rapidly by isolating him in a single room, restricting one team of HCWs to deal with him with strict personal protective measures. Supportive treatment was described, fever resolved and the patient ran a smooth course after that (Table 1).

The second patient was a 33-year-old male patient who underwent LDLT at 27/9/2020 for cryptogenic liver cirrhosis, repeated attacks of spontaneous bacterial peritonitis (SBP), MELD 23, CHILD 11, the patient was not diabetic or hypertensive, his donor was his 37-year-old-brother who was medically free. On day 5 post-transplantation, the patient developed agitation which was considered most likely to be Tacrolimus neurotoxicity (he was on 2 mg orally twice daily; trough level was 2.6 ng/ml). Tacrolimus was discontinued together with modification of his immunosuppression regimen resulting in marvelous improvement, followed by complete resolution of his agitation. The patient was maintained on prednisone 20 mg orally twice daily and mycophenolate mofetil 1500 mg orally twice daily. He is doing fine till the time of writing the manuscript (Table 2).

Table 1 Laboratory findings of the first patient

Date	Day 1 post-transplant	On discharge	Normal value
TLC	11.9	8.1	4–11 × 10^3/mm^3
Lymphocyte	12.8	50	20–45
Hb	12	9.6	12–15 g/dl
PLT	126	382	150–450 × 10^9/L
CRP	29.6	29	Up to 5 mg/l
Urea	30	18	7–50 g/dl
Creatinine	0.5	0.3	0.60–1.30 mg/dl
Na	137	136	136–145 mmol/l
K	4.1	4.2	3.5–5.1 mmol/l
AST	1104	70	Up to 32 u/l
ALT	1029	39	Up to 35 u/l
Albumin	3.8	2.8	3.5–5.2 g/dl
T. Bilirubin	5	0.6	0.3–1.2 mg/dl
D. Bilirubin	2.5	0.18	0.1–0.3 mg/dl
GGT	37	221	Up to 35 u/l
ALP	32	398	30–120 u/l
PC%	35	86	100%
INR	2.2	1.1	1

TLC total leucocytic count, *Hb* hemoglobin, *PLT* platelet count, *CRP* C-reactive protein, *Na* sodium, *K* potassium, *AST* aspartate transaminase, *ALT* alanine transaminase, *T. Bilirubin* total bilirubin, *D. Bilirubin* direct bilirubin, *GGT* gamma-glutamyl transferase, *ALP* alkaline phosphatase, *PC%* prothrombin concentration, *INR* international normalized ratio

Table 2 Laboratory findings of the second patient

Date	Day 1 post-transplant	On discharge	Normal value
TLC	7.1	8.7	4–11 × 10^3/cmm
Lymphocyte	1050	1110	20–45
Hb	9.1	8.2	12–15 g/dl
PLT	26	276	150–450 × 10^9/L
CRP	5	43	Up to 5 mg/l
Urea	175	62	7–50 g/dl
Creatinine	1.3	1.1	0.60–1.30 mg/dl
Na	139	133	136–145 mmol/l
K	4.2	4.3	3.5–5.1 mmol/l
AST	19	32	Up to 32 u/l
ALT	17	44	Up to 35 u/l
Albumin	2.4	3	3.5–5.2 g/dl
T. Bilirubin	1.5	1.1	0.3–1.2 mg/dl
D. Bilirubin	1.1	0.45	0.1–0.3 mg/dL
GGT	58	173	Up to 35 u/l
ALP	60	127	30–120 u/l
PC%	89%	66%	100%
INR	1.12	1.3	1

TLC total leucocytic count, *Hb* hemoglobin, *PLT* platelet count, *CRP* C-reactive protein, *Na* sodium, *K* potassium, *AST* aspartate transaminase, *ALT* alanine transaminase, *T. Bilirubin* total bilirubin, *D. Bilirubin* direct bilirubin, *GGT* gamma-glutamyl transferase, *ALP* alkaline phosphatase, *PC%* prothrombin concentration, *INR* international normalized ratio

Table 3 Laboratory findings of the third patient

Date	Day 1 post-transplant	On discharge	Normal value
TLC	9.5	3.2	4-11 × 10^3/cmm
Lymphocyte	11	11.9	20–45
Hb	9	9.5	12–15 g/dl
PLT	87	59	150–450 × 10^9/L
CRP	10.8	4.8	Up to 5 mg/l
Urea	56	48	7–50 g/dl
Creatinine	0.6	0.6	0.60–1.30 mg/dl
Na	136	136	136–145 mmol/l
K	4.4	4.2	3.5–5.1 mmol/l
AST	266	40	Up to 32 u/l
ALT	197	203	Up to 35 u/l
Albumin	3.2	3.5	3.5–5.2 g/dl
T. Bilirubin	13.4	7	0.3–1.2 mg/dl
D. Bilirubin	6.6	4.4	0.1–0.3 mg/dl
GGT	31	341	Up to 35 u/l
ALP	836	216	30–120 u/l
PC%	29	71	100%
INR	2.6	1.26	1

TLC total leucocytic count, *Hb* hemoglobin, *PLT* platelet count, *CRP* C-reactive protein, *Na* sodium, *K* potassium, *AST* aspartate transaminase, *ALT* alanine transaminase, *T. Bilirubin* total bilirubin, *D. Bilirubin* direct bilirubin, *GGT* gamma-glutamyl transferase, *ALP* alkaline phosphatase, *PC%* prothrombin concentration, *INR* international normalized ratio

The third one was a 10-year-old female patient, who underwent LDLT on 14/10/2020. She had biliary atresia and underwent a Kasai porto-enterostomy at the age of 2 months. Her donor was her 32-year-old mother who was medically free. On day 14, the patient developed sudden onset of deep jaundice with steep rise in liver enzymes. These changes were attributed to drug toxicity (sulphamethoxazole-trimethoprim/fluconazole/amoxacillin-clavulanate) vs. rejection. All suspected medications were discontinued and pulse steroid (solumedrol 10 mg/kg) was administered in a single daily dose for 3 successive days with improvement in total bilirubin and transaminases; steroids were changed to oral form (30 mg/day) with gradual withdrawal (Table 3).

All our donors did well and were discharged by day 3 post-transplant.

Before discharge, all our patients were instructed to follow strict social distancing, facial masks wearing, hand washing, and self-isolation measures.

Despite all these measures, one of our head nurses developed one attack of fever reaching 38 °C with bony pain and headache, nasopharyngeal swab tested positive for SARS-CoV-2 and was managed with self-isolation only.

During our early cases following reopening, we have faced the increased financial burden of transplantation including the shortage of PPE. A major problem we have faced was the difficulty to trace the source COVID-19 infections, as this requires an additional budget, to perform testing for all HCWs who got in contact with the patient.

Discussion

All healthcare delivery services were significantly disrupted by the global pandemic of COVID-19 [6]. Surely, SOT patients are the most vulnerable group subjected to severe infection, morbidity, and mortality. They also require a high level of care through pre-transplant evaluation, transplant surgery, and post-transplant management [6, 7].

Most of the organ transplantation centers worldwide have postponed all elective organ transplantation, and now we are in the process of resuming SOT. COVID-19 pandemic has created unprecedented circumstances and unique challenges for resuming SOT worldwide. Being a highly dynamic pandemic, our understanding continues to evolve. It remains difficult to provide strong unique recommendations given the paucity of robust data to inform guidance.

Being on immunosuppressive medications, the post-transplant patients are considered at high risk for COVID-19 infection, therefore with reopening care, every effort should be taken to protect them from exposure to the virus [6].

In order to prevent possible patient-to-patient and patient-to-personnel transmission, several aspects should be systematically taken into account. Overcrowding should be always avoided and an adequate air change per hour should be maintained [8].

Many transplant centers worldwide developed a COVID-19 donor and recipient clinical screening programs such as Canada, Switzerland, Italy, and Spain. Accordingly, the Japanese Society for Transplantation established a recommendation to screen donors for significant exposure to COVID-19, travel history to high-risk countries, and symptoms including fever and respiratory symptoms together with home or hospital isolation for 14 days prior to intervention in order to avoid COVID-19 exposure for both lung and liver living donors, in cases where transplantation can be postponed for 14 days. Also, the Korean Society for Transplantation published their recommendation on March 13, 2020, for testing both living and deceased donors for SARS-CoV-2 by a nasopharyngeal swab prior to appointment. However, there is still variation in approach to donation between different countries according to the burden of COVID-19 infection and availability of service resources [9].

Preventative strategies and social distancing measures should be reinforced in living donors, especially within 14 days prior to organ donation. Moreover, a high-risk living donor is either because of COVID-19 symptoms or exposure, postponement of organ donation for at least 28 days is a must. American Society of Transplantation recommends delaying the transplant for at least 14 days if the donor is of intermediate risk for COVID-19 such as those with exposure but no symptoms [10], the donor with resolved symptoms more than 28 days prior to organ donation, and with negative testing repeatedly with at least 24 h apart [10].

The aim of this article was to share our experience in resuming the LDLT program in the context of the COVID-19 pandemic and to report the obstacles that faced us.

In our study we reported three LDLT recipients once resuming the transplantation; unfortunately, one of them developed COVID-19 infection. We managed by isolating him in a single room, restricting one team of HCWs to deal with him with full PPE supplies. Finally, the patient improved and was discharged in a reasonable condition. The second patient ran a smooth course apart from FK neurotoxicity that was managed properly. The third patient experienced a sharp rise in bilirubin and transaminases on day 14 that was attributed to drug toxicity vs. rejection and managed by discontinuing the offending drugs and pulse steroids.

Unfortunately, we were unable to trace the source of COVID-19 infection in our first case, due to the lack of accessibility of performing the test to all HCWs. As for most centers, we are also facing the problem of the increased financial burden of transplantation including and the shortage of PPE.

There are no best practices in a pandemic; therefore, managing best practices in a pandemic requires bold decisions and frequent reassessment of rationales [11].

In Wuhan, the COVID-19 pandemic greatly slowed and then stopped organ donation and transplantation, but the decrease in the number of infections has allowed hospitals in Wuhan to carefully resume deceased donor organ donation and transplantation [12].

COVID-19 infection was reported in a 55-month-old girl, 5 months after undergoing liver transplantation; she recovered completely despite the high level of received immunosuppression [13]. Another case report, records living liver donation from a COVID-19 infected donor, the donor was apparently healthy with mild symptoms; lopinavir plus ritonavir were started to the recipient then shifted to hydroxychloroquine due to drug-drug interaction. Fortunately, the result of the serial COVID-19 RT-PCR test via both nasopharyngeal swab and serum was negative. Further information on the pathogenesis and transmissibility of COVID-19 in organ transplantation is still required [14].

Hyo-Lim Hong et al. [14] and Stephen Lagana et al. [15] have reported 2 cases of donor-derived transmission of COVID-19; therefore, a strategy is needed to prevent donor-derived transmission from all potential asymptomatic carriers.

In Italy, out of 17 liver transplanted patients, 2 developed COVID-19 on postoperative days 9 and 22 [16]. On the contrary, a center in China, among six liver transplants performed during COVID-19, no complications were reported [17].

It is still confusing whether the infection source is nosocomial, donor-derived, or just delayed diagnosis of asymptomatic recipients.

Hence, the recommendations for transplantation from donors diagnosed with COVID-19 are prudent, so it is of utmost importance to screen donors for COVID-19 by epidemiological investigations and clinical history for suspected COVID-19 as well as PCR within 3 days of procurement and CT, when feasible [18].

Currently, many SOT centers across the world recommend using CT to screen asymptomatic living donors for COVID-19 in the preoperative evaluation process;

however, the American Society of Transplantation is against this issue [6].

For the exclusion of asymptomatic infection in donors, most of the centers have already adopted real-time-PCR and CT scan screening along with serology. However, without complete isolation of the transplant process from cross-contamination and the capability for identification of all asymptomatic COVID-19 patients, the levels of transplantation will not reach their baseline level as it was in the pre-COVID-19 era [6].

Indeed, all the reopening measures should be considered in the context of the pandemic where the possibility of a second peak or even further peaks is still possible.

Furthermore, every effort should be made to maintain one full set of transplant armamentaria in a COVID-19 area, when still in place, in order to perform all SOT in an isolated clean environment with minimization of the risk of COVID-19 transmission.

Finally, strategic planning and coordination will be needed to ensure the robust enrolment of SOT patients in ongoing clinical trials once routine care in the COVID-19 era is reopened.

Conclusion

In this context during the COVID-19 pandemic, resuming transplantation under the umbrella of established infection control measures is a must. The pandemic has highlighted the utmost importance of working as a team and to share knowledge and experience for the benefit of patients. Indeed, many kinds of research for COVID-19 infection whether regarding outcomes, predictive diagnostics, and management strategies including the optimal approach for resuming SOT are largely needed.

Recommendations

- We recommend COVID-19 screening for both recipient and donor prior to transplantation.
- We recommend ensuring the availability of ICU beds, ventilators, and available donated blood prior to transplantation.
- We recommend strict prevention measures for post-transplant patients including frequent handwashing, cleaning frequently touched surfaces, staying away from large crowds, staying away from individuals who are ill, and not to travel during this pandemic.
- Reopening is considered in the context of the possibility of a second peak pandemic.

Abbreviations

CHILD: Child-Pugh score; CT: Chest computed tomography; HCWs: Healthcare workers; ICU: Intensive care unit; LDLT: Living donor liver transplantation; LT: Liver transplant; MELD: Model for end-stage liver disease; PPE: Personal protective equipment; RT-PCR: Reverse transcription-polymerase chain reaction; SARS-CoV-2: Severe acute respiratory syndrome coronavirus-2; SOT: Solid organ transplantation; WHO: World Health Organization.

Acknowledgements

We would like to acknowledge our great Kasr Al Ainy Hospital, and its workers, nurses, and staff members, for all the support and help in this study and throughout our careers.

Authors' contributions

ME, KH, and AS analyzed and interpreted the patient data regarding the liver disease and the transplant from the surgical point of view. HE analyzed and interpreted the patient data regarding the liver disease and the transplant from the pediatric point of view. SM, MS, NZ, MA, and AM analyzed and interpreted the patient data regarding the liver disease and the transplant from the medical point of view. EA and NA participated in revising the manuscript and general supervision of the research group. HG, AM, and DM participated in writing the manuscript and general supervision of the research group. AN and AG collected the data. AAA was a major contributor in writing the manuscript. All authors read and approved the final manuscript.

Declarations

Ethics approval and consent to participate

The study was approved by the institutional ethical committee and from the review board of Kasr Al Ainy hospital. Oral and written informed consents were obtained from the patient or from his eligible relatives.

Competing interests

The authors declare that they have no competing interests.

Author details

[1]Hepatogastroenterology, Liver Transplantation Unit, Internal Medicine Department, Kasr Al-Aini Hospitals, Cairo University, Kasr Al-Aini Street, Cairo PO: 11451, Egypt. [2]Department of General Surgery, Liver Transplantation Unit, Kasr Al-Ainy Hospital, Faculty of Medicine, Cairo University, Cairo, Egypt. [3]Pediatrics Department, Liver Transplantation Unit, Cairo University, Cairo, Egypt. [4]Endemic Medicine, Hepatogastroenterology, Liver Transplantation Unit, Kasr Al-Ainy Hospital, Faculty of Medicine, Cairo University, Cairo, Egypt. [5]Endemic Medicine Department, Liver Transplantation unit, Kasr Al-Ainy Hospital, Faculty of Medicine, Cairo University, Cairo, Egypt. [6]Endemic Hepatology and Gastroenterology, Liver Transplantation Unit, Kasr Al-Ainy Hospital, Faculty of Medicine, Cairo University, Cairo, Egypt. [7]General & HPB Surgery, Department of General Surgery, Unit of Hepatobiliary Surgery, Liver Transplantation Unit, Kasr Al-Ainy Hospital, Faculty of Medicine, Cairo University, Cairo, Egypt.

References

1. Zhu N, Zhang D, Wang W, Li X, Yang B, Song J et al (2020) A novel coronavirus from patients with pneumonia in China, 2019. N Engl J Med 382(8):727–733
2. Niriella MA, Siriwardana RC, Perera MTPR, Narasimhan G, Chan SC, Dassanayake AS (2020) Challenges for liver transplantation during recovery from the COVID-19 pandemic: insights and recommendations. Transplant Proc:S0041-1345(20)32572-0. https://doi.org/10.1016/j.transproceed.2020.05.032 Epub ahead of print. PMID: 32586665; PMCID: PMC7269961
3. Downes KJ, Danziger-Isakov LA, Cousino MK, Green M, Michaels MG, Muller WJ, Orscheln RC, Sharma TS, Statler VA, Wattier RL, Ardura MI (2020) Return to school for pediatric solid organ transplant recipients in the United States during the COVID-19 pandemic: expert opinion on

key considerations and best practices. J Pediatric Infect Dis Soc:piaa095. https://doi.org/10.1093/jpids/piaa095 Epub ahead of print. PMID: 32750142; PMCID: PMC7454776

4. Diagnosis and Treatment Protocol for Novel Coronavirus Pneumonia (Trial Version 7) (2020) Chin Med J (Engl) 133(9):1087–1095. https://doi.org/10.1097/CM9.0000000000000819
5. Expert group on prevention and control of new coronavirus pneumonia of Chinese Preventive Medicine Association (2020) New understanding of epidemiological characteristics of COVID-19. Chin J Epidemiol 41(2):139–144
6. Kapuria D, Bollipo S, Rabiee A, Ben Yakov G, Kumar G, Siau K, Lee HW, Congly S, Turnes J, Dhanasekaran R, Lui RN (2020) Global Online Alliance for Liver Studies (GOAL). Roadmap to resuming care for liver diseases after COVID-19. J Gastroenterol Hepatol. https://doi.org/10.1111/jgh.15178 Epub ahead of print. PMID: 32656794; PMCID: PMC7404933
7. Kates OS, Fisher CE, Stankiewicz-Karita HC, Shepherd AK, Church EC, Kapnadak SG, Lease ED, Riedo FX, Rakita RM, Limaye AP (2020) Earliest cases of coronavirus disease 2019 (COVID-19) identified in solid organ transplant recipients in the United States. Am J Transplant. https://doi.org/10.1111/ajt.15944 [Epub ahead of print]
8. Atkinson J, Chartier Y, Pessoa-Silva CL, Jensen P, Li Y, Seto WH. Editors. Natural ventilation for infection control in health-care settings. WHO Guidelines 2009. Availableat:https://www.who.int/water_sanitation_health/publications/natural_ventilation/en/
9. Kumar D, Manuel O, Natori Y, Egawa H, Grossi P, Han SH, Fernández-Ruiz M, Humar A (2020) COVID-19: A global transplant perspective on successfully navigating a pandemic. Am J Transplant. https://doi.org/10.1111/ajt.15876 [Epub ahead of print]
10. American Society of Transplantation. Recommendations and guidance for organ donor testing [Internet]. 2020 [cited 2020 May 23]. Available from: https://www.myast.org/sites/default/files/COVID19%20FAQ%20Donor%20Testing%2005.19.2020_0.pdf.
11. Friedman AL, Delli Carpini KW, Ezzell C, Irving H (2020) There are no best practices in a pandemic: organ donation within the COVID-19 epicenter. Am J Transplant. https://doi.org/10.1111/ajt.16157
12. Bian X, Fan X, Wang Y (2020) Influence of asymptomatic carriers with COVID-19 on transplantation resumption in Wuhan. Transplantation. https://doi.org/10.1097/TP.0000000000003356 Epub ahead of print. PMID: 32740319; PMCID: PMC7373358
13. Morand A, Roquelaure B, Colson P, Amrane S, Bosdure E, Raoult D, Lagier JC, Fabre A (2020) Child with liver transplant recovers from COVID-19 infection. A case report. Arch Pediatr. https://doi.org/10.1016/j.arcped.2020.05.004 [Epub ahead of print]
14. Hong HL, Kim SH, Choi DL, Kwon HH (2020) A case of coronavirus disease 2019-infected liver transplant donor. Am J Transplant. https://doi.org/10.1111/ajt.15997 [Epub ahead of print]
15. Lagana SM, De Michele S, Lee MJ et al (2020) COVID-19 associated hepatitis complicating recent living donor liver transplantation. Arch Pathol Lab Med. https://doi.org/10.5858/arpa.2020-0186-SA
16. Maggi U, De Carlis L, Yiu D et al (2020) The impact of the COVID-19 outbreak on liver transplantation programmes in Northern Italy. Am J Transplant 20:1840–1848 Available from: https://onlinelibrary.wiley.com/doi/abs/10.1111/ajt.15948
17. Wang Y, Liu H, Buhler LH, Deng S (2020) Strategies to halt 2019 novel coronavirus (COVID-19) spread for organ transplantation programs at the Sichuan Academy of Medical Science and Sichuan Provincial People's Hospital, China [Internet]. Am J Transplant 20:1837–1839. https://doi.org/10.1111/ajt.15972
18. Shah MB, Lynch RJ, El-Haddad H, Doby B, Brockmeier D, Goldberg DS (2020) Utilization of deceased donors during a pandemic: an argument against using SARS-CoV-2 positive donors. Am J Transplant. https://doi.org/10.1111/ajt.15969

Potential relation between non-alcoholic fatty liver disease and glycemic and metabolic parameters in subjects without diabetes

H. Naguib[1*] and H. Kassab[2]

Abstract

Background: Nonalcoholic fatty liver disease (NAFLD) is proved to be related to insulin resistance and type 2 diabetes, and it is also not rare in individuals without diabetes. The present study attempts to identify the metabolic risk factors of NAFLD among those individuals.

Results: ALT and HbA1c levels were independently associated with NAFLD development in individuals without diabetes. Receiver operating characteristic (ROC) analysis identified the optimal cutoff point of ALT (> 19 IU/ml) with AUC = 0.731, 95% CI 0.653–0.809. On the other hand, the optimal cutoff point of HbA1c was identified to be > 5.1% with AUC = 0.665, 95% CI 0.581–0.750.

Conclusions: Early identification of NAFLD among subjects without diabetes is crucial. In this study, ALT and HbA1c cutoff values had been identified, so we suggest that inclusion of both HbA1c and ALT levels may have significant implications for prediction of NAFLD among individuals without diabetes.

Keywords: Insulin resistance, Triglycerides to high-density lipoprotein ratio, Glycosylated hemoglobin, Nonalcoholic fatty liver disease

Background

Nonalcoholic fatty liver disease (NAFLD) became a major epidemiological burden worldwide with a predictable global occurrence of 20–30% [1]. It includes a considerable variety of illnesses ranging from hepatic inflammation to fibrosis, cirrhosis, and/or liver cancer. Moreover, NAFLD is at present the most common cause of elevated liver enzymes [2]. The association between NAFLD, diabetes, and obesity owing to insulin resistance (IR) has been well proven [3, 4]. Glycosylated hemoglobin (HbA1c) is one of the advanced glycation end-products (AGEs), resulting from non-enzymatic glycation of hemoglobin. The level of HbA1c reflects the duration and severity of hyperglycemia in diabetic and non-diabetic individuals [5]. Although earlier studies showed a link between HbA1c level and the prevalence of NAFLD [6, 7], their relationship is not yet well-established especially among individuals without diabetes. Dyslipidemia is a well-known influence factor of NAFLD [8, 9]. It has been reported in 20 to 80% of NAFLD cases [10]. Recent study showed the link between NAFLD and premature cardiovascular disease through atherogenic dyslipidemia which comes from IR [11]. Triglyceride to high-density lipoprotein ratio (TG/HDL-C) has been validated as a predictive indicator for IR, type 2 diabetes, cardiovascular disease, and hypertension [12–14]. TG/HDL-C is supposed to be associated with incident NAFLD [15]. To the best of our knowledge, studies focusing specifically on NAFLD among individuals without diabetes in the general population are limited [7, 16, 17]. Therefore, we aimed to evaluate their unique metabolic characteristics and to reveal

*Correspondence: hendnaguib88@yahoo.com
[1] Internal Medicine, Hepatobiliary Unit, Department of Internal Medicine, Faculty of Medicine, Alexandria University, 17 Champollion Street, El Messallah, Alexandria 21131, Egypt
Full list of author information is available at the end of the article

the independent factors associated with NAFLD among those individuals.

Methods

Study design and participant's selection

This is a case control study included 178 participants without diabetes recruited from Hepatology outpatient clinic in Alexandria Main University Hospital. We excluded patients with alcohol consumption, viral, autoimmune, neoplastic, or hereditary liver diseases, thyrotoxicosis or hypothyroidism, fasting plasma glucose (FPG) concentration ≥ 126 mg/dl or HbA1c $\geq 6.5\%$, and hemoglobin less than 12 g/dl.

Sample size

Sample size was calculated based on previous literature [18]; an expected difference of average HbA1c between NAFLD and the control group is 0.2, and the standard deviation is 0.3. Using the level of confidence of 95% (alpha = 0.05) and power of 90 (beta = 0.10) and allocation of 1:2, the minimal sample size required to reject the null hypothesis is 50 in the NAFLD group and 100 in the control group. We targeted 53 participants with NAFLD and 125 age and sex matched control subjects to compensate the missing data.

Clinical and biochemical data

All participants were subjected to clinical examination including blood pressure, weight (Wt), standing height (Ht), and waist circumference (WC) measurements. WC was measured according to the WHO recommendation at the end of normal expiration from the midpoint between highest point of the iliac crest and lowest point of the costal margin. Body mass index (BMI) was calculated as body Wt (kg) divided by body Ht squared (m^2). Overnight fasting blood samples were obtained from the antecubital vein for complete blood count, ALT, AST, total cholesterol (TC), triglycerides (TG), high-density lipoprotein (HDL-C), low-density lipoprotein (LDL-C), fasting insulin, plasma glucose, and HbA1c analysis. TG/HDL-C ratio was calculated by dividing serum TG level by serum HDL-C level. The Homeostasis Model Assessment 2 (HOMA2) calculator was used to estimate insulin resistance (HOMA-IR) according to the updated computer based HOMA2 mode [19].

Abdominal ultrasound examination

Abdominal ultrasonography was carried out by an expert radiologist. NAFLD was defined by the presence of at least two of four sonographic criteria: diffuse hyperechoic echo-texture (bright liver), increased echo-texture compared with the kidneys, vascular blurring, and deep attenuation [20].

Ethical statement

The study was performed in alignment with revised Declaration of Helsinki (2013) and with Good Clinical Practice guidelines. Our study was approved by the Ethical Committee of Faculty of Medicine, Alexandria University (IRB No. 0304901). Informed consent was obtained from all subjects included in the study.

Statistical analysis

Analysis was done using SPSS 20.0. Chi-square test was used to compare between groups for categorical variables. Student *t* test was used to compare two groups for normally distributed quantitative variables, while Mann-Whitney test was used to compare between two groups for not normally distributed quantitative variables. Logistic regression (univariate and multivariate) was used to analyze factors associated with NAFLD. Receiver operating characteristic curve (ROC) is plotted to predict the role of HbA1c in identifying NAFLD among subjects without diabetes. It showed the performance of the cutoff point in terms of sensitivity versus 1-specificity. The area under the curve (AUC) is an estimate of the accurateness of cutoff point. Area more than 50% gives acceptable performance. *P* value less than 5% level is considered significant.

Results

Baseline characteristics of participants are shown in Table 1. The NAFLD group has significantly higher BMI, WC, HbA1c, ALT, and GGT than the control group. Regarding lipid profile, total cholesterol, LDL-C, and TG/HDL-C ratio were significantly higher in NAFLD group than the control group (Table 1). Logistic regression analysis was used to evaluate the risk factors for NAFLD in subjects without diabetes. Eighteen variables were included into the analysis (Table 2). Our results showed that HOMA-IR, ALT, BMI, HbA1c, total cholesterol, LDL-C, and TG/HDL-C ratio were significantly associated with the risk of NAFLD. Upon them, ALT and HbA1c levels were independently associated with NAFLD development after performing the multivariate analysis. Receiver operating characteristic (ROC) analysis was plotted to study the ability of ALT level and HbA1c level for discrimination between those with and without NAFLD among non-diabetic individuals. The analysis identified the optimal cutoff point of ALT to be > 19 IU/ml. The corresponding sensitivity was 73.58%, specificity was 60.80%, and area under the curve was 0.731 (95% CI 0.653–0.809) (Fig. 1). On the other hand, the optimal cutoff point of HbA1c was identified to be > 5.1% with corresponding sensitivity and specificity being 79.25% and 41.60%, respectively.

Table 1 Comparison between the two studied groups according to different parameters

	Group I ($n = 53$) Mean ± SD.	Group II ($n = 125$) Mean ± SD.	Test of sig.	P
Age (years)	50.72 ± 4.24	51.1 ± 7	$t = 0.443$	0.658
Sex: number (%)				
Male	23 (43.4%)	74 (59.2%)	$\chi^2 = 3.749$	0.053
Female	30 (56.6%)	51 (40.8%)		
Hemoglobin (g/dl)	13.3 ± 1.2	13.5 ± 0.9	$t = 1.290$	0.201
Albumin (g/dl)	4.5 ± 0.5	4.55 ± 0.45	$t = 0.024$	0.981
Diastolic BP (mmHg)	77.9 ± 6.5	78.8 ± 5.8	$t = 0.901$	0.370
Systolic BP (mmHg)	120.3 ± 11.3	121.9 ± 11.7	$t = 0.853$	0.395
Fasting plasma glucose (mg/dl)	88.2 ± 7.2	88.2 ± 12	$t = 0.012$	0.990
Fasting insulin (IU/ml)	10.9 ± 8.0	10.6 ± 7.5	$U = 3305.0$	0.981
HOMA–IR	2.3 ± 2	1.7 ± 1.4	$U = 2755.0$	0.076
ALT (IU/L)	30.3 ± 12.2	21.1 ± 10.4	$U = 1782.0$*	< 0.001*
AST (IU/L)	25.8 ± 8.4	23.8 ± 5.1	$U = 2995.0$	0.311
GGT (IU/L)	43.7 ± 15.7	15.5 ± 3.6	$U = 17.0$*	< 0.001*
BMI (kg/m²)	28.7 ± 4.5	27.1 ± 4.3	$t = 2.280$*	0.024*
HbA1c (%)	5.5 ± 0.4	5.2 ± 0.5	$U = 2217.0$*	< 0.001*
Triglycerides (mg/dl)	127.74 ± 33.41	120.58 ± 43.03	$U = 2848.0$	0.139
Total cholesterol (mg/dl)	189.2 ± 21.4	171.8 ± 31.1	$t = 3.733$*	< 0.001*
HDL (mg/dl)	49.8 ± 10.3	51.5 ± 12.7	$t = 0.873$	0.384
LDL (mg/dl)	115.3 ± 23.5	93.1 ± 23.9	$t = 5.695$*	< 0.001*
Waist circumference (cm)	110.9 ± 13.5	94.3 ± 8.2	$t = 8.292$*	< 0.001*
TG/HDL	2.7 ± 1.0	2.65 ± 2.01	$U = 2666.5$*	0.040*

Table 2 Univariate and multivariate logistic regression analysis for the parameters affecting the NAFLD group

NAFLD group	Univariate		#Multivariate	
	P	OR (95%C.I)	P	OR (95%C.I)
Age (years)	**0.713**	0.990 (0.941–1.043)		
Sex	**0.054**	1.893 (0.988–3.625)		
Hemoglobin	**0.149**	0.779 (0.555–1.094)		
Albumin	**0.980**	0.991 (0.497–1.978)		
Diastolic blood pressure	**0.344**	0.974 (0.923–1.028)		
Systolic blood pressure	**0.393**	0.988 (0.961–1.016)		
Fasting blood glucose	**0.992**	1.000 (0.971–1.030)		
Fasting insulin	**0.862**	1.004 (0.963–1.046)		
HOMA–IR	**0.035***	1.229 (1.015–1.489)	**0.187**	1.172 (0.926–1.484)
ALT	**< 0.001***	1.070 (1.039–1.102)	**< 0.001***	1.085 (1.046–1.125)
AST	**0.057**	1.049 (0.999–1.102)		
BMI (kg/m²)	**0.026***	1.085 (1.010–1.167)	**0.306**	1.050 (0.956–1.152)
HbA1c	**< 0.001***	7.194 (2.759–18.758)	**0.002***	7.110 (2.102–24.052)
Triglycerides	**0.236**	1.005 (0.997–1.013)		
Total cholesterol	**0.001***	1.024 (1.010–1.037)	**0.675**	1.006 (0.979–1.033)
HDL	**0.382**	0.988 (0.963–1.015)		
LDL	**< 0.001***	1.041 (1.024–1.058)	**0.281**	1.020 (0.984–1.057)
TG/HDL (> 2.23)	**0.037***	2.004 (1.041–3.855)	**0.622**	1.262 (0.500–3.185)

OR Odd`s ratio, *C.I* Confidence interval, *BMI* Body mass index

All variables with $P < 0.05$ were included in the multivariate analysis

*Statistically significant at $P \leq 0.05$

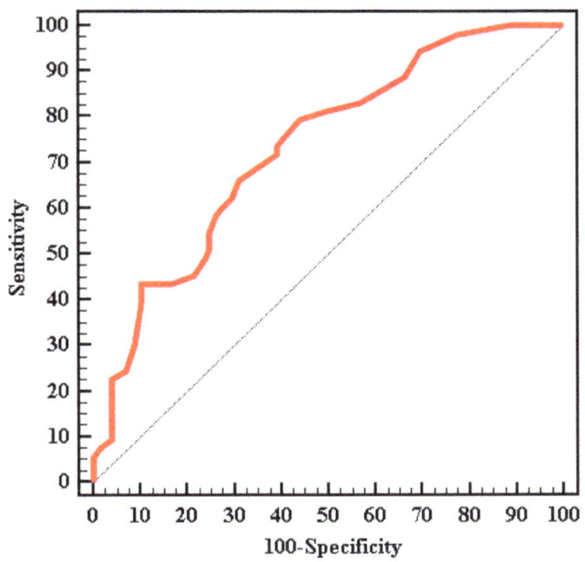

Fig. 1 ROC curve for ALT to diagnose NAFLD patients ($n = 53$ vs. 125). Cutoff value 19 IU/L, sensitivity 73.58%, specificity 60.80%, and area under the curve 0.731 (95% CI 0.653–0.809)

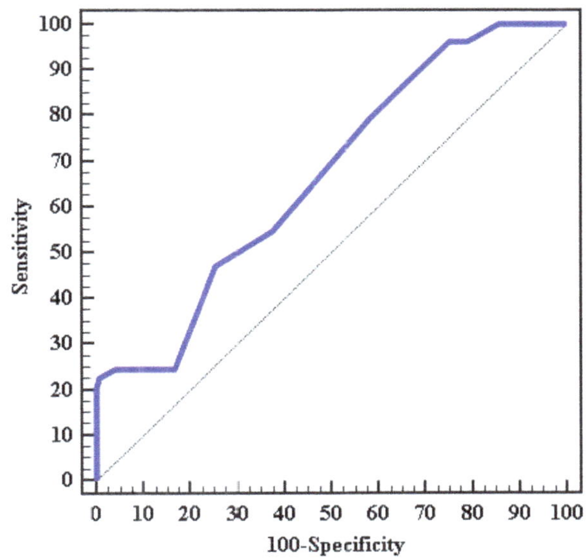

Fig. 2 ROC curve for HbA1c to diagnose NAFLD patients ($n = 53$ vs. 125). Cutoff point > 5.1%, sensitivity 79.25%, specificity 41.60%, and area under the curve 0.665 (95% CI 0.581–0.750)

The area under the curve was 0.665 (95% CI 0.581–0.750) (Fig. 2).

Discussion

Due to the high occurrence and important medical consequences of NAFLD, early diagnosis and intervention are crucial for termination of progression and even reversal of the disease [21]. Most NAFLD patients are asymptomatic and usually identified when abnormal liver studies particularly liver enzymes are noted. However, these enzymes may not be elevated in all NAFLD cases [22]. The present study showed that ALT is significantly higher in NAFLD patients than non NAFLD. In addition, our study revealed that the cutoff point of ALT > 19 IU/ml can independently predict NAFLD development among individuals without diabetes. Similarly, Wong et al. [23] revealed that raising liver enzyme levels, chiefly ALT, may predict incident diabetes and NAFLD. Similar observations were also obtained by a study among Montenegrin population, found that ALT was independent predictor for NAFLD but with a higher cutoff point of 22 IU/L [24]. These results are also consistent with that of Al Humayed et al. [25] who identified that ALT is a predictor for NAFLD with a threshold cutoff value of 22.1 nmol/L. Our lower ALT cutoff point might be explained by that the present study was done among individuals without diabetes while the participants of other studies had diabetes.

HbA1c and HOMA-IR are considered screening tools for insulin resistance [26]. The relationship between NAFLD and insulin resistance is obscure. Previous studies declared that insulin resistance is a well-established driver for NAFLD [27, 28], while another study showed that presence of NAFLD is an important marker of multi-organ insulin resistance [29]. The present study revealed that HbA1c level was independently associated with NAFLD in individuals without diabetes. These results are consistent with that of Chen et al. [7] who confirmed an association between the levels of HbA1c and NAFLD in metabolically intact patients with HbA1c levels of 5.6% or less. Similar results were obtained by Masroor et al. [16]. Independent association of NAFLD with HbA1c was also observed by Sharma et al. [17] who showed hepatic gluconeogenesis derangement in non-diabetic and non-obese subjects with NAFLD. Moreover, hemoglobin glycation index showed its ability to identify the non-diabetic individuals at risk of developing NAFLD [30]. In addition, our study showed that insulin resistance assessed by HOMA-IR is significantly positively correlated with NAFLD. These results go hand in hand with the findings of Bae et al. [31]. The question about whether or not glycemic derangement is a spectator, a cause, or a consequence of NAFLD is still unsettled. This relationship might be explained by one of the following two mechanisms. The first one is that it impaired hepatic lipid settling and increased oxidative stress in liver cells, played a crucial role in the hepatic insulin signaling, impaired insulin inhibition of hepatic glucose production, and affected insulin sensitivity in muscle and adipose tissue resulting in insulin resistance [32]. The other possible mechanism is that the insulin resistance plays an important role in NAFLD pathogenesis by allowing storage of free fatty acids in the liver [33]. Recent study showed that the activation of receptor for advanced glycation end products pathway (AGEs/RAGE) triggers further inflammation and oxidative stress and impairs insulin signaling and thus provokes the development and progression of NAFLD [34].

Obesity represents an essential risk factor for NAFLD development and progression, and weight loss can improve lipid metabolism in the liver [35]. Our study showed that high BMI is significantly associated with NAFLD. These results go hand in hand with the findings of Masroor et al. [16]. These findings can be also explained by that obesity may lead to an imbalanced production of pro- and anti-inflammatory adipokines, which contributes to NAFLD development. The other justification is that obesity is usually associated with insulin resistance and increase in HbA1c [36].

Deranged carbohydrate metabolism affects lipid metabolism and results in increased production of TG that deposits in various tissues including liver leading to fatty liver [37]. One of main features of NAFLD is dyslipidemia including increased TG, increased LDL-C, and decreased HDL-C [38].

In agreement with the results of the present study, Fukuda et al. [39] found a significant positive correlation between TG/HDL-C ratio and NAFLD, but on the other hand, Fukuda et al. [39] and Fan et al. [15], in discordance with the results of the current study, reported that TG/HDL-C ratio was an independent predictor of NAFLD. This difference could be attributed to the difference in study population and the small sample size of the current study compared to the other studies.

Though the relationship between TG/HDL-C and NAFLD has not been fully decoded, insulin resistance is a potential mediator. Compared with other lipid parameters, TG/HDL-C was declared to be strongly correlated with insulin resistance [40]. Experimentally, insulin resistance was shown to increase the secretion of TG over-enriched VLDL particles and decrease the level of HDL-C [41]. In conclusion, our results showed that serum ALT and HbA1c levels were independently associated with NAFLD in individuals without diabetes and may be used as surrogates for NAFLD in this cohort.

Conclusions

Our study had some limitations that should be taken into account. First, the diagnosis of NAFLD was performed by ultrasonography. Although ultrasonography is non-invasive, reasonably accurate, and widely used in clinical practice and epidemiological studies of NAFLD, it is not sensitive enough to identify mild steatosis. Second, the detection of the degree of steatosis and fibrosis in NAFLD patients by fibroscan is highly recommended nowadays. Unfortunately, it was not performed in the current study since it is expensive, needs special experts, and is not available in our institute. Third, there were no follow-up to confirm the results. Despite these study limitations, our study was unique in describing the predictors connected to NAFLD among individuals without diabetes in Alexandria, Egypt. Furthermore, this study highlights that the inclusion of both HbA1c and ALT levels may have significant clinical implications for prediction of NAFLD in individuals without diabetes. Thus, we suggest that individuals without diabetes with ALT values of >19 IU/ml and HbA1c>5.1% should be referred for ultrasound examination for the possibility of NAFLD.

Abbreviations

NAFLD: Nonalcoholic fatty liver disease; IR: Insulin resistance; HbA1c: Glycosylated hemoglobin; AGEs: Advanced glycation end-products; TG/HDL-C: Triglyceride to high-density lipoprotein ratio; FPG: Fasting plasma glucose; Wt: Weight; Ht: Height; WC: Waist circumference; BMI: Body mass index; ALT: Alanine transaminase; AST: Aspartate transaminase; TC: Total cholesterol; TG: Triglycerides; HDL-C : High-density lipoprotein; LDL-C: Low-density lipoprotein; HOMA: Homeostasis Model Assessment; GGT: Gamma-glutamyltransferase; ROC: Receiver operating characteristic; VLDL: Very low-density lipoprotein.

Acknowledgements

Not applicable

Authors' contributions

HN and HK have conceived and designed the study, participated in researching and analyzing data, wrote the manuscript, and approved the final version to be published.

Declarations

Competing of interests

The authors declare that they have no potential competing interests.

Ethics approval and consent to participate

The study was performed in alignment with revised Declaration of Helsinki (2013) and with Good Clinical Practice guidelines. Our study was approved by the Ethical Committee of Faculty of Medicine, Alexandria University (IRB No. 0304901). Informed consent was obtained from all subjects included in the study.

Author details

[1]Internal Medicine, Hepatobiliary Unit, Department of Internal Medicine, Faculty of Medicine, Alexandria University, 17 Champollion Street, El Messallah, Alexandria 21131, Egypt. [2]Internal Medicine, Diabetes and Metabolism Unit, Department of Internal Medicine, Faculty of Medicine, Alexandria University, Alexandria, Egypt.

References

1. Marchesini G, Day CP, Dufour JF et al (2016) EASL–EASD–EASO Clinical Practice Guidelines for the management of non-alcoholic fatty liver disease. J Hepatol. 64(6):1388–1402. https://doi.org/10.1016/J.JHEP.2015.11.004
2. Vernon G, Baranova A, Younossi ZM (2011) Systematic review: the epidemiology and natural history of non-alcoholic fatty liver disease and non-alcoholic steatohepatitis in adults. Aliment Pharmacol Ther. 34(3):274–285. https://doi.org/10.1111/J.1365-2036.2011.04724.X
3. Chalasani N, Younossi Z, Lavine JE et al (2018) The diagnosis and management of nonalcoholic fatty liver disease: practice guidance from the American association for the study of liver diseases. Hepatology. 67(1):328–357. https://doi.org/10.1002/HEP.29367
4. Association AD (2020) 4. Comprehensive medical evaluation and assessment of comorbidities: standards of medical care in diabetes—2020. Diabetes Care. 43(Supplement 1):S37–S47. https://doi.org/10.2337/DC20-S004
5. Chamberlain JJ, Rhinehart AS, Shaefer CF, Neuman A (2016) Diagnosis and management of diabetes: synopsis of the 2016 American diabetes association standards of medical care in diabetes. Ann Intern Med. 164(8):542–552. https://doi.org/10.7326/M15-3016
6. Tanaka K, Takahashi H, Hyogo H et al (2019) Epidemiological survey of hemoglobin A1c and liver fibrosis in a general population with non-alcoholic fatty liver disease. Hepatol Res. 49(3):296–303. https://doi.org/10.1111/HEPR.13282
7. Chen C, Zhu Z, Mao Y et al (2020) HbA1c may contribute to the development of non-alcoholic fatty liver disease even at normal-range levels. Biosci Rep. 40(1). https://doi.org/10.1042/BSR20193996
8. Yang SH, Du Y, Li XL et al (2017) Triglyceride to high-density lipoprotein cholesterol ratio and cardiovascular events in diabetics with coronary artery disease. Am J Med Sci. 354(2):117–124. https://doi.org/10.1016/J.AMJMS.2017.03.032
9. Wu L, Parhofer KG (2014) Diabetic dyslipidemia. Metabolism. 63(12):1469–1479. https://doi.org/10.1016/J.METABOL.2014.08.010
10. MR de A S, M de FF de M D, de JEM M-F, de MST A (2012) Metabolic syndrome and risk factors for non-alcoholic fatty liver disease. Arq Gastroenterol. 49(1):89–96. https://doi.org/10.1590/S0004-28032012000100015
11. Akhtar DH, Iqbal U, Vazquez-Montesino LM, Dennis BB, Ahmed A (2019) Pathogenesis of insulin resistance and atherogenic dyslipidemia in nonalcoholic fatty liver disease. J Clin Transl Hepatol. 7(4):362–370. https://doi.org/10.14218/JCTH.2019.00028
12. Murguía-Romero M, Jiménez-Flores JR, Sigrist-Flores SC et al (2013) Plasma triglyceride/HDL-cholesterol ratio, insulin resistance, and cardiometabolic risk in young adults. J Lipid Res. 54(10):2795–2799. https://doi.org/10.1194/JLR.M040584
13. Turak O, Afşar B, Ozcan F et al (2016) The role of plasma triglyceride/high-density lipoprotein cholesterol ratio to predict new cardiovascular events in essential hypertensive patients. J Clin Hypertens. 18(8):772–777. https://doi.org/10.1111/JCH.12758
14. Onat A, Can G, Kaya H, Hergenç G (2010) "Atherogenic index of plasma" (log10 triglyceride/high-density lipoprotein−cholesterol) predicts high blood pressure, diabetes, and vascular events. J Clin Lipidol. 4(2):89–98. https://doi.org/10.1016/J.JACL.2010.02.005
15. Fan N, Peng L, Xia Z et al (2019) Triglycerides to high-density lipoprotein cholesterol ratio as a surrogate for nonalcoholic fatty liver disease: a cross-sectional study. Lipids Heal Dis 181(1):1–6. https://doi.org/10.1186/S12944-019-0986-7
16. Masroor M, Haque Z (2021) HbA1C as a biomarker of non-alcoholic fatty liver disease: comparison with anthropometric parameters. J Clin Transl Hepatol. 9(1):15. https://doi.org/10.14218/JCTH.2019.00046
17. Sharma R, Sinha S, Danishad KA et al (2009) Investigation of hepatic gluconeogenesis pathway in non-diabetic Asian Indians with non-alcoholic fatty liver disease using in vivo (31P) phosphorus magnetic resonance spectroscopy. Atherosclerosis. 203(1):291–297. https://doi.org/10.1016/J.ATHEROSCLEROSIS.2008.06.016
18. Lin TC, Lee HM, Seo HN et al (2018) Correlation between non-alcoholic fatty liver disease and hemoglobin A1c level in adult males without diabetes. Korean J Fam Pract. 8(1):131–135. https://doi.org/10.21215/KJFP.2018.8.1.131
19. Diabetes Trials Unit: HOMA Calculator News archive. Accessed July 26, 2021. http://www.dtu.ox.ac.uk/generic/newsarchive.php?Study=91
20. Gore RM, Levine MS. Textbook of Gastrointestinal Radiology (NEED PHYSICAL COPY). Published online 2008. Accessed 26 Jul 2021. http://ucs.cirqahosting.com/HeritageScripts/Hapi.dll/retrieve2?SearchTerm0=001x000157079&Dispfmt=F
21. Cai J, Zhang X-J, Li H (2019) Progress and challenges in the prevention and control of nonalcoholic fatty liver disease. Med Res Rev. 39(1):328–348. https://doi.org/10.1002/MED.21515
22. Paschos P, Paletas K (2009) Non alcoholic fatty liver disease and metabolic syndrome. Hippokratia 13(1):9 Accessed 26 Jul 2021. /pmc/articles/PMC2633261/
23. Wong CA, Araneta MRG, Barrett-Connor E, Alcaraz J, Castañeda D, Macera C (2008) Probable NAFLD, by ALT levels, and diabetes among Filipino-American Women. Diabetes Res Clin Pract. 79(1):133–140. https://doi.org/10.1016/J.DIABRES.2007.07.012
24. Klisic A, Kavaric N, Ninic A (2019) Predictive values of serum uric acid and alanine-aminotransferase for fatty liver index in Montenegrin population. J Med Biochem. 38(4):407. https://doi.org/10.2478/JOMB-2019-0001
25. SM Al H, AA Al S, Mahfouz AA, Awadalla NJ, Musa MJ, Patel A (2020) Clinical and biochemical predictors of nonalcoholic fatty liver disease among type 2 diabetes mellitus patients at primary health care level in South Western Saudi Arabia. Diagnostics 10:809 https://doi.org/10.3390/DIAGNOSTICS10100809
26. Önal Z, Atasayan V, Gürbüz T, Hepkaya E, Nuhoğlu C (2014) Association of glycosylated hemoglobin (HbA1c) levels with Iinsulin resistance in obese children. Afr Health Sci. 14(3):533–538. https://doi.org/10.4314/ahs.v14i3.6
27. Kitade H, Chen G, Ni Y, Ota T (2017) Nonalcoholic fatty liver disease and insulin resistance: new insights and potential new treatments. Nutr 9:387. https://doi.org/10.3390/NU9040387
28. Stephen S, Baranova A, Younossi ZM et al (2014) Nat Rev Dis Primers 6(2):163–171. https://doi.org/10.1586/EGH.11.97
29. Bugianesi E, Gastaldelli A, Vanni E et al (2005) Insulin resistance in non-diabetic patients with non-alcoholic fatty liver disease: sites and mechanisms. Diabetol 48((4):634–642. https://doi.org/10.1007/S00125-005-1682-X
30. Hu DS, Zhu SH, Li X et al (2019) Association between hemoglobin glycation index and NAFLD in Chinese nondiabetic individuals. *Can.* J Gastroenterol Hepatol. 2019. https://doi.org/10.1155/2019/8748459
31. Bae JC, Cho YK, Lee WY et al (2010) Impact of nonalcoholic fatty liver disease on insulin resistance in relation to HbA1c levels in nondiabetic subjects. Am J Gastroenterol. 105(11):2389–2395. https://doi.org/10.1038/AJG.2010.275
32. D'Adamo E, Giannini C, Chiavaroli V et al (2011) What is the significance of soluble and endogenous secretory receptor for advanced glycation end products in liver steatosis in obese prepubertal children? Antioxid Redox Signal 14(6):1167–1172. https://doi.org/10.1089/ARS.2010.3719 https://home.liebertpub.com/ars
33. Fracanzani AL, Valenti L, Bugianesi E et al (2008) Risk of severe liver disease in nonalcoholic fatty liver disease with normal aminotransferase levels: a role for insulin resistance and diabetes. Hepatology. 48(3):792–798. https://doi.org/10.1002/HEP.22429
34. Palma-Duran SA, Kontogianni MD, Vlassopoulos A et al (2018) Serum levels of advanced glycation end-products (AGEs) and the decoy soluble receptor for AGEs (sRAGE) can identify non-alcoholic fatty liver disease in age-, sex- and BMI-matched normo-glycemic adults. Metabolism. 83:120–127. https://doi.org/10.1016/J.METABOL.2018.01.023
35. Cantero I, Abete I, JM del B et al (2018) Changes in lysophospholipids and liver status after weight loss: the RESMENA study. Nutr Metab 15(1):1–11. https://doi.org/10.1186/S12986-018-0288-5
36. Polsky S, Ellis SL (2015) Obesity, insulin resistance, and type 1 diabetes mellitus. Curr Opin Endocrinol Diabetes Obes. 22(4):277–282. https://doi.org/10.1097/MED.0000000000000170
37. Speliotes EK, Massaro JM, Hoffmann U et al (2010) Fatty liver is associated with dyslipidemia and dysglycemia independent of visceral fat: the Framingham heart study. Hepatology. 51(6):1979–1987. https://doi.org/10.1002/HEP.23593

38. Foster T, Anania FA, Li D, Ronit Katz, Budoff M. The prevalence and clinical correlates of nonalcoholic fatty liver disease (NAFLD) in African Americans: the multiethnic study of atherosclerosis (MESA). doi:https://doi.org/10.1007/s10620-013-2652-7
39. Fukuda Y, Hashimoto Y, Hamaguchi M et al (2016) Triglycerides to high-density lipoprotein cholesterol ratio is an independent predictor of incident fatty liver; a population-based cohort study. Liver Int. 36(5):713–720. https://doi.org/10.1111/LIV.12977
40. Zhou M, Zhu L, Cui X et al (2016) The triglyceride to high-density lipoprotein cholesterol (TG/HDL-C) ratio as a predictor of insulin resistance but not of β cell function in a Chinese population with different glucose tolerance status. Lipids Heal Dis 15(1):1–9. https://doi.org/10.1186/S12944-016-0270-Z
41. Lucero D, Miksztowicz V, Macri V et al (2015) Overproduction of altered VLDL in an insulin-resistance rat model: Influence of SREBP-1c and PPAR-α. Clín Invest Arterioscler. 27(4):167–174. https://doi.org/10.1016/J.ARTERI.2014.11.002

17

Role of plasma von Willebrand factor antigen in prediction of esophageal varices in pediatric and adolescent patients with portal hypertension

Lerine B. El Shazli[1], Dina A. Ragab[2], Karim A. Abdelhady[3] and Asmaa W. Abdelaziz[1*]

Abstract

Background: Ruptured esophageal varices (EVs) are a leading cause of death in Portal hypertension (PHT), it has been a big concern of research to screen EVs through non-invasive approaches. This study aimed to evaluate the role of plasma von Willebrand factor antigen (VWF-Ag) assay for early detection of EVs in patients with portal hypertension. This was a cross-sectional study, done on 47 portal hypertensive children and adolescents who were collected from the Pediatrics Hepatology Clinic, Children Hospital, Ain Shams University. All patients were subjected to comprehensive history taking, thorough clinical examination, routine investigations, abdominal ultrasound, upper GI endoscopy, and measurement of plasma VWF-Ag level. The patients were divided based on their endoscopic findings into two groups; a varices group which included 37 patients, and a non-varices group which included 10 patients.

Results: VWF-Ag rise significantly in patients with EVs, revealing a direct positive association with the degree of EVs.

Conclusion: The plasma VWF-Ag can be applied as a non-invasive evidence of the presence and grading of EVs.

Keywords: Portal hypertension, von Willebrand factor antigen, Esophageal varices

Background

Portal hypertension (PHT) is an extremely dangerous consequence of liver cirrhosis with its effects, e.g., hepatorenal syndrome, hepatic encephalopathy, ascites, and varices [1].

Ruptured esophageal varices (EVs) are a main cause of mortality in patients with liver cirrhosis and 30% may experience as a minimum one episode of variceal hemorrhage within a year of detection of varices [2].

So, searching for its markers is a matter to be considered carefully, as it might help in early detection, early treatment, or prevention of the progression of the condition [3].

VWF is a big multimeric protein with a vital function in the hemostasis process, as proven by the serious hemorrhage tendency combined with entire VWF insufficiency [4]; on the other hand, higher values of VWF are linked to thrombosis in arteries [5].

This work aimed to compare plasma VWF-Ag levels between variceal and non-variceal groups to assess its reliability as a predictor of varices presence, in addition, to assess if plasma VWF-Ag in variceal cases directly correlates with variceal grade.

Methods

This is a cross-sectional study that was conducted over 1 year, from December 2018 to December 2019, on pediatric and adolescent patients diagnosed with portal hypertension collected from hepatology clinic, Children Hospital, ain Shams University.

*Correspondence: dr.asmaa.wafeeq@gmail.com
[1] Pediatrics Department, Faculty of Medicine, Ain Shams University, Cairo, Egypt
Full list of author information is available at the end of the article

We included 47 portal hypertensive pediatric cases (diagnosis was based on clinical, laboratory, and radiological investigations) who were divided according to endoscopic findings into two groups: (varices group: which included 37 cases with EVs, and non-varices group: which included 10 cases without EVs).

Patients older than 18 years, and those with disorders of VWF as heart failure, renal failure, acute Infection on time of sampling, diabetes mellitus., hypertension, hyperlipidemia, malignancy, and patients on anticoagulant or antiplatelet therapy therapy, patients with active bleeding were excluded from the study. Written informed consent from the care giver of the participants was attained before being engaged in the study after getting approval from the Research Ethics Committee at the Faculty of Medicine.

Demographic data of the patients were recorded including age and sex, they were examined for clinical signs of liver disease and portal hypertension, size of liver, spleen, and presence of ascites. Patients were subjected to routine laboratory investigations including complete blood count, liver enzyme: alanine transaminase (ALT), aspartate aminotransferase (AST), serum alkaline phosphatase, albumin, bilirubin, international normalized ratio (INR)). Child-Pugh classification was used to classify the severity of liver disease [6].

Abdominal ultrasonography was done to detect size of liver and spleen, presence of cirrhosis, portal vein diameter [for children younger than 10 years, the normal diameter was 8.5 mm (± 2.7). For those whose age between 10 and 20 years, the normal diameter was 10 mm (± 2)], and presence of collaterals [7]. Moderate splenomegaly was considered if the largest dimension was 11–20 cm and marked splenomegaly if the largest dimension was more than 20 cm [8].

Upper GIT endoscopy was done using disinfected upper gastrointestinal video scope (OLYMPUS model) after good preparation of the patient. Patients were advised to fast for at least 6 h before the upper endoscopy. Complete evaluation of the esophagus, stomach and the duodenum down to the second part of the duodenum. Upper GIT endoscopy was performed in all cases to detect and grade the presence of EVs, they were graded according to the Japanese Research for Portal Hypertension Classification System as follows: grade (Gr) I: small EVs, Gr-II: moderated sized varices with slight obscuring of the gastroesophageal junction, Gr-III: large varices displaying luminal prolapse markedly obscuring the gastroesophageal junction and Gr IV: very large EVs, entirely obscuring the gastroesophageal junction and do not flattens on insufflation [9]. Portal hypertensive gastropathy was detected and categorized according to the classification proposed by Tanoue and his associates [10] into mild, moderate, and severe.

VWF-Ag measurement using VWF-Ag ELISA:vWF: Ag detection is a sandwich ELISA through subsequent processes including dilution, incubation, washing, and quantification. It runs on the automated VIDAS® immunoanalyzers (VIDAS, Biomerieux, France). Patient vWF Ag in comparative percent intensity is settled alongside a curve based on the reference plasma provided with the kit.

Data analysis

The collected data were coded, and analyzed using the SPSS (Statistical Package for Social Sciences) version 22 for Windows® (IBM SPSS Inc., Chicago, IL, USA). Qualitative data were signified as frequencies and relative percentages. The chi-square test ($\chi 2$) was utilized to determine the difference between qualitative variables as indicated. Continuous data were expressed as mean ± SD or median (min-max).

. Independent samples *t* test was used to compare between two independent groups of normally distributed variables while Mann-Whitney *U* test was used for non-normally distributed data. Comparison between three or more groups with normally distributed quantitative data was performed using the one-way ANOVA test. Pearson's correlation was used to test the correlation between two variables with parametric quantitative data. The receiver operator characteristic (ROC) curve was tested to calculate the diagnostic ability of quantitative variable (Von Willebrand factor) in the prediction of categorical outcome (varices). For all the above-mentioned tests, the level of significance was expressed as the probability of (p value) and the results were explained as following: non-significant if the p value is > 0.05, significant if the p value is ≤ 0.05, highly significant if the p value < 0.001.

Results

Demographic data

The mean age of the included cases was 8.5 and 7.5 years in the non-varices and varices groups, respectively. Six males and four females were included in the non-varices group, whereas the other group had 27 males and 10 females. Both ages, gender, and duration of the disease were statistically insignificant between the two groups, most recruited patients have classified as class A Child-Pugh score, with no significant difference between the two study groups ($p = 0.911$). The variceal group was receiving significantly higher doses of Inderal compared to the non-variceal group ($p = 0.001$).

Table 1 Analysis of laboratory parameters in the two groups

	Groups		*Test of significance*	*P*
	No varices (N = 10)	*Varices (N = 37)*		
Total serum bilirubin (mg/dl)	0.6 (0.2–6.3)	0.4 (0.1–8.6)	$z = -1.503$	0.137
Hemoglobin (gm/dl)	9.89 ± 1.05	9.56 ± 1.71	$t = 0.264$	0.527
WBCs (10^6/ml)	5.85 (4.3–9.1)	4.6 (2–11.6)	$z = -1.209$	0.231
PLTs(10^6lml)	159.5 (74–273)	105 (62–492)	$z = -0.702$	0.497
ALT (U/L)	29 (10–46)	19 (10–221)	$z = -0.247$	0.808
AST (U/L)	45.5 (28–83)	41 (17–311)	$z = -0.507$	0.612
Albumin (g/dl)	3.78 ± 0.61	3.78 ± 0.43	$t = 0.010$	0.992
PTT	31.21 ± 5.41	30.94 ± 7.37	$t = 0.109$	0.914
INR	1.31 ± 0.24	1.27 ± 0.25	$t = 0.422$	0.675
Serum creatinine (mg/dl	0.4 (0.1–0.8)	0.4 (0.1–0.6)	$z = -0.093$	0.929

Continuous data expressed as mean ± SD or median (min–max)

P probability

T = independent samples *t* test

Z = Mann-Whitney test

Laboratory parameters

CBC, liver functions, and renal functions were not significantly different between the two groups ($p > 0.05$) (Table 1).

Ultrasonographic findings

Liver size was not significantly different between the two groups ($p = 0.104$). However, marked splenic enlargement was significantly more observed in the variceal group ($p < 0.001$) (Table 2).

Endoscopic findings: In this study, variceal grades among the variceal group were as follows; grade I (13.5%), grade II (32.4%), grade III (37.8%), and grade IV (16.2%). There was a significant difference between the two groups regarding PHG ($p = 0.035$). Severe PHG was detected more in the variceal group (35.1%) compared to the non-varices group (10%) (Table 2).

Von Willebrand factor: VWF was significantly higher in the variceal group compared to the non-variceal cases (mean ± SD = 212.88 ± 25.53 vs. 147.65 ± 16.90%–$p < 0.001$) (Fig. 1). It was evident that VWF level increased as variceal grades increases ($p = 0.003$) (Fig. 2) with a strong positive correlation between VWF levels and variceal grade ($p < 0.001$) (Fig. 3). Using a cut-off value of 176.8%, VWF showed sensitivity and specificity of 96 and 100% respectively as a predictor of varices presence with a diagnostic accuracy was 95% (Fig. 4).

Discussion

Ruptured EVs resulting from portal hypertension is believed one of the main triggers of fatality in cirrhotic patients and 30% of those patients will experience an episode of variceal hemorrhage during the first year of variceal diagnosis [11]. Various predictors for the EVs presence with different levels of precision were weighed, involving laboratory and radiological procedures [12].

Comparison between the two groups as regards their demographic, Child score revealed no significant

Table 2 Analysis of US and endoscopic grading of portal vein gastropathy findings in the two study groups

	Groups				*Test of significance*
	No varices (N = 10)		*Varices (N = 37)*		
Liver size by US					
Large	4	40%	21	56.8%	$\chi 2 = 2.006$ $P = 0.104$
Moderate	1	10%	4	10.8%	
Normal	5	40%	12	32.4%	
Spleen size by US					
Markedly enlarged	2	20%	33	89.2%	$\chi 2 = 9.352$ $P < 0.001$*
Moderate enlarged	5	50%	3	8.1%	
Normal	3	30%	1	2.7%	
Endoscopic grading of portal vein gastropathy					
Mild	7	70%	8	21.6%	$\chi 2 = 5.631$ $P = 0.035$*
Moderate	2	20%	16	43.2%	
Severe	1	10%	13	35.1%	
Endoscopic grading of varices					
Grade 1	–		5	13.5%	
Grade 2	–		12	32.4%	
Grade 3	–		14	37.8%	
Grade 4	–		6	16.2%	

Categorical data expressed as number (%)

P probability

$\chi 2$ = chi-square test

*Statistically significant ($p < 0.05$)

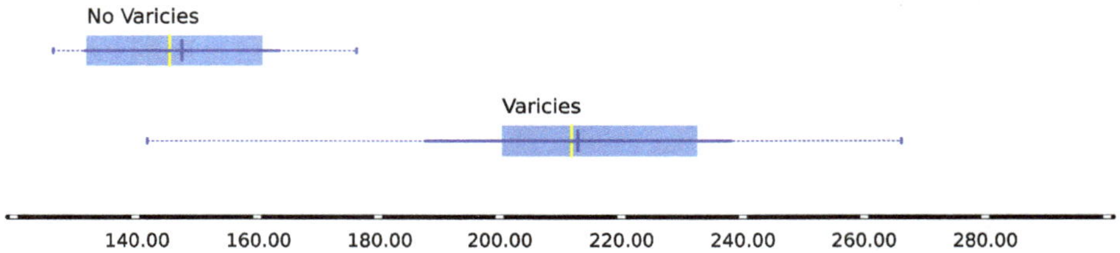

Fig. 1 Von Willebrand factor levels between the two groups

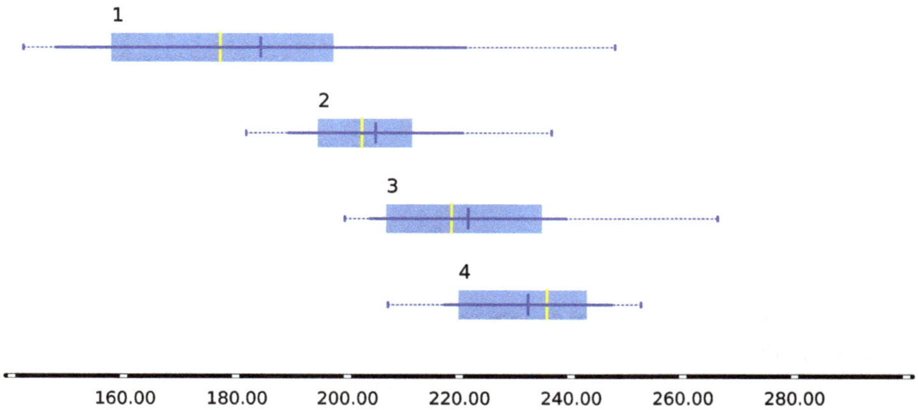

Fig. 2 Von Willebrand factor in different grades of varices

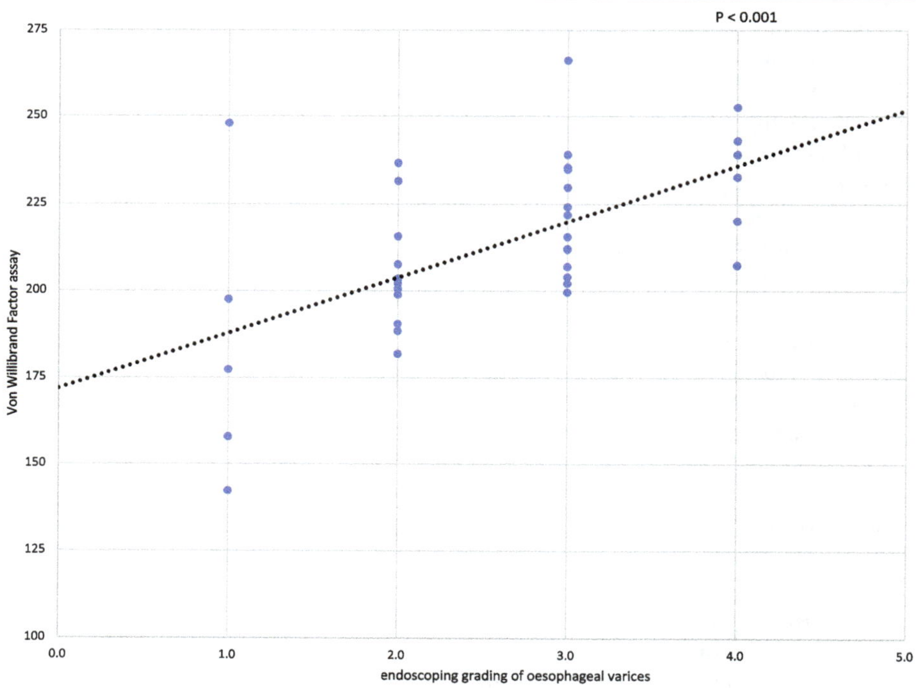

Fig. 3 Correlation between variceal grade and von Willebrand factor level

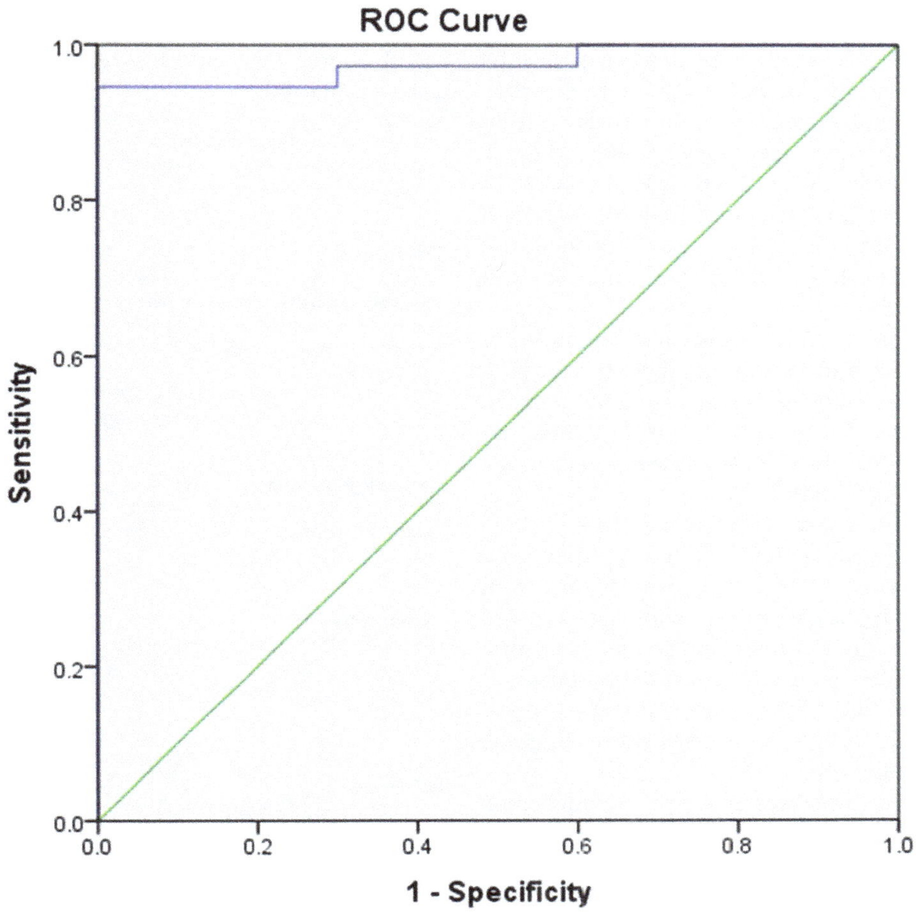

Fig. 4 ROC curve for von Willebrand factor as a predictor of variceal presence

differences as regards any of these data. This comes in favour of abolishing the effects of possible confounding factors.

As regards clinical and routine laboratory parameters no significant differences were found between the two studied groups except the spleen size, marked enlargement was diagnosed in 89.2% of cases in the variceal group, while it was present only in 20% of cases in the other group ($p < 0.001$).

Another study verified the same findings, as the spleen long axis was significantly increased in the variceal group (17.9 vs 15.1 cm in no varices group–$p = 0.0012$) [13]. Also, Agha et al. [14] stated that a greater mean spleen span was noticed in patients with varices when compared to patients without varices (14.7 cm versus 10.9 cm, $P = 0.0006$). This also coincides with Kedar et al. [15] who assumed that splenomegaly (> 12 cm) may be the mere indication of high portal pressures.

As regards the occurrence of gastropathy in this study, severe gastropathy was more found in the variceal group (35.1%), but mild gastropathy was the only finding in the no varices group, with a significant difference between the two groups ($p = 0.035$). Consistent with our results, an additional study described that the occurrence of PHG was more obvious in the variceal group (64.4% vs. 8.6% in the non-variceal group–$p = 0.001$) [9].

Coming to the level of vWF in the current study, it was significantly increased in the varices group 212.88 % when compared to 147.65% in the no varices group $p < 0.001$. Applying a cut-off level of 176.8%, it revealed a sensitivity of 96% and sensitivity of 100%, with an accuracy of 95% to expect the occurrence of varices. These results are supported by several adult studies that reported that vWF was significantly higher in patients with EVs, compared to patients without EVs, but with different cut off values [13, 16, 17].

In the variceal group, varices were represented as follows: grade I 13.5%, grade II 32.5%, grade III 37.8%, and grade IV 16.2%, the level of vWF antigen was significantly positively correlated with the variceal grade ($p < 0.001$). Mahmoud and his associates also reported that serum VWF was also positively correlated with variceal grade and size. It had a mean level of 1.635, 2.50, and 3.216 in cases with grades I, II, and III, respectively. Furthermore, it had a mean of 1.453 and 2.858 in cases with small and large varices respectively ($p < 0.001$) [16], this comes in line with our results.

The high levels of vWF in cirrhosis may be owing to stimulation of vWF production in the cirrhotic liver [18], or decreased liver-facilitated removal due to reduced level or activity of vWF-Ag splitting protease that can lead to additional elevation of VWF-Ag levels in cirrhotic patients complicating with PHT [19].

The preceding studies recommend that a cirrhotic liver could add to the elevated VWF, but in this study, most of recruited PHT patients were from the child a, and b classification who also showed increased VWF, this could be simplified as in normal conditions VWF is eliminated from the circulation at the levels of liver and spleen. The shifting of blood via portal-systemic collaterals causes increasing the levels of such factor [20].

Additional research indicates that vWF is implicated in the formation of blood vessels, that could clarify why certain people with vWF disease have vascular malformations mainly in the gastrointestinal system which may bleed terribly [21].

Conclusion

Based on the results of the current study, VWF-Ag can be used as a non-invasive neutral predictor for the discovery of EVs. Besides, it can be used to predict the variceal grade.

Limitation of this study

The main limitation of this study is that it included comparatively small sample size. Correlation between VWF level in different etiologies of portal hypertension and its relation to portal hypertensive gastropathy might be another limitation.

Abbreviations

PHT: Portal hypertension; VWF-Ag: Von Willebrand factor antigen; PV: Portal vein; EV: Esophageal varices; Gr: Grade; PHG: Portal hypertensive gastropathy; EVL: Endoscopic variceal ligation; CBC: Complete blood count; ALT: Alanine aminotransferase; AST: Aspartate aminotransferase; ALP: Alkaline phosphatase; ELISA: Enzyme-linked immunosorbent assay.

Acknowledgements

Not applicable.

Authors' contributions

LE designed and directed the study. AA and KA conducted the study and analyzed the data. DR contributed to the pathological studies and interpretation of the results LE, AA, and KA wrote the manuscript. All authors have read and approved the final manuscript.

Declarations

Ethics approval and consent to participate

Written informed consents were obtained from the parents of participating children, also ethical approval was obtained from the Research Ethics Committee at the Faculty of Medicine, Ain Shams University Hospital (FWA000017585) in the Declaration of Helsinki (FMASU REC) The study was approved in October 2016 by pediatric department committee.

Competing interests

The authors declare that they have no known competing financial interests or personal relationships that could have appeared to influence the work reported in this paper.

Author details

[1]Pediatrics Department, Faculty of Medicine, Ain Shams University, Cairo, Egypt. [2]Clinical Pathology Department, Faculty of Medicine, Ain Shams University, Cairo, Egypt. [3]Ministry of health, Cairo, Egypt.

References

1. Iwakiri Y (2014) Pathophysiology of portal hypertension. Clin Liver Dis 18(2):281–291. https://doi.org/10.1016/j.cld.2013.12.001 Epub 2014 Feb 25. PMID: 24679494; PMCID: PMC3971388
2. Haq I, Tripathi D (2017) Recent advances in the management of variceal bleeding. Gastroenterol Rep 5(2):113–126. https://doi.org/10.1093/gastro/gox007
3. Berzigotti A (2017) Advances and challenges in cirrhosis and portal hypertension. BMC Med 15(1):200. https://doi.org/10.1186/s12916-017-0966-6
4. Sadler JE, Mannucci PM, Berntorp E, Bochkov N, Boulyjenkov V, Ginsburg D, Meyer D, Peake I, Rodeghiero F, Srivastava A (2000) Impact, diagnosis and treatment of von Willebrand disease. Thromb Haemost 84(2):160–174 PMID: 10959685
5. Reiner AP, Siscovick DS, Rosendaal FR (2001) Hemostatic risk factors and arterial thrombotic disease. Thromb Haemost 85(4):584–595 PMID: 11341490
6. Child CG, Turcotte JG (1964) Surgery and portal hypertension. Major Probl Clin Surg 1:1–85 PMID: 4950264
7. Soyupak S, Gunesli A, Seydaoğlu G, Binokay F, Celiktas M, Inal M (2010) Portal venous diameter in children: normal limits according to age, weight, and height. Eur J Radiol 75(2):245–247. https://doi.org/10.1016/j.ejrad.2009.03.052
8. Poulin EC, Mamazza J, Schlachta CM (1998) Splenic artery embolization before laparoscopic splenectomy. An update. Surg Endosc 12(6):870–875
9. Ghweil A, Arafa UA, Khodeary A, Salem AN (2014) Predictors of bleeding from esophageal varices: the role of factor VII and von Willebrand Factor (vWF). Open J Gastroenterol 4(04):152. https://doi.org/10.4236/ojgas.2014.44023
10. Tsugawa K, Hashizume M, Migou S, Kishihara F, Kawanaka H, Tomikawa M, Sugimachi K (2000) Role of vascular endothelial growth factor in portal hypertensive gastropathy. Digestion 61:98–106. https://doi.org/10.1159/000007741
11. Păunescu V, Grigorean V, Popescu C (2004)Factori de risc in evoluţia imediată a hemoragiei digestive la cirotici. Risk factors for the immediate

outcome of gastrointestinal bleeding in patients with cirrhosis, Chirurgia (Bucur). 99(5):311–322 Romanian. PMID: 15675285

12. Mahmoud HS, Mostafa EF, Mohammed MA (2014) Role of portal haemodynamic parameters in prediction of oesophageal varices in cirrhotic patients. Arab J Gastroenterol 15(3-4):130–134. https://doi.org/10.1016/j.ajg.2014.09.001 Epub 2014 Dec 8. PMID: 25499211
13. Abdelmaksoud MA, Jouda A, Fathy T, Ibrahim AMA, Soliman AS, Baraka A et al (2019) Role of plasma von Willebrand factor-antigen in predicting the presence of esophageal varices and occurrence of its bleeding in cirrhotic patients. Afro-Egypt J Infect Endemic Dis 9(2):139–149. https://doi.org/10.21608/aeji.2019.12190.1020
14. Agha A, Abdulhadi MM, Marenco S, Bella A, Alsaudi D, El-Haddad A, Inferrera S, Savarino V, Giannini EG (2011) Use of the platelet count/spleen diameter ratio for the noninvasive diagnosis of esophageal varices in patients with schistosomiasis. Saudi J Gastroenterol 17(5):307–311. https://doi.org/10.4103/1319-3767.84483 PMID: 21912056; PMCID: PMC3178917
15. Kedar RP, Merchant SA, Malde HH, Patel VH (1994) Multiple reflective channels in the spleen: a sonographic sign of portal hypertension. Abdom Imaging 19(5):453–458. https://doi.org/10.1007/BF00206939 PMID: 7950827
16. Mahmoud HS, Ghweil A, Bazeed SE, Fayed HM, Meguid MMA (2015) Reliability of plasma Von Willebrand factor antigen in prediction of esophageal varices in patients with liver cirrhosis. Open J Gastroenterol 5(06):49. https://doi.org/10.4236/ojgas.2015.56010
17. El-Toukhy N, Issa H (2019) Predictive and prognostic value of von Willebrand factor in patients with cirrhosis and esophageal varices. Afro-Egypt J Infect Endemic Dis 9(1):67–73. https://doi.org/10.21608/aeji.2019.29119
18. Hollestelle MJ, Geertzen HG, Straatsburg IH, van Gulik TM, van Mourik JA (2004) Factor VIII expression in liver disease. Thromb Haemost 91(2):267–275. https://doi.org/10.1160/th03-05-0310
19. Lisman T, Bongers TN, Adelmeijer J, Janssen HL, de Maat MP, de Groot PG, Leebeek FW (2006) Elevated levels of von Willebrand Factor in cirrhosis support platelet adhesion despite reduced functional capacity. Hepatology. 44(1):53–61. https://doi.org/10.1002/hep.21231 PMID: 16799972
20. Denis CV, Christophe OD, Oortwijn BD, Lenting PJ (2008) Clearance of von Willebrand factor. Thromb Haemost 99(2):271–278. https://doi.org/10.1160/TH07-10-0629 PMID: 18278174
21. Randi AM, Laffan MA (2017) Von Willebrand factor and angiogenesis: basic and applied issues. J Thromb Haemost 15(1):13–20. https://doi.org/10.1111/jth.13551 PMID: 27778439

18

Medicinal plants with hepatoprotective potentials against carbon tetrachloride-induced toxicity

Chidiebere Emmanuel Ugwu* and Stephen Monday Suru

Abstract

Background: Carbon tetrachloride (CCl_4) is a well-characterized hepatotoxic agent. With rising cases of liver diseases, the identification, assessment, and development of hepatoprotective agents from plants source has become imperative.

Main body: With arrays of literature on plants with hepatoprotective potentials, this review sourced published literatures between 1998 and 2020 and systematically highlighted about 92 medicinal plants that have been reported to protect against CCl_4-induced liver injury in animal models. The results show that herbal plants provide protection for the liver against CCl_4 by downregulation of the liver marker enzymes and activation of antioxidant capacity of the liver cells with the restoration of liver architecture. We also provided the traditional and accompanying pharmacological uses of the plants. A variety of phytochemicals mostly flavonoids and polyphenols compounds were suggested to offer protection against liver injuries.

Conclusion: It can be concluded that there are a variety of phytochemicals in plant products with hepatoprotective activity against CCl_4-induced toxicity in animal models.

Keywords: Carbon tetrachloride, Medicinal plants, Hepatoprotective, Silymarin, Folkloric medicine

Background

The liver being an important organ is often exposed to array of threats [1]. Injury to the liver can lead to deterioration of its functions and may culminate in organ failure [2]. The likely risk factors for the development of the liver diseases have been suggested to include pathogenic microorganisms and viruses, hepatotoxins, overdose and duration of drugs, obesity and malnutrition, alcohol, autoimmune disorders, type-2 diabetes, and genetic factors [1]. The diseases of the liver are of public health concern because orthodox remedies for liver diseases produce limited results with attendant side effects. As such, utilization of complementary and alternative herbal medicine has attracted research interest for novel plausible hepatoprotective agents capable of ameliorating or reversing liver injury with little side effects [3, 4]. Over the years, this search has gained impetus with many studies focusing on hepatoprotective potentials of plant drugs.

Carbon tetrachloride (CCl_4) is a known hepatotoxicant in humans and animal models [5]. It has been successfully used in hepatotoxicity research as a model and to appraise hepatoprotective agents [6, 7]. With reports on the rise of liver diseases and numerous literature reports on plants with potential hepatoprotective activity, this review highlighted the mechanism of CCl_4 toxicity, the significance, effectiveness, and underlying mechanisms of herbal plant extracts on CCl_4-induced toxicity in experimental animal models.

*Correspondence: ce.ugwu@unizik.edu.ng
Department of Human Biochemistry, Faculty of Basic Medical Sciences, College of Health Sciences, Nnamdi Azikiwe University (Nnewi Campus), Nnewi, Anambra State, Nigeria

Main text

Insight on the mechanism of carbon tetrachloride hepatotoxicity

Prior to the Montreal Protocol, CCl_4 was formerly and widely used as a fire suppressant, as a precursor to refrigerants, propellants for aerosol cans, as a cleaning agent, a widely used solvent in organic chemistry, as a pesticide, and anesthetics [8, 9]. However, it is rarely used today because of adverse health effects and environmental safety concerns. Symptoms associated with acute inhalation of low–medium doses include headache, weakness, lethargy/general anesthesia, nausea, vomiting, and respiratory arrest. For medium to high oral exposure, the liver is known to be the primary site of CCl_4-induced toxicity beginning with acute but progressive centrilobular injury that may culminate in cell death [10].

Experimental deductions

Due to the complex nature of CCl_4-induced liver damage, there have emerged several independent mechanisms to explain each of the facets of the associated changes. The interrelationship among diverse mechanisms proposed for each of these associated changes has not been well-established/outlined. This is primarily because early and later changes associated with the hepatotoxic development have been mixed up. As a result, a harmonized understanding of the intricate mechanisms involved in hepatic damage has become partly elusive. However, this has not obscured the following experimental deductions (Fig. 1):

- Changes in endoplasmic reticulum (ER) function due to decrease in glucose-6 phosphatase [11], which may not be unconnected with CCl_4-induced glycogen depletion and attendant protection from carbohydrate-rich diets [12, 13]. Besides, CCl_4-induced disruption and disassociation of polyribosomes from ER alters its anabolic function as manifested in decreased incorporation of amino acids into proteins such as albumin and fibrinogen [14]. Additionally, CCl_4-induced hypomethylation of 2′-O-ribose moieties in rRNA might have resulted from transient increase in cytosolic Ca^{2+}. This increase may activate the selective destruction of rRNA methylases via

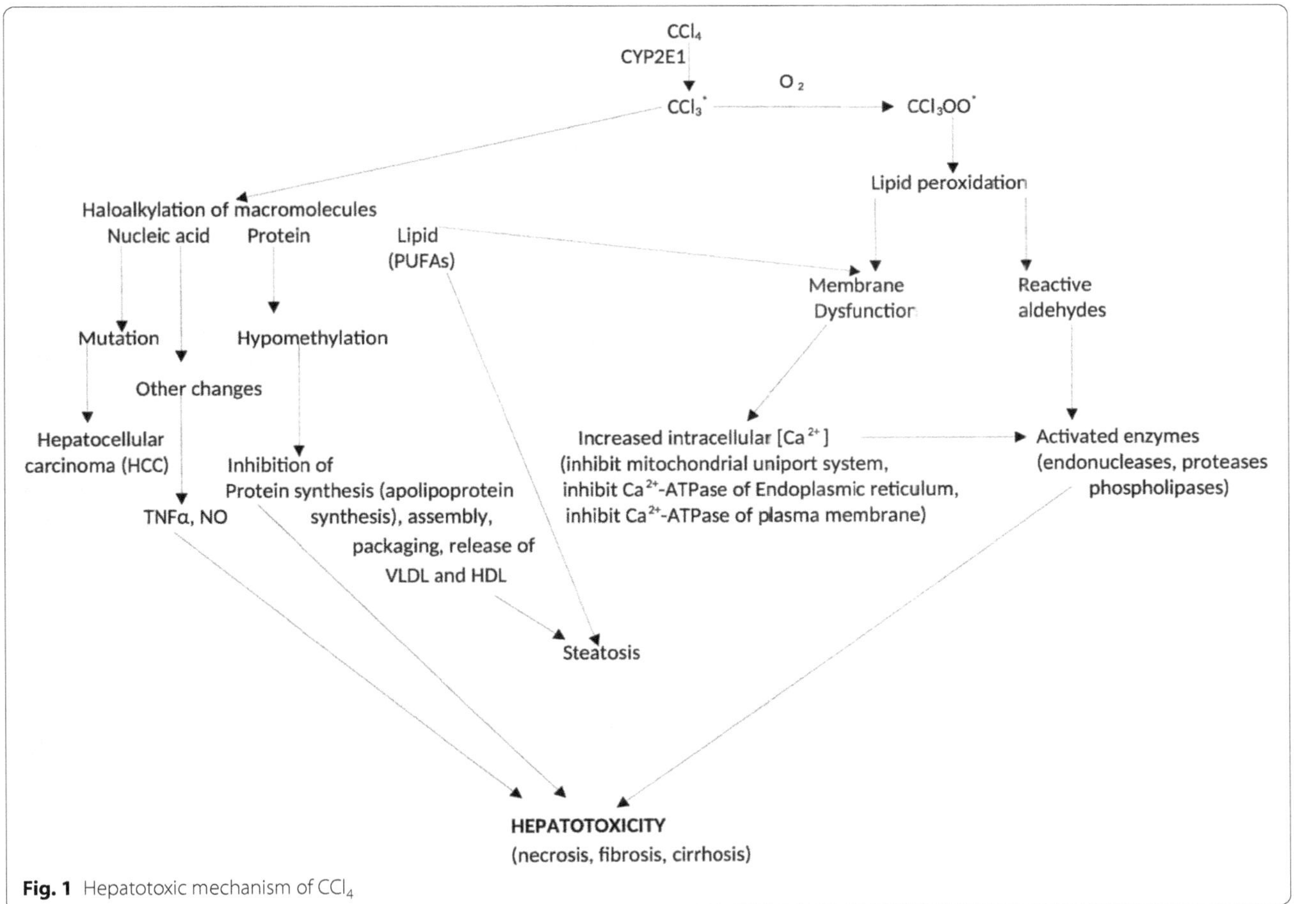

Fig. 1 Hepatotoxic mechanism of CCl_4

the action of demethylases or proteases. Overall, the protein synthetic function of ER in the centrilobular region may be hampered with an attendant defects in the ability of the liver to effectively respond to additional insults [10].

- Calcium homeostasis underlies some aspects of CCl_4 hepatotoxicity (plasma membrane blebbing and fatty accumulation- steatosis); CCl_4 may elicit dramatic redistribution of intracellular Ca^{2+} stores, albeit no total cellular change [10]. Calcium ion (Ca^{2+}) homeostasis is maintained by 3 mechanisms: (i) Ca^{2+} extrusion by plasma membrane ATPase, (ii) Ca^{2+} sequestration by mitochondria, and (iii) Ca^{2+} sequestration by liver ER. So, CCl_4 may cause decreased Ca^{2+} sequestration by ER and mitochondria, decreased extrusion by plasma membrane ATPase, as well as blockage of gap junctional intercellular communication may favor increase cytosolic Ca^{2+}. An ATP-dependent Ca^{2+} sequestration by hepatic ER has been shown to be disrupted by CCl_4 [15]. Endoplasmic reticulum membrane permeability may also be altered, being one indicator of impending cell death [16].
- Rapid destruction/decrease in cytochrome P_{450} in centrilobular regions (suggesting that CCl_4 was metabolized by ER mixed-function oxidase system), which is orchestrated by low levels of reduced glutathione (GSH) and low oxygen tension. In turn, low level oxygen tension may limit competition between O_2 and CCl_4 for cytochrome P_{450} binding (i.e., CCl_4 may readily bind to cytochrome P_{450}).
- Metabolic products [trichloromethyl (CCl_3^*) or peroxytrichloromethyl (CCl_3-OO^*) free radical] elicit damage: lipid peroxidation of vulnerable unsaturated fatty acids in membrane phospholipids and destruction of haem moiety of cytochrome P_{450}.
- Blockage of gap junctional communication by CCl_4 thereby shutting down intercellular communication.
- Changes in mitochondrial function: disruption of oxidative phosphorylation due partly to chelation of calcium [17].

Making sense out of experimental deductions

The hepatic biotransformation of CCl_4 primarily involves metabolic activation to transient reactive intermediates. Under low oxygen partial pressure, cytochrome P_{450} catalyzes the reductive de-halogenation of CCl_4 resulting in predominant formation of CCl_3^* and $CHCl^*$ radicals [18, 19]. These reactive intermediates may bind covalently to cellular components (membranes, microsomes) and impinge on mostly lipid metabolism (increased synthesis, decreased transport out of the hepatocyte) thereby culminating in hepatic steatosis (fatty liver) [20, 21].

Dianzani [22] reported that covalent modification of lipoproteins occurs prior to their decreased transport out of hepatocytes. Intracellular maturation of lipoproteins in the Golgi apparatus is dependent on galactosylation which is catalyzed by glucosyl- and galactosyltransferases [23]. The CCl_4-induced damage of Golgi apparatus and eventual reduction in the activities of these enzymes may explain the observed decrease in lipoprotein secretion associated with CCl_4 intoxication. Thus, CCl_4-induced inhibition of lipoprotein secretion, and its attendant hepatic steatosis mainly result from covalent binding of CCl_4 metabolites to cell constituents, but not due to lipid peroxidation.

Under high oxygen partial pressure, however, CCl_3^* may interact with oxygen to form CCl_3-OO^*. The peroxy radicals may elicit the peroxidation of unsaturated fatty acids especially in membrane phospholipids of intracellular and plasma membranes [24]. Some of the lipid peroxidative products may inflict further damage leading to increased membrane permeability and a comprehensive loss in membrane integrity [25]. Thus, both covalent binding of CCl_4 metabolites and lipid peroxidation work in tandem to elicit the hallmark of damage seen in CCl_4-induced hepatotoxicity.

The consequences of loss of membrane integrity are enormous and may lead to cascade of events culminating in liver necrosis. These events may include disturbed Ca^{2+} homeostasis/dramatic redistribution of Ca^{2+} in hepatocytes, leakage/efflux of K^+, and influx of Na^+ [10, 26].

Beside the peroxidative action, CCl_4-derived free radicals and their attendant oxidative stress have been shown to enhance NF-kB expression, which in turn initiates the synthesis of cytotoxic cytokines, which may be partly responsible for liver injury [27]. Tumor necrosis alpha (TNF-α) has been implicated in CCl_4-induced hepatocellular damage [28]. At lower doses of CCl_4, inflammatory responses prevail. Healthy hepatocytes are insensitive to tissue necrosis factor alpha (TNF-α) action, but become sensitive once protein and RNA synthesis are inhibited [29].

Summarily, CCl_4 hepatotoxicity may be due to a combination of factors such as the thorough inhibition of protein synthesis, the severe derailment of intracellular Ca^{2+} sequestration, and the effect on membrane integrity. These factors may result and progress through a series of steps that contribute to various extents to the ultimate damage: reductive dehalogenation, covalent binding of resulting radicals; inhibition of protein synthesis (in particular, apolipoprotein synthesis), assembly, packaging and release of VLDL and HDL, fat accumulation;

Table 1 List of traditional plants with anti-hepatotoxic potential against acute carbon tetrachloride hepatotoxicity

s/n.	Botanical name	Family	Plant part/extract	Folkloric use	Pharmacological use	Reference
1	*Abelmoselius manihot* (L) *medic*	*Malvaceae*	Flower, ethanol	Treatment of jaundice and hepatitis, control of fertility, easing of child birth and stimulation of lactation.	Anti-inflammatory, antioxidant, antibacterial, anticonvulsant, cardioprotective, and neuroprotective actions	[32]
2	*Acacia mellifera*	*Fabaceae*	Leaves, acetate/aqueous/n-butanol	Treatment of cold, malaria, syphilis, and bowel problems.	Antimalarial, antimicrobial, antiviral activity against HIV-1, and herpes simplex virus	[33]
3	*Aegle marmelos correa ex Roxb*	*Rutaceae*	Pulp/seed, aqueous	Treatment of jaundice, hepatitis, piles, tuberculosis and antidiarrheal. Used as stomach tonic.	Antidiarrhoeal, anti-inflammatory, and wound healing effects	[34]
4	*Aegle marmelos correa ex Roxb with piperine*	*Rutaceae*	Leaves, 70% ethanol	Used as astringent, laxative and expectorant. Treatment of inflammation, cataract, diabetes, diarrhea, and asthma.	Antifungal, ulcer healing, anti-inflammatory, antidiabetic, diuretic, anticancer, and antioxidant properties	[35]
5	*Alangium salviifolium* .	*Alangiacea*	Stem bark, methanol.	Treatment of rheumatism, cancer and hemorrhoids. Root used to manage skin diseases, diarrhea, fever, carminative, and purgative expectorant.	Antiarthritic, androgenic, anthelmintic, antidiabetic, hepatoprotective, and anti-inflammatory effects	[36]
6	*Alhagi maurorum (camel thorn)*	*Fabaceae*	Leaves, methanol	As a remedy for rheumatic pains, bilharziasis, liver disorders, and urinary tract infection.	Antioxidant, antidiarrheal, and antiulcerrogenic activities.	[37]
7	*Alhagi maurorum Medikus.*	*Fabaceae*	Aerial parts, 90% ethanol	Treatment of liver problems, migrane and cataract. As tonic, digestive, antipyretic, laxative, diuretic, and aphrodisiac	Antiulcer, antibacterial, antioxidant, anti-inflammatory, analgesic, antipyretic, antifungal, and hepatoprotective effects	[38]
8	*Allium sativum (Single clove garlic)*	*Amaryllidace*	Garlic bulbs, 70% ethanol	Used as nutraceuticals	Antidiabetic, anticancer, antioxidant, immune modulation activities, and lowering of blood pressure.	[39]
9	*Amaranthus spinosus*	*Amaranthaceae*	Whole plant, 50% ethanol	Prevent swelling around the stomach. Used in the treatment of jaundicc	Anti-inflammatory, antimalarial, antibacterial, antidiuretic, antiviral, immunostimulatory, and antioxidant effects	[40]
10	*Amorphophallus campanulatus (Roxb)*	*Araceae*	Tubers, aqueous	Treatment of piles, abdominal pain, tumors, enlargement of spleen, asthma, and rheumatism	Antibacterial, antifungal, and cytotoxic activities	[41]
11	*Arqemone Mexicana L*	*Papaveraceae*	Crude powder leaf	Treatment of malaria, fever, abdominal pains, and jaundice	Antibacterial, anti-inflammatory, wound-healing, antifertility, antistress, anti-allegic, cytotoxic, antidiabetic, and antihepatotoxic activities	[42]
12	*Artemisia iwayomogi*	*Comppositae*	Aqueous	Treatment of hepatic disorders	Antioxidant, cytoprotection, choleretic, hepatoprotection, antimicrobial, anti-inflammatory and antifibrotic effects.	[43]

Table 1 (continued)

s/n.	Botanical name	Family	Plant part/extract	Folkloric use	Pharmacological use	Reference
13	*Bauhinia variegate*	*Leguminasea.*	Stem bark, alcohol	Treatment of bronchitis, leprosy, diarrhea, piles, and tumor. Used as astringent	Hypoglycaemic, haemagglutinating, antibacterial, and antifungal effects	[44]
14	*Bougainullra spectabillis*	*Nyctaginaceae.*	Esculetin	Treatment of liver damage, cough, pertussis, and bronchitis	Antimicrobial, anticancer, antidiabetic, anti-inflammatory, antihyperlipidaemic, antioxidant, antiulcer, and antihepatotoxic activities	[45]
15	*Bryonia diocia Jacq*	*Cucurbitaceae*	Leaves, 80% ethanol	Treatment of various inflammatory conditions, brochial complaints, asthma, intestinal ulcer, hypertension, and arthritis. Applied as a rubefacient to muscular pains. Treatment of fever and bronchitis	Antinociceptive, antimicrobial, antioxidant, hepatoprotective, anticancer, hypercholesterolemia, analgesic, anti-inflammatory, cytotoxic, and hepatoprotective	[46]
16	*Brysocarpus coCClneus Schum*	*Connaraceae*	Leaves, aqueous	Mouth and skin sores, swellings, tumors, earache, muscular pain, and jaundice	Antioxidant and hepatoprotection	[47]
17	*Cajanus cajan*	*Leguminosae .*	Aerial, 70% ethanol	Jaundice and stomach disorders	Anthelmintic, antioxidant and protection against alcohol-induced liver damage	[48]
18	*Calotropis gigantean R.Br*	*Asclepiadaceae*	Stem, 50% ethanol.	In tooth ache and ear ache, sprain, anxiety, pain, epilepsy, and in mental disorders	Antidiarrheal, analgesic, CNS activity, and pregnancy interceptive properties	[49]
19	*Camellia ntidissima Chi*	*Theaceae*	Leaves, 10 % ethanol	Treatment of dysentery, hypertension, diarrhea, faucitis, hepatitis, jaundice, liver cirrhosis and sores	Leaves show antioxidative, antitumor, antibacterial, anti-inflammatory, hypoglycaemic, hypolipdemic, antidepressant, antillergic, and immunomodulatory activities	[1]
20	*Canna indica L*	*Cannaceae*	Aerial part, methanol	Treatment of diuresis, fever, dropsy, earaches, and eye disease	Analgesic, antioxidant, and hepatoprotective effects	[50]
21	*Capparis spinosa*	*Capparidaceae*	Root bark, 80% ethanol	Treatment of hepatic diseases. Reducing flatulence, treatment of rheumatism, anemia, and gout. Used as diuretics	Antidiabetic, hypoglycaemic, antioxidant, antiapoptotic, antibacterial, anti-inflammatory, antifungal, and hepatoprotective effects	[51]
22	*Capsella busa-pastoris (L.) Medik*	*Brassicaceae*	Aerial parts, 90% ethanol	Remedy for liver, hemorrhages, respiratory problem, and as diuretic	Antimicrobial, antioxidant, anticancer, anti-inflammatory, and sedative effects	[38]
23	*Carissa opaca*	*Apocynaceae*	Leaves, 95% methanol	Treatment of asthma, cardiac disorder and cough	Antioxidant, membrane stabilization, antipyretic and aperient activities	[52]
24	*Carthamus tinctorius L*	*Asteraceae*	Flower, hydroxysafflor yellow A	Treatment of dysmenorrhea, amenorrhea, postpartum abdominal pains, and pains of the joints. As antidote to poisoning and purgative	Antioxidant, antidiabetic, hepatoprotective, anti-inflammatory, antifungal, antimicrobial, and hepatoprotective effects	[53]

Table 1 (continued)

s/n.	Botanical name	Family	Plant part/extract	Folkloric use	Pharmacological use	Reference
25	*Carthamus tinctorius. L*	*Asteraceae*	Flower, Na_2CO_3	Treatment of gynecological diseases, osteoporosis, cardiovascular diseases, and angiitis	Nutraceutical, hepatoprotective, antioxidant, promoting blood circulation, and inhibiting platelet aggregation, anti-inflammatory, antipyretic, antitumor, and antidiabetic activities	[54]
26	*Carum carvil*	*Apiaceae*	Fruit, aqueous	Treatment of jaundice, indigestion and pneumonia. As appetizer, diuretic and gastric stimulant	Anti-inflammatory, spasmolytic, antimicrobial, antioxidant, caminative, antidiabetic, immunomodulatory, anticancer, and hypolipidaemic properties	[55]
27	*Cassia angustifolia Vahl*	*Caecalpiniaceae*	Leaves, ethanol.	Used in jaundice, rheumatoid arthritis, blood disease, diarrhea, ringworm, skin diseases, dysentery and as laxatives	Hepatoprotection and antioxidant activities	[56]
28	*Cassia angustofolia vahl*	*Leguminosea*	Leaves, 90% alcohol	Used as laxative, febrifuge, treatment of anemia, typhoid, cholera, jaundice and tumors	Hepatoprotection and antioxidant activities	[57]
29	*Cassia fistula Linn*	*Caesalpinacea*	Leaves, 90% ethanol	Treatment of Jaundice and rheumatism. Used as a laxative.	Hepatoprotective and antioxidant properties	[58]
30	*Cichorium intybus*	*Asteraceae*	Esculetin	Treatment of acne, inflammation of throat, jaundice, enlargement of spleen, diarrhea, vomiting, and rheumatism	Hepatoprotection, antihelminthic, antimicrobial, antidiabetic, and analgesic effects	[45]
31	*Cichorium intybus*	*Asteraceae*	Seed, ethanol	Treatment of acne, inflammation of throat, jaundice, enlargement of spleen, diarrhea, vomiting, and rheumatism.	Hepatoprotection, antihelminthic, antimicrobial, antidiabetic, and analgesic effects	[59]
32	*Cichorium intybus*	*Asteraceae*	Seed, 0.03% methanol.	Treatment of acne, inflammation of throat, jaundice, enlargement of spleen, diarrhea, vomiting, and rheumatism	Hepatoprotection, antihelminthic, antimicrobial, antidiabetic, and analgesic effects.	[59]
33	*Cichorium intybus*	*Asteraceae*	Leaves, hydroethanol (1:1)	Treatment of acne, inflammation of throat, jaundice, enlargement of spleen, diarrhea, vomiting, and rheumatism	Hepatoprotection, antihelminthic, antimicrobial, antidiabetic and anal gesic effects.	[60]
34	*Cinnamomum verum*	*Lauraceae*	Cinnamon powder, 95% ethanol	Treatment of diabetes, respiratory, and gynecological ailments	Enhancement of glycogen synthesis, antioxidant, antidiabetic, hypolidemic, antipyretic, and analgesic activities	[61]

Table 1 (continued)

s/n.	Botanical name	Family	Plant part/extract	Folkloric use	Pharmacological use	Reference
35	*Cinnamomum verum*	*Lauraceae*	Bark essential oil, dichloromethane	Preventing heart diseases, reduction in cholesterol and as an antidiabetic	Antioxidant, boosting cognitive activity, antiangiogenesis, anti-inflammatory, antimicrobial, and protection against Parkinson' disease	[62]
36	*Cinnamomum zeylanicum L*	*Lauraceacea*	Bark, 80% ethanol	Flavoring for foods and in traditional medicine to treat variety of health conditions	Antimicrobial, insecticidal, antityrosinease, antioxidant, antimutagenic, anti-inflammatory, hypotensive, and cholesterol-lowering effects.	[63]
37	*Citrus aurantium (essential oil)*	*Rutaceae*	Peel skin, aqueous oil	Diaphoretic and antiseptic	Analgesic, anti-inflammatory, antifungal, and antibacterial activities	[64]
38	*Citrus limon(L.) Burm.F*	*Rutaceae*	Fruit, 70% ethanol	Treatment of liver ailment and jaundice. Treatment of sluggish liver, rheumatism, fever, and febrile diseases	Chemoprevention, lipid peroxidation inhibitor, hypocholesterolemic, and antioxidant effects.	[65]
39	*Clerodendrum volubile*	*Verbenaceae*	Leaves, 50% methanol.	Treatment of diabetes, ulcer, arthritis, and rheumatism	Antidiabetic, antihypertensive, antioxidant, and anticancer effects	[66]
40	*Clitoria ternatea L*	*Fabaceae*	Leaves, ethanol	Treatment of liver diseases, insect bites, asthma, leukoderma, and inflammation	Antihelmintic, antihistaminic, antimicrobial, cytotoxic, anti-inflammatory, wound healing, proteolytic, hypoglycemic, and antioxidant activities	[56]
41	*Corianderum sativum. L*	*Apiaceae*	Leaves, ethanol	Treatment of jaundice	Anxiolytic, antidepressant and sedative-hypnotic effects. Neuroprotective, antibacterial, anti-inflammatory, analgesic, antidiabetic, antifungal, and hypolipidaemic effects	[67]
42	*Corianderum sativum. L. (essential oil)*	*Apiaceae*	Fruits, aqueous	Recommended for spastic condition of the gastro intestinal oral tract, flatulence, fullness and loss of appetite due to their antispasmodic, and antimicrobial activities	Anxiolytic, antidepressant and sedative-hypnotic effects. Neuroprotective, antibacterial, anti-inflammatory, analgesic, antidiabetic, antifungal, and hypolipidaemic effects	[55]
43	*Coriandrum sativum*	*Umbelifera*	Leaves/stem, 70% ethanol	Treatment of ailments like spasm, rheumatism, neuralgia, gastric complaint, bronchitis, diarrhea, carminative and diuretic tonic	Hypoglycemic, antibacterial, antifungal, free radical scavenging, and lipid peroxidation properties	[68]
44	*Cortex dictamni*	*Rutaceae*	Whole plant, aqueous	Treatment of Jaundice, chronic hepatitis, cough rheumatism and some skin diseases. To clear heat, dry dampness, dispel wind, treatment of arthritis, eczema, rubella, and urticarial	Good scavenger of free radicals and inhibition of lipid peroxide	[69]

Table 1 (continued)

s/n.	Botanical name	Family	Plant part/extract	Folkloric use	Pharmacological use	Reference
45	*Curcuma longa. L*	*Zingiberacae*	Rhizome(root), 50% ethanol and curcumin	Used for the treatment of chronic diseases like diabetes mellitus, dermatological infection, and depression	Anti-inflammatory, immunoregulatory, and antioxidant effects	[70]
46	*Cytisus scoparius L*	*Leguminosae*	Aerial, 70% ethanol	As a diuretic hypnotic, sedative, and antidiabetic	Used as diuretic, hypnotic, sedative, antidiabetic, and hepatoprotector	[71]
47	*Dicoma anomala Sond*	*Asteraceae*	Root, aqueous	Treatment of cold and cough, fever, ulcer, and dermatosis	Antisplasmodial, antibacterial, anthelmintic, antiviral, antioxidant, and anti-inflammatory effects	[72]
48	*Dioscorea alata peel*	*Dioscoreaceae*	Peel, aqueous	To strengthen stomach function, anorexia, and to eliminate diarrhea	Anti-inflammatory effect	[73]
49	*Eclipta alba(L) Hassk*	*Asteracea*	Leaves, aqueous	Treatment of Jaundice. Juice used in treatment of hair problem, typhoid, dysentery, and skin diseases	Hepatoprotection, antidiabetic, analgesic, antimicrobial, antioxidant, anticancer, anti-inflammatory, and immunoregulatory activities	[74]
50	*Emblica officinalis (Gaertn)*	*Euphorbiaceae*	Fruit, methanol	Relieving cough and skin diseases	Antidiabetic, cytoprotective, anti-ulcerogenic, immunomodulatory, antioxidant, and anticataractogenic effects	[75]
51	*Entada pursaetha DC*	*Fabaceae*	Stem, 85% ethanol	Used as narcotic. Treatment of jaundice. As an anthelmintic, in curing eye diseases, diarrhea, and skin diseases	Hepatoprotective and antioxidant effects	[76]
52	*Ephedra foliate Boiss*	*Ephedraceae*	Aerial parts, 90% ethanol	Treatment of allergies, asthma, lung congestion, chills and cold	Antidiabetic, anticancer, antimicrobial, antioxidant, anti-inflammatory, and hepatoprotective effects	[38]
53	*Euphorbia dracunculoides .L*	*Euphorbiaceae*	Aerial part, 95% methanol	Curing skin disorders and edema. Used as diuretic and laxative and in the treatment of rheumatism, snake bite and edema	Anti-inflammatory, analgesic and antioxidant activities. Hepatoprotection against hepatocyte cell lines	[5]
54	*Fagonia schweinfurthii(Hadidi) Hadidi*	*Zygophyllaceae .*	Whole plant, ethanol.	Treatment of Jaundice, diabetes, joint pains, asthma and dropsy.	Antioxidant, hepatoprotective, anti-inflammatory, wound healing and analgesic activities	[77]
55	*Fiscus carica Linn*	*Moraceae.*	Leaves, ethyl acetate.	Treatment of vitiligo, diabetes, cough, asthma, constipation and gingivitis.	Cytotoxic, hypoglycemic and anthelmintic activities.	[78]
56	*Flemingia macrophylla*	*Fabaceae/ Leguminosae.*	Root, aqueous.	Treatment of rheumatism, arthropathy, chronic nephritis, menalgia, and menopausal syndrome.	Antioxidative, anti-inflammatory, analgesic, hypotic-sedative and anxiolytic effects.	[79]

Table 1 (continued)

s/n.	Botanical name	Family	Plant part/extract	Folkloric use	Pharmacological use	Reference
57	*Ginko biloba*	*Ginkgoaceae*.	Leaves, aqueous.	Treatment of Alzheimer's dementia and other cognitive dysfunctions.	Antioxidant, cardioprotective, antiasthmatic, antidiabetic, management of cerebral insufficiency, and decreased gastric injury caused by ethanol.	[80]
58	*Glyphae brevis*	*Tiliaceae.*	Leaves, 50% methanol.	Treatment of hepatitis, jaundice and impotence.	Carminative, anticonvulsant effects, anti-inflammatory, antioxidant and improvement of lipid metabolism.	[81]
59	*Graptopetalum paraguayense E, Walther*	*Crassulaceae*	Leaves, aqueous	Regulation, alleviation of hepatic disorders, relief of pain, detumescence and carbuncles	Antioxidant, anti-inflammatory, neuroprotective, hypertension regulation, antioxidant activity, and inhibition of cancer cells	[82]
60	*Hibiscus sabdariffa. L*	*Malvaceae.*	Aerial parts, 90% ethanol	Used to prepare herbal drinks and as a flavoring agent. As diuretic and choleretic	Antibacterial, antioxidant, nephroprotective, antidiabetic and antihypertensive effects	[38]
61	*Hippophaerhamnoides L*	*Elaegnaceae*	Seabuckthorn berry polysaccharide, alcohol.	Treatment of asthma and circulatory disorders	Antioxidative, antimicrobial, antiatherogenic, cardioprotective, hepatoprotective, radioprotective, and anti-inflammatory effects	[83]
62	*Indigofera oblongifolia*	*Leguminaceae*	Whole plant, 90% ethanol	Treatment of hepatic diseases and dysentery, enlargements of liver and spleen. An antidote of poison	Antimicrobial, anti-inflammatory and analgesic activities	[84]
63	*Launaea procumbens*	*Asteraceae*	Aerial parts, chloroform	Treatment of kidney disorders, hormonal imbalance, and sexual diseases	Spasmogenic, cardiovascular, anticarcinogenic, anti-inflammatory, hepatoprotective, and antioxidant properties	[85]
64	*Lawson inermis L (Henna)*	*Lythraceae*	Leaves, 99% methanol	Used as astringent, hypotensive, sedative against headache. Treatment of jaundice, leprosy, and nervous disorder	Antimicrobial, anti-tumorigenic, anti-inflammatory, anti-apoptotic, antihyperglycaemic, antilipidaemic, antidiabetic, antiviral, and hepatoprotective effects	[86]
65	*Lawsonia inermis Linn*	*Lythraceae*	Leaves, aqueous	Treatment of liver diseases, jaundice, and burn	Anti-inflammatory, antipyretic, analgesics, antimicrobial, anticancer, and hepatoprotective properties	[87]
66	*Leucas cephalotes Linn.*	*Labiatae*	Whole plant, methanol	Treatment of liver disease, snake bite, and bronchitis, inflammation and jaundice.	Antifilarial and antidiabetic activities.	[88]
67	*Lobularia maritima*	*Brassicaceae*	Leaves, 10% ethanol	Antiscorbutic, diuretic, and as an astringent	Antioxidant and anti-inflammatory effects	[7]

Table 1 (continued)

s/n.	Botanical name	Family	Plant part/extract	Folkloric use	Pharmacological use	Reference
68	*Luffa acutangula (Var) amara*	*Cucurbitaceae*	Leaves, ethanol	As a laxative and carminative digestible. Treatment of anemia, jaundice, biliousness bronchitis, asthma, and piles	CNS depressant, antioxidant, and larvicidal activities	[89]
69	*Lygodium flexuosum(L.) Sw*	*Lygodiaceae*	Whole plant, n-hexane	Treatment of jaundice and liver disorders	Hepatoprotection against CCl_4	[90]
70	*Madhuca indica Syn*	*Sapotaceae*	Bark, methanol	Used as stimulants, demulcent, astringents, remedy of itching, and swelling	Anti-inflammatory, analgesic, hepatoprotective, antipyretic, antihyperglycaemic, antiulcer, and antidiabetic effects	[91]
71	*Madhuca indica Syn*	*Sapotaceae*	Leaves, 70% ethanol, 90% ethanol	Treatment of piles, emetic, laxative tonic, anti –burn, and wound healing	Antidiabetic, anti-inflammatory, analgesic, anti-pyretic, antiashmatic, antiulcer, anticancer, hepatoprotective, and antibacterial effects	[92]
72	*Mahonia oiwaken Hayata*	*Berberidaceae*	Root , 90% ethanol	Rheumarthritis, dysentery, hepatitis, antidote, and antiphylogistic agent	Hepatoprotection, antioxidant, and anti-inflammatory	[3]
73	*Mallotus philippensis Muell-Arg*	*Euphorbiaceae*	Leaves, methanol	Treatment of jaundice, threadworm, hookworm, and roundworm infections. As a purgative and carminative	Anticestodal, antibacterial, wound healing, antifilarial, antioxidant, anti-inflammatory, and immunoregulatory effects	[93]
74	*Memondica tuberosa Cogn*	*Cucurbitaceae*	Tubers, 70% ethanol	Used as abortifacient	Antioxidant, antihyperglycemic, anticonvulsant, anti-inflammatory, antiovulation, antidiarrhoeal, and nephroprotective activities	[94]
75	*Mentha piperita L*	*Lamiaceae*	Leaves (essential oil)	Treatment of nausea, bronchitis, flatulence, liver complaints, ulcerative colitis, and as carminative	Antioxidant and anti-inflammatory effects	[95]
76	*Menthe arvensis Linn*	*Lamiaceae*	Leaves, aqueous, chloroform, ethanol	Carminative, antispasmodic, and anti-peptic ulcer agent	Radioprotective, antispasmodic, antibacterial, anthelmintic, antifertility, hepatoprotective, antiulcer, and anti-inflammatory	[96]
77	*Mimosa pudica 2009*	*Fabaceae/Leguminosae.*	Leaves, methanol	Treatment of piles, fistula, insomnia, traumatic injury and jaundice	Hyperglycemic, antioxidant, anti-hepatotoxic, antidiabetic, wound healing, anti-inflammatory, and antimicrobial effects	[97]
78	*Mimosa pudica Linn*	*Fabaceae/Leguminosae.*	Leaves, ethanol	Treatment of wound, oedema, allergy, fever, diabetes, and indigestion	Hyperglycemic, antioxidant, anti-hepatotoxic, antidiabetic, wound healing, anti-inflammatory, and antimicrobial effects	[98]
79	*Momordica dioica Roxb*	*Cucurbitaceae*	Leaves, ethanol	Treatment of Jaundice, hepatic diseases, fever, asthma, and as anthelmintic. Used as stomach laxative	Hypoglycemic, gastroprotective, ulcer healing, and hepatoprotective effects	[99]

Table 1 (continued)

s/n.	Botanical name	Family	Plant part/extract	Folkloric use	Pharmacological use	Reference
80	*Nerium oleander Linn*	*Apocynaceae*	Flower, methanol	Treatment of malaria and venereal diseases. Used as diuretic, insecticide, abortifacient, and cardiotonic. Relieves Indigestion	Cardiac insufficiency, anticonvulsant, antitumor, and antioxidant effects	[100]
81	*Nicotiana plumbiginifolia .L*	*Solanaceae*	Whole plant, methanol	Treatment of cuts, wounds, toothache, and rheumatic swelling	Antispasmodic, leaves are effective lavicide, antioxidant, and antimicrobial	[101]
82	*Nymphaea alba. L*	*Nymphaeceae*	Leaves, 76% ethanol	Used as antiseptic, an astringent and as a rubefacient in insomnia	Antioxidant, anti-inflammatory, and hepatoprotective effects.	[6]
83	*Olea europaea .L.*	*Oleaceae*	Leaves, 20% oleuropein	Treatment of malaria and associated fever	Antimicrobial, anti-inflammatory, antioxidant, blood pressure lowering, lipid lowering, anticancer, and cardioprotective activities	[102]
84	*Origanum vulgare.*	*Lamiaceae*	Leaves, aqueous	Treatment of respiratory disorders, indigestion, and rheumatoid arthritis	Antihyperglycaemic, anti-inflammatory, cytotoxic, antioxidant, antithrombin, antimutagenic, and anti-carcinogenic effects	[103]
85	*Persea Americana mill*	*Lauraceae*	Leaves, aqueous	Remedy for pyorrhea. Toxic to silkworms	Antifungal, hypotensive, anti-inflammatory, anticonvulsant, antidiabetic, antioxidant, and vasorelaxant effects	[104]
86	*Phyllanthus niruri*	*Phyllanthaceae*	Aerial part, 80% ethanol	Treatment of urinary and bladder disorders, hepatic disorders, dyspepsia, influenza jaundice, and kidney stone	Hepatoprotective, antioxidant, antihyperuricemic, and lipid lowering effects	[105]
87	*Physalis peruviana (Golden berry)*	*Solanaceae*	Leaves, 50% methanol	Used as antispasmodic, diuretic, antiseptic, sedative, analgesic, and hepatitis	Antiulcer, antimicrobial, anti-inflammatory and antihypercholesterolemic activities	[106]
88	*Pleiogynium timorense (DC) Leenh*	*Anacardiaceae*	Bark, 70% methanol	–	Antimicrobial, hepatoprotective, antioxidant, anti-inflammatory, hypoglycemic, and cytotoxic effects	[107]
89	*Pleurotus ostreatus*	*Pleurotaceae*	Whole mushroom, 95% ethanol	Preventing heart disease, reduction in cholesterol, and treatment of diabetes	Inhibition of platelet aggregation, reduction of blood glucose and cholesterol, antibacterial, viral, and parasitic pathogens, and antioxidant activities	[108]
90	*Polygonum cuspidatum sieb et Zucc*	*Polygonaceae*	Rhizome, methanol	Treatment of jaundice, and to clear heat toxin, to promote blood circulation. Dispel stasis, suppress cough, and treat snake bites	Antidiabetic, anti-hepatitis B virus, antibacterial, anti-inflammatory, and antioxidant properties	[4]
91	*Premna esculenta Roxb*	*Verbenaceae*	Leaves, 95% ethanol	Treatment of hepatocellular jaundice, gout, hook worm infection, and snake bite	Antihyperlipidemic, hepatoprotective, antioxidant, analgesic, and anti-inflammatory activities	[109]

Table 1 (continued)

s/n.	Botanical name	Family	Plant part/extract	Folkloric use	Pharmacological use	Reference
92	*Raphanus sativus*	*Brassicaceae*	Leaves, aqueous and ethanol	Treatment of indigestion, abdominal bloating, diarrhea, bronchitis, intestinal parasites, and asthma	Antimicrobial, anticancer, antidiabetic, gastrointestinal, uterine tone modulatory, and cardio-modulatory activities	[110]
93	*Rourea induta planch*	*Connaraceae.*	Leaves, 99% ethanol	Treatment of respiratory and kidney diseases. Treatment of blood diarrhea, and as diuretics	Anti-inflammatory, hepatoprotective, antioxidant, and antipyretic activities	[111]
94	*Rubia cordifolia Linn*	*Rubiaceae.*	Root, 50% ethanol	Treatment of jaundice	Potent antioxidant property, inhibit lipid peroxidation, anti-inflammatory, immunomodulatory, anticonvulsant, anxiolytic and antitumor activities	[112]
95	*Rumex vasicarius L*	*Polygonaceae.*	Whole plant, methanol	Aperients, diuretic and cooling agent. Treatment of jaundice and dysentery. Curing stomach heat, toothache, and to promote appetite	Antimicrobial, anti-inflammatory, antioxidant, wound healing, and antitumor activities	[113]
96	*Semen celosia Cristatae.L*	*Amaranthaceae.*	Dry seeds, 60% ethanol	Treatment of hypertension, palsy, cataract, keratitis, diabetes, iridocyclitis, caligo corneal, and sarcoptidosis	Antibacterial, anticancer, antidiarroheal and anti-inflammatory effects	[114]
97	*Solanium trilobatum Linn*	*Solanaceae.*	Whole plant, 90% ethanol	Used as an expectorant in the treatment of respiratory diseases, asthma, tuberculosis, and liver diseases	Broad spectrum antibiotic, antibacterial, antimitotic, anticancer, and antioxidant properties	[115]
98	*Solanium xantholarpum*	*Solanaceae.*	Fruit, 50% ethanol	Laxative, treatment of enlargement of liver, anthelmintic, antipyretic, anti-inflammatory, antiasthmatic, and aphrodisiac activities.	Antiasthmatic, anti-nociceptive, antifungal, molluscicide, antispasmodic, antitumor, cardiotonic, hypotensive, antianaphylactic, and anti-urolithiatic activities	[116]
99	*Spondias mombim*	*Anacardiaceae*	Leaves and stem, 50% methanol	Treatment of hepatitis	Antimicrobial, antiviral, anti-inflammatory, anthelmintic, hematinic sedative, antioxidant, and hepatoprotective effects	[117]
100	*Stachys pilifera Benth*	*Lamiaceae*	Leaves, 70% ethanol	Treatment of asthma, rheumatoid arthritis, and asthma	Anti-inflammatory, antioxidant, antibacterial, antitumor, and antimicrobial effects	[118]
101	*Vitis thunbergii Var*	*Vitaceae*	Aerial part, ethanol	Treatment of hepatitis, jaundice, diarrhea, and arthritis	Antioxidant, anti-inflammatory, antihypertensive, neuroprotective, antibacterial, and inhibition of adipocyte differentiation	[119]
102	*Xylaria nigripes(Koltz) Sacc*	*Xylariaceae*	Solid cultured mycelia, aqueous	Treatment of insomnia, trauma, diuretic, and nerve tonic	Antioxidant and hepatoprotective effects	[120]

Table 1 (continued)

s/n.	Botanical name	Family	Plant part/extract	Folkloric use	Pharmacological use	Reference
103	*Zingiber officinale(Roscoe) rhizome (ginger)*	*Zingiberaceae*	Rhizome, 90% methanol	Nutraceutical. Treatment of stomach aches, nausea, diarrhea, as carminative, appetite stimulant, and choleretic	Antioxidant, anti-inflammatory, antitumor, antidiabetic, antimicrobial, neuro-protective, and gastro-protective potentials	[121]
104	*Zizyphus jujube Mill*	*Rhaminaceae*	Fruit, 70% ethanol	Invigorating the spleen, treatment of anorexia, lassitude, and control of hepatitis	Antioxidant and anti-inflammatory activities	[122]

Table 2 In vivo studies on medicinal plants with hepato protection against acute tetrachloride toxicity

s.no.	Botanical name	Animal model.	Maximum extract dose/route of administration	CCL4 dose/route of administration	Standard drug administered/route of administration	Result.	Active components.	Reference
1	*Abelmoschus manihot (L) medic*	Ku-Ming mice.	500mg/kg/b.w. (oral).	0.1 ml/kg/bw(0.12% v/v olive oil), i.p.	Biphenyl dicarboxylate (BDP) 150 mg/kg/b.w., oral.	ALT, AST, ALP, γ-GT, TNF-α, IL-1β, NO, MDA↓, GSH, SOD, GPx, CAT, GST↑.	Flavonoids, quercetin, hyperin, isoquercetin, quercetin-3′-0-glucoside, hibifolin, myricetin	[32]
2	*Acacia mellifera*	Wistar rats	500mg/kg/ b.w.	1.25 ml/kg/ b.w. (1:1 liquid paraffin) i.p	Silymarin, 100 mg/kg/bw	ALT, AST, GGT, ALP, T.B↓,T.P↑,MDA, NP-SH, T-chol, TG↓, NP-SH↑. (Nonprotein sulfhydryl)	Flavonoids, saponin, tannins, triterpenoids	[33]
3	*Aegle marmelos correa ex Roxb*	Albino Wistar rats	- (oral)	0.2 ml/100g/b.w. (olive oil), i.p.	–	AST, ALT, ALP, T.B↓	Flavonoids	[34]
4	*Aegle marmelos correa ex Roxb*	Wistar albino rats	50mg/kg/b.w. (oral)	3ml/kg/b.w., i.p.	Silymarin 200 mg/kg/b.w., (oral)	ALP, ALT, AST, T.B, LDH, MDA↓, SOD, CAT, GR, GSH, GST, GPx, G6PD, T.P↑, IL-10, TNF-α↓.	Rutin, piperine	[35]
5	*Alangium salviifolium*	Swiss albino mice	50mg/kg/b.w. (oral)	1 ml/kg/b.w. (1:1 in olive oil).	–	AST, ALT, ALP, MDA, LDH, CYT-P450 reductase, cyt b5 reductase↓, SOD, CAT, DT-diaphorase, glutathione-s-transferase↑	Piperine, γ-sistosterol	[36]
6	*Alhagi maurorum (camel thorn)*	Wistar rats	660 mg/kg/b.w. (oral)	1 ml/kg/b.w. (maize oil) oral.	–	ALT, AST↓	Flavonoids, phenols	[37]
7	*Alhagi maurorum Medikus*	Wistar rats	500 mg/kg/b.w.	0.125 ml/kg (liquid paraffin, 1:1), i.p	Silymarin, 10 mg/kg (oral)	SGOT, SGPT, ALP, T.B.	Flavonoids, tannins.	[38]
8	*Allium sativum (Single clove garlic)*	Male rabbits	0.8 g (oral)	3 ml/kg/b.w. (1:1, olive oil)	–	ALT, AST, ALP, T.B↓, T.P↑, MDA↓, CAT, GST, SOD↑	–	[39]
9	*Amaranthus spinosus*	Sprague-Dawley rats	400 mg/kg/b.w. (oral)	1 ml /kg/ b.w. (v/v olive oil) i.p.	–	AST, ALT, ALP, T.B, MDA↓, GSH, SOD, CAT↑	Flavonoids, phenols, betalains.	[40]
10	*Amorphophallus campanulatus (Roxb)*	Wistar albino rats and mice	500 mg/kg/b.w. (oral)	1 ml/kg/b.w., oral.	Silymarin, 50 mg / kg/b.w., (oral)	MDA, Hydroperoxides↓, GSH, SOD, CAT↑	Flavonoids	[41]
11	*Argemone Mexicana L*	Wistar rats	500 mg/kg/b.w. (oral)	0.5 ml/kg/b.w., i.p.	Silymarin, 100mg/kg (oral)	SGOT, SGPT, ALP, Total bilirubin↓	Leutolin, quercetin, quercetrin	[42]
12	*Artemisia iwayomogi*	Sprague-Dawley rats.	500 mg/ kg/b.w. (oral)	2 ml/kg/b.w. (50% oliveoil) i.p.	–	ALT, AST, ALP, MDA↓, TAC, GSH, SOD↑, Hydroxy proline↓	Scoparone	[43]
13	*Bauhinia variegate*	Sprague-Dawley rats	200 mg/kg/b.w. (oral)	1 ml/kg/b.w. (liquid paraffin, 1:1) subcutaneous.	–	AST, ALT, ALP, GGT↓, T.P↑, Total lipid↓	–	[44]
14	*Bougainullra spectabillis*	Wistar rats.	6 mg/kg/b.w. (oral)	1.5 ml/kg, oral.	–	AST, ALP, ALT↓	Esculetin	[45]
15	*Bryonia diocia Jacq*	Wistar albino rats	250 mg/kg/b.w. (gavage)	1 ml/kg/b.w. (corn oil,1:1v/v).	–	AST, AST↓	Flavonoids, terpenoids	[46]

Table 2 (continued)

s.no.	Botanical name	Animal model.	Maximum extract dose/route of administration	CCL4 dose/route of administration	Standard drug administered/route of administration	Result.	Active components.	Reference
16	*Brysocarpus coCClneus.*	Albino rats	1000 mg / kg /b.w. (oral).	0.7 ml/kg/b.w. (1:1 in olive oil) i.p.	livolin®, 200 mg/kg/b.w., (oral)	ALT, AST, ALP, MDA↓, T.P, Albumin, CAT, SOD, GPx, GSH↑	Alkaloids, flavonoids	[47]
17	*Cajanus cajan.*	Wistar albino rats	400 mg/kg/b.w. (oral)	2 ml/kg/b.w. (1:1 liquid paraffin), oral.	Liv 52, 100 mg/kg/b.w. (oral)	AST, ALT↓, T.P↑	Alkaloid, flavonoids	[48]
18	*Calotropis gigantean R.Br.*	Wistar rats	500 mg/kg/b.w. (oral)	2 ml/kg/b.w. (1:1 olive oil), subcutaneous.	Silymarin, 100 mg/kg/bw., (oral)	AST, ALT, LPO↓, GSH, SOD, GPX, CAT↑	Calotropin DI and DII, calotropin FI and FII.	[49]
19	*Camellia ntidissima Chi.*	Sprague-Dawley rats	160 mg/kg/day (i.p)	2 ml/kg (50% v/v, olive oil), i.p.	Thiopronin 20 mg/kg/day, (i.p)	AST, ALT, MDA↓, GSH, SOD↑, TNF-α, IL-6, IL-1β, NF-kβ signaling↓, NrF2 signaling partway, HO-1, SOD, GSH↑	Polyphenols, flavonoids	[1]
20	*Canna indica L.*	Sprangue-Dawley rats	200 mg/kg/b.w. (oral)	1.0 ml/kg(liquid paraffin,1:2) i.p.	Silymarin, 25 mg/kg, (i.p)	SGPT, SGOT, ALP, T.B, L.P↓, GSH, CAT, T.P↑	Lutein	[50]
21	*Capparis spinosa.*	Mice	400 mg/kg/b.w. (oral)	0.2 ml/kg (olive oil 1:1), oral.	–	ALT, AST↓	Flavonoids, phenols, rutin, quercetin-3-O-glucoside, kaempherol, 3-O-rutinoside	[51]
22	*Capsella busa-pastoris (L.) Medik.*	Wistar rats	500 mg/kg/b.w.	0.125 ml/kg (liquid paraffin, 1:1), i.p	Silymarin, 10 mg/kg, (oral)	SGOT, SGPT, ALP, T.B	–	[38]
23	*Carissa opaca*	Sprague-Dawley rats	200 mg/kg/b.w. (intragastrically)	0.5 ml/kg/b.w. (20% v/v olive oil), i.p.	Silymarin, 50 mg/kg/b.w., (intragastrically)	AST, ALT, ALP, LDH, ɤ-GT↓, GSH-Px, GSR, SOD, GST, CAT, Peroxidase, Quinone reductase(QR) ↑, TBARS, GSH, H2O2↓, T.P↑	Isoquercetin, hyperoside, vitexin, myicetin, kaempherol	[52]
24	*Carthamus tinctorius L*	Sprangue-Dawley rats.	5 mg/kg/day	1.0 ml/kg (olive oil).	–	ALT, AST, Hydroxy proline↓	Hydroxysafflor yellow A, isocarthamidin, carthamin, luteolin	[53]
25	*Carthamus tinctorius. L*	Sprague-Dawley rats	20 mg/kg/b.w. (oral)	2 ml/kg/b.w. (1:1 olive oil), i.p.	Silymarin, 50 mg/kg/b.w., (oral).	ALT, AST, ALP, T.P↓, NrF2, GSTα, NQOI expression, GSH↑, TBARS↓, SOD, CAT↑.	Carthamin, carthamidin, polyphenols, carthamus red, flavonoids	[54]
26	*Carum carvil*	NMRI mice	0.13 g/kg/b.w. (oral)	2 ml/kg/b.w. (olive oil, 1:2), i.p.	–	AST, ALT, L.P↓, GSH, GSH-Px↑, Px, XOD↓, Protein↑	Carvon	[55]
27	*Cassia angustifolia Vahl*	Wistar albino rats	300 mg/kg/bw (oral)	2.5 ml/kg/b.w.	Silymarin, 100 mg/kg/bw, (oral)	AST, ALT, ALP, Acid phosphatase(ACP), LDH, T.B↓, T.P↑	Flavonoid, terpenoids, tannin, steroid	[56]
28	*Cassia angustofolia vahl*	Wistar rats	500 mg/kg/b.w. (oral)	4 ml/kg/b.w. (50% olive oil) oral	–	T.B, GOT, GPT↓, T.P, GSH↑, LPO↓	Flavonoids	[57]

Table 2 (continued)

s.no.	Botanical name	Animal model.	Maximum extract dose/route of administration	CCL4 dose/route of administration	Standard drug administered/route of administration	Result.	Active components.	Reference
29	*Cassia fistula Linn*	Wistar albino rats	500 mg/kg/ b.w. (oral)	0.1 ml/kg/b.w. (liquid paraffin)	–	MDA, AST, ALT, GSH, ALP, LDH, γ-glutamyltranspeptidase↓	Flavonoids	[58]
30	*Cichorium intybus*	Wister rats	6 mg/kg/b.w. (oral)	1.5 ml/kg(oral)	–	AST, ALP, ALT↓	Esculetin	[45]
31	*Cichorium intybus*	Albino wistar rats	500 mg/kg/b.w. (oral)	1.5 ml/kg(olive oil 50%), i.p.	Silymarin 10 mg/kg (oral)	SGOT, SGPT, ALKP↓, T.P, albumin↑	Cichotyboside	[59]
32	*Cichorium intybus*	Albino wistar rats	500 mg/kg/b.w. (oral)	1.5 ml/kg olive oil50%), i.p.	Silymarin 10 mg/kg (oral)	SGOT, SGPT, ALKP↓, T.P, albumin↑	Cichotyboside	[59]
33	*Cichorium intybus*	Albino rats	500mg/kg/b.w. (oral)	1.0 ml/kg olive oil 50%), i.p.	–	AST, ALP, ALT, T.B↓, T.P, albumin↑	Esculetin and cichotyboside	[60]
34	*Cinnamomum verum*	Wistar albino rats	100 mg/ kg/ b.w. (oral)	1 ml/kg/b.w. (olive oil), subcutaneous.	–	AST, ALT, MDA↓, SOD, CAT↑	–	[61]
35	*Cinnamomum verum*	Wistar albino rats.	100 mg/kg/ b.w. (oral)	1 ml/ kg/ b.w. (olive oil), i.p.	Silymarin 50 mg/ kg/b.w. (oral)	ALT, AST, ALP, γ-glutamyl transferase, LDH, TBARS↓		[62]
36	*Cinnamomum zeylanicum L.*	Wister rats	0.1 g/kg(oral)	0.5 ml/kg/b.w. (50% olive oil).	–	AST, ALT, MDA↓, SOD, CAT↑	Flavonoids	[63]
37	*Citrus aurantium (essential oil)*	Sprangue-Dawley rats	0.8 ml/kg/b.w. (i.p)	0.8 ml/kg(olive oil 1:1), i.p.	Silibinin 50 mg/kg (i.p).	AST, ALT↓.	Limonene, alpa-pinene	[64]
38	*Citrus limon(L.) Burm.F.*	Wistar rats	500 mg/kg/b.w. (oral)	1 ml/kg (olive oil,50:50).	Silymarin 100 mg/kg (oral).	ALT, AST, ALP, T, B, MDA↓, SOD, GSH, CAT, albumin↑	Coumarins, limonoids, flavonoids, eriocitrin, C-glycosyl flavones 6,8-di-C-β-glucosyl-diosmin	[65]
39	*Clerodendrum volubile.*	Wistar albino rats	500 mg/ kg/bw.(oral)	1 ml/kg/b.w. (olive oil), i.p.	–	ALT, AST, ALP, LDH ↓, HDL, GSH, CAT, SOD, GPx↑	Phenols	[66]
40	*Clitoria ternatea L.*	Wistar albino rats	300 mg/kg/bw (oral)	2.5 ml/kg/b.w.	Silymarin, 100 mg/kg/ bw, (oral)	AST, ALT, ALP, Acid phosphatase(ACP), LDH, T.B↓, T.P↑	Flavonoid, terpenoids, tannin, steroid, quericimetrin, rutin, scutellarein	[56]
41	*Corianderum sativum. L*	Wistar albino rats	300 mg/kg(i.p)	1 ml/kg/b.w. (liquid parafin, 1:1), oral.	Silymarin, 50 mg/kg (i.p)	SGOT, SGPT, ALP↓, T.B↑	Caffeic acid, quercetin, gallic acid, flavonoids, essential oil	[67]
42	*Corianderum sativum. L. (essential oil)*	NMRI mice	0.03 g/kg/b.w. (oral)	2 ml/kg/b.w. (olive oil, 1:2), i.p.	-	AST, ALT, L.Px, XOD, Px↓, GSH, GSH-Px, Protein↑	Carvon	[55]

Table 2 (continued)

s.no.	Botanical name	Animal model.	Maximum extract dose/route of administration	CCL4 dose/route of administration	Standard drug administered/route of administration	Result.	Active components.	Reference
43	*Coriandrum sativum*	Wistar albino rats	200 mg/kg/ b.w. (i.p)	1 ml/kg b.w. (1:1 olive oil), i.p.	Silymarin, 25 ml/ kg/b.w., (i.p)	ALP, AST, ALT↓, T.P↑, T.B, MDA↓, SOD, CAT, GPx↑	Caffeic acid, ferulic acid, Isoquercitrin, rutin, quercetin 3-glucuronide, Quercetin, hyperin, quercetin-3-0-β-xyloside, quercetin-3-0-α-arabinose	[68]
44	*Cortex dictamni*	Sprague-Dawley rats	320 mg/kg/b.w. (oral)	2 ml/kg/b.w., i.p.	-	AST, ALT, ALP↓, SOD, CAT, GSH-Px, GSH↑, MDA↓	Limonoids, furoquinoline, flavonoids, fraxinellone	[69]
45	*Curcuma longa. L.*	Sprague-Dawley rats	300 mg/kg/b.w. (intragastrically)	0.1 ml/kg/b.w., i.p.	Curcumin, 200 mg/ kg/b.w., (intragastrically)	AST, ALT, TBARS↓, SOD, GPx↑.	Curcumin, memethoxy curcumin, bisdemethoxy curcumin	[70]
46	*Cytisus scoparius L.*	Wistar albino rats	500 mg/kg/b.w. (oral)	5 ml/kg(50% olive oil), i.p.	Silymarin, 25 mg/ kg/b.w., (oral)	SGOT, SGPT, LDH↓, GSH, SOD, CAT, GPx, GRD, GST↑, TBARS↓	Rutin, quercetin, quercitrin, isorhamnetin, kaempferol	[71]
47	*Dicoma anomala Sond*	Wistar rats; Rattus norvegicus	500 mg/kg/b.w. (oral)	1 ml/kg/b.w. (1:1, olive oil), i.p.	Silymarin, 100 mg/ kg.b.w., (oral)	AST, ALT↓, SOD, CAT, GPx↑	Total flavonoid and phenol contents	[72]
48	*Dioscorea alata peel*	Wistar albino rats	433.42 mg/kg/b.w.	1 ml/kg (20% olive oil)	Silymarin, 200 mg/ kg/b.w.	ALT, ALP, AST, TBARS↓, SOD, CAT, GSH-Px↑, NO, TNF-α, TNF-Kb, iNOS, COX-2 expression↓	Hesperetin, quercetin, hesperidin	[73]
49	*Eclipta alba(L) Hassk*	Male albino rats	500 mg/kg/b.w. (oral)	2 ml/kg/b.w. (olive oil), i.p.	Silymarin, 50 mg / kg/b.w., (i.p).	ALT, AST, ALP, T.B↓, T.P↑	Flavonoids, luteolin, demethylivedelolactone.wedelolactone	[74]
50	*Emblica officinalis (Gaertn)*	–	200 mg/kg/b.w.	1 ml/kg/b.w. (corn oil), oral.	–	SGOT, SGPT, LDH, MDA↓, GSH, GST, GPx, GRx, T.P↑, DNA synthesis↓	Quercetin, ascorbic acid, ellagic acid	[75]
51	*Entada pursaetha*	Colony bred male Wistar rats	300 mg/kg/b.w. (oral)	2 ml/kg/b.w. (1:1 olive oil).	Silymarin, 50 mg / kg/b.w. (2% polysorbate 80), (oral).	ALT, AST, ALP, T.B↓, T.P↑, LDH, MDA, Nitrate-nitrite, myeloperoxidase↓, SOD, CAT, GSH↑	Flavonoids	[76]
52	*Ephedra foliate Boiss*	Wistar rats	500 mg/kg/b.w.	0.125 ml/kg (liquid paraffin, 1:1), i.p.	Silymarin, 10 mg/kg, (oral).	SGOT, SGPT, ALP, T.B	Flavonoids, tannins	[38]
53	*Euphorbia dracunculoides L.*	Sprague-Dawley rats	400 mg/kg/b.w. (oral)	1 ml/kg/b, w (30% olive oil), i.p.	Silymarin 50 mg/ kg/b.w.	AST, ALT, ALP↓, CAT, Peroxidase, SOD, GST, GSH↑, Lipid peroxides, TBARS, nitrite, hydrogen peroxide, DNA damage↓	Catechin, rutin, caffeic acid, mricetin, coumarins, flavonoids	[5]

Table 2 (continued)

s.no.	Botanical name	Animal model.	Maximum extract dose/route of administration	CCL4 dose/route of administration	Standard drug administered/route of administration	Result.	Active components.	Reference
54	*Fagonia schweinfurthii(Hadidi) Hadidi*	Wistar albino rats	400 mg/kg/ b.w. (oral)	1 ml/kg/b.w., i.p.	Silymarin 100 mg/kg/b.w., (oral).	ALT, AST, ALP, T.B, MDA↓, SOD, CAT, GSH↑	Flavonoids, phenolic compounds, quinines and, coumarin	[77]
55	*Fiscus carica Linn*	Wistar rats	100 mg/kg/b.w. (oral)	1 ml/kg/bw(v/v olive oil), i.p.	–	SGOT, SGPT, T.B. ↓	Psoralen, bergapten, xantho toxin, calotropenyl acetate, lupeol acetate	[78]
56	*Flemingia macrophylla*	Male SD rats	1.0 g/kg/b.w. (oral)	15 ml/kg/b.w. (20% olive oil), i.p.	Silymarin, 25 mg/kg/b.w. in carboxy methyl cellulose.	ALT, AST, MDA↓, SOD, CAT, GSH-PX, GSH↑, NO, TNF-α, IL-1β↓.	Genistein, lupeol, rutin, flavonoids, isoflavones	[79]
57	*Ginko biloba*	Sprague-Dawley rats	150 mg/ kg/ b.w. (oral)	1 ml/kg/b.w. (1:1 liquid paraffin).	-	ALP, ALT, AST, MDA↓, T.P, HDL-c, GSH↑	Kaempferol, quercetin, isorhamnetin, diterpene lactones	[80]
58	*Glyphae brevis*	Swiss albino mice	490 mg/kg/ b.w. (oral)	2 ml/kg/b.w. (liquid paraffin) i.p.	Silymarin, 100 mg/kg (oral)	GSH, CAT, SOD↑, TBARS, ALT, AST, ALP, T-chol, LDL, TG↓, T.P↑	Flavonoids	[81]
59	*Graptopetalum paraguayense E, Walter*	Sprague-Dawley rats	300 mg/kg/b.w. (oral)	0.5 ml/kg/b.w. (1:4 olive oil) oral.	Silymarin, 200 mg/kg/b.w., (oral).	AST, ALT, MDA↓, GSH, SOD, GR, SOD, CAT↑, TNF-α↓	Gallic acid, genistin, daidzin, quercetin	[82]
60	*Hibiscus sabdariffa. L.*	Wistar rats	500 mg/kg/b.w.	0.125 ml/kg (liquid paraffin, 1:1), i.p.	Silymarin, 10 mg/kg (oral)	SGOT, SGPT, ALP, T.B	–	[38]
61	*Hippophaerhamnoides L*	C57BL/6 mice	200 mg/kg/b.w. (oral)	5 ml/kg/b.w. (20% in peanut oil), i.p.	–	ALT, AST, T.B↓, PALB, SOD, GSH-Px, GSH↑, MDA, TNF-α, IL-1β, iNOS, NO, TLR4, p38MAPK, p-ERK, p-JNK, NF-KB↓	Isorhamnetein, quercetin, chlorogenic acid, myricetin, kaempferol, catechins	[83]
62	*Indigofera oblongifolia*	Wistar albino rats	300 mg/kg/ b.w. (oral)	1 ml /kg/ b.w. (30% olive oil), i.p.	–	ALT, AST, ALP, TBARS↓, GSH, SOD, CAT, GPX↑	Flavonoids, coumarins, indirubin	[84]
63	*Launaea procumbens*	Sprague-Dawley rats	200 mg/kg/b.w. (oral)	3 ml/kg/b.w. (30% olive oil), i.p.	Silymarin 100 mg/kg/b.w., (oral)	AST, ALT, ALP, LDH↓, GST, GSR, GSH, CAT, POD, SOD, GSH-Px↑	Salicylic acid, vanillic acid, synergic acid, 2-methyl-resorcinol, and gallic acid	[85]
64	*Lawson inermis L (Henna)*	Albino rats	200 mg/kg/b.w. (oral)	2 ml/kg/bw (1:1 olive oil).	Silymarin, 25 mg/kg/b.w. (oral).	ALT, AST, ALP, T.B↓, T.P↑	Flavonoids	[86]
65	*Lawsonia inermis Linn*	Wistar albino rats	400 mg/kg/b.w. (i.p.)	1.25 ml/kg(1:1 liquid paraffin), i.p.	Silymarin, 100 mg/kg/b.w. (i.p)	SGOT, SGPT, MDA↓, T.P, GSH. ↑	Flavonoids	[87]
66	*Leucas cephalotes Linn*	Wistar albino rats	200 mg/kg/ b.w. (liquid paraffin) (i.p).	1.25 mg/kg (1:1 liquid paraffin), i.p.	Silymarin, 200 mg/kg (i.p).	SGOT, SGPT, Alkaline phosphatase (ALKP), T.B↓, T.P, TC. ↑.	Flavonoids	[88]

Table 2 (continued)

s.no.	Botanical name	Animal model.	Maximum extract dose/route of administration	CCL4 dose/route of administration	Standard drug administered/route of administration	Result.	Active components.	Reference
67	*Lobularia maritima*	Mice	500 mg/kg/b.w. (i.p)	1 ml/kg/b.w. (1:1 olive oil), i.p.	–	ALT, AST, MDA, ROS, TNF-α, IL-1β, IL-6↓, SOD, CAT, GPx↑	p-coumaric acid	[7]
68	*Luffa acutangula (Var) amara*	Colony bred strain of Wistar rats	600 mg/kg/ b.w. (oral)	1 ml/kg/b.w., oral	Silymarin, 25 mg/kg/b.w. (oral)	SGOT,S GPT, ALP, TC, TB ↓, TP, GPx, GST, GSH, SOD, CAT↑, LPO ↓ , Vit E, Vit C.↑	Flavonoids	[89]
69	*Lygodium flexuosum(L.) Sw*	Wistar rats	200 mg/kg/b.w.	150 µl /100 g (1:1 corn oil)	Silymarin, 50 mg/kg	AST, ALT, LDH, MDA↓, GSH↑	Β-sitosterol, stigmasterol, kaempferol, tectoquinone	[90]
70	*Madhuca indica Syn*	Wistar rats	400 mg/kg/b.w (oral)	2 ml/kg/b.w. (olive oil), (i.p)	Silymarin, 100 mg/kg/b.w.	T.B, SGOT, SGPT, ALP↓	Flavonoids	[91]
71	*Madhuca indica Syn*	Wistar rats	300 mg/ kg/ b.w.	0.5 ml/kg/b.w., i.p.	Silymarin, 100 mg/kg/bw.	SGOT, SGPT, ALP, T.B↓	Flavonoids	[92]
72	*Mahonia oiwaken Hayata*	Wistar albino rats	500 mg/kg/b.w (oral)	1 ml/kg/b.w. (50% olive oil), i.p.	Silymarin, 200 mg / kg/b.w, (oral)	ALT, AST, MDA↓, SOD, GP-x, GR↑, TNF-α, NO↓	Berberine, palmatine, jatrorrhizine	[3]
73	*Mallotus philippensis Muell-Arg*	Wistar albino rats	200 mg/kg/b.w (oral)	600 mg/kg/ml, oral	Silymarin, 25 mg/kg/b.w. (oral)	SGPT, SGOT, ALP, T.B↓, T.P, CAT, SOD↑, LPO↓	Flavonoids, phenols, isocoumarins, bergenin	[93]
74	*Memondica tuberosa Cogn*	Wistar rats	400 mg/kg/bw (oral)	2 ml/kg/b.w(1:1 liquid paraffin), subcutaneous	Silymarin, 100 mg/kg, (oral)	SGOT, ALPT, T.B, Cholesterol, TAG, MDA↓, GSH↑	Vitamin C, saponins, triterpenoids	[94]
75	*Mentha piperita L.*	Wistar rats	40 mg/kg/b.w (oral)	1 ml/kg (olive oil), i.p.	Silymarin, 50 mg / kg/b.w, (oral)	ALT, AST, ALP, LDH, γ-GT↓, SOD, CAT, GPx↑, TBARS↓	Spathulenol, cadinene, caryophyllene, caryophyllene oxide	[95]
76	*Menthe arvensis Linn*	Albino wistar rats	375 mg/kg/b.w (oral)	0.5 ml/kg/b.w., i.p.	Silymarin, 100 mg/kg/b.w. (oral)	SGPT, SGOT, SALP, T.B↓	Luteolin, menthoside, rutin, hesperidin, phenolic acid, quercetin, isorhoifolin	[96]
77	*Mimosa pudica 2009*	Wistar albino rats	200 mg/kg/b.w (oral)	1.25 ml/kg/b.w. (1:1 liquid paraffin), i.p.	Silymarin, 100 mg/kg/b.w.	SPGT, SGOT, ALP, TBL, T chol↓, T.P, albumin↑	Flavonoids, alkaloids, glycosides	[97]
78	*Mimosa pudica Linn*	Wistar albino rats	400 mg/kg/b.w. (oral)	1 ml/kg/b.w (1 : 2 liquid paraffin), subcutaneous.	Silymarin, 10 mg/kg/b.w, (oral)	SGOT, ALP, T.B, SGPT↓	Flavonoids, phenols, gallic acid	[98]
79	*Momordica dioica Roxb*	Wistar albino rats	200 mg/kg/b.w. (oral)	2 ml/kg/b.w(1:1 liquid araffin).	Silymarin, 5 mg/kg/b.w. (oral)	AST, ALT, ALP, T.B, MDA↓, SOD, CAT, GSH↑, Hydroperoxides↓	Flavonoids, phenolic compounds	[99]
80	*Nerium oleander Linn*	Wistar rats	400 mg/kg/b.w. (oral)	1 ml/kg/b.w(1;1 olive oil), i.p.	Silymarin, 100 mg/kg/b.w (oral).	AST, ALT, ALP, T.B, MDA↓, SOD↑	Oleandrin, Oleanolic acid	[100]
81	*Nicotiana plumbiginifolia .L.*	Male chicks	200 mg/kg/b.w. (oral)	1 ml/kg/b.w (30% olive oil), i.p.	Silymarin , 100 mg/kg/b.w, (gavage).	CAT, Peroxidase, SOD, GP-X, GRS↑, TBARS, LDH, TAG, T.Chol, LDL↓, HDL↑	Rutin, chlorogenic acid, quercetin	[101]

Table 2 (continued)

s.no.	Botanical name	Animal model.	Maximum extract dose/route of administration	CCL4 dose/route of administration	Standard drug administered/route of administration	Result.	Active components.	Reference
82	*Nymphaea alba. L.*	Wistar albino rats	200 mg/kg/b.w. (oral)	0.5 ml/kg/b.w, i.p.	Silymarin, 100 mg/kg/b.w(oral).	MDA↓, GSH, CAT, SOD, TAC↑, TNF-α, Caspase-3↓	Phenols, flavonoids, quercetin, ellagic acid, gallic acid, kaempferol	[6]
83	*Olea europaea .L.*	Sprague-Dawley rats	80 mg/kg/b.w. (oral)	0.2 ml/kg/b.w, i.p.	–	ALP, AST, ALP↓, CAT, SOD↑	Caffeic acid, diosmetin, verbascoside, oleuropein, luteolin 7-O-glucoside, rutin, leuteolin 4′-O-glycoside, P-coumaric acid, vanillin	[102]
84	*Origanum vulgare.*	Wistar albino rats	150 mg/kg/b.w. (oral)	2 ml/kg/b.w (1:1 olive oil)	–	ALT, ALP, AST↓, LPO, GST, CAT, SOD, GP x, GR, GSH↑	Carvacrol, thymol	[103]
85	*Persea Americana mill*	Wistar albino rats	200 mg/kg/day	3 ml/kg(1:1 olive oil) subcutaneous	reducdyn®, 100 mg/kg/day	ALT, AST, ALP, T.B↓, CAT, SOD, GPx, GST↑, Protein carbonyl↓	Flavonoids	[104]
86	*Phyllanthus niruri*	Wistar rats	100 mg/kg/b.w. (oral)	1 ml/kg/b.w(50% in corn oil), i.p.	Silymarin, 1mg/ml, (i.p).	AST, ALT, ALP, LDH, T-chol, T.B↓, T.P↑, TNF-α, NF-Kβ, IL-6, IL-8, IL-10↓, GR, GP↑, MDA↓, GSH↑, ROS↓.	Quercetin, gallic acid, corilagin, isocorilagin, rhamnoside, brevifolin carboxylic acid	[105]
87	*Physalis peruviana*	Wistar albino rats	500 mg/ kg/ b.w (oral)	0.5 ml/kg/bw (olive oil), i.p.	legation®100 mg/kg/b.w, (oral).	MDA↓, SOD↑, NO, AST↓, ALT↑, ALP↓, T.B, T.P↓	Flavonoids, lupeol, ursoli acid	[106]
88	*Pleiogynium timorense (DC) Leenh*	Sprague-Dawley rats	300 mg/kg/b.w.	0.5 ml/kg(10% olive oil).	Silymarin 50 mg/kg/b.w.	AST, ALT↓, TAC↑	Catechin, gallic acid, kaempferol, quercetin, rutin, quercetrin, β-sitosterol, lupeol	[107]
89	*Pleurotus ostreatus*	Wistar albino rats	200 mg/ kg/ b.w. (i.p)	2 ml/kg/b.w (olive oil), i.p.	–	SGOT, SGPT, ALP, MDA↓, GSH, CAT, SOD, GPx↑	–	[108]
90	*Polygonum cuspidatum sieb et Zucc*	Male ICR mice	100 mg/kg/day (oral)	50 µl/kg (olive oil) i.p.	Bifendate, 150 mg/kg/b.w, (oral)	AST, ALT, MDA, TNF α, IL 1β, COX-2, iNOS, NF-kβ↓, SOD, GST, GSH, CAT, GPx, TGF-β1↑	Polydatin, resveratrol, quercetin, emodin, citreorosein	[4]
91	*Premna esculenta Roxb*	Long-Evans rats (Rattus norvegicus)	400 mg/kg/day (oral)	1 ml/kg/bw. (1:1 olive oil), i.p.	Silymarin, 100 mg/kg/day, (oral)	SGPT, SGOT, SALP↓, T.P, ALB↑	Phenols, tannins, flavonoids	[109]
92	*Raphanus sativus*	Albino rats	300 mg/kg/b.w. (oral)	1 ml/kg/b.w (1:1 olive oil)	Silymarin, 50 mg/kg/b.w, (oral)	AST, ALT, ALP, T.B↓, CAT, GSH↑, MDA↓	Flavonoids, polyphenols	[110]
93	*Rourea induta planch*	Wistar albino rats	500 mg/kg/b.w. (oral)	2 ml/kg/b.w, i.p.	Legalon, 50 mg/kg/b.w, (oral)	AST, ALT, T.B↓, CAT, SOD, GPx, GSH↑, TBARS↓	Hyperin, quercetin-3-O-β-xyloside, quercetin-3-D-α-arabinofuranoside, quercetin	[111]

Table 2 (continued)

s.no.	Botanical name	Animal model.	Maximum extract dose/route of administration	CCL4 dose/route of administration	Standard drug administered/route of administration	Result.	Active components.	Reference
94	*Rubia cordifolia Linn*	Sprague-Dawley rats	200 mg/kg/b.w (oral)	0.1 ml/kg/b.w, i.p.	Silymarin, 100 mg/kg/b.w, (oral).	SGPT, SGOT, SAKP, γ-GT↓, GST, GR, GSH↑, MDA↓	Rubiadin	[112]
95	*Rumex vasicarius L*	Wistar albino rats	200 mg/kg/ b.w (oral)	1.5 ml/kg /b.w (1% tween 80) i.p.	Silymarin 50 mg/kg/b.w.	SGOT, SGPT, ALP↓, T.P↑, T.B↓, CAT, SOD↑, MDA↓	Phenols, flavonoids	[113]
96	*Semen celosia Cristatae.L*	Kunming mice	4.0 mg/kg/b.w (oral)	0.1% (edible oil), i.p.	Bifendate	AST, ALT, ALP, MDA↓, GSH-Px, CAT, SOD↑	Semenoside	[114]
97	*Solanium trilobatum Linn*	Wistar Albino rats	250 mg/ kg/ b.w (i.P)	1 ml/kg/bw(30% olive oil), i.p.	–	ALT, AST, ALP, LDH,↓T.P, GSH, GPx, CAT, SOD↑, Lipid peroxide↓	Sobatum, solasodine, β-solamarine, solaine	[115]
98	*Solanium xantholar-pum*	Sprague-Dawley rats	400 mg/kg/bw (oral)	1 ml/kg (1:1 liquid paraffin)	Silymarin, 100 mg/kg/b.w, (oral)	AST, ALT, ALP, T.B, MDA↓, CAT, GSH, SOD↑	Flavonoids, quercetin	[116]
99	*Spondias mombim*	Wistar rats	1000 mg/kg/b.w (oral)	2 ml/kg/b.w. (1:1 liquid paraffin)	Silymarin, 100 mg/kg/b.w, (oral)	ALT, AST, ALP, T.B↓, GSH, CAT, SOD↑, TBARS↓	Flavonoids, phenols	[117]
100	*Stachys pilifera Benth*	Wistar rats	400 mg/kg/day (oral)	1 ml/kg/b.w. (50% olive oil)	–	AST, ALT, ALP, MDA↓, T.P, T.B↑.	Flavonoids, phenyle-thanoid glycosides, diterpenes, terpenoids	[118]
101	*Vitis thunbergii var*	Male SD rats	400 mg/kg/b.w.	1.5 ml/kg/b.w. (20% olive oil) i.p.	Silymarin, 200 mg / kg/b.w. in carboxy methylcellulose	ALT, AST, MDA↓, SOD, CAT, GPX, GSH↑, TNF-α, IL-1β, NO, INOS, COX-2↓	Resveratrol deriva-tives, polyphenols compounds, quercetin, oligostibenes	[119]
102	*Xylaria nigripes(Koltz) Sacc*	ICR mice	100 mg/kg/b.w. (intra-gastrically)	2 ml/kg/b.w. (40% olive oil). Subcutaneously	Silymarin, 100 mg/kg/b.w., (intragastri-cally)	SGOT, SGPT, TBARS↓, SOD, CAT, GPX, ↑	Epicatechin, P-cou-maric acid, catechin	[120]
103	*Zingiber officinale (Roscoe) rhizome (ginger)*	Wistar rats	400 mg/kg/b.w. (oral)	0.7 ml/kg/b.w. (1:1, olive oil)	Livolin fort®, 5.2 mg/kg/b.w., (oral)	AST, ALT, ALP↓, T.P, GSH, CAT↑.	Flavonoids, 6-gingerol, shogaols	[121]
104	*Zizyphus jujube*	Male ICR mice	200 mg/kg/b.w. (intra-gastrically)	2 ml/kg/b.w. (40% v/v olive. oil), subcutane-ously	Bifendate, 7.5 mg/kg/b.w., (intragastri-cally)	ALT, AST, MDA↓, SOD, CAT, GSH-Px, GSH↑	Flavonoids	[122]

↓ decrease in effect/activity; ↑ increase in effect/activity

formation of CCl_3^* and $CHCl_2^*$ and CCl_3-OO^* radicals, lipid peroxidation, membrane damage, the severe derailment of intracellular Ca^{2+} sequestration, apoptosis, and fibrosis [10, 30, 31].

Traditional plants with anti-hepatotoxic potential

In this review, numerous experimental studies on the medicinal plants effectiveness to ameliorate CCl_4-induced hepatotoxicity in animal models were presented. The botanical names, ethnopharmacological and pharmacological uses of plants traditionally used to treat liver-related diseases were presented in Table 1. The comprehensive details on in vivo studies of medicinal plants with hepatoprotection against CCl_4-induced hepatotoxicity alongside the active phytochemicals and their probable mechanisms of action are presented in Table 2.

Discussion

For about three decades, extracts from different natural products have been identified to be hepatoprotective at varied doses against CCl_4-induced toxicity by reducing oxidative stress on liver enzymes. The findings from this review show that only few studies tested these natural products on hepatic cell lines (Table 2). Without separating the whole extract to identify the active components, a large number of hepatoprotective products will increase without corresponding clinical relativity [123]. There is an urgent need to study individual components of the plant extract especially in experimental animal models. The major drawback of herbal medicine is its potential hepatotoxicity in man which could cause acute to chronic liver injury with underlining mechanism of toxicity not clearly understood due to factors such as the synergistic and multi-organ targeted nature of the various components [124–127].

The protection provided by herbal plants against CCl_4-induced hepatotoxicity is basically due to the inhibitory nature of the phytochemicals present in them [70, 101]. These phytochemicals are able to inhibit the microsomal enzymes to restrict the generation of free radicals and stop lipid peroxidation through its antioxidant ability [66]. They can also enhance the regeneration of liver cells, radical scavenging, and stimulation of the anti-inflammatory ability of the liver cells against the inflammation induced by CCl_4 [102].

The treatment of the animal models with these herbal extracts showed beneficial effects through several biochemical and histological results. From the results in Table 2, it is clear that these plants extract downregulated serum liver marker enzymes like aspartate transaminase (AST), alanine transaminase (ALT), alkaline phosphatase (ALP), total bilirubin, and malondialdehyde (MDA) while upregulating the activity of antioxidant enzymes and total protein. The medicinal plants also downregulated the inflammatory markers expression in the hepatic cells. Some of these reported studies confirmed the hepatoprotective effectiveness of these medicinal plant products through histological reports [43, 54]. This review also reported numerous phytochemicals with possible hepatoprotective potentials ranging from flavonoids (quercetin, kaempferol), phenols, sobatum, courmarins, gallic acid, rutin, alkaloids, saponins, vitamin C, caffeic acid, etc. This review presented a number of plant species with ethnopharmacological relevance in the treatment of liver injury and their medicinal/pharmacological uses from literature.

Conclusion

We, therefore, conclude that there are a variety of phytochemicals in plant products with hepatoprotective activity against CCl_4-induced toxicity by downregulation of liver marker enzymes, and activation of antioxidative capacity of the liver cells that leads to the restoration of the liver architecture.

Future perspectives

There is need to validate the efficacy of some of the reported active components which can be likely candidate for therapeutic purposes. Research should move from whole plant extract experiment to isolation of bioactive components and testing the extract on culture cell lines.

Abbreviations

ALT: Alanine transaminase; AST: Aspartate transaminase; ALP: Alkaline phosphatase; γ-GT: Gamma glutamyltransferase; LDH: Lactate dehydrogenase; MDA: Malondialdehyde; GSH: Glutathione; GPx: Glutathione peroxidase; CAT : Catalase; SOD: Superioxide dismutase; POD: Peroxidase; GST: Glutathione S-transferase; GSTα: Glutathione S-transferase alpha; GR: Glutathione reductase; TBARS: Thiobarbituric acid reactive substance; NO: Nitric oxide; H_2O_2: Hydrogen peroxide; TNF-α : Tumor necrosis factor alpha; NF-kb: Nuclear factor-kappa B; INOS: Inducible nitric oxide synthase: COX-2: Cyclo oxygenase-2; IL-1β: Interlukin-1 beta; NrF-2: Nuclear factor erythroid-2-related factor 2; TGF-β(1): Hepatic growth factor-beta 1; IL-6: Intherleukin-6; IL-8: Interleukin-8; IL-10: Interleukin-10; HO-1: Heme oxygenase-1; NP-SH: Nonprotein sulfhydryls; NQO1: Quinine oxidoreductase; TLR4: Hepatic toll-like receptor 4; P38MAPK: P38 mitogen-activated protein kinase; p-ERK: Extracellular signal-regulated kinase; p-JNK: C-jun N-terminal kinase; CYT: Cytochrome; DTdiaphorase: A phase II enzyme; T-cho: Total cholesterol; TG: Triglycerides; LDL: Low-density lipoprotein; TAG: Triacylglycerol; HDL: High-density lipoprotein; TP: Total protein; TB: Total bilirubin; XOD: Xanthine oxidase; Vit. A: Vitamin A; Vit. E: Vitamin E; Vit. C: Vitamin C; CNS: Central nervous system

Acknowledgements

Not applicable.

Authors' contributions

CEU conceived the idea and wrote the initial draft. SMS did the literature search and data collection. Both authors proof read the final manuscript.

Declarations

Ethics approval and consent to participate
Not applicable.

Competing interests
The authors declared no competing interests.

References

1. Zhang X, Feng J, Su S, Huang L (2020) Hepatoprotective effects of *Camellia nitissima* aqueous ethanol extract CCl_4-induced acute liver injury in SD rats related to Nrf2 and NF-kB signaling. Pharm Biol 5(1):239–246
2. Wang S, Luan JJ, Lv XW (2019) Inhibition of endoplasmic reticulum stress attenuated ethanol-induced exosomal miR-122 and acute liver injury in mice. Alcohol Alcohol 54:465–471
3. Chao J, Lee M-S, Amagaya S, Liao J-W, Ho L-K, Peng W-H (2009) Hepatoprotective effect of *Shidagonlo* on acute liver injury induced by carbon tetrachloride. Am J Chin Med 37(6):1085–1097
4. Zhang H, Yu C-H, Jiang Y-P, Peng C, He K, Tang J-Y, Xin H-L (2012) Protective effects of polydatin from *Polygonum cuspidatum* against carbon tetrachloride-induced liver injury in mice. PLoS One 7(9):e46574. https://doi.org/10.1371/Journal.pone.0046574
5. Batool R, Khan MR, Majid M (2017) *Euphobia dracunculoides L.* abrogates carbon tetrachloride induced liver and DNA damage in rats. BMC Complement Altern Med 17:23. https://doi.org/10.1186/s12906-01744-x
6. Bakr RO, El-Naa MM, Zaghlou SS, Omar MM (2017) Profile of bioactive compounds in *Nymphaea alba L.* leaves growing in Egypt: hepatoprotective, antioxidant and anti-inflammatory activity. BMC Complement Altern Med 17:52. https://doi.org/10.1186/s12906-017-156/-2
7. Hsouna AB, Dhibi S, Dhifi W, Saad RB, Brini F, Hfaidh N, da Silva Almeida JRG, Mnif W (2020) *Lobularia maritima* leave extract, a neutraceutical agent with antioxidant activity, protects against CCl_4-induced liver injury in mice. Drug Chem Toxicol. https://doi.org/10.1080/01480545.2020.1742730
8. Jones I (1983) Chloroform anaesthesia in Liverpool. Anaesthesia 38:578–580
9. Agency for Toxic Substances and Disease Registry (ATSDR) (2005) Toxicological profile for carbon tetrachloride. U.S. Department of Health and Human Services, Public Health Service, Atlanta
10. Clawson GA (1989) Mechanism of carbon tetrachloride toxicity. Pathol Immunopathol Res 8:104–112
11. Recknagel R, Lombardi B (1961) Studies of biochemical changes in subcellular particles of rat liver and their relationship to a new hypothesis regarding the pathogenesis of carbon tetrachloride fat accumulation. J Biol Chem 236:564–569
12. Judah J (1969) Biochemical disturbances in liver injury. Br Med Bull 25:274–277
13. de Vries J (1983) Induction and prevention of biochemical disturbances in hepatic necrosis. Trends Pharmacol Sci 4:393–394
14. Smuckler E, Iseri O, Bendit E (1962) An intracellular defect in protein synthesis induced by carbon tetrachloride. J Exp Med 116:55–72
15. Moore L, Chen J, Knapp H, Landon E (1975) Energy-dependent calcium sequestration activity in rat liver microsomes. J Biol Chem 250:4562–4568
16. Fulceri R, Benedetti A, Comporti M (1984) On the mechanisms of the inhibition of calcium sequestering activity of liver microsomes in bromothrichloromethane intoxication. Res Commun Chem Pathol Pharmacol 46:235–243
17. Christie G, Judah J (1954) Mechanism of action of CCl_4 on liver cells. Proc R Soc Lond Ser 142:241–257
18. De Groot H, Littauer A, Hugo-Wissemann D, Wissemann P, Noll T (1988) Lipid peroxidation and cell viability in isolated hepatocytes in a redesigned oxystat system: Evaluation of the hypothesis that lipid peroxidation , preferentially induced at low oxygen partial pressure, is decisive for CCl_4 liver cell injury. Arch Biochem Biophys 264:591–599
19. Masuda Y, Nakamura Y (1990) Effects of oxygen deficiency and calcium omission on carbon tetrachloride hepatotoxicity in isolated perfused livers from phenobarbital-pretreated rats. Biochem Pharmacol 40:1865–1876
20. Kiezcka H, Kappus H (1980) Oxygen dependence of CCl_4-induced lipid peroxidation *in vitro* and *in vivo*. Toxicol Lett 5:191–196
21. Dianzani MU, Poli G (1985) Lipid peroxidation and haloalkylation in CCl_4-induced liver injury. In: Poli G, Cheeseman KH, Dianzani MU, Slater TF (eds) Free Radicals in Liver Injury. IRL Press, Oxford
22. Dianzani MU (1984) Lipid peroxidation and haloalkylation: Two distinct mechanisms for CCl_4 -induced liver damage. In: Calandra S, Carulli N, Salvioli G (eds) Liver and Lipid Metabolism. Excerpta Medica, Elsevier, Amsterdam, New York, Oxford
23. Marinari UM, Pronzato MA, Cottalasso D, Zicca-Cadoni A, Nanni G, Poli G, Chiarpotto E, Albano E, Biasi F, Dianzani MU (1985) CCl_4-induced early functional impairments of rat liver Golgi apparatus. In: Poli G, Cheeseman KH, Dianzani MU, Slater TF (eds) Free Radicals in Liver Injury. IRL Press, Oxford
24. Cheeseman KH, Albano EF, Tomasi A, Slater TF (1985) Biochemical studies on the metabolic activation of halogenated alkanes. Environ Health Perspect 64:85–101
25. Boll M, Weber LWD, Becker E, Stampfl A (2001a) Mechanism of carbon tetrachloride-induced hepatotoxicity. Hepatocellular damage by reactive carbon tetrachloride metabolites. Z Naturforsch C. J Biosci 56(7-8):649–659
26. Ozaki M, Masuda Y (1993) Carbon tetrachloride-induced cell death in perfused livers from phenobarbital-pretreated rats under hypoxic conditions and various ionic milieu. Further evidence for calcium-dependent irreversible changes. Biochem Pharmacol 46:2039–2049
27. Liu SL, Degli Esposti S, Yao T, Diehl AM, Zern MA (1995) Vitamin E therapy of acute CCl_4 -induced hepatic injury in mice is associated with inhibition of nuclear factor Kappa B binding. Hepatology 22:1474–1481
28. Czaja MJ, Xu J, Alt E (1995) Prevention of carbon tetrachloride-induced rat liver injury by soluble tumor necrosis factor receptor. Gastroenterol 108:1849–1854
29. Kull FC, Cuatrecasas P (1981) Possible measurements of internalization in the mechanism of *in vitro* cytotoxicity of tumor necrosis serum. Cancer Res 41:4885–4890
30. Boll M, Weber LWD, Becker E, Stampfl A (2001b) Pathogenesis of carbon tetrachloride-induced hepatocyte injury. Bioactivation of CCl_4 by cytochrome P_{450} and effects on lipid homeostasis. Z Naturforsch 56c:111–121
31. Boll M, Weber LWD, Becker E, Stampfl A (2001c) Hepatocyte damage induced by carbon tetrachloride. Inhibited lipoprotein secretion and altered lipoprotein composition. Z Naturforsch 56c:283–290
32. Ai G, Liu Q, Hua W, Huang Z, Wang D (2013) Hepatoprotective evaluation of the total flavonoids extracted from flowers of *Abelmoschus manihot (L) Medic*: *In vivo* and *in vivo* studies. J Ethnopharmacol 146:794–802
33. Arbab AH, Parvez MK, Al-Dosari MS, Al-Rehaily AJ, Al-Sohaibani M, Zaroug EE, Alsaid MS, Rafatullah S (2015) Hepatoprotective and antiviral efficacy of *Acacia mellifera* leaves fractions against Hepatitis B virus. Biomed Res Int. https://doi.org/10.1155/2015/929131
34. Singh R, Rao HS (2008) Hepatoprotective effect of the pulp/seed of *Aegle marmelos correa ex Roxb* against carbon tetrachloride induced liver damage in rats. Inter J Green Pharm:232–234
35. Rathee D, Kamboj A, Sidhu S (2018) Augmentation of hepatoprotective potential of *Aegle marmelos* in combination with piperine in carbon tetrachloride model in wistar rats. Chem Cent J 12:94. https://doi.org/10.1186/s/3065-018-0463-9
36. Dhruve P, Nauman M, Kale KR, Singh RP (2020) A novel hepatoprotective activity of *Alangium salviifolium* in mouse model. Drug Chem Toxicol. https://doi.org/10.1080/01480545.2020.1733593

37. Gargoum HM, Muftah SS, Shalmani SA, Mohammed HA, Alzoki AN, Debani AH, Fituri OA, Shari FE, Barassi IE, Meghil SE, Abdellatif AW (2013) Phytochemical screening and investigation of the effect of *Alhagi maurorum (camel thorn)* on carbon tetrachloride, acetaminophen and Adriamycin induced toxicity in experimental animals. J Sci Innov Res 2(6):1026–1033
38. Salah IA, Adnan JA, Abdulmalik MA, Maged SA (2008) Evaluation of hepatoprotective effect of *Ephedra foliate, Alhagi maurorum, Capsella bursa-pastoris* and *Hisbiscus sabdariffa* against experimentally induced liver injury in rats. Nat Prod Sci 14(2):95–98
39. Naji KM, Al-Shaibani ES, Alhadi FA, Al-Soudi SA, D'souza MR (2017) Hepatoprotective and antioxidant effects of single clove garlic against CCl_4-induced hepatic damage in rabbits. BMC Complement Altern Med 17:411. https://doi.org/10.1186/s12906-017-1916-8
40. Zeashan H, Amresh G, Singh S, Rao CV (2008) Hepatoxicity activity of *Amaranthus spinosus* in experimental animals. Food Chem Toxicol 46:3417–3421
41. Jain S, Dixit VK, Malviya N, Ambawatia V (2009) Antioxidant and hepatoprotective activity of ethanol and aqueous extracts of *Amorphophallus cmpanulatus Roxb.* tubers. Acta Pol Pharm Drug Res 66(4):423–428
42. Sourabie TS, Ouedraogo N, Sawadogo WR, Yougbare N, Nikiema JB, Guissou IP, Nacoulma OG (2012) Evaluation of the anti-iceterus effect of crude powdered leaf of *Argemone Mexicana L. (Papaveraceae)* against CCl_4-induced liver injury in rats. IJPSR 3(10):491–496
43. Wang J-H, Choi M-K, Shin J-W, Hwang S-Y, Son C-G (2012) Antifibrotic effects of *Artemisia capillaris* and *Artemisia iwayomagi* in a carbon tetrachloride-induced chronic hepatic fibrosis animal model. J Ethnopharmacol 140:179–185
44. Surenda HB, Apana R (2007) Hepatoprotective properties of *Bauhinia variegate* bark extract. Yakugaku Zasshi 127(9):1503–1507
45. Gilani AH, Janbaz KH, Shah BH (1998) Esculetin prevents liver damage induced by paracetamol and CCl_4. Pharm Res 37(1):31–35
46. Enas JK (2014) Phytochemicals investigation and hepato-protective studies of Iraqi *Bryonia* (Family *Cucubitaceae*). IJPSR 6(4):187–190
47. Akindele AL, Ezenwanebe KO, Anunobi CC, Adeyemi OO (2010) Hepatoprotective and *in vivo* antioxidant effects of *Byrscocarpus coC-Clneus Schum.* and *Thonn (Connaraceae)*. J Ethnopharmacol 129:40–52
48. Singh S, Mehta A, Mehta P (2011) Hepatoprotective activity of *Cajanus cajan* against carbon tetrachloride induced liver damage. IJPSR 3(sup 2):146–147
49. Lodhi G, Singh HK, Pant KK, Hussain Z (2009) Hepatoprotective effects of *Calotropis gigantean* extract against carbon tetrachloride induced liver injury in rats. Acta Pharm 59:89–96
50. Josi YM, Kadam VJ, Patil YV, Kaldhone PR (2009) Investigation of hepatoprotective activity of aerial parts of *Canna indica L.* on carbon tetrachloride treated rats. J Pharm Res 2(12):1879–1882
51. Nasrin A, Iran R, Amir M (2007) Hepatoprotective activity of *Capparis spinosa* root bark against CCl_4 induced hepatic damage in mice. Iranian J Pharm Res 6(4):285–290
52. Sahreen S, Khan MR, Khan RA (2011) Hepatoprotective effects of methanol extract of *Carissa opaca* leaves on CCl_4-induced damage in rat. BMC Complement Altern Med 11:48 www.biomedcentral.com/1472-6882/11/48
53. Zang Y, Guo J, Dong H, Zhao X, Zhou L, Li X, Liu J, Niu Y (2011) Hydroxysafflor yellow A protects against chronic carbon tetrachloride-induced liver fibrosis. Eur J Pharmacol 660(2-3):438–444
54. Wu S, Yue Y, Tian H, Li Z, Li X, He W, Ding H (2013) Carthamus red from *Carthamus tinctorius L.* exerts antioxidant and hepatoprotective effect against CCl_4-induced liver damage in rats via the NrF2 pathway. J Ethnopharmacol. https://doi.org/10.1016/j.jep.2013.04.054
55. Samojlik L, Lakic N, Mimica-Dukic N, Dakovic-Svajcer K, Bozin B (2010) Antioxidant and hepatoprotective potential of essential oils of (*Coriandrum sativum L*) and caraway (*Carvum carvi L.*) (*Apiaceae*). J Agric Food Chem 58:8848–8853
56. Shanmugasundaran R, Devi VK, Tresina PS, Maruthupandian A, Mohan VR (2010) Hepatoprotective activity of ethanol extracts of *Clitoria ternatea L.* and *Cassic angustifolia vahl* leaf against CCl_4 induced liver toxicity in rats. IJRP 1(1):201–205
57. Ilavarasan R, Mohideen S, Vijayalakshmi M, Manonmani G (2001) Hepatoprotective effect of *Cassia angustofolia Vahl.* Indian J Pharm Sci 63(6):504–507
58. Pradeep K, Mohan CVR, Anand KG, Karthikeyan S (2005) Effect of pretreatment of *Cassia fistula Linn.* leaf extract against subacute CCl_4 induced hepatotoxicity in rats. Indian J Exp Biol 43:526–530
59. Ahmed B, Khan S, Masood HM, Siddique AH (2008) Anti-hepatotoxic activity of Cichotyboside, a sequiterpene glycoside from seeds of *Cichorium intybus*. J Asian Nat Prod Res 10(3):218–223
60. Sadeghi H, Reza NM, Izadpanah G, Sohailla S (2008) Hepatoprotective effect of *Cichorium intybus* on CCl_4-induced liver damage in rats. Afr J Biochem Res 2(6):141–144
61. Moselhy SS, Ali HKH (2009) Hepatoprotective effect of Cinnamon extracts against carbon tetrachloride induced oxidative stress and liver injury in rats. Boil Res 42:93–98
62. Bellassoued K, Hamed H, El Feki A, Ghrab F, Kallel R, van Pelt J, Lahyani A, Ayadi FM (2019) Protective effect of essential oil of *Cinnamomum verum* bark on hepatic and renal toxicity induced by carbon tetrachloride in rats. Appl Physiol Nutr Metab 44(6):606–618
63. Eidi A, Mortazvi P, Bazargan M, Zaringhalam J (2012) Hepatoprotective activity of *Cinnamon ethanolic* extract against CCl_4-induced liver injury in rats. EXCLI J 11:495–507
64. Karaca M, Iihan F, Altan H, Him A, Tutuncu M, Ozbek H (2005) Evaluation of hepatoprotective activity of *Bergamot orange* in rats. Eastern J Med 10:1–4
65. Bhavsar SK, Joshi P, Shah MB, Santani DD (2007) Investigation of hepatoprotective property of *Citrus limon*. Pharm Biol 45(4):303–311
66. Molehin OR, Oloyede OL, Idowu KA, Adeyanju AA, Olowoyeye AO, Tubi OI, Komolafe OE, Gold AS (2017) White butterfly (*Clerodendrum volubile*) leaf extract protect against carbon tetrachloride-induced hepatotoxicity in rats. Biomed Pharmacother 96:924–929
67. Pandey A, Bigoniya P, Raj V, Patel KK (2011) Pharmacological Screening of *Coriandrum sativum Linn.* for hepatoprotective activity. J Pharm Bio allied Sci 3(3):435–441
68. Sreelatha S, Padma PR, Umadevi M (2009) Protective effects of *Coriandrum sativum* extracts on carbon tetrachloride-induced hepatotoxicity in rats. Food Chem Toxicol 47:702–708
69. Li L, Zhou Y-F, Li Y-L, Wang L-L, Arai H, Xu Y (2017) *In vitro* and *in vivo* antioxidative and hepatoprotective activity of aqueous extract of *Cortex dictamni*. World J Gastroentrol 23(16):2912–2927
70. Lee G-H, Lee H-Y, Choi M-K, Chung M-K, Kim S-W (2017) Protective effect of *Curcuma longa L.* extract on CCl_4-induced acute hepatic stress. BMC Res Notes:10:77. https://doi.org/10.1186/s13104-017-2409-z
71. Raja S, Nazeer Ahamed KFH, Kumar V, Mukherjee K, Bandyopadhyay A, Mukherjee PK (2007) Antioxidant effect of *Cytisus scoparius* against carbon tetrachloride treated liver injury in rats. J Ethnopharmacol 109:41–47
72. Balogun FO, Ashafa AOT (2016) Antioxidant and hepatoprotective activities of *Dicoma anomala Sond.* aqueous root extract against carbon tetrachloride-induced liver damage in Wistar rats. J Tradit Clin Med 36(4):504–513
73. Yeh Y-H, Hsieh Y-L, Lee Y-T (2013) Effects of yam peel extract against carbon tetrachloride-induced hepatotoxicity in rats. J Agric Food Chem 61:7387–7396
74. Beedimani RS, Shetkar S (2015) Hepatoprotective activity of *Eclipta alba* against carbon tetrachloride-induced hepatotoxicity in albino rats. Inter J Basic Clin Pharm 4(3):404–409
75. Sultana S, Ahmad S, Khan N, Jahangir T (2005) Effect of *Emblica officinalis (Gaertn)* on CCl_4 induced hepatic toxicity and DNA synthesis in Wistar rats. Indian J Exp Biol 43:430–436
76. Gupta G, More AS, Kumari RR, Lingaraju MC, Kumar D, Kumar D, Mishra SK, Tandan SK (2014) Protective effect of alcoholic extract *of Entada pursaetha DC.* against CCL_4 induced hepatotoxicity in rats. Indian J Exp Biol 52:207–214
77. Pareek GA, Issarani R, Nagori BP (2013) Antioxidant hepatoprotective activity of *Fagonia schweinfurthii (Hcdidi) Hadidi* extract in carbon tetrachloride induced hepatotoxicity in HepG2 cell line and rats. J Ethnopharmacol 150:973–981
78. Sharma M, Abid R, Ahmad Y, Nabi NG (2017) Protective effect of leaves of *Fiscus carica* against carbon tetrachloride-induced hepatic damage in rats. UK J Pharm Biosci 5(1):6–11

79. Hsieh PC, Ho YL, Huang GJ, Huang MH, Chiang YC, Huang SS, Hou WC, Chang YS (2011) Hepatoprotective effect of the aqueous extract of *Flemingia macrophylla* on carbon tetrachloride-induced acute hepatotoxicity in rats through anti-oxidant activities. Am J Chin Med 39(2):349–365
80. Khattab HAH (2012) Effect of *Ginkgo biloba* leaves aqueous extract on carbon tetrachloride induced acute hepatotoxicity in rats. Egypt J Hosp Med 48:483–495
81. Nwidu LL, Oboma YI, Elmorsy E, Carter WG (2018) Alleviation of carbon tetrachloride-induced hepatocellular damage and oxidative stress with a leaf extract of *Glyphae brevis (Tiliaceae)*. J Basic Clin Physiol Pharmacol 29(6):609–619
82. Duh P-D, Lin S-L, Wu S-C (2011) Hepatoprotection of *Graptopetalum paraguayense E.* Walther on CCl_4-induced liver damage and inflammation. J Ethnopharmacol 134:379–385
83. Zhang W, Zhang X, Xie J, Zhao S, Liu J, Liu H, Wang J, Wang Y (2017) Seabuckthorn berry pollysacharide protects against carbon tetrachloride-induced hepatotoxicity in mice via anti-oxidative and anti-inflammatory activities. Food Funct. https://doi.org/10.1039/C7FO00399D
84. Shahjahan M, Vani G, Shyamala Devi CS (2005) Protective effect of *Idigofolia oblongifolia* in CCl4- induced hepatotoxicity. J Med Food 8(2):261–265
85. Khan RA, Khan MR, Ahmed M, Sahreen S, Shah AN, Shah MS, Bokhari J, Rashid U, Ahmed B, Jan S (2012) Hepatoprotection with a chloroform extract of *Launea procumbens* against CCl_4-induced injuries in rats. BMS Compl Altern Med 12:114 http://www.biomedcentral.com/1472-6882/12/114
86. Mohamed MA, Eldin IMT, Mohammed AH, Hassan HM (2016) Effects of *Lawsonia inermis L. (Henna)* leaves' methanolic extact on carbon tetrachloride-induced hepatotoxicity in rats. J Intercult Ethnopharmacol 5(1):22–26. https://doi.org/10.5455/jice.20151123043218
87. Hossain CM, Maji HS, Chakraborty P (2011) Hepatoprotective activity of *Lawsonia inermis Linn*, warm aqueous extract in carbon tetrachloride induced hepatic injury in Wistar rats. Asian J Pharm Clin Res 4(3):106–109
88. Sailar GU, Dudhrejiya AV, Seth AK, Maheshwari R, Shah N, Aundhia C (2010) Hepatoprotective effect of *Leucas cephalotes spreng* on CCl_4 induced liver damage in rats. Pharmacology Online 1:30–38
89. Ulaganathan I, Divya D, Radha K, Vijayakumar TM, Dhanaraju MD (2010) Protective effect of *Luffa acurangula (Var) amara* against carbon tetrachloride-induced hepatotoxicity in experimental rats. Res J Biol Sci 5(9):615–624
90. Wills PJ, Asha VV (2006) Protective effect of *Lygodium flexuosum (L.) Sw.* extract against carbon tetrachloride-induced acute liver injury in rats. J Ethnopharmacol 108:320–326
91. Chaudhary A, Bhandari A, Pandurangan A (2011) Hepatic activity of methanolic extract of *Madhuca indica* on carbon tetrachloride- induced hepatotoxicity in rats. Pharmacology Online 1:873–880
92. Patel PK, Sahu J, Prajapati NK, Dubey BK, Alia A (2012) Hepatoprotective effect of ethanolic and hydro alcoholic leaf extract of *Madhuca indica* in carbon tetrachloride intoxicated rat. Res J Pharmacol Pharmacodynamics 4(5):311–314
93. Ramakrishna S, Geetha KM, Bhaskargopal PVVS, Ranjit Kumar P, Charan Madav P, Umachandar L (2011) Effect of *Mallotus philippensis Muell-Arg* leaves against hepatotoxicity of carbon tetrachloride in rats. IJPSR 2(2):74–83
94. Pramod K, Deval RG, Lakshmayya RSS (2008) Antioxidant and hepatoprotective activity of tubers of *Momordica tuberosa Cogn*. against CCl_4 induced liver injury in rats. Indian J Exp Biol 46:510–513
95. Bellassoued K, Hsouna AB, Athmouni K, Pelt J, Ayadi FM, Rebai T, Elfeki A (2018) Protective effects of *Mentha piperita L.* leaf essential oil against CCl_4 induced hepatic oxidative damage and renal failure in rats. Lipids Health Dis 17:9. https://doi.org/10.1186/s12944-017-064S-9
96. Patil K, Mall A (2012) Hepatoprotective activity of *Mentha arvensis Linn.* leaves against CCl_4 induced liver damage in rats. Asian Pac J Trop Dis 2(1):S223–s226
97. Rajendran R, Hemalatha S, Akasalai K, Madhakrishna CH, Vittal BS, Sundaram RM (2009) Hepatoprotective activity of *Mimosa pudica* leaves against carbon tetrachloride induced toxicity. J Nat Prod 2:116–122
98. Purkayastha A, Chakravarty P, Dewan B (2016) Evaluation of hepatoprotective activity of the ethanolic extract of leaves of *Mimosa pudica Linn.*in carbon tetrachloride induced hepatic injury in albino rats. Inter J Basic Clin Pharmacol 5(2):496–501
99. Jain A, Soni M, Deb L, Jain A, Rout SP, Gupta VB, Krishna KL (2008) Antioxidant and hepatoprotective activity of ethanolic and aqueous extracts of *Momordica dioica Roxb*. leaves. J Ethnopharmacol 115:61–66
100. Singhal KG, Gupta GD (2012) Hepatoprotective and antioxidant activity of methanolic extract of flowers of *Nerum oleander* against CCl_4-induced liver injury in rats. Asian Pac J Trop Med 5(9):677–683
101. Abdus SS, Rahmat AK, Mushtaq A, Nawshad M (2016) Hepatoprotective role of *Nicotiana plumbaginifolia Linn*. against carbon tetrachloride-induced injuries. Toxicol Ind Health 32(2):292–298. https://doi.org/10.1177/0748233713498448
102. Ustuner D, Colak E, Dincer M, Tekin N, Donmez DB, Akyuz F, Colak E, Kolac UK, Entok E, Ustuner MC (2018) Post treatment effects of *Olea europaea L.* leaf extract on carbon tetrachloride-induced liver injury and oxidative stress in rats. J Med Food 00(0):1–6
103. Sikander M, Malok S, Parveen K, Ahmad M, Yadav D, Hafeez ZB, Bansal M (2013) Hepatoprotective effect of *Origanum vulgare* in Wistar rats against carbon tetrachloride-induced hepatotoxicity. Protoplasma 250:483–493
104. Brai BIC, Adisa RA, Odetola AA (2014) Hepatoprotective properties of aqueous leaf extract of *Persea Americana, Mill (Lauraceae)* 'avocado' against CCl_4-induced damage in rats. Afr J Tradit Complement Altern Med 11(2):237–244
105. Ezzat MI, Okba MM, Ahmed SH, El-Banna AP, Mohamed SO, Ezzat SM (2020) In-dept hepatoprotective mechanisistic study of *Phyllanthus niruri*: *in vitro* and *in vivo* studies and its chemical characterization. PLoS One 15(1):e0226185. https://doi.org/10.1371/journal.pone.0226185
106. Khalaf-Allah AM, El-Gengahi SE, Hamed MA, Zahran HG, Mohammed MA (2016) Chemical composition of golden berry leaves against hepato-renal fibrosis. J Diet Suppl 13(4):378–392
107. Abdel Raoof GF, Said AA, Mohamed KY, Gomaa HA (2020) Phytoconstituents and bioactivities of the bark of *Pleiogynium timorense (DC) Leenh (Anacardiaceae)*. J Herbmed Pharmacol 9(1):20–27
108. Jayakumar T, Ramesh E, Geraldine P (2006) Antioxidant activity of the oyster mushroom, *Pleurotus ostreatus*, on CCl_4-induced liver injury in rats. Food Chem Toxicol 44:1989–1996
109. Mahmud ZA, Bachor SC, Qais N (2012) Antioxidant and hepatoprotective activities of ethanolic extracts of leaves of *Preruna esculenta Roxb* against carbon tetrachloride-induced liver damage in rats. J Young Pharm 4(4). https://doi.org/10.4103/0975-1483-104360
110. Syed SN, Rizvi W, Kumar A, Khan AA, Moin S, Ahsan A (2014) *In vitro* antioxidant and *in vivo* hepatoprotective activity of leave extract of *Raphanus sativus* in rats using CCl_4 model. Afr J Tradit Complement Altern Med 11(3):102–106
111. Kalegari M, Gemin CAB, Araujo-silva N, de Brito NJ, Lopez JA, Tozetto S, Almeida M, Migue IMD, Stien D, Miguel OG (2014) Chemical composition, antioxidant activity and hepatoprotective potential of *Rourea induta planch (Connaraceae)* against CCl_4-induced liver injury in female rats. Nutr 30:713–718
112. Rao GMM, Rao CV, Pushpangadan P, Shirwaikar A (2006) Hepatoprotective effects of rubiadin, a major constituent of *Rubia cordifolia Linn*. J Ethnopharmacol 103:484–490
113. Tukaappo NK, Londonkar RL, Nayaka HB, Kumar SCB (2015) Cytotoxicity and hepatoprotective attributes of methanolic extract of *Rumex vesicarius L.* Biol Res 48(19). https://doi.org/10.1186/s40659-015-0009-B
114. Sun ZL, Gao GL, Xia YF, Qiao ZY (2011) A new hepatoprotective saponin from *Semen celosia cristatate*. Fitoterapia 82(4):591–594
115. Shahjahan M, Sabitha KE, Jainu M, Shyamala Devi CS (2004) Effect of *Solanum trilobatum* against carbon tetrachloride induced hepatic damage in albino rats. Indian J Med Res 120:194–198
116. Gupta RK, Hussain T, Panigrahi G, Das A, Singh GN, Sweety K, Faiyazuddin MD, Rao CV (2011) Hepatoprotective effect of *Solanum xanthocarpum* fruit extract against CCl_4-induced acute liver toxicity in experimentals. Asian Pac J Trop Med 4(12):964–968
117. Nwidu LL, Elmorsy E, Oboma YI, Carter WG (2018) Hepatoprotective and antioxidant activities of *Spondias mombin* leaf and stem extracts against carbon tetrachloride-induced hepatotoxicity. J Taibah Univ Med Sci 13(3):262–271
118. Kokhdan EP, Ahmadi K, Sadeghi H, Dadgary F, Danaei N, Aghamaali MR (2017) Hepatoprotective effect of *Stachys pilifera* ethanol extract

in carbon tetrachloride-induced hepatotoxicity in rats. Pharm Biol 55(1):1389–1393

119. Deng J-S, Chang Y-S, Wen C-L, Liao J-C, Hou W-C, Amagaya S, Huang S-S, Huang G-J (2012) Hepatoprotective effect of the ethanol extract of *Vitis thunbergii* on carbon tetrachloride-induced acute hepatotoxicity in rats through anti-oxidative activities. J Ethnopharmacol 142:795–803
120. Song A, Ko HJ, Lai MN, Ng LT (2011) Protective effects of Wu-Liang-Shen (*Xylaria nigtipes*) on carbon tetrachloride-induced hepatotoxicity in mice. Immunopharmacol Immunotoxicol 33(3):453–460
121. Oke GO, Abiodun AA, Imafidon CE (2019) *Zingiber officinale (Roscoe)* mitigates CCl_4- induced liver histology and biochemical derangements through antioxidant, membrane-stabilizing and tissue-regenerating potential. Toxicol Rep 6:416–425
122. Shen X, Tang Y, Yang R, Yu L, Fang T, Duan J (2009) The protective effect of *Zizyphus jujube* fruit on carbon tetrachloride-induced hepatic injury in mice by anti-oxidative activities. J Ethnopharmacol 122:555–560
123. Chang L, Xu D, Zhu J, Ge G, Kong X, Zhou Y (2020) Herbal therapy for the treatment of acetaminophen-associated liver injury: recent advances and future perspectives. Front Pharmacol 11:313. https://doi.org/10.3389/fphar.2020.00313
124. Stickel F, Shouval D (2015) Hepatotoxicity of herbal and dietary supplements: an update. Arch Toxicol 89(6):851–865
125. Janghel V, Patel P, Chandel SS (2019) Plants used for the treatment of icterus (jaundice) in Central India: A review. Ann Hepatol 18:658–672
126. Zhu J, Chen M, Borlak J (2019) The landscape of hepatobiliary adverse reactions across 53 herbal and dietary supplements reveals immune-mediated injury as a common cause of hepatitis. Arch Toxicol 94(1):273–279
127. Shakya AK (2020) Drug-induced hepatotoxicity and hepatoprotective medicinal plants: a review. Indian J Pharm Edu Res 54(2):234–247

19

Arctigenin attenuates CCl_4-induced hepatotoxicity through suppressing matrix metalloproteinase-2 and oxidative stress

Ghalia Mohamed Kanawati[1], Iqbal Hassan Al-Khateeb[1] and Yasser Ibrahim Kandil[1,2*]

Abstract

Background: In spite of the huge advances in recent medicine, there is no effective drug that completely protects the liver from toxic materials. This study was conducted to investigate the hepatoprotective effect of arctigenin from burdock (*Arctium lappa*) against carbon tetrachloride (CCl_4)-induced liver injury.

Results: Arctigenin pre-administration reduced hepatotoxicity markers significantly as compared to CCl_4 group. In addition, both silymarin and arctigenin declined matrix metalloproteinase-2 (MMP-2) in the serum (1177 ± 176), (978 ± 135) significantly as compared to CCl_4 group (1734 ± 294). The hepatic antioxidant parameters (total glutathione, superoxide dismutase, and glutathione reductase) were significantly decreased after CCl_4 injection, an effect that has been prevented by pre-administration of both silymarin and arctigenin. Histological examinations illustrated that arctigenin reduced CCl_4 damage, where it decreased inflammation, congestion, and ballooning.

Conclusions: Arctigenin exerted a hepatoprotective effect against CCl_4-induced liver damage in terms of suppressing MMP-2 and oxidative stress comparative to that of silymarin.

Keywords: Arctigenin, CCl_4, Hepatoprotective, Matrix metalloproteinase-2, Silymarin

Background

An organ as complex as the liver can be susceptible to a variety of problems. However, in an unhealthy or malfunctioning liver, the outcomes can be dangerous or even fatal. Liver cirrhosis is one of liver serious problems; it is a frequent consequence of the long clinical course of all chronic liver diseases and is characterized by tissue fibrosis and the conversion of normal liver architecture into structurally abnormal nodules [1, 2].

Liver diseases were the 10th leading cause of death for men and the 12th for women in the USA, killing about 27,000 people each year. Also, the cost of liver diseases in terms of human suffering, hospital costs, and lost productivity is very high [3].

The extracellular matrix (ECM), formed by the complex network of proteins and sugars surrounding cells in all solid tissues, is among the most important regulators of cellular and tissue functions in the body [4]. In addition to providing structural support for cells, ECM regulates various cellular functions, such as adhesion, migration, differentiation, proliferation, and survival. Cellular responses are context-dependent, and dysregulation of ECM production and proteolysis is often associated with the development of liver pathology [5]. Matrix metalloproteinases (MMPs) are a family of over 24 zinc-dependent endopeptidases capable of degrading virtually any component of the ECM. MMPs have emerged as essential mediators in defining how cells interact with their surrounding microenvironment in normal liver [6].

Many plants have important roles in human health care. There are some plants that are consumed habitually by humans and that have been proven as

* Correspondence: Kandil.yasser@azhar.edu.eg
[1]Pharmacological and Diagnostic Research Centre, Faculty of Pharmacy, Al-Ahliyya Amman University, Amman 19328, Jordan
[2]Biochemistry and Molecular Biology Department, Faculty of Pharmacy, Al-Azhar University, Cairo 11884, Egypt

hepatoprotective capacity, for example, artichoke [7–9], milk thistle [10, 11], grapefruit, and chamomile [12, 13].

Arctigenin (AG) is an aglycon of arctiin [14]. It is a bioactive lignan isolated from the seeds of burdock (*Arctium lappa*) [15], acts as an antioxidant. The phenolic content of burdock is antioxidant too [16, 17]. As previous studies confirmed that *Arctium lappa* extract has hepatoprotective effect [18], there is no survey related to AG alone (which is one of the constituents of *Arctium lappa*), has the same effect, knowing that AG has an antioxidant [19], anti-inflammatory [20], and gastroprotective properties [21]. This study was aimed to investigate the hepatoprotective effect of AG on CCl_4-induced liver toxicity in experimental rats, in terms of hepatic markers, MMP-2, oxidative stress, and histopathological changes.

Methods

This study was conducted in the Experimental Animal Laboratory of the Faculty of Pharmacy, Al-Ahliyya Amman University, and ethically approved by ethical committee for the care and use of laboratory animals (ethical approval no. AAU-1/14/2017-2018).

Chemicals, reagents, and kits

Arctigenin (Item No. 270652), glutathione (GSH) kit (Item No.703002), superoxide dismutase (SOD) kit (Item No. 706002), and glutathione reductase kit (Item No. 703202) were purchased from (Cayman chemicals, USA). CCl_4 (> 99.9%, Item No. 270652), carboxymethylcellulose (CMC) (Item No. C9481), and metphosphoric acid (MPA) (Item No. 79613) from Sigma Aldrich, USA.

Total MMP-2 ELISA kit (Item No. MMP200) and lysis buffer (Item No. 895347) were supplied by RnD Systems, USA. Alanine aminotransferase (ALT) (Item No. 11533), aspartate aminotransferase (AST) (Item No. 11531), alkaline phosphatase (ALP) (Item No.11592), and bilirubin (Item No. 11515) assay kits were purchased from BioSystems S.A., Barcelona (Spain). Silymarin (Legalon® 70 mg) was kindly provided by Chemical Industries Development CID, Egypt.

Animals

A total of 24 male Wistar rats (age 6-8 weeks, weight 210-240 g) were provided from the Jordanian University of Science and Technology (JUST), Irbid, Jordan. All animals were kept under observation in Al-Ahliyya Amman University animal house, for 2 weeks prior to the study with free access to commercial rat diet and water *ad libitum*. Rats were housed at 22 ± 2 °C with a 12 h light-dark cycle. All animals' handling and treatment were in adherence to the ARRIVE guidelines.

Experimental design

The rats were randomly divided into 4 equal groups (n = 6 rats). Group A (control) and B (toxic), animals were administered the vehicle daily (1% CMC, 4 mL/kg, i.p.). Group C (standard), rats were daily administered silymarin (200 mg/kg, 4 mL/kg, i.p.) [22]. Group D (treatment), rats were daily administered AG (15 mg/kg, 4 mL/kg, i.p.) [19] (Fig. 1). All animals were treated for 6 weeks. The experimental design was approved by the ethical committee in Al-Ahliyya Amman University.

Induction of hepatotoxicity

A single dose of CCl_4 (1 mL/kg, i.p.) was chosen according to Kandil et al. [23]. Diluted CCl_4 solution was prepared by dissolving CCl_4 in olive oil (1:1) to prevent its evaporation. On the last day of the designated period, animals were overnight fasted before the injection with diluted CCl_4 (groups of B, C, and D) or olive oil (2 mL/kg, group A). One hour later, they were provided with food. On the next day, animals were fasted for 4 h, lightly anesthetized then sacrificed by cervical dislocation after taking the blood samples.

Blood samples

Twenty-four hours after CCl_4 injection, blood samples were withdrawn by heparinized capillary tubes from a

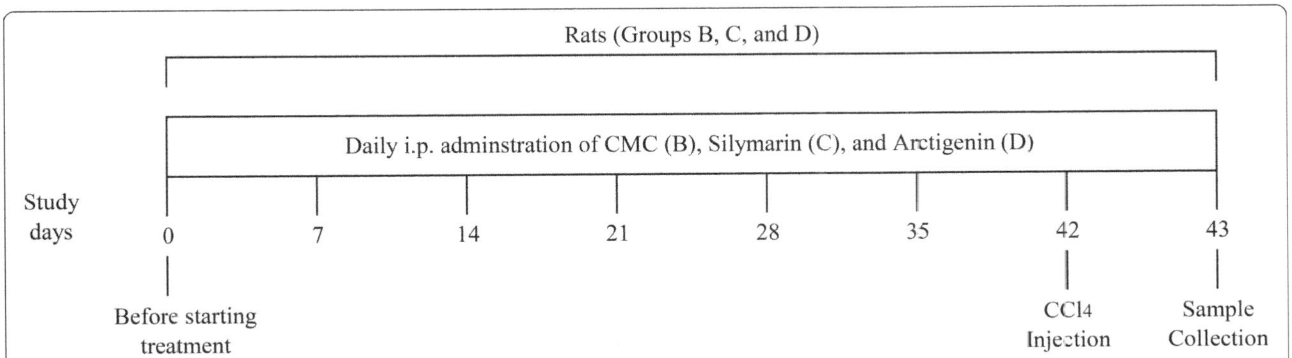

Fig. 1 Experimental design

retro-orbital vein under light anesthesia using a piece of cotton immersed in diethyl-ether [24], allowed to clot for 30 min, sera were separated by centrifugation at RCF 1000×*g* for 10 min. Four aliquots were prepared from each serum and stored at −20 °C until analysis.

Liver tissue specimens

After blood samples collection, animals were sacrificed by cervical dislocation, livers were taken using histological scissors, rinsed with cold saline, dried on a filter paper, and photographed. A portion of each liver was excised, put in 10% formalin solution, and processed as for routine histological evaluation. The remaining part of each liver was stored at −80 °C for later oxidative stress analyses [23].

Liver tissue homogenization

Around 50 mg sample was excised from each liver and homogenized in 1 ml of cell lysis buffer using Teflon homogenizer in ice. The lysate was then cold-centrifuged at RCF 10,000×*g* for 15 min at 4 °C. Supernatants were distributed into four Eppendorf tubes and stored at −80 °C to be analyzed later.

Histological investigation

Five-micrometer sections were stained with hematoxylin-eosin, examined using a light microscope (Leica). and photographed using MC 170 HD Leica Camera (Switzerland) and LAS EZ software. The histological sections were investigated by 2 of the authors in a blinded fashion.

Serum parameters

Serum ALT, AST, ALP, total bilirubin, and total MMP-2 were analyzed 24 h after induction of hepatotoxicity according to manufacturer instructions.

Oxidative stress

Hepatic total protein was determined in the tissue homogenate according to Lowry method [25], total GSH was assayed according to Eyer et al. [26] method. Briefly, the clear supernatant obtained from the homogenate was first deproteinized using 5% MPA then Ellman's reagent (5,5′-dithiobis-2-nitrobenzoic acid) was added which is reduced by sulfhydryl group of GSH to yield a yellow color with a maximum absorbance at 405-412 nm. The concentration was expressed as nM/mg tissue.

Superoxide dismutase activity was analyzed according to Spits and Oberley [27] utilizing a tetrazolium salt for the detection of superoxide radicals generated by xanthine oxidase and hypoxanthine. One unit of SOD is defined as the amount of enzyme needed to exhibit 50% dismutation of the superoxide radical.

Glutathione reductase activity was measured by measuring the rate of NADPH oxidation which is accompanied by a decrease in absorbance at 340 nm [28].

Statistical analyses

All descriptive statistics, analyses, and graphics were performed using GraphPad Prism version 6 (GraphPad Software, San Diego. USA). Data passed the Shapiro-Wilk normality test and were expressed in tables as mean, standard deviation, and standard error of the mean. One-way analysis of variance (ANOVA) followed by Tukey-Kramer post-analysis procedure was used to compare the means of all groups. Differences between means were considered statistically significant at $P \leq 0.05$.

Results

Hepatotoxicity markers

As shown in Table 1, a single injection of CCl_4 significantly increased all hepatotoxicity markers as compared to control group, an effect that was inhibited by pre-administration of both silymarin and AG.

Serum total MMP-2

Serum total MMP-2 (ng/ml) was significantly higher (1734 ± 294) in CCl_4 group than the control group. Both silymarin and AG maintained the level of MMP-2 close to the control group (1177 ± 176), (978 ± 135), (844 ± 178), respectively (Fig. 2).

Hepatic oxidative stress markers (Fig. 3)

Hepatic total GSH level (nM/mg tissue) after CCl_4 injection was significantly lower (0.75 ± 0.20) as compared to the control group (1.26 ± 0.07). On the contrary, both silymarin (1.08 ± 0.13) and AG (1.18 ± 0.13) showed

Table 1 Hepatotoxicity markers in all studied groups

	Control	CCl_4	Silymarin	Arctigenin
ALT (U/L)	27.2 ± 8.67	920 ± 137^{a****}	644 ± 128^{a****b**}	658 ± 144^{a****b**}
AST (U/L)	42.1 ± 9.41	1390 ± 262^{a****}	805 ± 194^{a****b***}	753 ± 185^{a****b****}
ALP (U/L)	71.5 ± 26.4	169 ± 20.7^{a****}	106 ± 18.9^{b***}	119 ± 26.5^{a*b**}
Total bilirubin (mg/dl)	0.61 ± 0.18	1.82 ± 0.27^{a****}	1.03 ± 0.25^{a*b****}	1.11 ± 0.21^{a**b***}

[a] Significantly different from the control group
[b] Significantly different from CCl_4 group *P* values: $^{*}P \leq 0.05$, $^{**}P \leq 0.01$, $^{***}P \leq 0.001$, $^{****}P \leq 0.0001$

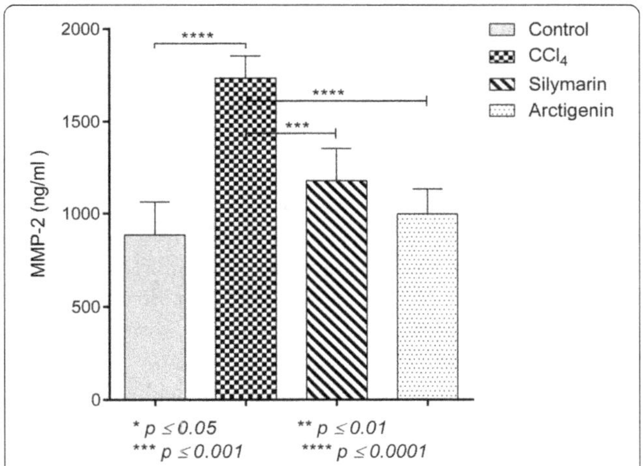

Fig. 2 Serum level of total MMP-2 (ng/ml) in the studied groups

higher GSH levels in the hepatic tissues. However, AG and silymarin GSH levels were close to each other and lied between those of control and CCl_4.

Hepatic SOD activity (U/mg protein) of CCl_4 group was diminished significantly (1.65 ± 0.48) when compared to the control group (3.60 ± 0.25). AG injected-group showed SOD activity (2.34 ± 0.17) higher than that of CCl_4 but lower than the control group. Also, silymarin pretreatment induced SOD activity (2.71 ± 0.38).

Single CCl_4 injection lowered the glutathione reductase activity in the hepatic tissues (2.90 ± 1.35) significantly as compared to the control group (6.78 ± 1.55); this effect of CCl_4 was prevented by the administration of both silymarin (5.49 ± 1.46) and AG (4.59 ± 0.78).

Histopathological results

Figure 4a shows a section in control liver tissue which demonstrates normal histology; central vein and each

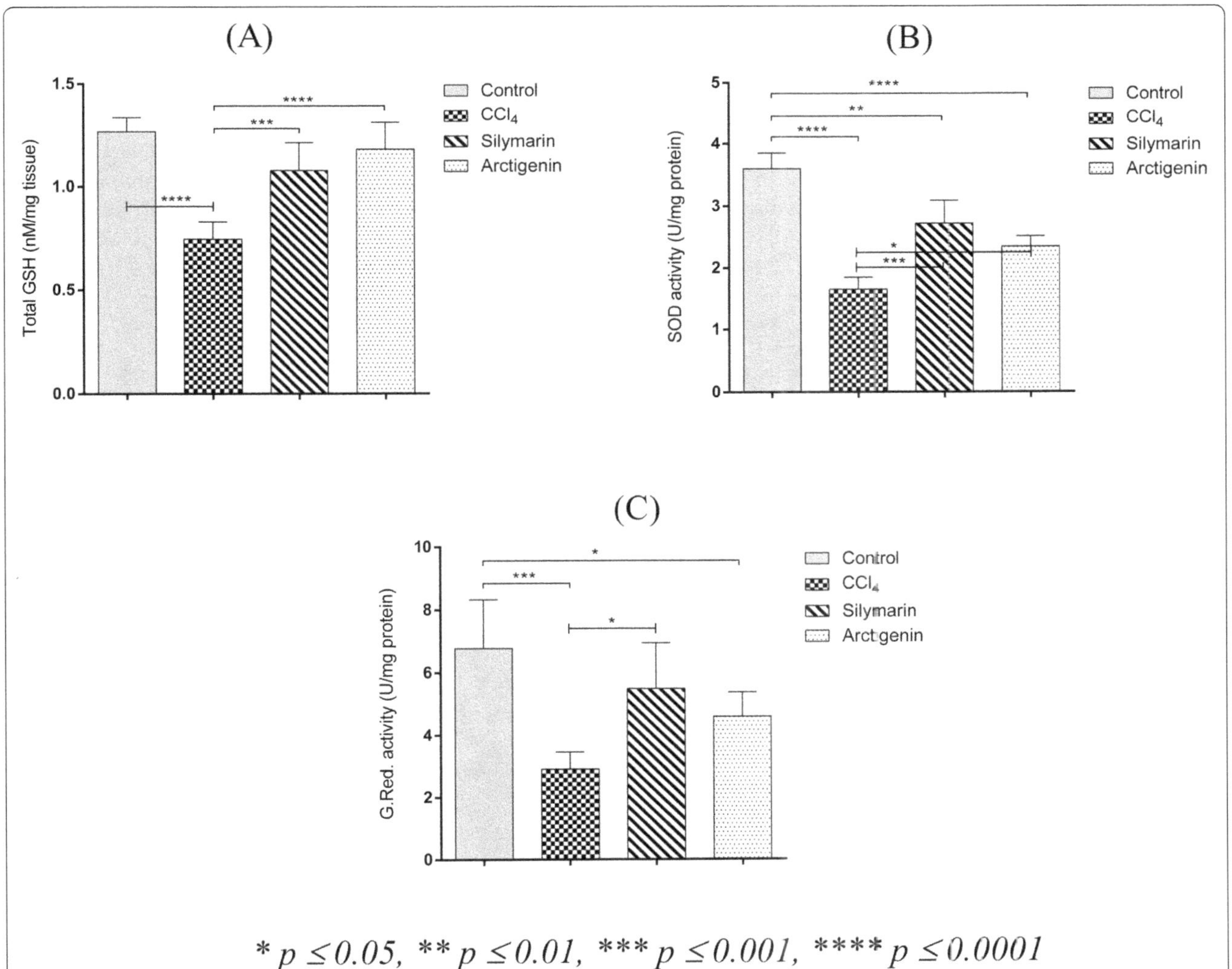

Fig. 3 Hepatic oxidative stress markers **a** Total GSH (nM/mg tissue), **b** SOD activity (U/mg protein), **c** glutathione reductase (U/mg protein)

lobule are bordered by the "portal triad" consisting of a (branch of the hepatic artery, portal vein, and bile duct), in addition to hepatocytes surrounding it which are in sinusoids.

Ballooning (degeneration of hepatocytes) is obvious in CCl_4-injected group section (Fig. 4b). Cells are pale (lightly stained); parenchymal cells show necrotic and apoptotic alterations, in addition to an increase in the number of inflammatory cells (WBCs), and congestion (RBCs).

Figure 4c shows that silymarin repaired some of the damage which is caused by CCl_4 when they were injected respectively. Silymarin group section shows less inflammation and less ballooning. AG also protected the liver tissue from CCl_4 damage (Fig. 4d); it is obvious that ballooning, congestion, and inflammation were reduced.

Discussion

Due to its large size, exclusive structure, and essential roles in maintaining homeostasis, the liver is subjected to many types of diseases and toxic agents [1]. CCl_4 is commonly used for free radical-induced liver injury as many experimental and clinical studies consider it as a classical hepatotoxic agent that induces liver cirrhosis, fibrosis, and necrosis [29]. People may easily be exposed to it by inhalation or skin absorption due to its various usage such as in fire extinguisher and in refrigerant gas [30].

It is now generally accepted that CCl_4 toxicity results from bioactivation of CCl_4 into trichloromethyl free radical by cytochrome P_{450} system in liver microsomes and consequently causes lipid peroxidation of membranes that leads to liver damage. The free radicals generated by CCl_4 metabolism attack polyunsaturated fatty acids in cell membranes forming (fatty acid) free radicals and induce lipid peroxidation with the production of reactive aldehydes, which lead to oxidative stress [31]. Lipid peroxidation causes cell membrane disruption leading to increased cell membrane permeability and enzyme leakage. This, in turn, activates cellular proteases, phospholipid, and protein degradation leading to cytotoxicity and inflammatory response [32]. Antioxidants and anti-inflammatory agents play a critical role against CCl_4 intoxication by scavenging active oxygen and free radicals and neutralizing lipid peroxides [33].

We have used CCl_4 rat model to investigate the hepatoprotective effect of AG in terms of hepatotoxic markers, antioxidant activities, MMP-2, and histopathological outcomes. Male Wistar rats were the animals of choice due to their higher ability to withstand CCl_4-induced hepatotoxicity and to avoid any hormonal changes that may interfere with study outcomes when use females [23]. Silymarin (200 mg/kg) was used as a standard drug due to its reported hepatoprotective benefits [34].

Inflamed or injured hepatocytes leak high amounts of its contents including enzymes into the bloodstream;

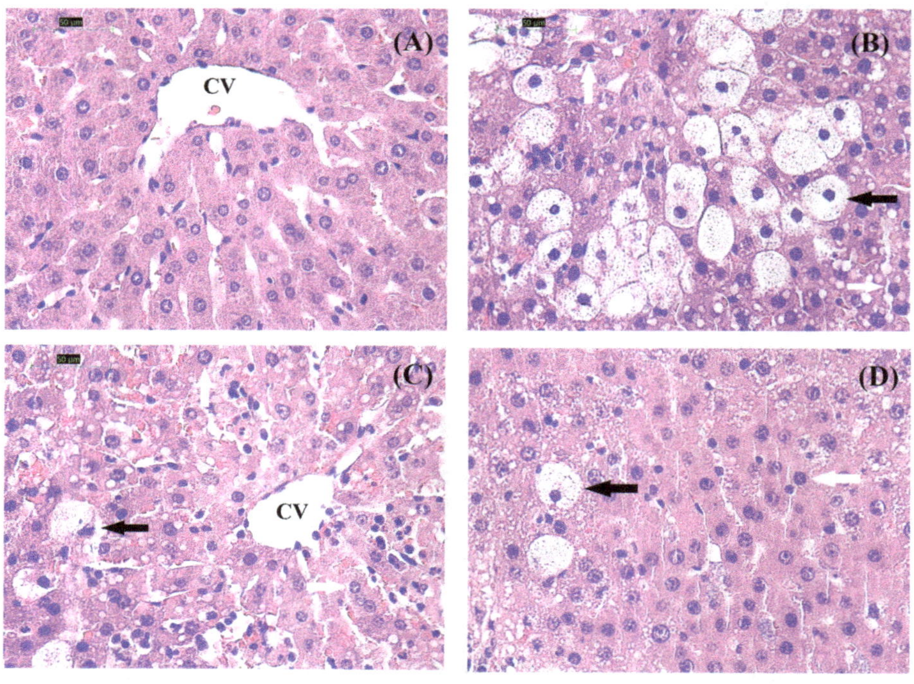

Fig. 4 Histology of the liver from rats receiving only vehicle **a**, CCl_4 **b**, silymarin **c**, AG **d** (H & E stain). CV, central vein; ballooning degeneration (black arrow); infiltration of inflammatory cells (white arrow)

these enzymes are perfect indicators for diagnosis of hepatocellular damage [35].

After injection of CCl_4, hepatotoxicity parameters ALT, AST, ALP, and bilirubin, were significantly increased as compared to the control group. Results that are supported by many previous studies [36, 37]. In our study, previous silymarin and AG administration demonstrated decreased levels in ALT, AST, ALP, and bilirubin. The same results were obtained by Lee *et al.* and Talwar et al. [37, 38] when they tested silymarin efficacy and found that it suppressed CCl_4 damage and normalized hepatotoxicity markers due to its free radical scavenging effect.

According to oxidative stress parameters, there was a significant drop in GSH, SOD, and glutathione reductase in the liver of CCl_4-injected animals compared to the control group. This effect agrees with Abdel-Moneim et al.'s study, when they investigated CCl_4 efficacy on rat models too [36]. On the other hand, pretreatment with AG or silymarin expressed higher levels in these main liver antioxidant parameters. GSH, SOD, and glutathione reductase were normalized by silymarin which could diminish oxidative stress produced by ethanol gavage in mice. It was able to enhance mitochondrial metabolic processes and electron transport chain, to increase intracellular SOD activity, which led to the drop of intracellular ROS levels to improve mitochondrial function [34].

Matrix metalloproteinase-2 is also an important indicator of liver impairment. Our results elucidated the upregulation of this enzyme in rats injected with CCl_4. Liang et al. proved this effect after the application of CCl_4 in rats too, owing that to the activation of hepatic stellate cells (HSCs) by CCl_4 which in turn increases MMP-2 expression. This enzyme increase resulted in hepatocytes matrix degradation, which ends in basement membrane destruction and initiating inflammatory cells to recruit to the injured site [39]. Feher and Lengyel found that silymarin has a beneficial effect on liver carcinogenesis explained by attenuating MMP-2 which is involved in invasion and angiogenesis [40].

When AG and silymarin were injected into rats in the current study, MMP-2 level was declined; findings that are supported by Kara et al. where silymarin lowered total MMP-2 activity knowing that total MMP-2 activity increases in hepatic decay [41]. In addition, Clichici et al. reported that administration of silymarin reduced inflammatory mediators including MMP-9 and liver fibrosis [42].

Conclusion

In conclusion, this study emphasized that AG played an obvious protective role from the harmful effect of CCl_4 on rats' liver. In addition to that, AG protective efficacy with a dose of 15 mg/kg/day, is very close to that of silymarin 200 mg/kg in the term of hepatotoxicity markers, oxidative stress parameters, MMP-2, and histopathological observations.

Abbreviations

AG: Arctigenin; ALP: Alkaline phosphatase; ALT: Alanine aminotransferase; ANOVA: Analysis of variance; AST: Aspartate aminotransferase; CCl_4: Carbon tetrachloride; CMC: Carboxymethylcellulose; ECM: Extracellular matrix; GSH: Glutathione; HSCs: Hepatic stellate cells; JUST: Jordan University of Science and Technology; MMP: Matrix metalloproteinase; MPA: Metphosphoric acid; $NADP^+$: Nicotinamide adenine dinucleotide phosphate; RBCs: Red blood corpuscles; RCF: Relative centrifugal force; ROS: Reactive oxygen species; SD: Standard deviation; SE: Standard error; SOD: Superoxide dismutase; WBCs: White blood cells

Acknowledgements

This work was conducted with the support of Al-Ahliyya Amman University.

Authors' contributions

GK performed the analytical methods. IA contributed in the proposal and manuscript writing. YK was a major contributor in performing the analytical methods, collecting and analyzing data, and writing the manuscript. All authors have read and approved the manuscript.

Ethics approval and consent to participate

This study was ethically approved by ethical committee for the care and use of laboratory animals at Al-Ahliyya Amman University (ethical approval no. AAU-1/14/2017-2018).

Competing interests

The authors declare that they have no competing interests.

References

1. Tarantino G, Citro V, Capone D (2019) Nonalcoholic fatty liver disease: a challenge from mechanisms to therapy. J Clin Med 9(1). https://doi.org/10.3390/jcm9010015
2. Zeng F, Zhang Y, Han X, Weng J, Gao Y (2019) Liver buds and liver organoids: new tools for liver development, disease and medical application. Stem Cell Rev Rep 15(6):774–784. https://doi.org/10.1007/s12015-019-09909-z
3. Anushiravani A, Ghajarieh Sepanlou S (2019) Burden of liver diseases: a review from Iran. Middle East J Dig Dis 11(4):189–191 10.15171/mejdd.2019.147
4. Li L, Zhao Q, Kong W (2018) Extracellular matrix remodeling and cardiac fibrosis. Matrix Biol 68-69:490–506. https://doi.org/10.1016/j.matbio.2018.01.013
5. Friedman SL, Maher JJ, Bissell DM (2000) Mechanisms and therapy of hepatic fibrosis: report of the. AASLD Single Topic Basic Res Conf 32(6):1403–1408. https://doi.org/10.1053/jhep.2000.20243
6. Hamada T, Fondevila C, Busuttil RW, Coito AJ (2008) Metalloproteinase-9 deficiency protects against hepatic ischemia/reperfusion injury. Hepatology (Baltimore, Md) 47(1):186–198. https://doi.org/10.1002/hep.21922
7. Elsayed Elgarawany G, Abdou AG, Maher Taie D, Motawea SM (2019) Hepatoprotective effect of artichoke leaf extracts in comparison with silymarin on acetaminophen-induced hepatotoxicity in mice. J Immunoass Immunochem:1–13. https://doi.org/10.1080/15321819.2019.1692029

8. Panahi Y, Kianpour P, Mohtashami R, Atkin SL, Butler AE, Jafari R, Badeli R, Sahebkar A (2018) Efficacy of artichoke leaf extract in non-alcoholic fatty liver disease: a pilot double-blind randomized controlled trial. Phytotherapy research : PTR 32(7):1382–1387. https://doi.org/10.1002/ptr.6073
9. Tang X, Wei R, Deng A, Lei T (2017) Protective effects of ethanolic extracts from artichoke, an edible herbal medicine, against acute alcohol-induced liver injury in mice. Nutrients 9(9). https://doi.org/10.3390/nu9091000
10. Jung HA, Abdul QA, Byun JS, Joung EJ, Gwon WG, Lee MS, Kim HR, Choi JS (2017) Protective effects of flavonoids isolated from Korean milk thistle *Cirsium japonicum* var. maackii (Maxim.) Matsum on tert-butyl hydroperoxide-induced hepatotoxicity in HepG2 cells. J Ethnopharmacol 209:62–72. https://doi.org/10.1016/j.jep.2017.07.027
11. Abenavoli L, Izzo AA, Milic N, Cicala C, Santini A, Capasso R (2018) Milk thistle (*Silybum marianum*): a concise overview on its chemistry, pharmacological, and nutraceutical uses in liver diseases. Phytotherapy research : PTR 32(11):2202–2213. https://doi.org/10.1002/ptr.6171
12. Ebada ME (2018) Essential oils of green cumin and chamomile partially protect against acute acetaminophen hepatotoxicity in rats. An Acad Bras Cienc 90(2 suppl 1):2347–2358. https://doi.org/10.1590/0001-3765201820170825
13. Madrigal-Santillán E, Madrigal-Bujaidar E, Álvarez-González I, Sumaya-Martínez MT, Gutiérrez-Salinas J, Bautista M, Morales-González Á, MG-L YG-R, Aguilar-Faisal JL, Morales-González JA (2014) Review of natural products with hepatoprotective effects. World J Gastroenterol 20(40):14787
14. Hayashi K, Narutaki K, Nagaoka Y, Hayashi T, Uesato S (2010) Therapeutic effect of arctiin and arctigenin in immunocompetent and immunocompromised mice infected with influenza A virus. Biol Pharm Bull 33(7):1199–1205. https://doi.org/10.1248/bpb.33.1199
15. Lou C, Zhu Z, Zhao Y, Zhu R, Zhao H (2017) Arctigenin, a lignan from Arctium lappa L., inhibits metastasis of human breast cancer cells through the downregulation of MMP-2/-9 and heparanase in MDA-MB-231 cells. Oncol Rep 37(1):179–184. https://doi.org/10.3892/or.2016.5269
16. Ferracane R, Graziani G, Gallo M, Fogliano V, Ritieni A (2010) Metabolic profile of the bioactive compounds of burdock (Arctium lappa) seeds, roots and leaves. J Pharm Biomed Anal 51(2):399–404. https://doi.org/10.1016/j.jpba.2009.03.018
17. Romualdo GR, Silva EDA, Da Silva TC, Aloia TPA, Nogueira MS, De Castro IA, Vinken M, Barbisan LF, Cogliati B (2019) Burdock (Arctium lappa L.) root attenuates preneoplastic lesion development in a diet and thioacetamide-induced model of steatohepatitis-associated hepatocarcinogenesis. Environ Toxicol. https://doi.org/10.1002/tox.22887
18. Lin SC, Lin CH, Lin CC, Lin YH, Chen CF, Chen IC, Wang LY (2002) Hepatoprotective effects of *Arctium lappa* Linne on liver injuries induced by chronic ethanol consumption and potentiated by carbon tetrachloride. J Biomed Sci 9(5):401–409. https://doi.org/10.1007/BF02256533
19. Ming Wu R, Yan Sun Y, Ting Zhou T, Yuan Zhu Z, Jing Zhuang J, Tang X, Chen J, Hong Hu L, Shen X (2014) Arctigenin enhances swimming endurance of sedentary rats partially by regulation of antioxidant pathways. Acta Pharmacol Sin 35(10):1274–1284. https://doi.org/10.1038/aps.2014.70
20. Kang HS, Lee JY, Kim CJ (2008) Anti-inflammatory activity of arctigenin from Forsythiae Fructus. J Ethnopharmacol 116(2):305–312. https://doi.org/10.1016/j.jep.2007.11.030
21. Li XM, Miao Y, Su QY, Yao JC, Li HH, Zhang GM (2016) Gastroprotective effects of arctigenin of Arctium lappa L. on a rat model of gastric ulcers. Biomed Rep. https://doi.org/10.3892/br.2016.770
22. Navidi-Shishaone M, Mohhebi S, Nematbakhsh M, Roozbehani S, Talebi A, Pezeshki Z, Eshraghi-Jazi F, Mazaheri S, Shirdavani S, Gharagozloo M, Moaeidi BA (2014) Co-administration of silymarin and deferoxamine against kidney, liver and heart iron deposition in male iron overload rat model. Int J Prev Med 5(1):110–116
23. Kandil YI, Maraqa AD, Oriquat GA, Shraideh ZA (2017) Resveratrol pretreatment reduces circulating inflammatory interleukins in CCl4-induced hepatotoxicity rats. Bull Faculty Pharmacy Cairo Univ 55(2):319–323. https://doi.org/10.1016/j.bfopcu.2017.09.005
24. Parasuraman S, Raveendran R, Kesavan R (2010) Blood sample collection in small laboratory animals. J Pharmacol Pharmacother 1(2):87–93. https://doi.org/10.4103/0976-500X.72350
25. Lowry OH, Rosebrough NJ, Farr AL, Randall RJ (1951) Protein measurement with the Folin phenol reagent. J Biol Chem 193(1):265–275. https://doi.org/10.1016/0304-3894(92)87011-4
26. Eyer P, Podhradsky D (1986) Evaluation of the micromethod for determination of glutathione using enzymatic cycling and Ellman's reagent. Anal Biochem 153(1):57–66. https://doi.org/10.1016/0003-2697(86)90061-8
27. Spitz DR, Oberley LW (1989) An assay for superoxide dismutase activity in mammalian tissue homogenates. Anal Biochem 179(1):8–18. https://doi.org/10.1016/0003-2697(89)90192-9
28. Mannervik B (2001) Measurement of glutathione reductase activity. Curr Protoc Toxicol Chapter 7:Unit7 2. https://doi.org/10.1002/0471140856.tx0702s00
29. Liu H, Zhang Z, Hu H, Zhang C, Niu M, Li R, Wang J, Bai Z, Xiao X (2018) Protective effects of Liuweiwuling tablets on carbon tetrachloride-induced hepatic fibrosis in rats. BMC Complement Altern Med 18(1):212. https://doi.org/10.1186/s12906-018-2276-8
30. Yehye WA, Rahman NA, Ariffin A, Abd Hamid SB, Alhadi AA, Kadir FA, Yaeghoobi M (2015) Understanding the chemistry behind the antioxidant activities of butylated hydroxytoluene (BHT): a review. Eur J Med Chem 101: 295–312. https://doi.org/10.1016/j.ejmech.2015.06.026
31. Manibusan MK, Odin M, Eastmond DA (2007) Postulated carbon tetrachloride mode of action: a review. J Environ Sci Health C Environ Carcinog Ecotoxicol Rev 25(3):185–209. https://doi.org/10.1080/10590500701569398
32. Kim DH, Kwack SJ, Yoon KS, Choi JS, Lee BM (2015) 4-Hydroxynonenal: a superior oxidative biomarker compared to malondialdehyde and carbonyl content induced by carbon tetrachloride in rats. J Toxicol Environ Health A 78(16):1051–1062. https://doi.org/10.1080/15287394.2015.1067505
33. Ohta Y, Ohashi K, Matsura T, Tokunaga K, Kitagawa A, Yamada K (2008) Octacosanol attenuates disrupted hepatic reactive oxygen species metabolism associated with acute liver injury progression in rats intoxicated with carbon tetrachloride. J Clin Biochem Nutr 42(2):118–125. https://doi.org/10.3164/jcbn.2008017
34. Federico A, Dallio M, Loguercio C (2017) Silymarin/silybin and chronic liver disease: a marriage of many years. Molecules 22(2). https://doi.org/10.3390/molecules22020191
35. Limdi JK, Hyde GM (2003) Evaluation of abnormal liver function tests. Postgrad Med J 79(932):307–312. https://doi.org/10.1136/pmj.79.932.307
36. Abdel-Moneim AM, Al-Kahtani MA, El-Kersh MA, Al-Omair MA (2015) Free radical-scavenging, anti-inflammatory/anti-fibrotic and hepatoprotective actions of taurine and silymarin against CCl4 induced rat liver damage. PLoS One 10(12):e0144509. https://doi.org/10.1371/journal.pone.0144509
37. Lee CP, Shih PH, Hsu CL, Yen GC (2007) Hepatoprotection of tea seed oil (*Camellia oleifera* Abel.) against CCl4-induced oxidative damage in rats. Food Chem Toxicol 45(6):888–895. https://doi.org/10.1016/j.fct.2006.11.007
38. Talwar S, Jagani HV, Nayak PG, Kumar N, Kishore A, Bansal P, Shenoy RR, Nandakumar K (2013) Toxicological evaluation of *Terminalia paniculata* bark extract and its protective effect against CCl4-induced liver injury in rodents. BMC Complement Altern Med 13:127. https://doi.org/10.1186/1472-6882-13-127
39. Liang B, Guo XL, Jin J, Ma YC, Feng ZQ (2015) Glycyrrhizic acid inhibits apoptosis and fibrosis in carbon-tetrachloride-induced rat liver injury. World J Gastroenterol 21(17):5271–5280. https://doi.org/10.3748/wjg.v21.i17.5271
40. Feher J, Lengyel G (2012) Silymarin in the prevention and treatment of liver diseases and primary liver cancer. Curr Pharm Biotechnol 13(1):210–217. https://doi.org/10.2174/138920112798868818
41. Kara E, Coşkun T, Kaya Y, Yumuş O, Vatansever S, Var A (2008) Effects of silymarin and pentoxifylline on matrix metalloproteinase-1 and-2 expression and apoptosis in experimental hepatic fibrosis. Curr Ther Res 69(6):488–502
42. Clichici S, Olteanu D, Filip A, Nagy AL, Oros A, Mircea PA (2016) Beneficial effects of silymarin after the discontinuation of CCl4-induced liver fibrosis. J Med Food 19(8):789–797. https://doi.org/10.1089/jmf.2015.0104

20

NS34A resistance-associated substitutions in chronic hepatitis C in Upper Egypt and regression of liver fibrosis after direct-acting antiviral therapy

Nahed A. Makhlouf[1], Mohamed Farouk[2*], Hanan Mohamed Nafeh[1], Ahmad Farooq Alsayed Hasanain[1], Mohamed Ahmed El-Mokhtar[3], Helal F. Hetta[3], Mohamed A. Mekky[1], Mohamed A boraie[4], Hussein ELamin[2,5] and Ahmed Medhat Nasr[1]

Abstract

Background: Viral resistance-associated substitutions (RASs) can develop in the setting of DAAs therapy (i.e., emerging RASs). Long-term monitoring of fibrosis regression after achieving SVR to simiprevir (SMV)/sofosbuvir (SOF) is essential. The aim of this study was to determine the prevalence of baseline and emerging NS34A RASs in chronic HCV patients in Upper Egypt and to assess the impact of SMV/SOF therapy on liver stiffness.

Results: The enrolled 59 patients had HCV genotype 4a without any baseline RASs in the NS34A region. 96.6% (57/59) of patients achieved sustained virological response (SVR12). Of the two patients who failed to achieve SVR12, one of them developed emerging RASs Q80K in the NS34A region. Seventy-two weeks after SMV/SOF therapy, the percentage of patients with liver fibrosis stage (F2, F3, and F4) decreased from 75.4% before treatment to 42.1% after treatment. The combination of SOF and SMV appeared to be well tolerated.

Conclusions: All patients had HCV genotype 4a without any baseline RASs in the NS34A region. In addition, there was improvement of non-invasive measures of liver fibrosis in patients who achieved SVR, 72 weeks after SMV/SOF therapy.

Keywords: SMV/SOF, RASs, Fibrosis regression, HCV

Background

In Egypt, the seroprevalence of hepatitis C virus (HCV) infection was about 10% in 2015. Since HCV infection is the main cause of liver cirrhosis, hepatocellular carcinoma (HCC), and liver transplantation globally, those patients with HCV are in a need for effective antiviral therapy to overcome the progression to these complications and to reduce mortality [1, 2].

HCV is a small, 9500-nucleotide, plus-stranded ribonucleic acid (RNA) virus that replicates in the cytoplasm with a single open reading frame. The plus-stranded viral RNA is first translated into a large polyprotein containing about 3000 amino acids which is then cleaved by host and viral proteases into structural and non-structural proteins [3].

Directly acting antivirals (DAAs) were designed to directly inhibit viral enzymes and proteins. The NS proteins NS3/4A protease–helicase and NS5B and the NS5A protein all perform crucial activities for the viral life cycle and by far have been the favorite targets for the development of new DAAs [4]. Sofosbuvir (SOF) is a pyrimidine nucleotide analog inhibitor of NS5B and simeprevir (SMV) is an NS3/4A protease inhibitor [5, 6].

* Correspondence: dr.mfarouk.git@hotmail.com
[2]Assiut Center for Management of Viral Hepatitis, Assiut 71515, Egypt
Full list of author information is available at the end of the article

The high rate of HCV replication allows rapid response to selective immune or drug-induced pressure, which may select for resistant variants [7]. Viral resistance-associated substitutions (RASs) have been detected in patients naïve in HCV treatment (i.e., pre-existing, baseline RASs), and RASs can occur with DAAs therapy (i.e., emerging RASs). Natural polymorphism Q80K, responsible for the reduced response of HCV to protease inhibitor simeprevir, is the most studied RAS [8, 9].

A huge number of patients with advanced chronic liver disease are achieving sustained virological response (SVR), highlighting the importance of monitoring fibrosis regression. Non-invasive methods such as transient elastography (TE), Fib-4 index, and APRI score may be useful for monitoring these changes [10, 11].

According to recommendations of the National Committee for Control of Viral Hepatitis (NCCVH) in 2015 guided by recommendations of EASL 2015, 12 weeks of treatment with SMV/SOF combination therapy was recommended for patients with chronic HCV genotype4 [12]. Till the time of our study conduction, real-life data regarding the safety profile, tolerability, and effectiveness of SMV/SOF combination therapy in chronic HCV patients in Upper Egypt were still limited.

The aims of the work are (1) to determine the prevalence of baseline and emerging NS34A RASs in chronic HCV patients in Upper Egypt and (2) to assess the impact of SMV/SOF combination therapy on liver stiffness in patients with chronic HCV infection.

Methods

It was a prospective, open-label study that was conducted at the National Center for the Management of Viral Hepatitis. It took about 2 years' duration, from 1st of December 2015 to 30th of November 2017. All patients were subjected to detailed medical history, complete clinical examination, abdominal ultrasonography, fibroscan examination, routine laboratory investigations, AST to Platelet Ratio Index (APRI) score, and Fibrosis-4 (Fib-4 index) (in addition to HCV RNA PCR, HCV genotyping, and RAS testing).

Fibroscan examination was done at baseline and 72 weeks after the end of treatment. Fifty-nine patients with chronic HCV infection with and without compensated cirrhosis were enrolled.

The study population received a 12-week regimen of simeprevir 150 mg (Olysio® produced by Janssen company) in combination with sofosbuvir 400 mg (Sovaldi® produced by Gilead Sciences company) once daily, in treatment-naïve or INF-experienced patients. The cost of this combination therapy was about 4000 L.E per month for each patient, and it was covered by the Egyptian government as a part of the national campaign for eradication of HCV in Egypt held by the National Committee for Control of Viral Hepatitis, The Egyptian Ministry of Health. Patients were advised to avoid sun exposure and to use sunscreen cream locally on sun-exposed areas as possible. Patients also were advised not to take any other medication for any comorbidity without our consultation to check for drug-drug interactions.

Molecular investigations

PCR, sequencing for genotyping, and amplification of NS34A were carried out in the Medical Research Center, Faculty of Medicine, Assiut University, and in Macrogen Korea Laboratory, South Korea. SVR12 is sustained virological response with HCV RNA negative at 12 weeks after the end of therapy.

APRI score [13] and *Fib-4 index* [14] were calculated at baseline and 12 weeks after the end of therapy (EOT).

Fibroscan examination was performed in the Assiut Center for Management of Viral Hepatitis. The median value of ten successful measurements was considered representative of the liver stiffness (LS), according to the manufacturer's recommendations (IQR less than 30% of the median value and success rate of more than 60%) [15]. Based on the baseline LSM, patients were stratified according to estimated METAVIR fibrosis score into F0, F1, F2, F3, and F4 groups. Liver stiffness measurement (LSM) was used to estimate the METAVIR fibrosis stage as follows: F1 ≥ 6.5 kPa [16], F2 ≥ 7.1 kPa, F3 ≥9.5 kPa, and F4 ≥ 12.5 kPa [17].

Statistical analysis

Statistical tests were performed using SPSS 16.0 (SPSS Inc., Chicago, USA) for Windows. Results were reported as the absolute value, mean ± standard deviation, and range. Continuous variables were compared using Student's *T* test or Mann-Whitney *U* test as appropriate. Nominal or ordinal variables were analyzed by the chi-square test and Fisher's exact test. $P < 0.05$ was considered statistically significant. Variables with p value < 0.05 were then tested in a logistic regression model. The ability of Fib-4 index improvement in predicting LSM improvement was assessed by specificity, sensitivity, positive and negative predictive values, and positive and negative likelihood ratios, and accuracy was calculated.

Results

Table 1 shows the demographic and baseline data of the study group. All patients had HCV genotype 4a, and we did not find any baseline RASs in the NS34A region.

Table 2 shows virological response in the study group, where 96.6% achieved sustained virological response (SVR12). SVR was 96.3% (52/54) in naïve patients and 100% (5/5) in INF experienced patients. Regarding patients who achieved SVR12, no one relapsed 72 weeks

Table 1 Demographic and baseline data of the study group

Item	Descriptive
1. Age "years" mean ± SD (range)	50.66 ± 9.80 (27.0–69.0)
2. Sex:	
• **Male**	41 (69.5%)
3. BMI "kg/m^2" mean ± SD (range)	27.84 ± 4.42 (19.4–39.1)
4. Diabetes mellitus:	
• **Yes**	14(23.7%)
5. Treatment status:	
• **Naïve**	54(91.5%)
• **INF experienced**	5(8.5%)
6. HCV genotype	Genotype 4a (100%)
7. Baseline NS34A RASs	0 (0%)

after the end of treatment (EOT). Patients with liver fibrosis F0–F2 (31/31) (100%) achieved SVR (the two patients who did not achieve SVR12; one of them was F3 and the other was F4).

Of the two patients who failed to achieve sustained virological response, one of them developed emerging RASs Q80K in the NS34A region [sequencing analysis revealed that in this patient, the cytosine nucleotide was replaced by adenine at position 238 of the triplet, forming the amino acid number 80, which resulted in the replacement of the glutamine (Q) amino acid with lysine (K)], and the other patient did not have any emerging RASs in the NS34A region.

Table 3 shows changes in the laboratory data of the study group. There was a significant decrease in the mean values of alanine aminotransferase (ALT) and aspartate amninotransferase (AST) level after treatment at week 4, week 8, at EOT, and 12 weeks after EOT (at SVR 12) (p value = 0.001 and < 0.001, respectively). There was no significant difference (p value > 0.05) between the mean platelet count before treatment and after 4 and 8 weeks. However, there was a significant increase (p value < 0.05) in the mean platelet count at EOT and at SVR 12. Regarding serum total bilirubin, there was a highly significant increase (p value = 0.001) in serum total bilirubin at week 4 and week 8 of treatment compared to baseline. However, there was a significant decrease (p value = 0.001) in serum total bilirubin at SVR 12 compared to baseline. There was a significant decrease in the mean Fib-4 index and APRI score post-treatment when compared to pretreatment.

As shown in Table 4 and Fig. 1, after SMV/SOF therapy, patients with liver fibrosis stage (F2, F3, and F4) decreased from 75.4% before treatment to 42.1% after treatment and the total percentage of patients with liver fibrosis (F0 and F1) increased from 24.6 to 57.9%.

Table 5 shows that the highest significant decrease in LSM, 72 weeks after EOT, was in patients with baseline liver fibrosis stage F2 and F3 (p value = 0.001). There was a significant difference between those with LSM improvement and those without LSM improvement, regarding treatment status before SMV/SOF therapy and Fib-4 index improvement status 12 weeks after EOT (at SVR 12) (p value = 0.042 and 0.035, respectively).

Multiple linear regression analysis showed that LSM improvement was significantly higher in patients who were naïve and patients who showed Fib-4 index improvement after SMV/SOF therapy. The sensitivity of Fib-4 index improvement in predicting LSM improvement was 81.6% and specificity was 55.6%. Its positive predictive value and negative predictive values were 88.6% and 41.7%, respectively. The overall accuracy was 76.6%.

Two patients suffered from headaches (3.4%), two patients developed photosensitivity reactions (3.4%), one patient developed bleeding gums (1.7%), and one patient developed fatigue (1.7%). Bilirubin level raised above 1.2 mg/dl in 32/59 patients during SMV/SOF therapy with a percentage of 54.2%. Among them, 9 patients (28%) raised to a level above or equal to 2 mg/dl.

There was a significant difference between those who developed an increase in serum bilirubin to a level ≥ 2 mg during SMV/SOF therapy and those who did not show this increase, regarding baseline platelet count and baseline LSM in kilo Pascal (kPa). Multiple linear regression analyses showed that the degree of rising in serum bilirubin levels significantly increased in patients who had higher baseline LSM (kPa). Six patients out of 9 (66.7%), whose bilirubin levels were elevated to a level equal to or above 2 mg/dl after receiving SMV/SOF combination therapy, had liver fibrosis F4.

Table 2 Virological response in the study group

Item	F3, F4	F0–F2	Total
Response:			
• **Patients who achieved SVR12**	92.9% (26/28)	100% (31/31)	57 (96.6%)
• **Patients who did not achieve SVR12**	7.1% (2/28)	0 (0%)	2 (3.4%)
***p* value**	0.001*	NA	0.001*

Total number = 59 patients
NA not applicable, *SVR12* sustained virological response with HCV RNA negative at 12 weeks after the end of therapy
* Statistically significant

Table 3 Changes in the laboratory data of the study group

Variable	ALT	AST	PLT	Bilirubin	Fib-4	APRI
Baseline	44.86 ± 21.34	51.41 ± 22.95	195 ± 68	0.93 ± 0.40	2.42 ± 1.69	0.821 ± 0.08
4 weeks	25.19 ± 9.07	32.46 ± 11.93	196 ± 66	1.29 ± 0.69		
Percent of change	– 43.84%	– 36.86%	0.41%	38.7%		
p value	0.001*	0.001*	ns	0.001*		
8 weeks	23.46 ± 9.33	27.64 ± 10.91	207 ± 74	1.26 ± 0.64		
Percent of change	– 47.70%	– 46.23%	5.80%	35.48%		
p value	0.001*	0.001*	ns	0.001*		
12 weeks (EOT)	26.68 ± 7.96	29.03 ± 7.14	215 ± 52	0.98 ± 0.44		
Percent of change	– 40.52%	– 43.54%	10.11%	5.37%		
p value	0.001*	0.001*	0.05*	ns		
12 weeks after EOT (SVR 12)	24.46 ± 7.63	29.53 ± 6.61	218 ± 64	0.77 ± 0.20	1.60 ± 0.61	0.407 ± 0.08
Percent of change	– 45.47%	– 42.55%	11.67%	– 17.2%	– 33.88%	– 50.42%
p value	0.001*	0.001*	0.05*	0.001*	0.001*	0.027*

Data were expressed as mean ± standard deviation
Percent of change = [(variable 12 weeks after EOT – variable at baseline)/variable at baseline] × 100
All *p* values compared the changes in the mean value of each parameter at a certain time in relation to the baseline, *Highly statistical significance
EOT endo of treatment, *SVR12* sustained virological response with HCV RNA negative at 12 weeks after the end of therapy, *ns* not statistically significant

Discussion

HCV genotype 4a has been reported as the predominant subtype in Egypt in some studies [18–20]. In a study conducted in Damietta, El-Tahan et al. [21] found that HCV genotype 4a represents 93.3% (28/30) and genotype 1 represents 6.7% (2/30). However, we found that all 59 patients were infected with genotype 4a without any baseline RASs at NS34A regions that reflect the high prevalence of HCV genotype 4a in Upper Egypt and the absence of baseline RASs in NS34A regions in Egyptian chronic hepatitis C (CHC) patients, and this is unlike other regions in the world, whereas the prevalence of Q80K in HCV genotype 1 in North America was 34% [9]. To the best of our knowledge, we had conducted the first study that reported the prevalence of baseline NS34A RASs in patients treated with DAAs in routine clinical practice in Upper Egypt.

In the present study, the virological response agrees with the results of another study conducted by El-Khayat et al. [22] who assessed SVR12 for 583 Egyptian patients with HCV genotype 4 infections after receiving SMV/SOF without ribavirin for 12 weeks, and the SVR12 rate in their study was 95.7% and was lower among cirrhotic patients (80.8%). Our results are also consistent with a study conducted by Eletreby et al. [23] who revealed the SVR12 rate achieved among a cohort of 6211 patients with genotype 4 HCV infection was 94%. Besides, we found that patients who achieved SVR12 were still a viremic 72 weeks after EOT.

RAS testing was done in the two patients who did not achieve SVR, and this revealed the presence of Q80K RAS in one patient (50%). Due to the small number of patients who did not achieve SVR12, only two patients, we could not discover the possible predictors of the development of emerging NS34A RASs. We just observed that the female patient who developed Q80K after SMV/SOF therapy had leucopenia at baseline [TLC (Total leucocytic count) = 2.5 K/cm] while the other male patient who did not develop Q80K had normal TLC (4.5 K/cm).

ALT is a biochemical marker for hepatocyte injury. Persistent ALT elevation is associated with chronic hepatitis C progression and increased risk for cirrhosis and an indication for treatment [24]. In the present study, there was a highly significant difference between ALT levels before treatment versus the ALT level after treatment at week 4, week 8, EOT, and 12 weeks after EOT (*p* value = 0.001). These results agree with De Pace et al. [25] who found that AST and ALT decreased during therapy: baseline mean AST = 52 (32–81) UI/mL and mean ALT = 52.5 (34–83.2) UI/mL vs EOT AST = 21 (18–28) UI/mL and ALT = 17 (13–24.2). These results show the rapid improvement of the inflammatory

Table 4 Fibrosis stage before and 72 weeks after SMV/SOF therapy in SVR patients

Liver fibrosis stage	Before treatment (baseline)	72 weeks after treatment	*P* value
F0	10 (17.5%)	20 (35%)	0.001*
F1	4 (7%)	13 (22.9%)	0.001*
F2	17 (29.8%)	7 (12.3%)	0.001*
F3	10 (17.5%)	2 (3.5%)	0.001*
F4	16 (28.2%)	15 (26.3%)	ns

Total cases = 57
*Statistically significant

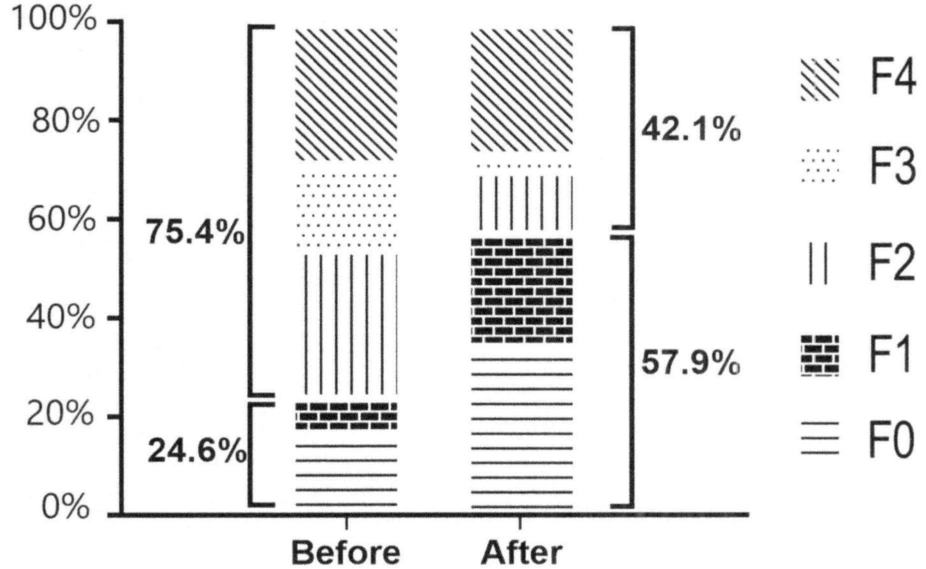

Fig. 1 Relation between fibrosis stage before and 72 weeks after SMV/SOF therapy

process and hepatocyte injury accompanying HCV infection.

Also, our study showed that non-invasive biomarkers of liver fibrosis as APRI score and FIB-4 index improved significantly in most of the patients. Unexpectedly, they improved in patients who did not achieve SVR. Also, we found that the possible predictors of APRI score improvement were lower baseline platelet, higher baseline AST, and higher baseline APRI score. In addition, we found that higher baseline AST was a possible predictor of Fib-4 index improvement. These results go in concordance with De Pace et al. [25] who found a significant dropping of APRI score and a moderate improvement in platelet values from baseline to EOT. In our study, platelet count increased significantly after treating patients with SMV/SOF combination therapy, and this agrees with Sayyar et al. [26]. Unexpectedly in our study, PLT count increased even in patients who did not achieve SVR.

Table 5 LSM before and 72 weeks after SMV/SOF therapy in SVR patients

Baseline liver fibrosis stage	Mean liver stiffness before treatment (baseline) (kPa), mean ± SD	Mean liver stiffness 72 weeks after treatment (kPa), mean ± SD	*P* value
F1 (*n* = 4)	6.4 ± 0.5	5.4 ± 0.9	0.088 ns
F2 (*n* = 17)	8.5 ± 0.5	6.1 ± 1.3	0.001*
F3 (*n* = 10)	10.7 ± 0.7	6.9 ± 2	0.001*
F4 (*n* = 16)	24.9 ± 6.9	20.7 ± 5.6	< 0.05*
Total (*n* = 47)	15.12 ± 0.54	10.27 ± 0.97	0.001*

*Statistically significant

Lower baseline platelet count, higher baseline APRI score, Fib-4 index, lower baseline prothrombin, and higher baseline AFP (alfa-fetoprotein) were associated with the increased PLT (platelet) count after treatment. Nevertheless, linear regression analysis showed that lower baseline platelet count is the main predictor of the platelet count increase after treatment. This result may be explained by Amer et al. who studied the relation between platelet viral load and the possible response after antiviral therapy; low baseline platelet count and low platelet viral load may explain the better response in platelet count after antiviral therapy [27].

Amer et al. were investigating platelets as a possible reservoir of HCV and predictor of response to treatment, and they found that the platelet count tended to be lower among those with rapid virological response (RVR) compared to those with non-RVR throughout the follow-up. In addition, they found that among individuals with RVR, platelet counts declined slightly by week 4 and week 12 then gradually increased to reach pretreatment levels by week 48, but there was no similar decline among patients who did not achieve RVR. Also, they found that platelet count remained almost constant over time, among non-SVR, but among SVR, it should have a steady small decline until week 12, then it started to increase to pre-treatment levels, and also, they found that platelet counts did not correlate with platelet or serum viral loads or treatment responses [27].

Regarding the effect of antiviral therapy on the degree of hepatic fibrosis in our cohort, there was a significant difference between the degree of liver stiffness by fibroscan before and after therapy. According to literatures, a more accurate evaluation of fibrosis regression using fibroscan needs longer duration after EOT. Liver stiffness measurement can be influenced by inflammatory activity. Transient elastography improves within a short period of time following SVR, likely reflecting resolution of inflammation rather than regression of fibrosis. However, for patients evaluated at later time points post-SVR, elastography appears to have good performance characteristics. Thus, delaying the post SVR assessment of liver stiffness for at least 1 year post SVR would seem prudent [28–30]. So we decided to choose a point of time which is of longer duration than 1 year for a better and more accurate evaluation of liver fibrosis regression.

Pons et al. [31] reported that the improvement of liver stiffness was found 4 weeks after starting DAAs therapy, which most probably reflects a reduction in inflammation rather than in fibrosis. We found that there was a significant difference between those patients who achieved liver stiffness improvement and those who did not achieve liver stiffness improvement regarding treatment status before treatment and the improvement occurring in the Fib-4 index after treatment. Patients who were naïve or who showed post-treatment Fib-4 improvement were more liable for improvement of LSM after SMV/SOF therapy. These parameters may be possible predictors of liver stiffness improvement.

Tag-Adeen et al. [32], in a study conducted in Qena University Hospital that enrolled 80 CHC patients who received different DAAs regimens, found that LSM dropped from 15.6 ± 10.8 to 12.1 ±8 .7 kPa post-SVR; the maximum change of − 5.8 occurred in F4 versus − 2.79, − 1.28, and + 0.08 in F3, F2, and F0–F1, respectively ($p < 0.0001$). Also, those patients showed significant improvement in the APRI score and Fib-4 index after achieving SVR. They found that younger age, male gender, raised baseline ALT, and raised AST were possible predictors of LSM improvement. Concerning the safety profile in this cohort, the combination of SOF and SMV appeared to be well tolerated in the majority of patients, where no deaths or serious side effects leading to the stoppage of the therapy had been reported. The incidence and degree of the adverse effects are comparable to those reported in the published international trials using the same regimen and with the same doses.

The safety profile seen in this study is in-line with the OPTIMIST-1 and OPTIMIST-2 studies [33]. Among the fifty-nine patients, minor clinical side effects as fatigue and bleeding gums were reported in one case for each (1.7%). Headache and photosensitivity were reported in 2 patients for each (3.4%). After EOT, all the dermatological manifestations gradually disappeared with a complete resolution with no residual sequels.

Raised bilirubin > 1.2 mg/dl was the most frequent adverse effect where it occurred in 32/59 (54.2%). Total serum bilirubin level exceeded 2 mg/dl in nine patients (9/59) (17.3%). This rise was reversible and the bilirubin level began to improve at week 8 of therapy, improved significantly at EOT, and returned to normal 12 weeks after EOT.

These findings came in agreement with the findings observed by El-Khayat et al. [22]; photosensitivity occurred in 18 patients among 583 patients (3%) and hyperbilirubinemia occurred in 44 patients (7.2%).

The current work had some limitations: (1) the small sample size was one of the drawbacks of the present cohort; (2) although the absence of baseline NS34A RASs is a good indicator of its low prevalence in Egypt, this made it difficult to study the effect of baseline NS34A RASs on the virological response after receiving the NS34A inhibitor-containing regimen (SMV/SOF combination therapy); (3) we could not study the efficacy of SMV/SOF combination therapy on other HCV genotypes because we found that all patients were infected with HCV genotype 4a only, although this is a good indicator of the high prevalence of genotype 4 in Egypt; and (4) another limitation is that our cohort is a Single Center Experience.

Conclusions

All patients had HCV genotype 4a without any baseline RASs in the NS34A region. One patient developed emerging RASs Q80K in the NS34A region. In addition, there was improvement of non-invasive measures of liver fibrosis in patients who achieved SVR, 72 weeks after SMV/SOF therapy.

Abbreviations

APRI: AST to Platelet Ratio Index; AST: Aspartate transferase; ALT: Alanine transferase; TLC: Total leucocytic count; LSM: Liver stiffness measurement; RASs: Resistance-associated substitutions; SIM/SOF: Simiprevir/sofosbuvir; SVR: Sustained virological response; EOT: End of therapy; HCV: Hepatitis C virus; RNA: Ribonucleic acid; DAAs: Directly acting antivirals; TE: Transient elastography; NCCVH: National Committee for Control of Viral Hepatitis

Acknowledgements

The research team would like to thank all physicians and nurses in Assiut Center for Management of Viral Hepatitis and laboratory technicians in the Medical Research Center, Faculty of Medicine, Assiut University, and in Macrogen Korea Laboratory, South Korea, for their patience and their help during this study.

Authors' contributions

MFA, MAM, and AFAH were responsible for data collection and were the operators of the fibroscan procedure. MA was the supervisor of the fibroscan procedure and analysis of its data. HFH and MAE were responsible of the laboratory testing including genotyping and RAS testing in collaboration with Macrogen Korea lab. NAM and HMN were responsible for writing and editing the manuscript. AMN and HE were the supervisors of the research work. All authors have read and approved the manuscript.

Ethics approval and consent to participate
Reviewing the proposal was carried out before starting data collection via the ethical review committee of Assiut Faculty of Medicine. Privacy and confidentiality of all the data were assured. The aim of the study was explained to each participant before enrollment. Informed written consent was obtained from those who agreed to participate in the study. All patients were informed clearly that refusal of participation does not interfere with receiving the optimum available medical care.
The committee's reference number is not applicable and not available.

Competing interests
There was no conflict of interest.

Author details
[1]Department of Tropical Medicine and Gastroenterology, Faculty of Medicine, Assiut University, Assiut, Egypt. [2]Assiut Center for Management of Viral Hepatitis, Assiut 71515, Egypt. [3]Department of Microbiology and Immunology, Faculty of Medicine, Assiut University, Assiut, Egypt. [4]Department of Internal Medicine, Al-Azhar University, Cairo, Egypt. [5]Department of Internal Medicine, Faculty of Medicine, Assiut University, Assiut, Egypt.

References
1. Shawkat H, Yakoot M, Shawkat T, Helmy S (2015) Efficacy and safety of a herbal mixture (Viron® tablets) in the treatment of patients with chronic hepatitis C virus infection: a prospective, randomized, open-label, proof-of-concept study. Drug Des Devel Ther 9:799–804
2. Elgharably A, Gomaa AI, Crossey MME, Norsworthy PJ, Waked I, Taylor-Robinson SD (2017) Hepatitis C in Egypt – past, present, and future. Int J Gen Med 10:1–6
3. Lindenbach BD, Rice CM (2005) Unravelling hepatitis C virus replication from genome to function. Nature 436:933–938
4. Kayali Z, Schmidt WN (2014) Finally sofosbuvir: an oral anti-HCV drug with wide performance capability. Pharmacogenomics Pers Med 7:387–398
5. AASLD American Association for the Study of Liver Diseases/ IDSA; Infectious Diseases Society of America (2015) Hepatitis C guidance: AASLD-IDSA recommendations for testing, managing, and treating adults infected with hepatitis C virus. Hepatology 62:932–954
6. Titusville NJ (2013) Janssen Therapeutics. Available from Drugs@FDA http://www.accessdata.fda.gov/drugsatfda_docs/label/2017/205123s012lbl.pdf. Accessed 17 Feb 2017.
7. Ahmed A, Felmlee DJ (2015) Mechanisms of hepatitis C viral resistance to direct acting antivirals. Viruses 7:6716–6729
8. Lawitz E, Sulkowski MS, Ghalib R, Rodriguez-Torres M, Younossi ZM, Corregidor A, DeJesus E, Pearlman B, Rabinovitz M, Gitlin N, Lim JK, Pockros PJ, Scott JD, Fevery B, Lambrecht T, Ouwerkerk-Mahadevan S, Callewaert K, Symonds WT, Picchio G, Lindsay KL, Beumont M, Jacobson IM (2014) Simeprevir plus sofosbuvir, with or without ribavirin, to treat chronic infection with hepatitis C virus genotype 1 in non-responders to pegylated interferon and ribavirin and treatment-naive patients: the COSMOS randomized study. Lancet 384:1756–1765
9. Sarrazin C, Lathouwers E, Peeters M, Daems B, Buelens A, Witek J (2015) Prevalence of the hepatitis C virus NS3 polymorphism Q80K in genotype 1 patients in the European region. Antiviral Res 116:10–16
10. Angulo P, Hui JM, Marchesini G, Bugianesi E, George J, Farrell GC, Enders F, Saksena S, Burt AD, Bida JP, Lindor K, Sanderson SO, Lenzi M, Adams LA, Kench J, Therneau TM, Day CP (2007) The NAFLD fibrosis score: a noninvasive system that identifies liver fibrosis in patients with NAFDL. Hepatology 45:846–854
11. Robic MA, Procopet B, Métivier S, Péron JM, Selves J, Vinel JP, Bureau C (2011) Liver stiffness accurately predicts portal hypertension-related complications in patients with chronic liver disease: a prospective study. J Hepatol 55:1017–1024
12. EASL; European Association for the Study of the Liver (2015) EASL recommendations on treatment of hepatitis C. J Hepatol 63:199–236
13. Borsoi Viana MS, Takei K, Collarile Yamaguti DC, Guz B, Strauss E (2009) Use of AST platelet ratio index (APRI Score) as an alternative to liver biopsy for treatment indication in chronic hepatitis C. Ann Hepatol 8:26–31
14. Kim BK, Kim DY, Park JY, Ahn SH, Chon CY, Kim JK, Paik YH, Lee KS, Park YN, Han KH (2010) Validation of FIB-4 and comparison with other simple noninvasive indices for predicting liver fibrosis and cirrhosis in hepatitis B virus-infected patients. Liver Int 30:1073–1081
15. Lucidarme D, Foucher J, Le Bail B, Vergniol J, Castera L, Duburque C et al (2009) Factors of the accuracy of transient elastography (fibroscan) for the diagnosis of liver fibrosis in chronic hepatitis C. Hepatology 49:1083–1089
16. Tsochatzis EA, Gurusamy KS, Ntaoula S, Cholongitas E, Davidson BR, Burroughs AK (2011) Elastography for the diagnosis of severity of fibrosis in chronic liver disease: a meta-analysis of diagnostic accuracy. J Hepatol 54:650–659
17. Castéra L, Vergniol J, Foucher J, Le Bail B, Chanteloup E, Haaser M, Darriet M, Couzigou P, De Lédinghen V (2005) Prospective comparison of transient elastography, Fibrotest, APRI, and liver biopsy for the assessment of fibrosis in chronic hepatitis C. Gastroenterology 128:343–350
18. Ray SC, Arthur RR, Carella A, Bukh J, Thomas DL (2000) Genetic epidemiology of hepatitis C virus throughout Egypt. J Infect Dis 182:698–707
19. Youssef A, Yano Y, Utsumi T, Serwah A-H, Hayashi Y, Abd El-alah EM (2009) Molecular epidemiological study of hepatitis viruses in Ismailia, Egypt. Intervirology 52:123–131
20. Fakhr AE, Pourkarim MR, Maes P, Atta AH, Marei A, Azab M, Ranst MV (2013) Hepatitis C virus NS5B sequence-based genotyping analysis of patients from the Sharkia Governorate, Egypt. Hepat Mon 13(12):e12706
21. El-Tahan RR, Ghoneim AM, Zaghloul H (2018) 5′UTR and NS5B-based genotyping of hepatitis C virus in patients from Damietta governorate. Egypt J Adv Res 10:39–47
22. El-Khayat HR, Fouad YM, Maher M, El-Amin H, Muhammed H (2017) Efficacy and safety of sofosbuvir plus simeprevir therapy in Egyptian patients with chronic hepatitis C: a real-world experience. Gut 66:2008–2012
23. Eletreby R, Elakel W, Said M, El Kassas M, Seif S, Elbaz T, El Raziky M, Abdel Rehim S, Zaky S, Fouad R (2017) Real-life Egyptian experience of efficacy and safety of Simeprevir/ Sofosbuvir therapy in 6211 chronic HCV genotype IV infected patients. Liver Int 37:534–541
24. Attar BM, Van Thiel DH (2015) Hepatitis C virus: a time for decisions. Who should be treated and when? World J Gastrointest Pharmacol Ther 7:33–40
25. De Pace V, Morelli MC, Ravaioli M, Maggi F, Galli S, Vero V, Re MC, Cescon M, Pistello M (2019) Efficacy, safety, and predictors of direct-acting antivirals in hepatitis C virus patients with heterogeneous liver diseases. New Microbiol 42:189–196
26. Sayyar M, Saidi M, Zapatka S, Deng Y, Ciarleglio M, Garcia-Tsao G (2019) Platelet count increases after viral elimination in chronic HCV, independent of the presence or absence of cirrhosis. Liver Int 39:2061–2065
27. Amer A, Abu Madi M, Shebi FM, Al Faridi D, ALkhinji M, Derbala M (2016) Platelets as a possible reservoir of HCV and predictor of response to treatment. J Virol Antivir Res 5:3
28. Terrault NA, Hassanein TI (2016) Management of the patient with SVR. J Hepatol 65:120–129
29. Andersen ES, Moessner BK, Christensen PE et al (2011) Lower liver stiffness in patients with sustained virological response 4 years after treatment for chronic hepatitis C. Eur J Gastroenterol Hepatol 23:41–44
30. Hezode C, Castera L, Roudot-Thoraval F et al (2011) Liver stiffness diminishes with antiviral response in chronic hepatitis C. Aliment Pharmacol Ther 34:656–663
31. Pons M, Santos B, Simón-Talero M, Ventura-Cots M, Riveiro-Barciela M, Esteban R, Augustin S, Genescà J (2017) Rapid liver and spleen stiffness improvement in compensated advanced chronic liver disease patients treated with oral antivirals. Ther Adv Gastroenterol 10:619–629
32. Tag-Adeen M, Sabra AM, Akazawa Y, Ohnita K, Nakao K (2017) Impact of hepatitis C virus genotype-4 eradication following direct-acting antivirals on liver stiffness measurement. Hep Med 9:45–53
33. Kwo P, Gitlin N, Nahass R, Bernstein D, Etzkorn K, Rojter S, Schiff E, Davis M, Ruane P, Younes Z, Kalmeijer R, Sinha R, Peeters M, Lenz O, Fevery B, De La Rosa G, Scott J, Witek J (2016) Simeprevir plus sofosbuvir (12 and 8 weeks) in hepatitis C virus genotype 1-infected patients without cirrhosis: OPTIMIST-1, a phase 3, randomized study. Hepatology 64:370–380

21

Evaluating lubiprostone for effective bowel preparation before colonoscopy

Yasser Hamada[1*], Ibrahim Emam[2], Rabab Maher[2] and Hassan El-Garem[1]

Abstract

Background: Colon preparation is a fundamental step for performing a successful colonoscopy. We aimed to evaluate the effectiveness of administering lubiprostone (LB) added to a single dose of oral polyethylene glycol (PEG) solution in achieving satisfactory colon cleanliness and decreasing the side effects.

Results: One-hundred percent of the control group patients reported that the experienced taste was worse than expected, while in the intervention group half of the patients (50%) said that the taste was natural and 48% experienced taste worse than expected ($p<0.0001$). Regarding Boston bowel preparation scale (BBPS), there was a significant difference in the overall Boston scale ($p=0.02$) with more efficacy in the intervention group as 66% of patients in the intervention group had good bowel preparation (5–7) and 24% excellent preparation (8–9). On the other hand, the overall Boston scale in the control group showed that 54% of patients were between 5 and 7, and only 16% of patients had overall Boston scale 8–9. In terms of the side effects of the preparation in both arms, the majority of cases in the intervention arm did not complain of any side effects (78%), while the majority of the complaints were vomiting in 16% of the intervention cases.

Conclusion: The current evidence suggested that adding LB to the colon preparation significantly improved the tolerability and efficacy.

Keywords: Colonoscopy, Lubiprostone, Polyethylene glycol, Bowel preparation, Comparative study

Background

Colon preparation before the colonoscopy is of crucial importance and is a major factor in the success of the procedure as it helps to ensure ideal polyp detection rates [1]. In the case of poor preparation, medical costs, missed lesions, and procedure times are increased, leading to decreased patient's satisfaction [2]. Before the colonoscopy, dietary restrictions and bowel lavage using a preparation of sodium picosulfate plus magnesium oxide or polyethylene glycol (PEG) are very critical. Osmotically balanced PEG was introduced in 1980, and nowadays, it is the most commonly used bowel preparations [3].

Many patients reported some complaints as the bad taste and the large volumes required [4, 5]. Moreover, in some cases, nausea, cramping, and vomiting were reported. All of these side effects directly influence the adherence of the patients [6]. It was reported that the compliance rates for colonoscopy screening were only 34% [7]. In order to decrease the side effects of PEG preparation and improve its efficacy, many investigators proposed the administration of lubiprostone (LB) prior to the usage of PEG solution [8, 9].

LB is an approved medication for chronic idiopathic constipation that activates the chloride type 2 channels of the apical epithelial membrane in a selective manner to enhance chloride efflux in the intestinal lumen, thus maintaining its absorptive capacity [10]. The resulting fluid softens stool and increases intestinal transit [11]. Most patients rapidly metabolize and tolerate LB very well, as it acts locally inside the intestinal tract, and has very low systemic bioavailability [12]. In this study, we aimed to evaluate the effectiveness of administering LB in addition to a single dose of oral PEG solution in

* Correspondence: Yass.tabakh@cu.edu.eg
[1]Endemic Medicine Department, Faculty of Medicine, Cairo University, Cairo, Egypt
Full list of author information is available at the end of the article

achieving satisfactory colon cleanliness and decreasing the side effects.

Methods

Study design

A parallel group randomized control study was conducted throughout a period of 6 months (May–November 2019), recruiting a total of 100 patients who were referred to the gastrointestinal endoscopy and liver unit Kasr El Aini (GIELUKA) for colonoscopic examination. By means of block randomization, patients were assigned into either of the two study groups. The first group (control group, n=50) received the standard bowel preparation, two doses of PEG (120 mg of polyethylene glycol 3350 powder plus ascorbic acid), each dose added to 1L of water [13], while the second group (intervention group, n=50) recieved lubiprostone-based preparation, lubiprostone (LB) (24 μg) tablets twice daily for 2 days, then only a single dose PEG 12 h before the colonoscopy. Both groups received only clear fluids for 24 h prior to colonoscopy. A written informed consent was obtained from all patients included.

Inclusion and exclusion criteria

Adult patients (18–65 years) of both genders, with average bodyweight, were included. Patients with chronic diarrhea, known or suspected ileus, gastrointestinal obstruction, gastric retention (gastro-paresis), rectal impaction, toxic colitis, toxic megacolon, uncontrolled inflammatory bowel disease presenting in severe activity, or bowel perforation were excluded. Moreover, we excluded pregnant or breastfeeding females, patients with previous significant gastrointestinal surgery, patients with uncontrolled pre-existing electrolyte abnormalities, patients with a severe renal impairment, and patients who require emergency colonoscopy without bowel preparation.

Data collection

Demographic data were obtained from all included patients, followed by complete colonoscopic examination with intravenous propofol sedation. The degree of bowel preparation was evaluated according to Boston bowel preparation scale (BBPS). Moreover, patients' feedback regarding tolerability and accessibility was also assessed using the 5-point Treatment Acceptability Questionnaire.

BBPS

The main objective of this scale was to evaluate specific issues that are influencing bowel preparation quality, as described by Kastenberg et al. [1]. According to the quality of the preparation, each colonic segment is graded from 0 to 3. By adding the score for all three segments, the overall score is obtained, resulting in a score between 0 and 9. A score below 4 is considered a bad preparation, resulting in a repeat procedure recommendation. The score of 5–7 is considered to be good preparation, whereas the score of 8–9 is considered to be excellent.

Statistical analysis

With a sample size of at least 78 (39/group), we had a power of 90% to assess whether the mean Boston scale was significantly higher in the lubiprostone group (~7.25 (1)) compared to its mean value in the control group of ~6.5 (1), using a two-sample means test and a significance level of 0.05. Descriptive analysis was performed using STATA 15 and was described as mean and standard deviation (SD). Categorical variables were defined as frequency and percentage. The difference between the two groups was made using the chi-square test for categorial variables and the Student t-test for quantitative variables. p-values of less than 0.05 were considered to be significant.

Ethics and consent to participate

Being conformed to the ethical guidelines of the 1975 Declaration of Helsinki and its later amendments revised in Seoul, Korea, October 2008 as reflected in previous approval by the institution's human research committee, the study protocol was approved by the research ethical committee of the endemic medicine department and the institutional review board of the faculty of medicine, Cairo University. All patients had signed a written informed consent before the start of any procedure related to the study. The personal data were concealed and replaced by numbers for patient's confidentiality.

Results

Table 1 shows the demographic data of the included patients. In the intervention group, 42 (84%) of included patients were aged 18–30, compared to 14 (28%) in the control group (p<0.0001). Both genders were

Table 1 Demographic characteristics of the included patients

	Control (n=50)	Intervention (n=50)	p-value
Age			
18–30	14 (28%)	42 (84%)	< 0.0001
30–40	11 (22%)	6 (12%)	
40–50	14 (28%)	2 (4%)	
50–60	8 (16%)	0	
> 60	3 (6%)	0	
Gender			
Male/female	36/14	32/18	0.40
First colonoscopy	32 (64%)	41 (82%)	0.02

represented in both groups (p=0.40). This was the first colonoscopy experience for the majority of the included patients (82% of the intervention and 64% of the control groups). Regarding comorbidities, 72% of the patients did not report any comorbidities; however, 18% of patients were hypertensive, and only 4% were diabetic.

The main concerns before colonoscopy in the intervention group were purgatives (72% vs. 20%, p<0.0001), sedation (38% vs. 70%, p=0.001), and colonoscopy (80% vs. 66%, p=0.10), compared to the control group. Interestingly, 100% of the control group reported that the experienced taste was worse than expected, while in the intervention group, half of the patients (50%) said that the taste was natural and 48% experienced a taste worse than expected (p<0.0001). When the patients were asked about the amount of liquid they can consume, their answers were comparable in both groups (p=0.70). The large liquid volume and bad taste are the main parameters that discouraged patients in the control group. In the intervention group, the patients reported bad taste and diarrhea as the main parameters that discouraged them. When we asked the patients about how easy it was to consume the study preparation, we found a significant difference between both groups (p<0.0001); 80% of the control group reported difficult or very difficult, while only 12% in the intervention group chose difficult and 66% tolerable. Therefore, all patients (100%) in the control group would have used a different purgative if they had the choice, compared to 26% in the intervention group (p<0.0001), (Table 2).

Regarding the side effects of the preparation in both arms, the majority of cases in the intervention group did not complain of any side effects (78%), while the majority of the complaints were vomiting in 16% of the cases. Only 22% reported no side effects from the preparation in the control group, but 34% complained of abdominal pain and vomiting (Table 3).

With respect to BBPS, there was a significant difference in the overall Boston scale (0.02) with more efficacy in the intervention group as 66% of patients had good bowel preparation (5–7) and 24% excellent preparation (8–9). On the other hand, the overall Boston scale in the

Table 2 Patient satisfaction

Parameters		Control (n=50)	Intervention (n=50)	p-value
What concerns you most before colonoscopy	Purgative	10	36	< 0.0001
	Sedation	35	19	0.001
	Colonoscopy	33	40	0.1
I experienced the taste as	Neutral	0	25	< 0.0001
	Worse than expected	50	24	
	Better than expected	0	1	
Maximum volume of liquid you would be able to consume	0.5 L	9	6	0.7
	1 L	27	27	
	2 L	14	16	
	3 L	0	1	
	Maximum volume (L) median (IQR)	1 (1–2)	1 (1–2)	0.3
What would discourage you most	Bad taste	47	48	0.6
	Bad smell	0	2	0.1
	Too large liquid volume	31	8	< 0.0001
	Diarrhea	7	19	0.006
How easy or difficult was it to consume the study drugs	Very difficult	11	0	< 0.0001
	Difficult	29	6	
	Tolerable	9	33	
	Easy	1	11	
If I had the choice, I would for next colonoscopy	Use a different purgative	50	13	< 0.0001
	Use this purgative	0	36	
The overall experience of the preparation	Poor	26	12	< 0.0001
	Bad	12	0	
	Fair	11	15	
	Good	1	23	

Table 3 Side effects

	Control (n=50)	Intervention (n=50)	p
Experiencing side effects	39 (78%)	11 (22%)	< 0.0001
Side effects			
No	11 (22%)	39 (78%)	< 0.0001
Abdominal pain	11 (22%)	1 (2%)	
Vomiting	9 (18%)	8 (16%)	
Abdominal pain and vomiting	17 (34%)	1 (2%)	
Abdominal pain and headache	1 (2%)	0	
Abdominal pain, vomiting and headache	0	1 (2%)	

control group showed that 54% of patients were between 5 and 7, and only 16% of patients had overall Boston scale 8–9 (Table 4).

Discussion

Diagnostic accuracy and therapeutic safety in colonoscopy are significantly impacted by the quality of bowel preparation [14–17]. In this prospective comparative study, we addressed the quality of PEG preparation and patient satisfaction in both groups. Our findings demonstrated that adding LB to the preparation significantly improved the tolerability of the preparation. Additionally, it was associated with a lower incidence of adverse events, except for some cases of vomiting. In terms of efficacy, and according to the BBPS, the overall good and excellent outcomes of the intervention group were much higher than the standard group (p=0.02). These findings indicate that the addition of LB produced a better colon cleansing, especially in the right colon. In addition, the

Table 4 BBPS

	Control (n=50)	Intervention (n=50)	p
Ascending colon score			
1	25	16	0.1
2	24	32	
3	1	2	
Transverse colon score			
1	15	6	0.02
2	29	29	
3	6	15	
Descending colon score			
1	8	0	<0.0001
2	30	24	
3	12	26	
Overall Boston scale			
< 4	15	4	0.02
5–7	27	33	
8–9	8	12	

reduced need to repeat procedures in the LB group showed the significant impact of LB in the bowel preparation regimens.

Previous studies reported a success rate of PEG-based preparations of 56 to 76% for bowel cleansing. In our study, bowel preparation with the addition of LB has been effective in up to 90% of participants [18]. The rapid and enhanced colonic passage time with LB, together with the enhanced duration of bowel movement, may have contributed to the efficacy [19]. At present, the greatest obstacle for patient tolerance and adherence is the large volume of PEG-based preparation and the associated distension, fever, nausea, and vomiting. Small volume PEG preparations provide an effective alternative to regular volume preparations to decrease bowel preparation pain and inconvenience [8].

Banerjee and colleagues evaluated the adequacy and efficacy of LB and PEG as a colonoscopy preparation. They found that excellent preparation was observed in 66.5% in the LB group and 38% in the standard group (p<0.01), according to the BBPS scale [8]. Stengel and Jones assessed the tolerability, safety, and efficacy of LB prior to a single dose of PEG preparation without dietary restriction. They found that the addition of LB enhanced the colon cleansing in the whole colon. They showed that the total procedure time and abdominal bloating were significantly decreased in the LB group compared to the second group. However, they could not find any significant reduction in nausea in both groups [9].

Split dosing to improve patient tolerance has been recommended [20, 21]. However, Ell et al. have demonstrated in the meta-analysis that more than 70% of the patients had only a single intake of dosing [22]. Therefore, the timing of the intake can be decided based on the convenience of the patient. Our findings appear similar. Furthermore, our study is noteworthy because we included all patients referred for colonoscopy and not only colorectal cancer screens. There have been no dietary restrictions.

This is the first study in Egypt to show that even lower doses of PEG will contribute to sufficient bowel cleaning by incorporating LB. The usage of a more practical single-day PEG regimen will certainly boost patient adherence in future with the CRC screening guidelines. In fact, a preparation for a better colonoscopy was recently recommended on that same day.

The present study has some limitations, as it is a single-center study where only outpatients were recruited. Compliance and the outcomes could be enhanced by fairly mobile patients with a clear clarification of the planning procedures prior to the treatment. Moreover, the lesion abnormality rate was not assessed. It was not possible for us to speculate on the relationship between enhanced bowel preparation and an improved adenoma detection rate. In earlier studies, however, improved BBPS scores were associated with increased polyp detection rate.

The incidence and mortality of colorectal cancer decreased by diagnostic colonoscopies with exclusion samples of adenomatous polyps. However, patient compliance and tolerability have been significantly impacted by the obstacles of a large volume bowel preparation and the pre-procedure dietary restrictions. Our study demonstrated that LB pre-treatment 2 days before colonoscopy would enhance bowel cleansing with a substantially reduced rate of repeat procedures. Even lower doses of PEG could be used without any effect on the overall preparation quality.

Conclusion

The current study shows a strong evidence that using lubiprostone is effective for sufficient bowel cleansing prior to colonoscopy, in comparison to the standard of care PEG preparation. Lubiprostone usage allowed reducing the volume of PEG solution needed during colon preparation which resulted in better patient satisfaction and tolerability of the preparation, while maintaining equivalent colon cleanliness results. Applying the same preparation strategy to a larger number of patients would allow better evaluation of the adenoma detection rate.

Abbreviations

PEG: Polyethylene glycol; LB: Lubiprostone; GIELUKA: Gastrointestinal endoscopy and liver unit Kasr El Aini; BBPS: Boston bowel preparation scale; SD: Standard deviation; BMI: Body mass index

Acknowledgements

For the patients and the authors for completing the study and manuscript

Authors' contributions

All listed authors have read and approved the manuscript. Y H: planning the study, colonoscopy of the studied patients, manuscript writing and editing. I E: patient recruitment and data analysis. R M: preparation of the manuscript and statistical analysis. H EG: revising and finalizing the manuscript

Declarations

Ethics approval and consent to participate

Being conformed to the ethical guidelines, the study protocol was approved by the research ethical committee of the endemic medicine department and the institutional review board of the faculty of medicine, Cairo University. All patients had signed a written informed consent before the start of any procedure related to the study. The personal data were concealed and replaced by numbers for patient's confidentiality.

Competing interests

The authors declare that they have no competing interest.

Author details

[1]Endemic Medicine Department, Faculty of Medicine, Cairo University, Cairo, Egypt. [2]Student Hospital, Cairo University Hospitals, Cairo, Egypt.

References

1. Kastenberg D, Bertiger G, Brogadir S (2018) Bowel preparation quality scales for colonoscopy. World J Gastroenterol 24(26):2833–2843. https://doi.org/10.3748/wjg.v24.i26.2833
2. Rex DK, Schoenfeld PS, Cohen J, Pike IM, Adler DG, Fennerty MB, Lieb JG II, Park WG, Rizk MK, Sawhney MS, Shaheen NJ, Wani S, Weinberg DS (2015) Quality indicators for colonoscopy. Gastrointest Endosc 81(1):31–53. https://doi.org/10.1016/j.gie.2014.07.058
3. Franco DL, Leighton JA, Gurudu SR (2017) Approach to incomplete colonoscopy: new techniques and technologies. Gastroenterol Hepatol (N Y) 13(8):476–483
4. Lee KJ, Park HJ, Kim HS, Baik KH, Kim YS, Park SC, Seo HI (2015) Electrolyte changes after bowel preparation for colonoscopy: a randomized controlled multicenter trial. World J Gastroenterol 21(10):3041–3048. https://doi.org/10.3748/wjg.v21.i10.3041
5. Adamcewicz M, Bearelly D, Porat G, Friedenberg FK (2011) Mechanism of action and toxicities of purgatives used for colonoscopy preparation. Expert Opin Drug Metab Toxicol 7(1):89–101. https://doi.org/10.1517/17425255.2011.542411
6. Kang SH, Jeen YT, Lee JH, Yoo IK, Lee JM, Kim SH, Choi HS, Kim ES, Keum B, Lee HS, Chun HJ, Kim CD (2017) Comparison of a split-dose bowel preparation with 2 liters of polyethylene glycol plus ascorbic acid and 1 liter of polyethylene glycol plus ascorbic acid and bisacodyl before colonoscopy. Gastrointest Endosc 86(2):343–348. https://doi.org/10.1016/j.gie.2016.10.040
7. Kherad O, Restellini S, Martel M, Barkun AN (2015) Polyethylene glycol versus sodium picosulfalte bowel preparation in the setting of a colorectal cancer screening program. Can J Gastroenterol Hepatol 29(7):384–390. https://doi.org/10.1155/2015/350587
8. Banerjee R, Chaudhari H, Shah N, Saravanan A, Tandan M, Reddy DN (2016) Addition of lubiprostone to polyethylene glycol (PEG) enhances the quality & efficacy of colonoscopy preparation: a randomized, double-blind, placebo controlled trial. BMC Gastroenterol 16(1):133. Published 2016 Oct 13. https://doi.org/10.1186/s12876-016-0542-0
9. Stengel JZ, Jones DP (2008) Single-dose lubiprostone along with split-dose PEG solution without dietary restrictions for bowel cleansing prior to colonoscopy: a randomized, double-blind, placebo-controlled trial. Am J Gastroenterol 103(9):2224–2230. https://doi.org/10.1111/j.1572-0241.2008.02053.x
10. Wilson N, Schey R (2015) Lubiprostone in constipation: clinical evidence and place in therapy. Ther Adv Chronic Dis 6(2):40–50. https://doi.org/10.1177/2040622314567678
11. Bijvelds MJC, Bot AG, Escher JC, de Jonge HR (2009) Activation of intestinal Cl- secretion by lubiprostone requires the cystic fibrosis transmembrane conductance regulator. Gastroenterology 137(3):976–985 Available from: https://doi.org/10.1053/j.gastro.2009.05.037

12. McKeage K, Plosker GL, Siddiqui MA (2006) Lubiprostone. Drugs 66(6):873–879. https://doi.org/10.2165/00003495-200666060-00015
13. ASGE Standards of Practice Committee, Saltzman JR, Cash BD, Pasha SF, Early DS, Muthusamy VR, Khashab MA, Chathadi KV, Fanelli RD, Chandrasekhara V, Lightdale JR, Fonkalsrud L, Shergill AK, Hwang JH, Decker GA, Jue TL, Sharaf R, Fisher DA, Evans JA, Foley K, Shaukat A, Eloubeidi MA, Faulx AL, Wang A, Acosta RD (2015) Bowel preparation before colonoscopy. Gastrointest Endosc 81(4):781–794. https://doi.org/10.1016/j.gie.2014.09.048
14. Harewood GC, Sharma VK, de Garmo P (2003) Impact of colonoscopy preparation quality on detection of suspected colonic neoplasia. Gastrointest Endosc 58(1):76–79. https://doi.org/10.1067/mge.2003.294
15. Froehlich F, Wietlisbach V, Gonvers JJ, Burnand B, Vader JP (2005) Impact of colonic cleansing on quality and diagnostic yield of colonoscopy: the European Panel of Appropriateness of Gastrointestinal Endoscopy European multicenter study. Gastrointest Endosc 61(3):378–384. https://doi.org/10.1016/S0016-5107(04)02776-2
16. Chokshi RV, Hovis CE, Hollander T, Early DS, Wang JS (2012) Prevalence of missed adenomas in patients with inadequate bowel preparation on screening colonoscopy. Gastrointest Endosc 75(6):1197–1203. https://doi.org/10.1016/j.gie.2012.01.005
17. Lebwohl B, Kastrinos F, Glick M, Rosenbaum AJ, Wang T, Neugut AI (2011) The impact of suboptimal bowel preparation on adenoma miss rates and the factors associated with early repeat colonoscopy. Gastrointest Endosc 73(6):1207–1214. https://doi.org/10.1016/j.gie.2011.01.051
18. Rostom A, Jolicoeur E (2004) Validation of a new scale for the assessment of bowel preparation quality. Gastrointest Endosc 59(4):482–486. https://doi.org/10.1016/S0016-5107(03)02875-X
19. Aoun E, Abdul-Baki H, Azar C, Mourad F, Barada K, Berro Z, Tarchichi M, Sharara AI (2005) A randomized single-blind trial of split-dose PEG-electrolyte solution without dietary restriction compared with whole dose PEG-electrolyte solution with dietary restriction for colonoscopy preparation. Gastrointest Endosc 62(2):213–218. https://doi.org/10.1016/S0016-5107(05)00371-8
20. Enestvedt BK, Tofani C, Laine LA, Tierney A, Fennerty MB (2012) 4-Liter split-dose polyethylene glycol is superior to other bowel preparations, based on systematic review and meta-analysis. Clin Gastroenterol Hepatol 10(11):1225–1231. https://doi.org/10.1016/j.cgh.2012.08.029
21. Park SS, Sinn DH, Kim YH, Lim YJ, Sun Y, Lee JH, Kim JY, Chang DK, Son HJ, Rhee PL, Rhee JC. Kim JJ (2010) Efficacy and tolerability of split-dose magnesium citrate: low volume (2 liters) polyethylene glycol vs. single-or split-dose polyethylene glycol bowel preparation for morning colonoscopy. Am J Gastroenterol 105(6):1319–1326. https://doi.org/10.1038/ajg.2010.79
22. Ell C, Bitoun A, Goerg K, Halphen M, Gruss H-J (2005) Meta-analysis to assess the influence of two different schedules of intake on the efficacy, acceptability and safety of a new 2 litre PEG + E gut cleansing solution. Gastrointest Endosc 61:AB151

22

Five-day outcome of hepatitis E-induced acute liver failure in the ICU

Debashis Chowdhury[1*], Farhana Mahmood[2], Cathryn Edwards[3] and Simon D. Taylor-Robinson[4]

Abstract

Background: Hepatitis E virus (HEV) is an important cause of acute liver failure (ALF) in Bangladesh with pregnant mothers being more vulnerable. As HEV occurs in epidemics, it limits medical capabilities in this resource-poor country. Cerebral oedema, resulting in raised intracranial pressure (ICP), is an important cause of morbidity and mortality. Practical treatments are currently few.

- To study the baseline characteristics and clinical outcome of HEV-induced ALF in a recent HEV epidemic
- To detect raised ICP clinically and observe response to mannitol infusion.

This was a prospective cohort study from June until August 2018 of 20 patients admitted to the intensive care unit (ICU) of a major Bangladeshi Referral Hospital with HEV-induced ALF. We diagnosed HEV infection by detecting serum anti-HEV IgM antibody. All were negative for hepatitis B surface antigen and hepatitis A IgM antibody. Data were collected on 5-day outcome after admission to ICU, monitoring all patients for signs of raised ICP. An intravenous bolus of 20% mannitol was administered at a single time point to patients with raised ICP.

Results: Twenty patients were included in the study. Ten (50%) patients, seven (70%) females, received mannitol infusion. HE worsened in eight (40%): seven female and three pregnant. Glasgow Coma scores deteriorated in six (30%): all (100%) females and three pregnant. Consciousness status was not significantly different between pregnant and non-pregnant subjects, nor between those who received mannitol and those who did not. Six patients met King's College Criteria for liver transplantation.

Conclusions: Female patients had a worse outcome, but pregnancy status was not an additional risk factor in our cohort. Mannitol infusion was also not associated with a significant difference in outcome.

Keywords: Hepatitis E, Acute liver failure, Intensive care unit, Hepatic encephalopathy, Mannitol

Background

Every year, more than 20 million people contract hepatitis E virus (HEV) infection, and among them, more than 70, 000 die from its complications, including acute liver failure (ALF) [1]. Most of these deaths occur in Asia, Africa and Latin America, where contaminated water from flooding of low-lying areas gives rise to epidemic of HEV infection almost every year [2].

HEV infection is common in Bangladesh; Sheikh and colleagues found IgM antibodies against HEV in 63.6% of patients with ALF, 83.3% of HBV carriers and in 7.3% of apparently healthy persons in their study [3]. According to another Bangladeshi study, in an epidemic of HEV infection, which affected more than 4000 people, most deaths occurred in pregnant women [4]. Moreover, women were more likely to die from the illness than male subjects. In a different study, HEV-induced ALF was found to result in mortality in more than 75% of subjects in their second and the third trimester of pregnancy in Bangladesh [5].

* Correspondence: debashis712003@yahoo.com
[1]Department of Gastroenterology and Hepatology, Chattogram Maa O Shishu Hospital (CMOSH) Medical College, Chattogram, Bangladesh
Full list of author information is available at the end of the article

Studies in Bangladesh and India have demonstrated that cerebral oedema resulting in raised intracranial pressure (ICP) is an important cause of morbidity and mortality in HEV-induced ALF [6–8]. Mannitol infusion is often chosen as the first option [9–11] followed by hypertonic saline and moderate hypothermia to manage raised ICP in ALF patients [12, 13]. Barbiturates, indomethacin and hyperventilation were also used as short-term salvage therapies in some refractory cases [10, 11, 14]. Mannitol acts by changing the viscoelasticity of blood and drawing fluid along an osmotic gradient from brain to blood [15]. A previous study [16] suggested that infusion of mannitol could reduce the water content and volume of normal brain tissue. However, mannitol cannot act once brain tissue is permanently damaged. Canalese and colleagues in a controlled trial demonstrated that mannitol can both decrease the raised ICP level and improve survival in ALF patients [9].

Acharya and co-workers in India found that outcome of ALF in pregnant subjects was similar to that in non-pregnant subjects, and one-third of ALF patients in their study survived with aggressive conservative management [6]. The authors also observed that two-thirds of deaths due to ALF occurred within 72 h of hospital admission. Shalimar and colleagues in their study observed that the model for end-stage liver disease (MELD), ALF study group model, and King's College Hospital criteria failed to predict outcome in HEV-induced ALF [8].

We did this study during an HEV epidemic in a major Bangladesh referral centre to audit treatment given to patients with HEV-induced ALF and to assess the effectiveness of intensive care support in the epidemic. We did this by using the clinical tools available in this resource-poor country:

- Examining the baseline characteristics and clinical outcome of HEV-induced ALF at 5 days
- Detecting raised ICP clinically and observing response to mannitol infusion, a key treatment given for HEV-associated cerebral oedema in Bangladeshi patients with ALF

Methods

This was a prospective cohort study on baseline characteristics and clinical outcomes of 20 patients admitted to the intensive care unit (ICU) of Chattogram Maa-O-Shishu Hospital (CMOSH) in Chattogram (Chittagong), Bangladesh, with hepatitis E-induced ALF during an epidemic from June 2018 until August 2018 [17].

ALF was diagnosed by clinical detection of encephalopathy and raised INR within 24 weeks of development of jaundice [18, 19]. ALF was diagnosed by increased INR with or without hepatic encephalopathy (HE). We took a history of onset, duration and clinical features from family members of subjects and consent from the next of kin before enrolment in the study.

HE grade was defined by West Haven Criteria as follows: grade 1, any alteration in mentation; grade 2, somnolent or obtunded, but easily rousable or presence of asterixis; grade 3, rousable with difficulty; and grade 4, unresponsive to deep pain [20, 21].

We diagnosed HEV by serum anti-HEV IgM antibody [22, 23]. All patients tested negative for hepatitis B surface antigen (HBsAg) and hepatitis A (anti-HAV) IgM antibody. Other causes of acute liver failure were excluded.

We selectively intubated subjects with Glasgow Coma Scale (GCS) ≤8 and/or respiratory acidosis in the setting of severe HE (encephalopathy grade ≥ 3) [24].

We collected data regarding treatment, monitoring and hemodynamic and laboratory values daily for the first 5 days after admission to ICU. We monitored all patients for oxygenation, vital signs and raised ICP. A diagnosis of raised ICP was made when neurological examination revealed either decerebrate posture or two of the following four criteria: (1) hypertension (supine blood pressure > 150/90 mmHg), (2) bradycardia (pulse rate < 10/min for the expected pulse rate for the given body temperature), (3) pupillary changes and (4) neurogenic hyperventilation (hyperventilation in the absence of metabolic or respiratory cause) [25].

We infused an intravenous bolus of 20% mannitol in ten patients with a clinical diagnosis of raised ICP. We corrected any metabolic derangement before mannitol infusion, and all patients received standard anti-coma and supportive measures [14, 26]. Only single infusions of mannitol were administered to those requiring treatment—the dose was not repeated in any patient at any time point.

We performed statistical analysis using the STATA software, version 13 (StataCorp, College Station, TX, USA), expressing continuous variables as mean, standard error, and confidence intervals, with categorical variables as frequencies and percentages. We compared continuous data using two-sample Wilcoxon rank-sum (Mann-Whitney) test and categorical data using Fisher's exact test. A p value of <0.05 was considered significant. We defined outcomes as HE deterioration and deterioration of GCS after 5-day stay in the ICU.

Results

A total of 20 subjects were included in the study. Table 1 shows the demographic and biochemical characteristics of our subjects. Figures 1 and 2 show HE grades from day 1 to day 5 and GCS scores from day 1 to day 5, respectively. Figure 3 shows a flow chart of the patient journey.

HE worsened in eight subjects (40%); seven among them (87.5%) were female, and of these, three (37.5%)

Table 1 Demographic and biochemical characteristics

Variable	Mean	Standard error	[95% Conf. Interval]	
Age (years)	36.7	3.23	29.92	43.48
Serum Bilirubin mg/dL	10.87	1.04	8.69	13.06
Serum ALT Units/L	1528	210	1087	1970
MELD Score	29.95	2.39	24.95	34.95
INR on Day 1	2.83	0.40	1.98	3.68
INR on Day 2	3.02	0.47	2.04	3.99
INR on Day 3	2.89	0.43	1.98	3.80
INR on Day 4	2.81	0.42	1.92	3.71
INR on Day 5	3.01	0.44	2.07	3.94
Serum Creatinine On Day 1 (mg/dL)	2.45	0.52	1.37	3.53
Serum Creatinine On Day 2 (mg/dL)	2.49	0.49	1.46	3.51
Serum Creatinine On Day 3 (mg/dL)	2.64	0.55	1.48	3.80
Serum Creatinine On Day 4 (mg/dL)	2.28	0.46	1.31	3.25
Serum Creatinine On Day 5 (mg/dL)	2.36	0.46	1.38	3.35

were pregnant individuals. GCS deteriorated in six (30%); of these, all (100%) were females, and of those, three (50%) were pregnant.

The majority (75%) among our subjects were female. Seven (46.67%) out of 15 females and one (20%) out of five male subjects developed HE deterioration. HE deterioration was not significantly different between male and female subjects (Fisher's exact=0.603).

Six (40%) out of 15 female subjects and none (0%) out of five male subjects developed deterioration of GCS. Deterioration of GCS was not significantly different between male and female subjects (Fisher's exact = 0.260).

Seven (35%) out of 20 subjects were pregnant. Three (42.86%) out of seven pregnant subjects and five (38.46%) out of 13 non-pregnant subjects developed HE deterioration. HE deterioration was not statistically significantly different between pregnant and non-pregnant subjects (Fisher's exact=1.000). Three (42.86%) out of seven pregnant subjects and three (23.08%) out of 13 non-pregnant subjects developed deterioration of GCS. Deterioration of GCS grades was not significantly different between pregnant and not pregnant individuals (Fisher's exact=0.613).

Six (30%) out of 20 subjects met King's College Criteria for liver transplantation. Six (40%) out of 15 female and none (0%) out of five male subjects met King's College Criteria for liver transplantation (p= 0.260). Three (42.86%) out of seven pregnant subjects and three (23.08%) out of 13 non-pregnant subjects met King's College Criteria for liver transplantation (Fisher's exact = 0.613). Four (66.67%) among these six subjects developed HE deterioration (p=0.018), and five (83.33%) developed deterioration of GCS (Fisher's exact=0.002).

One subject, a female, 30 years old, pregnant, serum bilirubin 17 mg/dL, ALT 3120 units/L, MELD score 45, HE grade IV, GCS <8, INR 4.12 and creatinine 5.1 mg/dL, died on the third day in the ICU.

Mannitol infusion requirements

Ten (50%) out of 20 subjects received mannitol infusion. Two patients (both female and one being pregnant) with raised ICP could not be given mannitol infusion because of renal impairment (serum creatinine more than 4.5 mg/dL). Seven (46.67%) out of 15 female and three (60%) out of five male subjects received a mannitol infusion. Three (42.86%) out of seven pregnant subjects received a mannitol infusion.

HE deteriorated in 2 (10%) out of 10 patients who received and 6 (30%) out of 10 patients who did not receive mannitol. HE deterioration was not significantly different between patients who received and those who did not receive mannitol (1-sided Fisher's exact = 0.085).

GCS deteriorated in 1 (5%) out of 10 patients that received a mannitol infusion and 5 (25%) out of 10 patients who did not receive a mannitol infusion. Deterioration of GCS was also not significantly different between subjects who received mannitol and those who did not receive mannitol (1-sided Fisher's exact = 0.070).

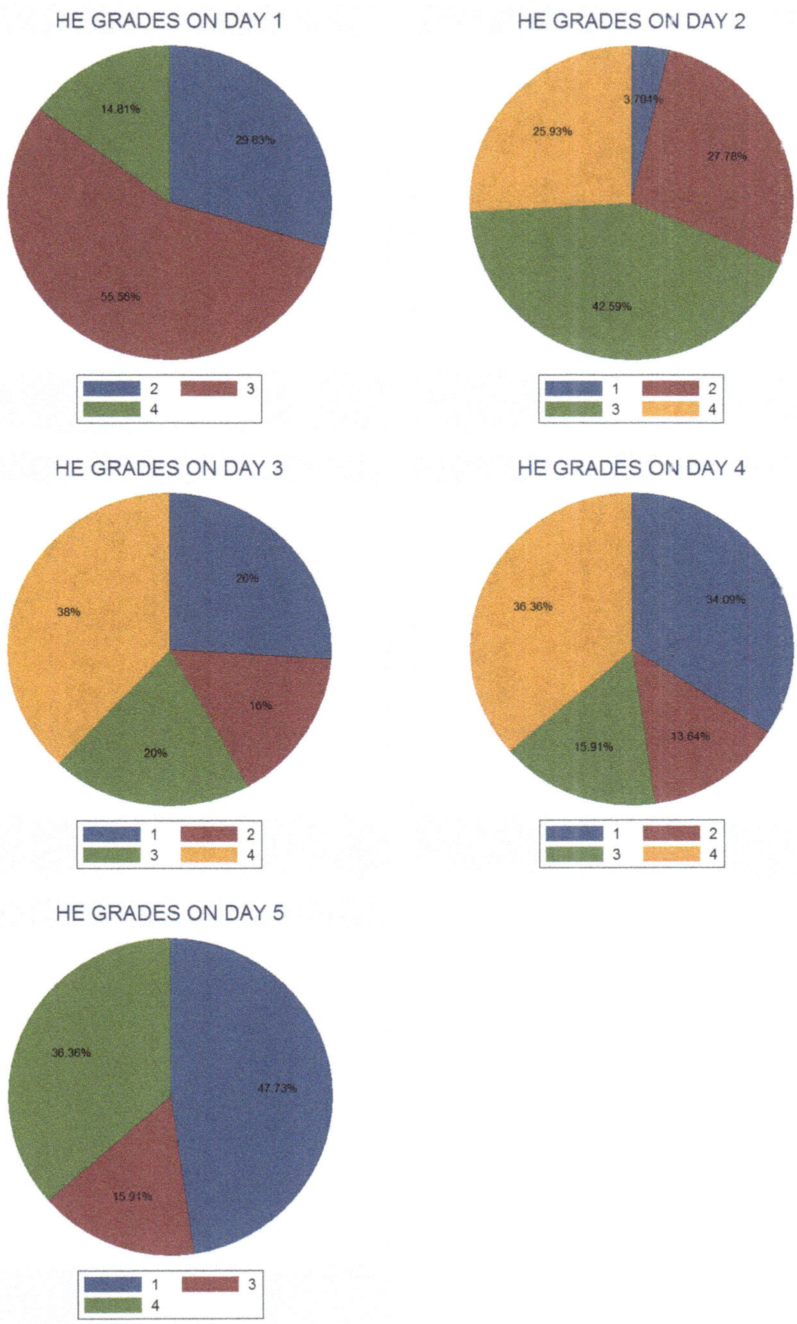

Fig. 1 Hepatic encephalopathy grades from day 1 to day 5

Mechanical ventilation requirement

Seven (35%) out of 20 subjects: three out of five males, four out of 15 females and of these, two out of seven pregnant subjects, received mechanical ventilation on day 1. Nine (55%) out of 20 subjects: three out of five males and six out of 15 females and out of these, three out of seven pregnant subjects, received mechanical ventilation on day 2. On day 3, nine out of 19 subjects: two out of four male subjects and seven out of 15 female subjects and of these, three out of seven pregnant subjects, received mechanical ventilation. On day 4, seven out of 17 subjects: two out of four male subjects and five out of 13 female subjects and of these, one out of five pregnant subjects, were ventilated. On day 5, seven out

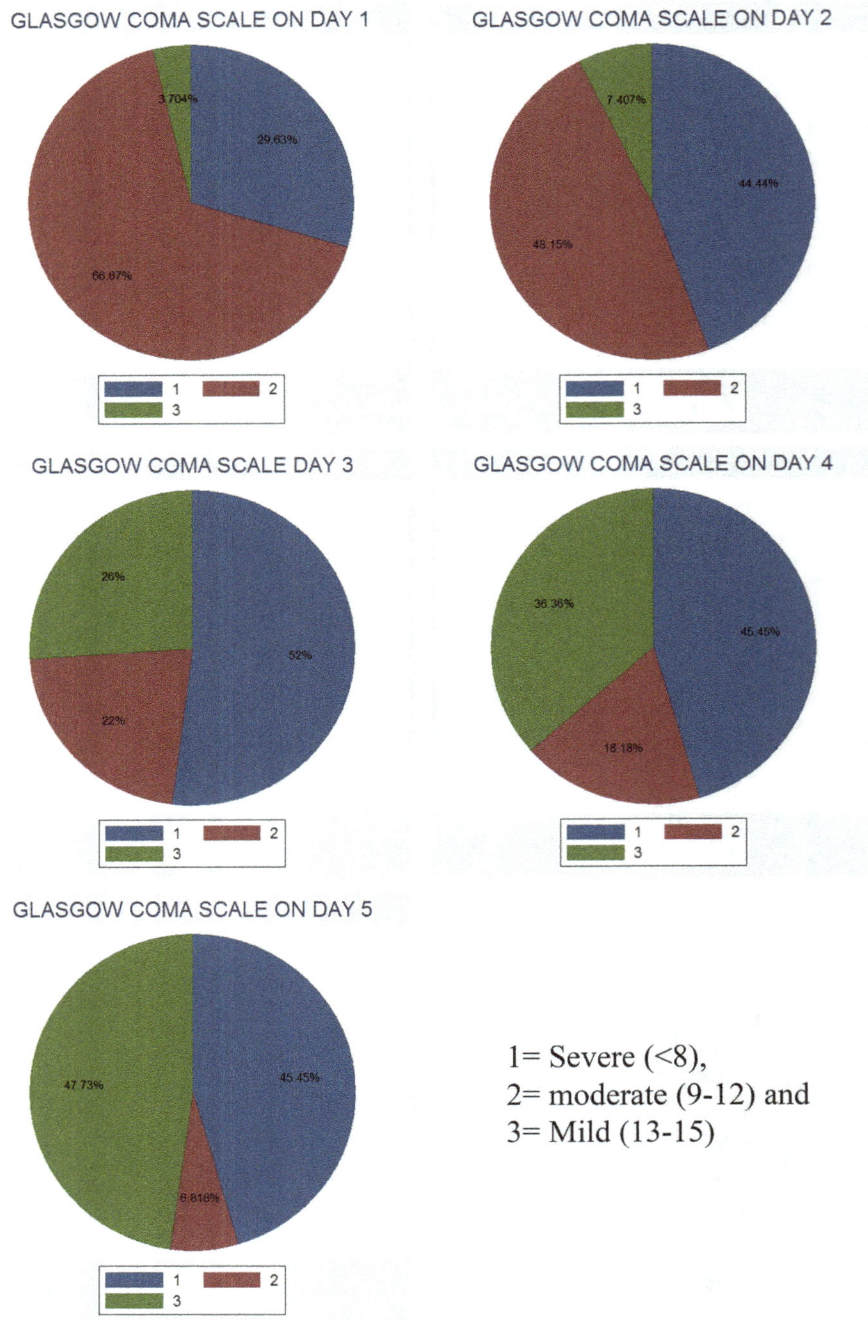

Fig. 2 Glasgow Coma Scale from day 1 to day 5

of 17 subjects: two out of four male subjects and five out of 13 female subjects and of these, one out of five pregnant patients, were ventilated.

Vasopressor requirements

From day 1 to day 3, a total of seven (2 males, 5 females and of these, 2 pregnant) subjects received vasopressor support. On day 4 and day 5, six (2 males, 4 females and of these, 1 pregnant) subjects received vasopressor support.

Haemodialysis requirements

Haemodialysis was started when subjects developed renal failure (urine output less than 300 mL/day; serum creatinine more than 400 micromol/L (4.52 mg/dL) with a normal central venous pressure: two subjects—a

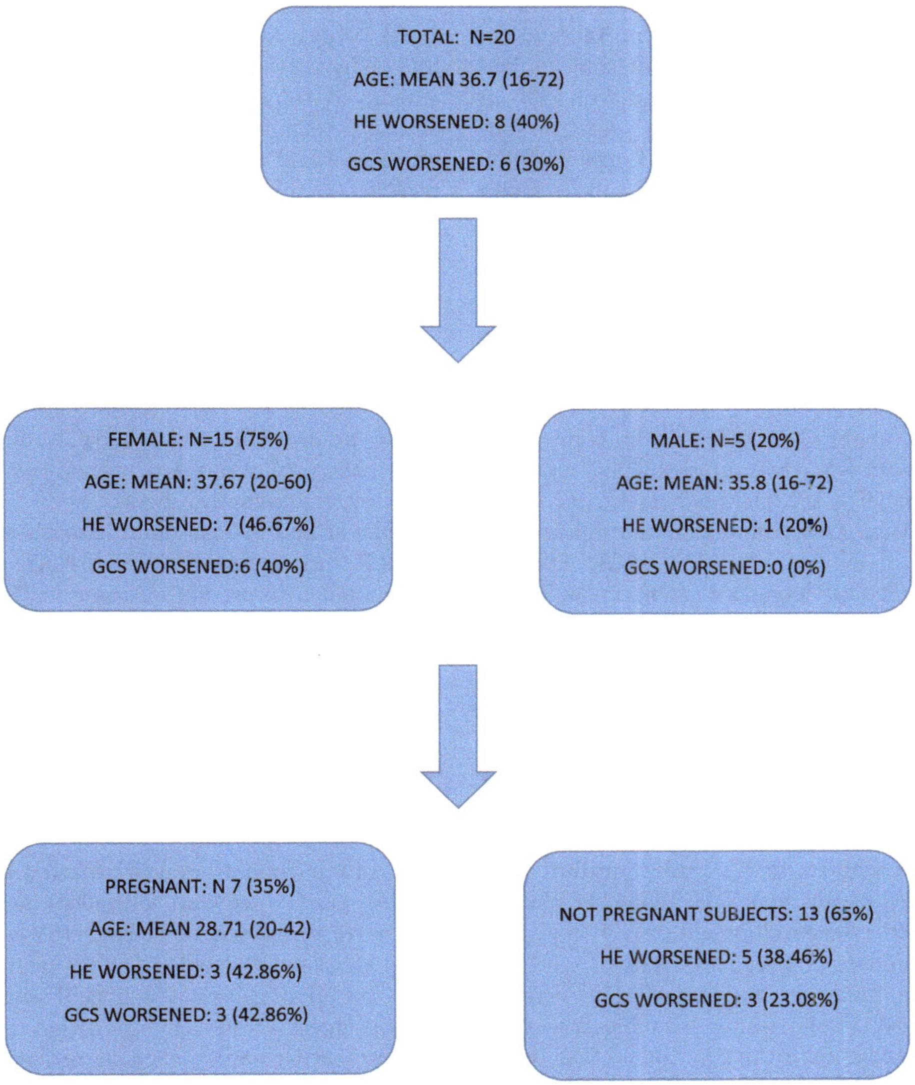

Fig. 3 Flow chart of the patient journey

female, 22 years (creatinine 8.2 mg/dL), second, a female, 60 years (serum creatinine 7.1 mg/dL)). Both received haemodialysis for 5 days in ICU.

Discussion

This study reports the acute outcomes in a typical resource-poor setting in Bangladesh. The majority (75%) of subjects were female. Seven (35%) patients in our study were pregnant. Three (42.86%) out of 7 pregnant subjects and 3 (23.08%) out of 13 non-pregnant subjects had worsening of HE. Deterioration of HE was not statistically significantly different between pregnant and non-pregnant subjects (Fisher's exact = 1.000).

In a previous study on this HEV epidemic in Chattogram (Chittagong), Bangladesh, we found that among 230 of our patients 24 (10.4%) had developed ALF. Four (1.8%) among them died due to multiorgan failure with acute kidney injury, and all were pregnant [17].

Other studies in Bangladesh also found that women, especially pregnant women, were more susceptible to HEV-induced ALF and had worse outcome when they developed ALF [4, 5]. Moreover, in another Bangladeshi study, the authors observed that mortality approached 75% when women in the second and third trimester of pregnancy developed HEV-induced ALF [5].

In prospective studies comparing HEV hepatitis and non-HEV hepatitis in India, the authors observed that 55–70% of pregnant subjects with HEV hepatitis and 10–20% of pregnant subjects with non-HEV hepatitis developed liver failure [27, 28]. Furthermore, a study in China also found that 15–60% of the pregnant subjects with acute HEV hepatitis developed ALF [29].

On the other hand, in a study in India, which included 20 years' data from a single tertiary centre, the authors observed that pregnant and non-pregnant subjects had equal chances of developing HEV-induced ALF [30]. In that study, which compared 249 (38.5%) pregnant subjects with 341 non-pregnant women and girls and 425 men and boys, aged 15 to 45 years, the authors found that the mortality rate of pregnant women and girls (53.8%) was similar to age-matched non-pregnant women and girls (57.2%), men and boys (57.9%) (P = 0.572). The authors also observed that the clinical and biochemical profile, disease intensity and sequelae were also comparable in those three study groups. Although a significantly higher percentage of ALF was attributable to HEV among pregnant subjects (59.4%) in comparison to both non-pregnant women and girls (30.4%) and men and boys (23.1%), ($P < 0.001$), the outcome of HEV-induced ALF had no association with the gender and pregnancy status of the subjects (P = 0.103). Furthermore, the mortality of pregnant subjects in HEV-induced ALF of 51% (74/145) and non-HEV-induced ALF of 54.7% (52/95) was not significant ($P > 0.1$). In addition, the authors also found that the outcome in HEV-induced ALF in pregnant subjects was not associated with the trimester of pregnancy.

Shalimar and colleagues in their study observed that the increased HEV-induced ALF and resulting mortality might be due to the increased susceptibility of women, especially pregnant women, to HEV infection during an epidemic in affected populations [31]. Moreover, the authors found that after the development of ALF, the prognosis was not dependent on pregnancy status.

According to a study in Bangladesh [7], cerebral oedema found in 48 (71.6%) among 67 subjects was the most important cause of death in the ALF patients. Acharya and co-workers in a study in India [25], which included 423 consecutive patients with ALF due to hepatotropic viruses (predominantly non-A, non-B), found that the presence of cerebral oedema was an independent predictor of adverse outcome.

We found that 12 (60%) among our 20 subjects showed clinical features of raised ICP. Ten (50%) subjects received mannitol infusion. HE deteriorated in two (10%) out of 10 subjects who received mannitol and 6 (30%) out of 10 subjects who did not receive mannitol. GCS deteriorated in one (5%) out of 10 subjects who received and 5 (25%) out of 10 subjects who did not receive mannitol. Although the outcome was not found to be statistically significant for either HE worsening (p= 0.085) or GCS deterioration (p= 0.070), the reason for this can be explained by the small sample size of the study.

Canalese and co-workers compared the effects of prophylactic dexamethasone and mannitol infusion to revert cerebral oedema in subjects with ALF with HE grade IV in a randomised controlled clinical trial. Cerebral oedema resolved significantly more frequently in 17 among 34 subjects who received mannitol and in 17 among 34 subjects who did not (p<0001) [9]. Survival was also found to be significantly better in subjects that received mannitol (p 0.008).

Acharya and colleagues [6] in India found that outcome of ALF in pregnant subjects was similar to that in non-pregnant subjects and one-third of ALF patients survived with aggressive conservative therapy. Our study also found that the outcome in pregnant and non-pregnant subject was not statistically significantly different. Moreover, HE worsened in 8 (40%) and GCS deteriorated in 6 (30%) of our subjects during the 5 days. More than 60% of our patients showed clinical improvement with conservative therapy.

Shalimar and his colleagues also observed that MELD, an ALF study group model, and King's College Hospital criteria failed to predict outcome in HEV-induced ALF. In our study, six patients (30%) met King's College Criteria for liver transplantation. Four (66.67%) among those 6 patients developed deterioration of their encephalopathy grades (Fisher's exact =0.018), and 5 (83.33%) developed deterioration of GCS (Fisher's exact=0.002) [8].

Limitations of our study

Most of our patients were transferred from different inpatient units—medicine, obstetrics and surgery when they were diagnosed as having HEV-induced ALF. We could not take a detailed history from the patients or look for other causes which could have modified the clinical illness in our subjects owing to cerebral obtundation. Furthermore, we could not test for HEV RNA and detect the HEV genotype in our subjects, owing to resource issues.

Moreover, we diagnosed raised ICP, based on clinical parameters, which may not be optimum in some cases, again owing to lack of resources. The sensitivity and specificity of clinical parameters for the diagnosis of raised ICP in the settings of ALF are low. Neurological examination and clinically establishing raised ICP in these patients can be challenging [24].

Conclusion

Most of our patients were female, and many among them were pregnant. Female patients developed worse outcome than male patients. Pregnancy status was not associated with worse outcome in our cohort. More than 50% of our subjects had cerebral oedema, as evidenced by clinical signs of raised ICP. Mannitol infusion, although not found to be statistically significant, was observed to improve outcome in them. Future directions should be early detection of cerebral oedema using more sophisticated imaging techniques and management of cerebral oedema using new therapeutic agents. Finally, HEV infection is common in Bangladesh, and HEV epidemics can result in significant morbidity and mortality in vulnerable populations, which include women and especially pregnant women. Aggressive conservative management with proper ICU protocols of HEV-induced ALF may save many lives.

Abbreviations

ALF: Acute liver failure; CMOSH: Chattogram Maa O Shishu Hospital; GCS: Glasgow Coma Scale; HE: Hepatic encephalopathy; HEV: Hepatitis E virus; ICP: Intracranial pressure; ICU: Intensive care unit; IRB: Institutional Review Board

Acknowledgements

All authors are grateful to CMOSH Medical college authority and ICU staff for their cooperation. CE is grateful to the British Society of Gastroenterology and the Bangladesh Gastroenterology Society for underpinning this UK-Bangladesh collaboration.

Authors' contributions

All authors contributed to the design of the study, data interpretation, manuscript preparation and manuscript editing. DC and FM were involved with data collection and data analysis. All authors have read and approved the final manuscript.

Declarations

Ethics approval and consent to participate

The study received local Institutional Review Board (IRB) ethics approval from the Medical Ethics Review Board in CMOSH Medical College, Chattogram, Bangladesh (ethics approval number: CMOSH 279-19). The outlined study conformed to the guidelines set out by the 1975 Declaration of Helsinki on Human Rights with participants providing informed, written consent. We took a short history of the onset, duration and clinical features including from the family members of the subjects and their next of kin, who also provided written, informed consent before patient enrolment in the study.

Competing interests

The authors declare that they have no competing interests.

Author details

[1]Department of Gastroenterology and Hepatology, Chattogram Maa O Shishu Hospital (CMOSH) Medical College, Chattogram, Bangladesh. [2]Department of Medicine, Chattogram Maa O Shishu Hospital (CMOSH) Medical College, Chattogram, Bangladesh. [3]Office of the President, British Society of Gastroenterology, St Andrew's Place, London, UK. [4]Department of Surgery and Cancer, Imperial College London, St Mary's Hospital Campus, London, UK.

References

1. Rein DB, Stevens GA, Theaker J, Wittenborn JS, Wiersma ST (2012) The global burden of hepatitis E virus genotypes 1 and 2 in 2005. Hepatology 55(4):988–997. https://doi.org/10.1002/hep.25505
2. Teshale EH, Hu DJ, Holmberg SD (2010) The two faces of hepatitis E virus. Clin Infect Dis 51:328–334. https://doi.org/10.1086/653943
3. Sheikh A, Sugitani M, Kinukawa N, Moriyama M, Arakawa Y, Komiyama K et al (2002) Hepatitis E virus infection in fulminant hepatitis patients and an apparently healthy population in Bangladesh. Am J Trop Med Hyg 66:721–724. https://doi.org/10.4269/ajtmh.2002.66.721
4. Gurley ES, Hossain MJ, Paul RC, Sazzad HMS, Islam MS, Parveen S et al (2014) Outbreak of hepatitis E in urban Bangladesh resulting in maternal and perinatal mortality. Clin Infect Dis 59(5):658–665. https://doi.org/10.1093/cid/ciu383
5. Krawczynski K, Hepatitis E (1993) Hepatitis E. Hepatology 17:932–941. https://doi.org/10.1002/hep.1840170525
6. Acharya SK, Panda SK, Saxena A, Gupta SD (2000) Acute hepatic failure in India: a perspective from the East. J Gastroenterol Hepatol 15:473–479. https://doi.org/10.1046/j.1440-1746.2000.02073.x
7. Alam S, Azam G, Mustafa G, Azad AK, Haque I, Gani S, Ahmad N, Alam K, Khan M (2009) Natural course of fulminant hepatic failure: the scenario in Bangladesh and the differences from the west. Saudi J Gastroenterol 15: 229–233. https://doi.org/10.4103/1319-3767.56094
8. Shalimar KS, Gunjan D, Sonika U, Mahapatra SJ, Nayak B, Kaur H, Acharya SK (2017) Acute liver failure due to hepatitis E virus infection is associated with better survival than other etiologies in Indian patients. Dig Dis Sci 62:1058–1066. https://doi.org/10.1007/s10620-017-4461-x
9. Canalese J, Gimson AE, Davis C, Mellon PJ, Davis M, Williams R (1982) Controlled trial of dexamethasone and mannitol for the cerebral oedema of fulminant hepatic failure. Gut. 23:625–629. https://doi.org/10.1136/gut.23.7.625
10. Lee WM, Stravitz RT, Larson AM (2012) Introduction to the revised American Association for the Study of Liver Diseases Position Paper on acute liver failure 2011. Hepatology 55:965–967. https://doi.org/10.1002/hep.25551
11. Stravitz RT, Kramer AH, Davern T, Shaikh AO, Caldwell SH, Mehta RL, Blei AT, Fontana RJ, McGuire BM, Rossaro L, Smith AD, Lee WM (2007) Intensive care of patients with acute liver failure: recommendations of the U.S. Acute Liver Failure Study Group. Crit Care Med 35:2498–2508. https://doi.org/10.1097/01.CCM.0000287592.94554.5F
12. Murphy N, Auzinger G, Bernel W, Wendon J (2004) The effect of hypertonic sodium chloride on intracranial pressure in patients with acute liver failure. Hepatology 39:464–470. https://doi.org/10.1002/hep.20056
13. Larsen F, Murphy N, Bernal W, Bjerring P, Hauerberg A, Wendon J (2011) The prophylactic effect of mild hypothermia to prevent brain oedema in patients with acute liver failure: results of a multicentre randomised controlled trial [Abstract]. J Hepatol 54(Supplement 1):S26
14. Ede RJ, Gimson AE, Bihari D, Williams R (1986) Controlled hyperventilation in the prevention of cerebral oedema in fulminant hepatic failure. J Hepatol 2: 43–51. https://doi.org/10.1016/S0168-8278(86)80007-1
15. Bruce DA, Berman WA, Schut L (1977) Cerebrospinal fluid pressure monitoring in children. Physiology pathology and clinical usefulness. Adv Pediatr 24:233–289 http://pascal-francis.inist.fr/vibad/index.php?action=getRecordDetail&idt=PASCAL7850276519
16. Videen TO, Zazulia AR, Manno EM, Derdeyn CF, Adams RE, Diringer MN, Powers WJ (2001) Mannitol bolus preferentially shrinks non-infarcted brain in patients with ischemic stroke. Neurology. 57:2120–2122. https://doi.org/10.1212/wnl.57.11.2120
17. Biswas RS, Hasan F, Sultana A, Uddin MK, Chowdhury D, Rosy S, Mamun S (2019) A documentation of hepatitis outbreak in Chittagong. Chattagram Maa-O-Shishu Hosp Med Coll J 17(2):2–5. https://doi.org/10.3329/cmoshmcj.v17i2.39768
18. Lee WM, Squires RH Jr, Nyberg SL, Doo E, Hoofnagle JH (2008) Acute liver failure: summary of a workshop. Hepatology. 47:1401–1415. https://doi.org/10.1002/hep.22177
19. Tandon BN, Bernauau J, O'Grady J (1999) Recommendations of the International Association for the Study of the Liver Subcommittee on nomenclature of acute and subacute liver failure. J Gastroenterol Hepatol 14:403–404. https://doi.org/10.1046/j.1440-1746.1999.01905.x

20. Conn HO, Lieberthal MM (eds) (1979) The hepatic coma syndromes and lactulose. Williams & Wilkins, Baltimore
21. Atterbury CE, Maddrey WC, Conn HO (1978) Neomycin-sorbitol and lactulose in the treatment of acute portal-systemic encephalopathy. A controlled, double-blind clinical trial. Am J Dig Dis 23(5):398–406. https://doi.org/10.1007/bf01072921
22. Clayson ET, Myint KS, Snitbhan R, Vaughn DW, Innis BL, Chan L, Cheung P, Shrestha MP (1995) Viremia, fecal shedding, and IgM and IgG responses in patients with hepatitis E. J Infect Dis 172:927–933. https://doi.org/10.1093/infdis/172.4.927
23. Favorov MO, Fields HA, Purdy MA, Yashina TL, Aleksandrov AG, Alter MJ, Yarasheva DM, Bradley DW, Margolis HS (1992) Serologic identification of hepatitis E virus infections in epidemic and endemic settings. J Med Virol 36:246–250. https://doi.org/10.1002/jmv.1890360403
24. Warrillow SJ, Bellomo R (2014) Preventing cerebral oedema in acute liver failure: the case for quadruple-H therapy. Anaesth Intensive Care 42:78–88. https://doi.org/10.1177/0310057X1404200114
25. Acharya SK, Dasarathy S, Kumer TL, Sushma S, Prasanna KS, Tandon A, Sreenivas V, Nijhawan S, Panda SK, Nanda SK (1996) Fulminant hepatitis in a tropical population: clinical course, cause, and early predictors of outcome. Hepatology. 23:1448–1455. https://doi.org/10.1002/hep.510230622
26. Polson J, Lee WM (2005) AASLD position paper: the management of acute liver failure. Hepatology. 41:1179–1197. https://doi.org/10.1002/hep.20703
27. Khuroo MS, Kamili S (2003) Aetiology and prognostic factors in acute liver failure in India. J Viral Hepat 10:224–231. https://doi.org/10.1046/j.1365-2893.2003.00415.x
28. Patra S, Kumar A, Trivedi SS, Puri M, Sarin SK (2007) Maternal and fetal outcomes in pregnant women with acute hepatitis E virus infection. Ann Intern Med 147:28–33. https://doi.org/10.7326/0003-4819-147-1-200707030-00005
29. Li XM, Ma L, Yang YB, Shi ZJ, Zhou SS (2005) Clinical characteristics of fulminant hepatitis in pregnancy. World J Gastroenterol 11:46003. https://doi.org/10.3748/wjg.v11.i29.4600
30. Bhatia V, Singhal A, Panda SK, Acharya SK (2008) A 20-year single-center experience with acute liver failure during pregnancy: is the prognosis really worse? Hepatology. 48:1577–1585. https://doi.org/10.1002/hep.22493
31. Shalimar ASK (2013 Sep) Hepatitis E and acute liver failure in pregnancy. J Clin Exp Hepatol 3(3):213–224. https://doi.org/10.1016/j.jceh.2013.08.009

Self-expandable metallic stents (SEMS) in esophageal varices post-band ulcer refractory bleeding: a retrospective study

Osama Elbahr[1*], Ahmad Kamal[1], Ayman Alsebaey[1], Mohamed Amin[1], Mohamed Abbasy[1], Ahmad Edris[1], Ali Nada[1], Alyaa Sabry[1], Sameh Afiffy[1], Abd El-Aleem Helal[1], Mohamad Abd El-aziz[2] and Abd El-naser Gad-Allah[3]

Abstract

Background: Post-variceal band ligation bleeding ulcer is a severe complication with considerable mortality. We tried evaluating self-expandable metallic stent (SEMS) with concern to the ulcer morphology not well studied.

Results: We did a retrospective analysis of patients with bleeding post-band ulcers and treated by SEMS with concern to control bleeding and 6 weeks survival. Twenty-eight patients studied had their age (mean ± S.D.) 57.8 ± 8.6 years, and 85.7% were males. The Child-Pugh score range was 5–12]. Control of bleeding by SEMS was achieved in 23 (82.1%) patients, and overall, 6-week survival was 75%. Both post-band ulcer types B (oozing blood and type C (active spurted) were a risk for 6 weeks mortality (P = 0.04, OR 1.58, CI 95% 1.12–2.23).

Conclusion: SEMS is considered an excellent choice to control esophageal post-banding ulcer bleeding and a definite treatment bridge.

Keywords: Liver cirrhosis, Portal hypertension, Varices, Post-band ulcer, Metallic stents, Bleeding

Background

Liver cirrhosis is a consequence of multiple etiologies that affect the liver. Chronic hepatitis C [1] and B viruses, non-alcoholic steatohepatitis, and alcoholic steatohepatitis are the most common leading causes of cirrhosis [2]. Patients with liver cirrhosis are classified into compensated or decompensated cirrhosis, according to Child-Pugh classification [3]. Further staging of cirrhosis depends on the development of varices, variceal bleeding, jaundice, hepatic encephalopathy, and ascites' development. The previous staging is the clinical presentation of portal hypertension that developed because of liver cirrhosis [4].

Esophageal varices are portosystemic venous channels and present in about half of patients diagnosed with cirrhosis. When portal pressure elevated to be clinically significant (hepatic vein portal gradient [HPVG] > 10 mmHg), portosystemic collaterals develop [5]. They at first create as little varices that continuously expand at a pace of 5% every year [6]. Screening for varices is an essential step in patients diagnosed with cirrhosis, and upper gastrointestinal endoscopy is the procedure of choice for defining, typing, and grading varices. Prophylaxis from 1st esophageal varices bleeding is achieved by either varices band ligation or non-selective beta-blocker administration [5, 7].

Acute variceal bleeding (AVB) is a well-known dangerous inconvenience in patients with cirrhosis. Current standard-of-care treatment incorporates the blend of vasoactive medications, band ligation, and anti-infection agents [8]. Endoscopic variceal band ligation (EVL) and pharmacological therapy for active esophageal variceal hemorrhage remain the first-line therapy. In most cases, band ligation outcomes are excellent, offering high initial hemostasis levels, low rebleeding rates, minimal side effects, and increased survival compared to sclerotherapy.

* Correspondence: osama.elbahr@liver.menofia.edu.eg; oelbahr@yahoo.com
[1]Hepatology and Gastroenterology Department, National Liver Institute, Menoufia University, Shebin Alkawm, Menoufia, Egypt
Full list of author information is available at the end of the article

Variceal ligation using an endoscope of diagnostic size can monitor excessive variceal bleeding with bands on active varix [9]. After EVL, the ligature bands stay in place for a range of 3 to 7 days. An ulcer remains that heals within 2 to 3 weeks. The thrombus formation is incomplete when the ligature band sloughs off, post-ligation ulcer bleeding occurs. Overall, the risk of post-EVL ulcer bleeding is 3.6 to 15% [5]. The placement of a transjugular intrahepatic portosystemic shunt (TIPS) is considered for patients with treatment failure or recurrent bleeding, but it is not applicable for all cases [10]. For 10–20% of cirrhotics refractory for medical and endoscopy therapy, alternative treatment options must mitigate the substantial morbidity and mortality associated with it [11]. Nevertheless, the 6-week mortality rate after an E.V. bleed index is approximately 20%. However, it varies from 0% among patients with Child-Pugh class A to roughly 30% among patients with Child-Pugh C disease [12].

Years ago, self-expanding metal stents (SEMS) were proposed in palliation for esophageal malignancy [13]. The fully covered SEMS is considered a rescue therapy in patients with refractory esophageal variceal bleeding. These stents can be deployed endoscopically in the lower esophagus with or without radiological assistance and easily removed later [14–16].

Methods

A retrospective study conducted on 28 patients with refractory bleeding post-band ulcers admitted to a specialized tertiary center (Hepatology and Gastroenterology Department), National Liver Institute, Menuofia University, Egypt, who received fully covered self-expandable metallic stents (FCSEMS) (NITI-S Mega stents-Tae Wong-S Korea) as a management of their refractory bleeding from post-variceal band ligation ulcer between January 2017 and December 2018.

During these 2 years, 1324 cases of hematemesis were admitted to our hospital, and 1096 cases had portal hypertensive cause of bleeding, and 612 had esophageal varices bleeding.

Prior endoscopic band ligation (EBL) treatments in the emergency setting, laboratory parameters, size of varices, and the bleeding episodes were recorded. The Child-Pugh score, MELD, MELD-Na, and ALBI were calculated. Rebleeding rates and mortality after SEMS placement were defined as primary efficacy endpoints within 6 weeks. Moreover, adverse events and the patients' clinical course were recorded. We recorded rates of successful bleeding control (≤ 5 days), early rebleeding (≤ 6 weeks), bleeding-related mortality (≤ 6 weeks), and overall mortality. Successful SEMS removal was defined as no rebleeding or death within 1 day after stent removal. Refractory acute variceal bleeding (failure-to-control bleeding) with vasoactive drugs and endoscopy was defined according to the Baveno IV and V guidelines [17, 18]: fresh hematemesis or aspiration of more than100 mL of new blood via the nasogastric tube beyond 2 h after the endoscopy and a 3 g/dL drop in hemoglobin without blood transfusion. According to the Baveno V guidelines, rebleeding was defined as evidence of rebleeding from portal hypertensive sources (hematemesis, melaena, aspiration of more than 100 mL of fresh blood in patients with a nasogastric tube or drop in hemoglobin of 3 g/dL without blood transfusion) [17, 18].

We classified post-banding ulcer endoscopically into (A) ulcer covered with clot; (B) ulcer oozing with blood; and (C) ulcer actively spurting.

We excluded patients with age < 18 years, intermediate and advanced HCC, the simultaneous presence of fundal varices, and previous attempts for balloon tamponade (B.T.) by sungestaken tube insertion management for refractory bleeding.

The technique of stent deployment

After sedation and adequate airway protection, the patient was placed in the left lateral position, the endoscope was passed into the esophagus, and a guidewire (0.035-in.) was established. The SEMS was loaded onto the guidewire and passed under fluoroscopic guidance. The radiopaque markers were helpful in the accurate positioning of the stent. Oral feeds with a liquid diet were started 12–24 h after the procedure, and patients were positioned at 45° in a supine position for 1 day.

No informed consent has been obtained in this retrospective study.

This study was conducted under the Declaration of Helsinki and approved by the ethics committees of our IRB.

Calculations

From online calculators

Child-Pugh

https://www.mdcalc.com/child-pugh-score-cirrhosis-mortality

ALBI

https://www.mdcalc.com/albi-albumin-bilirubin-grade-hepatocellular-carcinoma-hcc

MELD

https://www.mdcalc.com/meld-score-original-pre-2016-model-end-stage-liver-disease

MELD-Na

https://www.mdcalc.com/meldna-meld-na-score-liver-cirrhosis

Statistical analysis

Results were statistically analyzed using IBM SPSS version 21 for Windows. Variables were summarized as mean ± S.D., range, median, or frequency

(%), as appropriate. Student's t test was used to compare the results of all examined subjects in all groups under study. Odds ratio (OR) and 95% confidence interval (CI), and the chi-square test were used. Results were considered significant when $P \leq 0.05$.

Table 1 Demographic, clinical, and endoscopic characteristics of the patients:

Characteristics	Range	
Age, years (mean ± SD)	35–75	56.6 ± 9.4
Gender (male) NO %		24 (85.7%)
Cirrhosis aetiology (HCV/HBV) NO %		24 (85/7%)/4
Diabetes NO %		13 (46.4%)
Hypertension NO %		3 (10.7%)
Smokers NO %		9 (32.1%)
HCC NO %		5 (17.85%)
PVT NO %		6 (21.4%)
SBP at admission		12 (42.86%)
CTP class (A/B/C) NO %		3 (10.7%)/15 (53.6%)/10 (35.7%)
CTP score (mean ± SD)	5–12	8.6 ± 1.8/median 8
MELD at admission (mean ± SD)	8–42	15.7 ± 6.3
MELD Na at admission (mean ± SD)	10–42	20 ± 6.4
ALBI at admission (mean ± SD)	− 2.36 to − 0.14	− 1.36 ± 0.58
Post band bleeding presentation time	2–14 days	Median 10 days
Mean blood pressure (mean ± SD)	53–97	75 ± 10.8
Hemoglobin at admission g/dl (mean ± SD)	6.2–13.2	8.2 ± 1.45
Units of transfused blood (NO)	0–16	Median 2 units
Prophylactic antibiotics (NO)		
- 3rd cephalosporins		- 18
- Quinolones		- 4
- combined		- 6
Portal decompressive drugs (NO)		
- Sandostatin		- 14
- glypressin		- 14
OVs size (small:large) NO %		15 (53.57%)/ 13 (46.43%)
Post band ulcer NO %		
- Type A		- 9 (32.14%)
- Type B		- 7 (25%)
- Type C		- 12 (42.86%)

Results

Patients' characteristics

From our data, esophageal variceal bleeding was 46% of all cases of hematemesis present in our department, and refractory bleeding post-variceal band ligation was 4% of variceal bleeding cases.

As presented in Table 1, 28 patients studied had their age (mean ± S.D.) 57.8 ± 8.6 years, and 85.7% were males. Their Child score range 5–12 and the median was 8. Five patients had early-stage HCC. 21.4% of the patients had portal vein thrombosis (PVT). Patients presented with bleeding after previous band ligation either 1ry or 2ry prophylaxis for esophageal varices 2–14 days with 10 days median. On admission, their prognostic scores were MELD 15.7 ± 6.3, MELD Na 20 ± 6.4, and ALBI score − 1.36 ± 0.58. Patients needed 0–16 units of blood transfused with a mean of 2 units.

Bleeding post-banding ulcer (BPBU) classified endoscopically into (A) 32.14% ulcer covered with clot (9 patients); (B) 25% ulcer oozing blood (7 patients); and (C) 42.86% ulcer with active spurting (12 patients).

Post-SEMS placement outcomes (Table 2, Figs. 1 and 2, and Additional file 1)

Regarding control of bleeding, 3 (10.7%) patients had uncontrolled bleeding despite stent insertion, and all died. Two patients experienced early rebleeding after

Table 2 Outcome data

	N (%)
Control of bleeding	
Uncontrolled	3
Re-bleeding	2 (1 stent displaced-1 post-stent removal)
controlled	23 (82%)
6 weeks survival (deceased/alive)	7/21 (75%)
Stent displaced	6 (21.43%) (1 re-stent and 3 re-positioned)
Stent-related complications (no. 4)	2 aspiration
	2 aspiration bronchopneumonia
Development of encephalopathy post-endoscopy (no. 9)	9 (32.1%)
Covert	3
Overt	6
6 weeks cause related mortality (no. 7)	
Bleeding	4 (14.3%)
Sepsis	1
MOF	2
Rescue therapy	2 sungestaken tubes (1 deceased)

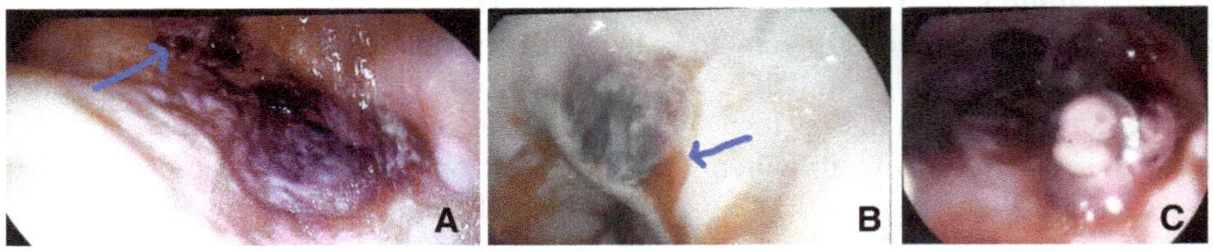

Fig. 1 **a** Type A ulcer with an adherent blood clot. **b** Type B ulcer with oozing blood. **c** Type C ulcer spurting blood

initial management. SEMS achieved bleeding control in 23 (82.1%) patients. From all patients, for 42 days follow-up, 14.3% of patients died due to bleeding. The mean days of survival were 34 (CI 95% 28–39) with 6 weeks survival 75%. Six (21.4%) patients' stents were displaced, and only one patient experienced rebleeding that was uncontrollable after sungestaken tube insertion, and he died. The others, one patient, undergone re-stenting, three stents repositioned, and one showed healed stable ulcers, so followed up. Successful stent removal was done in 20 (71.4%) patients from 23 who survived. At the same time, one patient had rebleeding after stent removal controlled by sungestaken tube insertion. Nine patients (32.1%) developed hepatic encephalopathy post-SEMS deployment. Two patients had aspirated, and another two patients developed aspiration pneumonia.

Identified risk factors for 6 weeks mortality after SEMS deployment

Univariate analysis was conducted (Tables 3 and 4) revealed that post-band ulcers other than type A, development of overt hepatic encephalopathy were a risk for 6 weeks mortality (P = 0.04, 0.02 respectively). Low baseline arterial blood pressure (65 ± 6.7, P = 0.003) and increased number of transfused blood units (5.4 ± 4.8, P = 0.006) were associated with 6 weeks mortality.

Discussion

Current guidelines recommend either balloon tamponade (B.T.), SEMS, or TIPS to manage refractory and endoscopically uncontrolled variceal bleeding [11, 19]. Nevertheless, the evaluation of SEMS in refractory bleeding post-band ulcers concerning ulcer morphology was not well studied.

In our study, we had a high rate of successful bleeding control in 82% of patients. Our rebleeding rate was so low that only one patient due to stent displacement and another after stent removal. A meta-analysis comprising n = 134 showed a failure-to-control bleeding rate of 14.2% [8]. Pfisterer and colleagues showed 1/3 of their cases achieved control of bleeding in their follow-up period. Also, they showed a higher overall rate of rebleeding, especially after stent removal (about 29.4%) [19]. In the previously mentioned meta-analysis, post-SEMS removal bleeding was 11% [8]. Another meta-analysis showed rebleeding rate was 13.2% [6]. This difference could be attributed to the type and diameter of SEMS used. In our study, a mega stent with a diameter of 28 mm that is fitting well on the esophageal wall.

Pfisterer stated that "bleeding-related mortality was as high as 47.1% (n = 16/34) of patients in our study, including 20.6% (n = 7/34) who deceased owing to uncontrolled bleeding" [19]. In our retrospective analysis, bleeding-related mortality was very low, 14.3 (n = 4/28), and this agrees with two recent meta-analyses, the first found 12% for mortality related to variceal bleeding, and

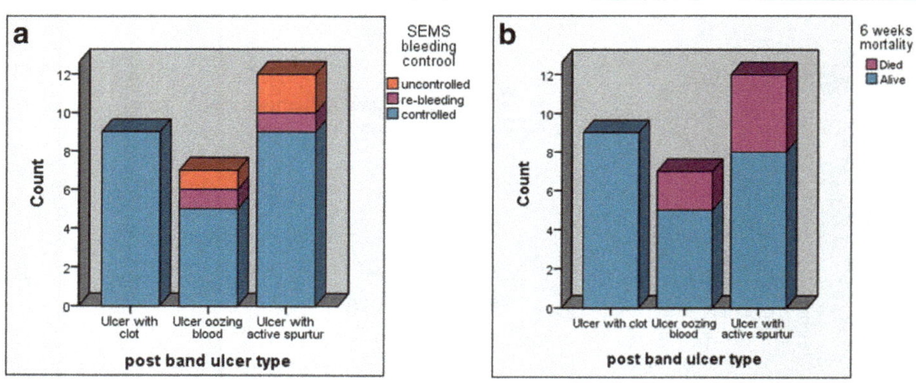

Fig. 2 **a** Control of bleeding. **b** Mortality after SEMS deployment according to ulcer type

Table 3 Univariate analysis for mortality 6 weeks follow-up

	6 weeks mortality Dead 7	6 weeks mortality Alive 21	Test	*P* value	CI 95%
Age, years	55.8 ± 10.38	58.5 ± 8.2	*T* **− 0.68**	0.5	(− 10.45–5.2)
CTP score	8.7 ± 1.8	8.5 ± 1.8	*T* **0.17**	0.86	(− 1.5–1.8)
MELD at admission	17.14 ± 11.45	15.24 ± 3.72	*T* **2.8**	0.008*	(− 3.8–7.6)
MELD Na at admission	22.86 ± 9.65	19.05 ± 4.9	*T* **3.1**	0.004**	(− 1.85–9.47)
Hemoglobin on admission g/dl	7.8 ± 1.2	8.4 ± 1.5	*T* **− 0.84**	0.4	(− 1.85–0.77)
Mean blood pressure on admission	65.14 ± 6.74	78.3 ± 9.88	*T* **− 3.2**	0.003***	(− 21.5 to − 4.5)
UNITS of blood	5.4 ± 4.8	2 ± 1.5	*T* **2.9**	0.006***	(1.05–5.8)
ALBI	− 1.16 ± 0.69	− 1.42 ± 0.54	*T* **1.03**	0.3	(− 0.25–0.77)

* means significant

18% for failure to control bleeding with SEMS [8], and the second found 12.6% of patients died from uncontrolled bleeding [6]. We think the possible explanation for this with our results is selecting patients with post-band ulcers only in our study.

A multicenter trial compared SEMS with balloon tamponade (B.T.) in a series of cirrhotic patients with variceal bleeding. This study showed a superior safety profile and higher efficacy in controlling bleeding with SEMS. However, the use of SEMS did not result in improved survival [20]. They had no patients who developed aspiration and aspiration pneumonia in the SEMS group. Still, in our study, we had two patients who had aspiration and another two who developed pneumonia, which could be due to the low number of participants in the Escorsell study (n = 13) [20].

Stent dislocations were found in n = 13 (38.2%) patients in Pfisterer study 2019. In our analysis, it was n = 6 (21.43%) patients. In a meta-analysis, the incidence of stent migration was 21.6% [6]. The different types and diameters of SEMS used in the study may be the explanation for this difference.

Six weeks of survival in our study was 75% (n = 21). In the Spanish clinical trial study, the survival was 54%, which is not different from the B.T. group 40% [20]. 47.1% of patients died within 6 weeks due to bleeding-related complications in Pfisterer study [19]. Pooled 30-day and 60-day survival rates were 68% and 64%, respectively, in a meta-analysis [11].

No previous studies specified post-band ulcer bleeding in their analysis and respect to the ulcers' morphology. In our research, the ulcer type has a significant impact on rebleeding and mortality after SEMS insertion. As we have all type A (ulcer with clot) patients that had 100% for both bleeding control and 6 weeks survival. So, we think the ulcer type can guide the intervention modality to be used. Jamwal and colleagues tried in their retrospective study to evaluate the impact of the morphology

Table 4 Clinical data related to 6 weeks mortality

		6 weeks mortality Dead 7		6 weeks mortality Alive 21		Test	*P* value	Odd's ratio	CI 95%
HCC	**Yes**	2	40%	3	60%	**Fisher 0.7**	0.57		
No	5	21.7%	18	78.3%					
SBP	**Yes**	3	25%	9	75%	**χ2 0.00**	0.6		
	No	4	25%	12	75%				
Post-band ulcer	**Type A**	0	0%	9	100%	**χ2 4.4**	0. 043*	1.58	(1.12–2.23)
	Type (B and C)	7	36.8%	12	63.2%				
Encephalopathy	**Overt**	4	66.7%	2	33.3%	**χ2 7**	0.02*	2.59	(0.8–8.1)
	Covert	3	13.6%	19	86.4%				

of post-band bleeding ulcers on the choice of treatment options, and they found that ulcers with clots could have a favorable outcome with repeated banding or SEMS insertion according to Child-Pugh class [21].

The most important limitation of our study is its uncontrolled retrospective design and the low number of cases.

Conclusion

SEMS is a very effective strategy when used appropriately in post-band ulcer bleeding. We should take into consideration the morphological picture of the ulcer and the general condition of the patient. So, we can get a high rate of bleeding control and survival benefits.

Abbreviations

SEMS: Self-expandable metallic stents; AVB: Acute variceal bleeding; HPVG: Hepatic vein portal gradient; EVL or EBL: Endoscopic variceal band ligation; TIPS: Transjugular intrahepatic portosystemic shunt; B.T.: Balloon tamponade; HCC: Hepato-cellular carcinoma; PVT: Portal vein thrombosis; MELD: Model of end-stage liver disease

Acknowledgements

The authors thank and acknowledge the endoscopy unit's role at the National Liver Institute, Menoufia University.

Authors' contributions

O.E.: data collection, endoscopist, statistical analysis, manuscript writing, AK: endoscopist, data collection, A.A.: endoscopist, manuscript writing, MA: endoscopist, data collection, MA: endoscopist, manuscript writing, A.E.: endoscopist, data collection, AIN: endoscopist, data collection, AS: endoscopist, data collection, S.A.: endoscopist, data collection, A.H.: data collection, MAE: endoscopist, data collection, AG: endoscopist, data collection. All authors have read and approved the final manuscript.

Declarations

Ethics approval and consent to participate

The Research Ethics Committee approved the study of our medical institute (National Liver Institute IRB00003621). All study procedures were carried out per the Declaration of Helsinki regarding research involving human subjects. Every patient filled a written consent form after a detailed explanation of the study and management plan.

Competing interests

The authors declare that they have no competing interests.

Author details

[1]Hepatology and Gastroenterology Department, National Liver Institute, Menoufia University, Shebin Alkawm, Menoufia, Egypt. [2]Internal medicine department, Alexandria University, Alexandria, Egypt. [3]Internal Medicine Department, Menoufia University, One, Meleeg Road, National liver Institute, Shebin Alkawm, Menoufia, Egypt.

References

1. Elbahr O, Saleh AA, Bakery LH (2020) PNPLA3 L148M (rs738409) polymorphism as a risk for new onset diabetes mellitus and obesity in non-NASH/cryptogenic living related donor liver transplant recipients. Gene Rep. 19:100607. https://doi.org/10.1016/j.genrep.2020.100607
2. Wiegand J, Berg T (2013) The etiology, diagnosis and prevention of liver cirrhosis: part 1 of a series on liver cirrhosis. Dtsch Arztebl Int. 110(6):85–91. https://doi.org/10.3238/arztebl.2013.0085
3. Ginés P, Quintero E, Arroyo V, Terés J, Bruguera M, Rimola A, Caballería J, Rodés J, Rozman C (1987) Compensated cirrhosis: natural history and prognostic factors. Hepatology. 7(1):122–128. https://doi.org/10.1002/hep.1840070124
4. D'Amico G, Garcia-Tsao G, Pagliaro L (2006) Natural history and prognostic indicators of survival in cirrhosis: a systematic review of 118 studies. J Hepatol. 44(1):217–231. https://doi.org/10.1016/j.jhep.2005.10.013
5. Nett A, Binmoeller KF (2019) Endoscopic management of portal hypertension-related bleeding. Gastrointest Endosc Clin N Am. 29(2):321–337. https://doi.org/10.1016/j.giec.2018.12.006
6. Shao X-D, Qi X-S, Guo X-Z (2016) Esophageal stent for refractory variceal bleeding: a systemic review and meta-analysis. Biomed Res Int. 2016: 4054513–4054510. https://doi.org/10.1155/2016/4054513
7. Bunchorntavakul C, Reddy KR (2019) Pharmacologic management of portal hypertension. https://doi.org/10.1016/j.cld.2019.06.004
8. Marot A, Trepo E, Doerig C, Moreno C, Moradpour D, Deltenre P (2015) Systematic review with meta-analysis: self-expanding metal stents in patients with cirrhosis and severe or refractory oesophageal variceal bleeding. Aliment Pharmacol Ther. 42(11-12):1250–1260. https://doi.org/10.1111/apt.13424
9. Kovacs TOG, Jensen DM (2019) Varices: esophageal, gastric, and rectal. Clin Liver Dis. 23(4):625–642. https://doi.org/10.1016/j.cld.2019.07.005
10. Fortune B, Garcia-Tsao G (2014) Current management strategies for acute esophageal variceal hemorrhage. Curr Hepatol Rep. 13(1):35–42. https://doi.org/10.1007/s11901-014-0221-y
11. McCarty TR, Njei B (2016) Self-expanding metal stents for acute refractory esophageal variceal bleeding: a systematic review and meta-analysis. Dig Endosc. 28(5):539–547. https://doi.org/10.1111/den.12626
12. Kovacs TOG, Jensen DM Varices esophageal, gastric, and rectal. https://doi.org/10.1016/j.cld.2019.07.005
13. Elbahr O, Kamal A, Amin M, et al. Cronicon EC GASTROENTEROLOGY AND DIGESTIVE SYSTEM Evaluation of Self Expandable Metal Stents (SEMS) in Upper Gastrointestinal Malignancies as a Palliative Treatment, a Single Center Experience "Evaluation of Self Expandable Metal Stents (SEMS) in Upper Gastrointestinal Malignancies as a Palliative Treatment, a Single Center Experience". EC Gastroenterology and Digestive System 5.4 (2018): 204-210.; 2018.
14. Zehetner J, Shamiyeh A, Wayand W, Hubmann R (2008) Results of a new method to stop acute bleeding from esophageal varices: implantation of a self-expanding stent. Surg Endosc Other Interv Tech. 22(10):2149–2152. https://doi.org/10.1007/s00464-008-0009-7
15. Hubmann R, Bodlaj G, Czompo M, Benkö L, Pichler P, al-Kathib S, Kiblböck P, Shamyieh A, Biesenbach G (2006) The use of self-expanding metal stents to treat acute esophageal variceal bleeding. Endoscopy. 38(9):896–901. https://doi.org/10.1055/s-2006-944662
16. Elbahr O, Kamal A, Alsebaey A et al (2019) Self-expandable metallic stents (SEMS) in esophageal varices post band ulcer refractory bleeding, a retrospective study. In: ESGE Days 2019, vol 51. Georg Thieme Verlag KG. https://doi.org/10.1055/s-0039-1681881
17. De Franchis R (2005) Evolving consensus in portal hypertension report of the Baveno IV Consensus Workshop on methodology of diagnosis and therapy in portal hypertension. J Hepatol. 43(1):167–176. https://doi.org/10.1016/j.jhep.2005.05.009
18. De Franchis R (2010) Revising consensus in portal hypertension: report of the Baveno V consensus workshop on methodology of diagnosis and therapy in portal hypertension. https://doi.org/10.1016/j.jhep.2010.06.004

19. Pfisterer N, Riedl F, Pachofszky T, Gschwantler M, König K, Schuster B, Mandorfer M, Gessl I, Illiasch C, Fuchs EM, Unger L, Dolak W, Maieron A, Kramer L, Madl C, Trauner M, Reiberger T (2019) Outcomes after placement of a SX-ELLA oesophageal stent for refractory variceal bleeding—a national multicentre study. Liver Int. 39(2):290–298. https://doi.org/10.1111/liv.13971
20. Escorsell A, Pavel O, Cardenas A et al (2016) Esophageal balloon tamponade versus esophageal stent in controlling acute refractory variceal bleeding: a multicenter randomized, controlled trial. Hepatology. 63(6):1957–1967. https://doi.org/10.1002/hep.28360
21. Jamwal KD, Maiwall R, Sharma MK, Kumar G, Sarin SK (2019) Case control study of post-endoscopic variceal ligation bleeding ulcers in severe liver disease: outcomes and management. https://doi.org/10.14218/JCTH.2018.00059

24

Norfloxacin with itopride versus norfloxacin alone in secondary prophylaxis of spontaneous bacterial peritonitis

Afaf Y. M. Younes[1], Sherief Abd-Elsalam[1*], Gehan F. Attia[2] and Mona A. H. Shehata[1]

Abstract

Background: Bacterial translocation is considered the pathophysiological hallmark in the development of spontaneous bacterial peritonitis (SBP). Prokinetics can increase gastrointestinal (GIT) motility, reduce small bowel transit time, decrease bacterial translocation, and the possibility of SBP. The aim of this work was to compare the effectiveness and safety of itopride and norfloxacin versus norfloxacin only in secondary prophylaxis for cirrhotic ascitic patients with spontaneous bacterial peritonitis.

Results: Regarding the baseline clinical manifestations and laboratory investigations, there was no significant difference between both groups. The incidence of a recurrent SBP in group I, who had received itopride plus norfloxacin, reduced with a significant difference than other group II (P=0.018). The median time for recurrence of SBP was highly longer in group I than group II with a significant difference (P=0.042).

Conclusions: The combined usage of itopride with norfloxacin in patients with cirrhosis and ascites can decrease the occurrence of a recurrent SBP and significantly improve the survival of patients.

Trial registration: ClinicalTrials.gov Identifier: NCT04161768.

Keywords: Spontaneous bacterial peritonitis, Cirrhosis, Ascites, Prokinetics, Norfloxacin, Itopride

Background

Spontaneous bacterial peritonitis (SBP) is an ascitic fluid infection that occurs spontaneously with no overt source that can be remedied surgically. It is a common complication in cirrhotic patients with ascites. All cirrhotic patients with ascites are at risk of SBP. The occurrence of SBP is 1.5–3.5% in outpatients and is about 10% in hospitalized patients [1].

The most common life-threatening complication in patients with cirrhosis and ascites is SBP and the mortality rate ranges between 30 and 50%; prompt diagnosis and treatment are the most common variable causes in reducing morbidity and mortality from SBP [2].

When the number of polymorph nuclear cells was> 250 cells/mm^3 in ascitic fluid in the absence of the source of intra-abdominal infection, the diagnosis of SBP is established [1].

Variable factors are associated with the development of SBP but bacterial translocation is considered the pathophysiological hallmark in immune-compromised hosts in the pathogenesis of SBP [3].

SBP treatment is based on the administration of broad-spectrum empiric antibiotics such as third-generation cephalosporins. For patients with beta-lactam allergy, alternatives include fluoroquinolones such as levofloxacin can be administered [4].

* Correspondence: sherif_tropical@yahoo.com
[1]Department of Tropical Medicine and Infectious Diseases, Faculty of Medicine, Tanta University, Elbahr Street, Tanta 35111, Egypt
Full list of author information is available at the end of the article

Recently, it was found that prokinetics could increase GIT motility, decrease small bowel transit time and decrease small intestinal bacterial overgrowth (SIBO), so could decrease bacterial translocation and the possibility of SBP [5].

The aim of the work was to compare the effectiveness and the safety of itopride with norfloxacin versus norfloxacin only in secondary prevention of spontaneous bacterial peritonitis in cirrhotic ascitic patients.

Methods

This randomized study was conducted on 80 cirrhotic patients with ascites and previous episode of SBP attending to the Tropical Medicine Department of Tanta University Hospital in a time of 1 year since December 2018 toward December 2019. The committee of ethics of scientific research of Tanta Faculty of Medicine approved the studied protocol and written consents were obtained from the studied groups for participation. The study was registered on clinicaltrials.gov with a registration number NCT04161768. For comparing the 2 groups, we adopted simple randomization through computer-generated random numbers with equal allocation ratio by referring to a table of random numbers.

Patients with cirrhosis and ascites and with previous events of SBP who were diagnosed by pelvi-abdominal ultrasound, liver function tests, and ascitic fluid aspiration, and analysis were included in the study and all patients included in our study did not receive prokinetices before. However, patients with ascites due to causes other than cirrhosis, patients with hepatocellular carcinoma or any other neoplastic disorder, pregnant and lactating women, patients with recent antibiotic therapy in the 2 weeks before or patients with allergy or other contraindications of the used drugs were excluded from the study.

Patients in our study were randomized into 2 groups: group 1, cases who received itopride 150 mg daily plus norfloxacin 400 mg daily; group 2, patients who received norfloxacin 400 mg daily alone. The two studied groups were followed up for 6 months, every 2 months for ascitic fluid analysis and when the clinical examination can be suggested SBP sings such as fever, tenderness, abdominal pain, or vomiting are present. The compliance was detected by asking the patients through their telephone numbers and by recovery of empty drug envelopes. Flow chart of the study is demonstrated in Fig. 1.

All patients were subjected for full history taking with attention on history of a previous attack of SBP, symptoms related to spontaneous bacterial peritonitis, history of treatment received through the 2 weeks before ascitic sample aspiration or history of the hepatic encephalopathy. Complete physical examination with attention on manifestations of advanced chronic liver disease. Laboratory investigations was performed for all the patients enrolled in the study including complete blood count (CBC), liver biochemical investigations, coagulation profile, kidney function assessments, serum C-reactive protein (CRP), ascitic fluid chemical, physical and cytological analysis and culture, and the serum-ascites albumin gradient (SAAG). Pelvi-abdominal ultrasound was done for all patients to asses liver conditions and aspiration of ascitic fluid sample can be performed.

The primary end point was the percentage of patients who developed a recurrent attack of SBP at the end of six months follow up. The secondary end points were the mortality rate in both groups.

Statistical analysis

The collected data statistically analyzed by usage of the statistical package for social studies (SPSS) program. These numerical variables included (mean±SD) were calculated. The analysis of variance (ANOVA) was used to parallel of mean values between both groups. When ANOVA (F) value was significant, post hoc test (LSD) test could be used to assess the difference between both groups. The comparison of both groups was done by usage (chi-square-test ($\chi 2$) to assess qualitative data; Student *t* test to carry out the significance of the difference in two means of parametric data; and Mann-Whitney *U* test to assess the significance of the difference in both variables of (numerical) non parametric data). The results were represented in tables and graphs. The level of significance was taken at p value of <0.05. P value is either non-significant (NS) if > 0.05, significant (S) if < 0.05, or highly significant (HS) if < 0.001 was calculated.

Results

Our study enrolled 80 patients, 46 men in addition to 34 women and their mean age was 57.50 ± 6.48 years for group I and 59.40 ± 6.16 years for group II (Table 1). As regard to the clinical manifestations which were present in both studied groups, there was no significant difference between both two groups. Regarding the laboratory investigations, there were no significant variances between both studied groups (Table 1).

The ascitic fluid culture of the two studied groups did not show significant difference between both groups. The most frequent organism in both groups was *E. coli* (Table 2).

Table 3 shows the incidence of recurrence of SBP and the cause of death in both groups. There was a significant increase in the occurrence of recurrent SBP in group II with P value (P=0.018*). Also, the number of deaths showed a significant increase in group II P= 0.043*and SBP was significantly considered the main factor of death. Table 4 shows the median time for recurrence of SBP in the studied groups which was

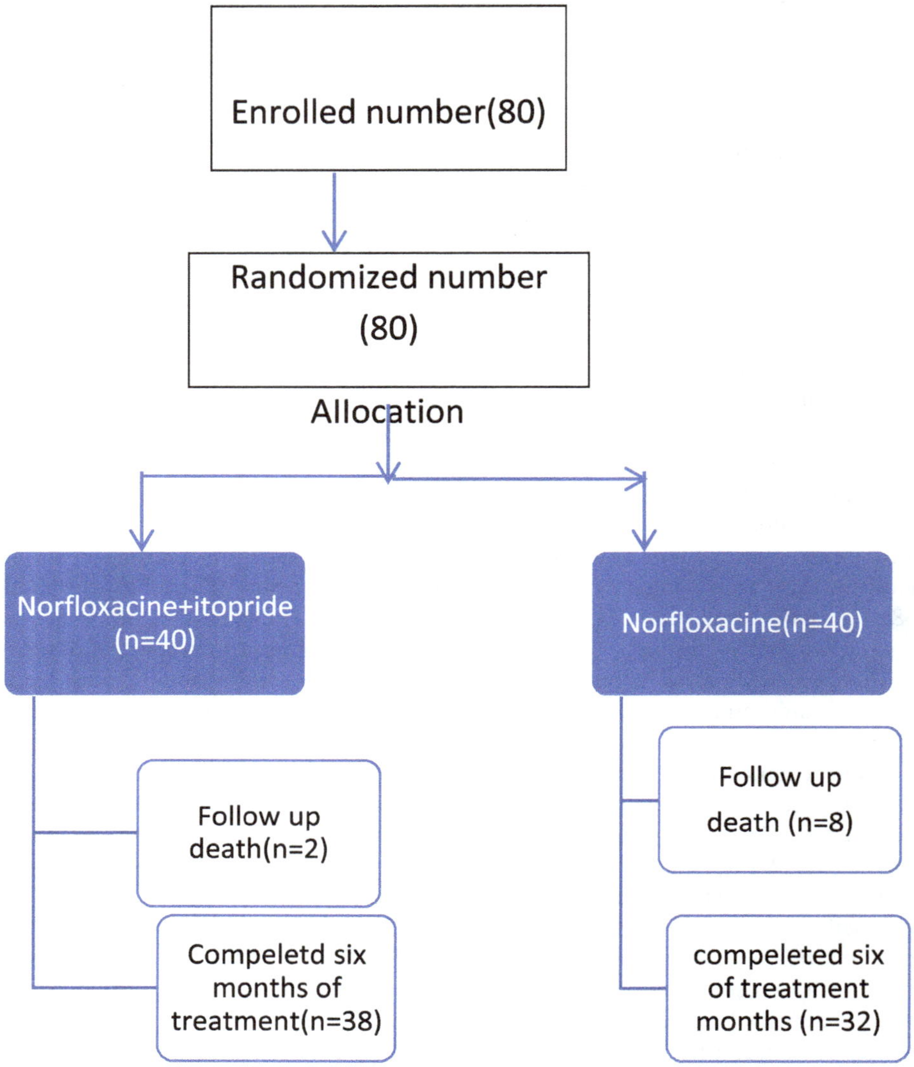

Fig. 1 Flow chart of the study: Flow chart shows Study analysis of cases. n, number of cases

significantly longer in group I P=0.042*. Figure 2 shows Kaplan–Meier survival curve which was used to assess the survival among the studied groups. Regarding the side effects of drugs, no side effects were reported by the included patients in both groups.

Discussion

The most common potential life-threatening complications in patients with cirrhosis and ascites is SBP where the mortality rate is alternating between 30 and 50%; hence, the prompt diagnosis and treatment are the most common variable causes in reducing morbidity and mortality of SBP. Bacterial translocation is considered the pathophysiological hallmark in developing spontaneous bacterial peritonitis (SBP). Prokinetics can increase GIT motility, decrease small bowel transit time, decrease bacterial translocation and the possibility of SBP.

Our study was conducted for evaluating the effectiveness and safety of itopride, as a prokinetic drug, in cirrhotic patients with spontaneous bacterial peritonitis to detect its role in secondary prophylaxis of SBP.

The major strength of this study is that it shed a light about the role of prokinetics in prevention of SBP in cirrhotic ascitic cases through its effect on decreasing the probability of a bacterial overgrowth via increasing the intestinal motility.

In our study, we enrolled 80 cirrhotic ascitic cases with a previous event of SBP who were classified into two groups, each of 40 cases. SBP was common in males in the two studied groups (21 and 25 patients respectively). The mean age was 57.50 ± 6.48 years in group I and

Table 1 Baseline demographic data, clinical manifestations, and the laboratory investigations of both groups

	Group I (itopride + norfloxacin) (number=40) No. (%)	Group II (norfloxacin) (number=40) No. (%)	Test of sig	P value
Age (years) (mean± SD)	57.50 ± 6.48	59.40 ± 6.16	t=1.34	0.183
Gender				
Male	21 (52.5)	25 (62.5)	χ^2= 0.81	0.366
Female	19 (47.5)	15 (37.5)		
Abdominal pain	39 (97.5)	37 (92.5)	FE=1.05	0.615
Fever	31 (77.5)	34 (85.0)	χ^2= 0.73	0.390
Hepatic encephalopathy	8 (20.0)	9 (22.5)	χ^2= 0.07	0.785
Hemoglobin (g/dl)	10.33 ± 1.34	9.83 ± 1.10	t=1.82	0.072
Platelets (cell× 103/mm^3)	122.67 ± 73.03	146.62 ± 77.41	U=1.54	0.122
Total leucocytic count (cell× 103/mm^3)	5.85 ± 3.42	6.51 ± 4.58	U=0.476	0.634
S. creatinine (mg/dl)	1.08 ± 0.58	1.16 ±0.40	U=1.61	0.106
S urea (mg/dl)	56.47 ± 41.81	52.19 ± 29.86	U=0.09	0.923
AST (u/l)	52.67 ± 36.43	50.70 ± 33.67	U=0.24	0.810
ALT (u/l)	41.82 ± 27.27	36.62 ±17.36	U=0.28	0.776
S. albumin (g/dl)	2.51 ± 0.50	2.61 ± 0.41	t=0.97	0.335
S. Bilirubin (mg/dl)	2.80 ± 2.68	3.82 ± 3.69	U=0.90	0.368
INR	1.56 ± 0.42	1.65 ± 0.45	t=0.86	0.389
CRP (mg/l)	38.86 ± 37.59	31.00 ±24.56	U=0.45	0.649

59.40 ± 6.16 years in group II without any a significant difference in both studied groups in age and sex distribution. The two groups were mostly cross-matched.

In this study, the most common symptoms of SBP which presented in both groups were abdominal pain in 39 patients (97.5%) in group I but in 37 cases (92.5%) in group II and fever presented in 31 patients (77.5%) through group I but 34 cases (85%) in group II then vomiting and hepatic encephalopathy (22.5% and 20% respectively) of group I and 40% and 22.5% respectively of group II without a significant differences in both studied groups as regards the clinical manifestations plus laboratory characteristics of our studied patients. This shows that the patients of both studied groups are cross matched.

In the current work, the degree of ascites in SBP patients was either moderate up or marked. Moderate ascites presented in 32 cases 80% (group I) while (group II) the moderate ascites was detected in 17 cases (42%), while marked ascites was reported in 20% and 57.5% of

Table 2 The patients' ascitic fluid culture analysis

	Group I Number of cases No. (%)	Group II Number of cases No. (%)	Test of sig	P value
Culture result			χ^2= 0.07	0.765
Positive	32 (80.0)	31 (77.5)		
Negative	8 (20.0)	9 (22.5)		
Organisms				
E. coli –G–ve	16 (50.0)	14 (45.2)	FE=0.27	0.965
Klebesiella- G–ve	8 (25.0)	9 (29.03)		
Proteous- G–ve	4 (12.5)	4 (12.9)		
Staph- G+ve	4 (12.5)	3 (9.6)		

χ^2 chi squared test, *FE* Fisher's exact test
*Significant

Table 3 Incidence of SBP recurrence and causes of death in both groups

Time	Group I number No. (%)	Group II number No. (%)	χ^2	P value
2nd month (n=80)				
SBP free	35 (87.5)	26 (65.0)	5.59	0.018*
SBP	5 (12.5)	14 (35.0)		
4th month (n=72)				
SBP free	34 (89.5)	25 (73.5)	3.08	0.079
SBP	4 (10.5)	9 (26.5)		
6th months (n=70)				
SBP free	34 (87.5)	23 (71.8)	2.49	0.094
SBP	4 (12.5)	9 (28.1)		
Fate (end study)				
Alive	38 (95.0)	32 (80.0)		0.043*
Dead	2 (5.0)	8 (20.0)	4.11	
Causes of death				
HRS	2 (5.0)	5 (12.5)	2.94	0.230
SBP	0 (0.0)	6 (15.0)		
HE	0 (0.0)	3 (7.5)		

*Significant

group I and II respectively with no statistically significant difference in group I and group II. These results corroborate the ideas of [6] who stated that ascitic fluid infection mostly developed when the ascitic fluid volume was at its maximum.

In the current study, patient groups showed low serum albumin level but high serum bilirubin, INR, AST, and ALT levels which mean the most reported cases of that disease (SBP) were Child-Pugh class C in both groups without a statistically significant variance in the studied groups [7].

Diagnostic paracentesis is the main stay in SBP diagnosis and can differ in SBP from secondary peritonitis [8]. It was performed to all cases in groups I and II included in this study. There was no statistically significant variance in the two patient groups according to the ascitic fluid analysis.

Table 4 Median time of recurrence of spontaneous bacterial peritonitis between both studied groups

Group	Mean time (month)			Log-rank test	P value
	Estimate	95% CI			
		Lower	Upper		
Group I (n=39)	5.76	5.41	6.12	4.14	0.042*
Group II (n=36)	5.42	4.90	5.94		
Overall	5.57	5.26	5.87		

*Significant

The mean value of serum-ascites albumin gradient (SAAG) in our current study was > 1.1 g/dl in both patient groups which confirmed that the etiology of ascites was portal hypertension in our SBP patients. Agarwal et al. [9] stated that SAAG levels of > 1.1 g/dl confirms that ascites is because of portal hypertension regardless the infection.

As regards to the ascitic fluid culture, the most reported cases of SBP, in both groups, were positive for gram-negative cocci without a statistical significant difference between both groups. These results did not match with Mostafa et al. [10] who found that the majority of their cases of SBP because of gram-positive cocci. In our study, we found that the most common and virulent organisms isolated from the cases were *Escherichia coli* species and Klebesiella but the less common was Staph-Gram-positive cocci, this matched with Novella et al. [11] who observed that of *E. coli* was isolated in 90% of their SBP patients.

In our study, on follow-up of the studied SBP patients, we observed, at the second month, a total of 14 episodes (35%) of recurrent SBP infections in group II (norfloxacin only) versus 5 episodes (12.5%) in group I (norfloxacin plus itopride) with an apparent statistically significant difference. The same variance was also detected in both studied groups in that fourth and sixth month follow-up; however, this difference was not significant. So the usage of both norfloxacin plus itopride (group I) showed a better SBP incidence free through the study follow-up period being 87.5%, 89.5, and 87.5% on the follow-up periods at second, fourth, and sixth month respectively, as compared to that, on usage of norfloxacin only as a SBP secondary prophylactic measure in group II. This accompanied with death of 20% of group II cases compared to death of only 5% of group I cases through the fourth and sixth months follow-up.

According to the present results, regarding the percentage of patients in group I (under treatment with norfloxacin plus itopride) who developed recurrent SBP which represented 12.5%, 10.5%, and 12.5% of cases through the follow-up period at the second, fourth, and sixth months respectively. As a probable explanation for the developing of SBP by the translocation of the bacteria from the intra (intestine) to extra (ascitic fluid) could not be the only route of infection, and the presence of ascitic bacterial DNA can support that condition [12].

In the present study, we reported a 65%, 73.5%, and 71.9% of SBP incidence free through the second, fourth, and sixth months follow-up period respectively in group II who received norfloxacin only. This result matched with Ghafar et al. [13] study that evaluated norfloxacin use in prophylaxis of SBP that established 40% decreasing in the frequency of SBP, among their patients. Also,

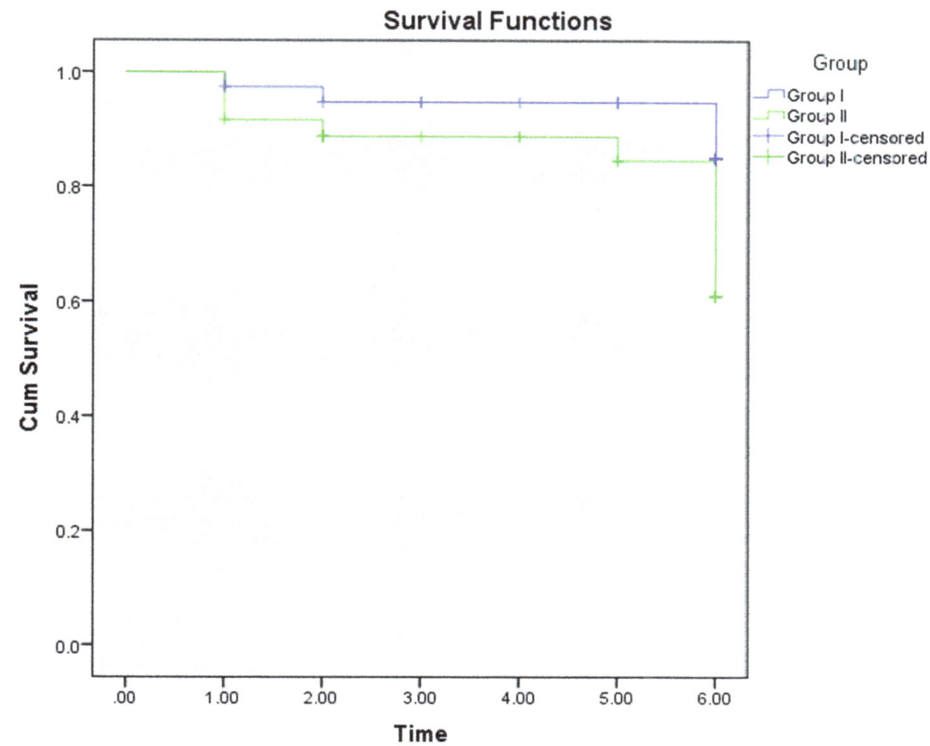

Fig. 2 Disease free (SBP free) survival (in months) by Kaplan-Meier analysis at 6 months

Hanouneh et al. [14] found 72% prevention rates of SBP in their study.

On the other hand, Fernandez et al.'s [15] work showed that 93% reducing in the SBP incidence cases, who received norfloxacin. This difference might be due to the type of patients included in our study or the prophylaxis of SBP with norfloxacin only becomes less active as before, because of increasing the incidence of quinolones bacterial resistance in cirrhotic patients flora in the stool due to over use of these drugs [16].

In the current study, the median time for recurrent SBP development was a highly significant prolonged in group I when we compared it by the group II. This was associated with a statistically significant improvement in patient survival rate. The recurrent SBP development rate was significantly decreased in group I (5%) when we compared that by the other group (II) (20%) and that difference in the incidence of SBP recurrence occurred in only in the first 2 months of follow-up due to the number of patient's death increased through the last 4 months that was mainly due to recurrent SBP (15%), HRS (12.5%), and hepatic encephalopathy (7.5%) in group II. While only HRS was reported as the only cause of death in 5% of group I. These results highlight the advantage of using the prokinetics agents (itopride) in combination with norfloxacin in SBP secondary prophylaxis.

The most common causes of mortality allover our study were hepatic encephalopathy, sepsis, and hepatorenal syndrome. And the results showed the beneficial effect of prokinetices (itopride) on group I cases that death in this group was 5% only compared to 20% death rate in group II.

On the same hand, PC Revaiah et al. [17] reported that combined use of prokinetics drugs could considerably reduce the possibility of small intestinal bacterial over growth because of increasing the intestinal motility, which lead to reduce bacterial translocation, the path of bacteria from the intra (intestine) to extra-intestinal such as ascitic fluid and this condition can be useful in SBP prophylaxis and treatment approach.

On other hand, Frazee et al. [18] found that long-term antimicrobial prophylaxis may be useful and has a benefit in cirrhotic patients. However, the magnitude of the benefits was less and the frequency of overall infections and mortality did not change [19].

In the current study, we did not report any side effects from usage of itopride which supported by Huang X (2012), [20] who found that itopride was the least prokinetics agent side effects through the incidence rate of its side effects. Also, itopride had an excitatory influence on the small and large intestine better than cisapride or mosapride [21].

The main limitation of this study is being a single center study with a problem of generalizing the findings. Therefore, larger multicenter studies are crucially needed to document the role of prokinetic drugs in prevention of SBP.

Conclusions

Norfloxacin plus itopride (alkapride) prophylaxis reduced the possibility of development of recurrent SBP in addition to hepatorenal syndrome (HRS) which can precipitated by SBP and that clue why combined therapy improved HRS. This regimen can improve the survival rate in cirrhotic ascitic patients.

Abbreviations

Alb: Albumin; ALT: Alanine transaminase; AST: Aspartate transaminase; BMI: Body mass index; CBC: Complete blood count; DM: Diabetes mellitus; Hb: Hemoglobin; HBV: Hepatitis B virus; HCV: Hepatitis C virus; HTN: Hypertension; No.: Number; PCR: Polymerase chain reaction; PLT: Platelets; SBP: Spontaneous bacterial peritonitis; SD: Standard deviation; SVR: Sustained virological response; WBCs: White blood cells

Acknowledgements

The authors acknowledge all patients participated in this study and take responsibility for all aspects of the reliability and freedom from bias of the data presented and their discussed interpretation.

Authors' contributions

SA designed the study. SA and MAHS developed the methodology, AYMY, MAHS, and SA wrote the manuscript. AYMY, MAHS, GFA, and SA collected the data. All the authors participated sufficiently in the work and approved the final version of the manuscript. The authors have read and approved the manuscript.

Declarations

Ethics approval and consent to participate

The research was approved from Tanta University Faculty of medicine Research ethical committee with approval code 30766/7/18. The research also was approved by the ministry of health research ethical committee. An informed written consent was taken from each patient. The study protocol complies with the ethical guidelines of the 1975 Declaration of Helsinki as reflected in prior approval by the institution's Human Research Committee.

Competing interests

The authors declare that there is no conflict of interest.

Author details

[1]Department of Tropical Medicine and Infectious Diseases, Faculty of Medicine, Tanta University, Elbahr Street, Tanta 35111, Egypt. [2]Department of Clinical Pathology, Faculty of Medicine, Tanta University, Tanta, Egypt.

References

1. European Association for the Study of the Liver (EASL) (2018). EASL recommendations on treatment of hepatitis C 2018. J Hepatol.2018.
2. Thevenot T, Cadranel JF, Nguyen- Khac E, Tilmant L, Tiry C (2004) Diagnosis of spontaneous bacterial peritonitis in cirrhotic patients by use of two reagent strips. Eur J Gastro enterol Hepatol 16(16):579–583
3. Wiest R, Krag A and Gerbes A.(2012): Spontaneous bacterial peritonitis: recent guidelines and beyond. Gut. 2012; 61:297–310, 2, doi: https://doi.org/10.1136/gutjnl-2011-300779.
4. Kim J, Tsukamoto M, Mathur A (2014) Delayed paracentesis is associated withincreased in-hospital mortality in patients with spontaneous bacterialperitonitis. Am J Gastroenterol 109(9):1436–1442. https://doi.org/10.1038/ajg.2014.212
5. Arroyo V, Garcia-Martinez R, Salvatella X (2014) Human serum albumin, systemic inflammation, and cirrhosis. J Hepatol 61(2):396–407. https://doi.org/10.1016/j.jhep.2014.04.012
6. Runyon BA (2002) Strips and tubes: improving the diagnosis of spontaneous bacterial peritonitis. Hepatology 37(4):745–747
7. Paul K, Kaur J, Kazal HL (2015) To study the incidence, predictive factors and clinical outcome of spontaneous bacterial peritonitis in patients of cirrhosis with ascites. J Clin Diagn Res 9(7):9–12
8. Green TE, Bandy SM. (2015): Spontaneous bacterial peritonitis work up (online accessed 11 April 2016) URL: http://emedicine.medscape.com/article/789105-workup.
9. Agarwal MP, Choudhury BR, Banerjee BD, Kumar A (2008) Ascitic fluid examination for diagnosis of spontaneous bacterial peritonitis in cirrhotic ascites. J Indian Acad Clin Med 9(1):29–32
10. Mostafa MS, El-Seidi EA, Kassem AM, Shemis MA, Saber M, Michael MN (2015) Detection of ascitic fluid infections in patients with liver cirrhosis and ascites. Arab J Gastroenterol 12(1):20–24
11. Novella M, Solà R, Soriano G, Andreu M, Gana J, Ortiz J et al (1997) Continuous vs. inpatient prophylaxis of the first episode of spontaneous bacterial peritonitis in cirrhotic patients with norfloxacin. Hepatology 25(3): 532–536. https://doi.org/10.1002/hep.510250306
12. Rogers GB, van der Gast CJ, Bruce KD, Marsh P (2013) Ascitic microbiota composition is correlated with clinical severity in cirrhosis with portal hypertension. Plos One 8(9):e74884. https://doi.org/10.1371/journal.pone.0074884
13. Ghafara AA, Salah R, Ahmed A (2019) Rifaximin plus norfloxacin versus norfloxacin alone in primary prophylaxis of spontaneous bacterial peritonitis in patients with variceal bleeding. Egypt J Intern Med 31(3):281–287. https://doi.org/10.4103/ejim.ejim_6_19
14. Hanouneh MA, Hanouneh IA, Hashash JG, Law R, Esfeh JM, Lopez R et al (2012) The role of rifaximin in the primary prophylaxis of spontaneous bacterial peritonitis in patients with liver cirrhosis. J Clin Gastroenterol 46: 709–715
15. Fernandez J, Navasa M, Planas R, Montoliu S, Monfort D, Soriano G et al (2007) Primary prophylaxis of spontaneous bacterial peritonitis delays hepatorenal syndrome and improves survival in cirrhosis. Gastroenterology 133(3):818–824. https://doi.org/10.1053/j.gastro.2007.06.065
16. Fernandez J, Navasa J, Colmenero J (2002) Bacterial infections in cirrhosis: epidemiological changes with invasive procedures and norfloxacin prophylaxis. Hepatol 35(1):140–148. https://doi.org/10.1053/jhep.2002.30082
17. Revaiah PC, Kochhar R, Rana SV, Berry N, Ashat M, Dhaka N et al (2018) Risk of small intestinal bacterial overgrowth in patients receiving proton pump inhibitors versus proton pump inhibitors plus prokinetics. J Gastroenterol Hepatol 33:47–53
18. Frazee LA, Marinos AE, Rybarczyk AM, Fulton SA (2005) Long-term prophylaxis of spontaneous bacterial peritonitis in patients with cirrhosis. Ann Pharmacother 39(5):908–912. https://doi.org/10.1345/aph.1E585
19. Assem M, Elsabaawy M, Abdelrashed M (2016) Efficacy and safety of alternating norfloxacin and rifaximin as primary prophylaxis for spontaneous bacterial peritonitis in cirrhotic ascites: a prospective randomized open-label comparative multicenter study. Hepatol Int 10:377–385
20. Huang X, Lv B, Zhang S, Fan YH, Meng LN (2012) "Itopride therapy for functional dyspepsia: a meta-analysis".World. J Gastroenterol 18(48):7371–7377
21. Lim HC, Kim YG, Lim JH, Kim HS, Park H (2008) Effect of itopride hydrochloride on the ileal and colonic motility in guinea pig in vitro. Yonsei Med J 49:3

Hepatic ischemia reperfusion injury: effect of moderate intensity exercise and oxytocin compared to L-arginine in a rat model

Amr H. ELKady, Bataa M. Elkafoury[1], Dalia A. Saad[1*], Doaa M. Abd el-Wahed[1], Walaa Baher[2] and Mona A. Ahmed[1]

Abstract

Background: Hepatic ischemia reperfusion (IR) injury is considered as a main cause of liver damage and dysfunction. The L-arginine/nitric oxide pathway seems to be relevant during this process of IR. Although acute intense exercise challenges the liver with increased reactive oxygen species (ROS), regular training improves hepatic antioxidant status. Also, oxytocin (Oxy), besides its classical functions, it exhibits a potent antistress, anti-inflammatory, and antioxidant effects. This study was designed to evaluate the hepatic functional and structural changes induced by hepatic IR injury in rats and to probe the effect and potential mechanism of moderate intensity exercise training and/or Oxy, in comparison to a nitric oxide donor, L-arginine, against liver IR-induced damage.

Results: Compared to the sham-operated control group, the hepatic IR group displayed a significant increase in serum levels of ALT and AST, plasma levels of MDA and TNF-α, and significant decrease in plasma TAC and nitrite levels together with the worsening of liver histological picture. L-Arg, Oxy, moderate intensity exercise, and the combination of both Oxy and moderate intensity exercises ameliorated these deleterious effects that were evident by the significant decrease in serum levels of ALT and AST, significant elevation in TAC and nitrite, and significant decline in lipid peroxidation (MDA) and TNF-α, besides regression of histopathological score regarding hepatocyte necrosis, vacuolization, and nuclear pyknosis. Both the moderate intensity exercise-trained group and Oxy-treated group showed a significant decline in TNF-α and nitrite levels as compared to L-Arg-treated group. The Oxy-treated group showed statistical insignificant changes in serum levels of ALT, AST, and plasma levels of nitrite, MDA, TAC, and TNF-α as compared to moderate intensity exercise-trained group.

Conclusion: The combination of both moderate intensity exercise and Oxy displayed more pronounced hepatoprotection on comparison with L-Arg which could be attributed to their more prominent antioxidant and anti-inflammatory effects but not due to their NO-enhancing effect.

Keywords: Liver, Ischemia reperfusion injury, L-arginine, Nitric oxide, Exercise, Oxytocin

Background

Hepatic ischemia reperfusion (IR) injury is considered as the main cause of liver damage and dysfunction or functional failure and contributes to a high morbidity and mortality [1, 2]. Hepatic IR injury is commonly seen in hepatic surgery, such as in hepatectomy, liver transplantation, and resuscitation after shock [3, 4]. Also, abdominal trauma, myocardial ischemia, stroke, and hemorrhagic shock can cause insufficient liver blood flow, resulting in liver IR injury after reperfusion [5, 6].

The pathophysiology of hepatic IR injury is complex and multifactorial as it involves interaction with hepatocytes, liver sinusoidal and endothelial cells, Kupffer cells (KCs), and hepatic stellate cells. Also, it results in

* Correspondence: Drdalia2009@med.asu.edu.eg
[1]Physiology Department, Faculty of Medicine, Ain Shams University, Cairo, Egypt
Full list of author information is available at the end of the article

infiltration of inflammatory cells, activation of platelets, generation of reactive oxygen species (ROS), and reactive nitrogen species due to ischemia as well as reperfusion, increased levels of adhesion molecules, and release of cytokines and chemokines [7, 8].

During hepatic IR, the role of nitric oxide (NO) is ambiguous, because it may protect from the lesion owing to its vasodilator, antiplatelet, and ROS scavenging effect, or it may be a deleterious agent due to its interaction with superoxide radicals, forming peroxynitrite radicals [9, 10].

Exercise has been considered an important therapeutic tool in preventing and treating many diseases including obesity, non-alcoholic fatty liver disease, insulin resistance, type 2 diabetes, metabolic cardiovascular, and gastrointestinal disorders [11–13]. On the other hand, exercise may represent a physical stress that result in transient disruption of homeostasis [14]. The liver is considered the remarkably important organ during exercise outcomes due to its contribution in the modulation of ROS and inflammatory mediators [15]. Although acute intense exercise was found to challenge the liver with increased ROS and inflammation onset, regular exercise was found to induce hepatic antioxidant and anti-inflammatory improvements [16].

Oxytocin (Oxy), the hormone released from the posterior pituitary, besides its classical functions, was reported to exhibit a wide spectrum of central and peripheral activities [17]. Oxy has been shown to stimulate social behaviors and exert a potent anti-stress effect by reducing the activity in the hypothalamic-pituitary adrenocortical axis and sympathetic nervous system, and possess antioxidant and anti-inflammatory effects [18, 19]. Hekimoglu et al. [20] observed that Oxy protect against renal IR-induced remote liver injury by increasing NO synthase activity and releasing NO from vascular endothelium, suppression of inflammation, and regulation of oxidant-antioxidant status.

This study was carried out to investigate hepatic functional and structural changes induced by hepatic IR and to evaluate the effect and potential mechanisms of moderate intensity exercise training and Oxy, together or separately, in comparison to, a NO donor, L-arginine (L-Arg) in protecting the liver function from the damage induced by hepatic IR.

Methods

This study was carried out on 60 adult male albino rats, initially weighing 250–300 g. Rats were purchased from an animal farm in Helwan and were housed in the Faculty of Medicine, Ain Shams Research Institute (MASR I), under standard conditions of boarding at room temperature 22–25°C, 12-h light/dark cycle with free access to food and water. Regular meals were introduced daily at 8 am. Rats were fed standard rat diet. Rats were kept for 7 days before the experimental procedures for acclimatization. Animals included in the study were adult males after successful induction of the designated experiment and no animals were excluded.

Animal experiments were conducted in accordance to the Guide for Care and Use of Laboratory Animals, and the study protocol was approved by the Research Ethical Committee of Faculty of Medicine, Ain Shams University (FMASU, MD 100/2018).

Experimental animals

Rats were randomly allocated into the following six groups:

Group I: Sham-operated control (sham group) (n=10)

In the first 3 weeks, rats were kept undisturbed in their cages. In the fourth week, rats received L-Arg solvent daily, at 9 am, by oral gavage. At the end of the 4 weeks, rats were subjected to the same surgical procedures as the hepatic IR group without portal triad clamping.

Group II: Hepatic ischemia-reperfusion group (hepatic IR group) (n=10)

In the first 3 weeks, rats were kept undisturbed in their cages. In the fourth week, rats received L-Arg solvent daily, at 9 am, by oral gavage. At the end of the fourth week, rats underwent hepatic IR procedure (30 min of partial hepatic ischemia (70%) followed by 2 h of reperfusion) [21].

Group III: L-arginine-treated hepatic ischemia-reperfusion group (L-Arg + IR group) (n=10)

In the first 3 weeks, rats were kept undisturbed in their cages. In the fourth week, rats received L-Arg daily, at 9 am, by oral gavage in a dose of 100 mg/kg (7 days) [22].

Group IV: Exercise-trained hepatic ischemia-reperfusion group (Ex + IR group) (n=10)

Rats in this group were studied after 4 weeks of exposure to swim exercise 2 h daily (from 10 am to 12 pm) and 6 days/week [23]. In the fourth week, rats received distilled water as in sham group. At the end of the fourth week, rats underwent hepatic IR procedure.

Group V: Oxytocin-treated hepatic ischemia-reperfusion group (Oxy + IR group) (n=10)

In the first 3 weeks, rats were kept undisturbed in their cages. In the fourth week, rats received distilled water as in the sham group together with Oxy, daily at 9:30 am, by subcutaneous (S.C.) injection in a dose of 3.6 μg/100 g BW [24]. At the end of the fourth week, rats underwent hepatic IR procedure.

Group VI: Exercise-trained and oxytocin-treated hepatic ischemia-reperfusion group (Ex + Oxy + IR group) (n=10)
Rats in this group were studied after 4 weeks of exposure to swim exercise as in Ex + IR group. In the fourth week, rats received daily distilled water and S.C. Oxy as in Oxy + IR group. At the end of the fourth week, rats underwent hepatic IR procedure.

Experimental procedures

L-arginine treatment
L-Arg was supplied as powder by the Qualikems Fine Chemicals (New Delhi, India). A 100 mg of L-Arg was dissolved in 2-ml distilled water to make the final concentration of 50 mg/ml. At the beginning of fourth week of the study, rats received L-Arg, daily at 9 am by oral gavage in a dose of 100 mg/kg for 7 days [22].

Exercise Swim Training Program
At the beginning of the program, the aquatically naive rats were given the chance to stay in the water bath for 30 min in order to become familiar with water. This period was progressively increased everyday by 30 min till it reached 2 h per day, and this duration was maintained throughout the exercise period [25].

The dimensions of the swimming tank used were 70 cm in depth, 100 cm in length, and 70 cm in width. The tank was filled with water to a depth of 50 cm. Swimming water temperature was maintained at a thermoneutral temperature of 31 ± 1°C. The tank is equipped with a fan with strong motor (1425 revolutions per minute) that stir strong water currents. This equipment acts as a helping force to the rats to swim actively all the time and ensure uniformity of temperature. After each swimming session, the water was emptied from the tank and the tank was thoroughly cleaned.

The protocol of swimming consisted of one session of 2 h (from 10 am to 12 pm), 6 days/week for 4 weeks, which is considered a moderate intensity aerobic exercise [23].

Oxytocin treatment
Oxy was in the form of ampoules (10 IU/ml) supplied by the Novartis Pharmaceuticals (Switzerland). At the beginning of fourth week of the study, Oxy was administered daily at 9:30 am, by S.C. injection in a dose of 3.6 μg/100 g BW for 7 days [24].

Hepatic ischemia-reperfusion procedure
Hepatic IR in the present study was a model of partial hepatic ischemia (70% of liver mass) performed according to the method described by Shibamoto et al. [21]. The overnight fasted rats were weighed and anesthetized by intraperitoneal (i.p.) injection of ketamine (EPICO) in a dose of 50 mg/kg and xylazine HCl (ADWIA) in a dose of 10 mg/kg [26].

A midline longitudinal laparotomy was performed, followed by section of the falciform ligament. Then, by delicate digital maneuvers, the median hepatic lobe was pushed upwards in cranial direction to allow the exposure of the hepatic pedicle. Partial hepatic ischemia was induced by clamping the portal vein, hepatic artery, and bile duct (portal triad) supplying the median and left lobes with an atraumatic vascular clamp. In this method, the blood supply to the right and caudate lobes remained uninterrupted, attenuating intestinal congestion through portal flow bypass. Successful induction of the hepatic IR procedure was determined by visually comparing the ischemic lobes of liver (the median and left lobes) which turned pale denoting establishment of ischemia compared to non-ischemic lobes (right and caudate lobes), and also, successful reperfusion was observed by turning the color of ischemic lobes back to their pre-ischemic period and the non-ischemic lobes.

The abdomen was humidified with a saline solution in order to avoid fluid loss through evaporation, and the muscular layer was approximated with single stitches. After 30 min of ischemia, reperfusion was initiated by removing the clamp, and the abdomen was closed in a single layer. The animals were, then, allowed to recover. The reperfusion was allowed for 2 h.

The time of each procedure done was fixed throughout the study. All other groups—sham group, hepatic IR group, Ex + IR group, Oxy + IR group, and Ex + Oxy + IR group, also, received distilled water (L-Arg solvent) orally by gavage at 9 am for the same duration given to L-Arg + IR group in order to exclude the effect of the solvent and the maneuver of gavage. In addition, at the end of the study, the sham-operated control group was subjected to the same surgical steps of hepatic IR procedure without clamping of the portal triad, to exclude the effect of anesthesia, surgical incision, and the maneuver of hepatic pedicle exposure on the results obtained from rats that underwent hepatic IR.

Animals were not exposed to unnecessary pain or stress and animal manipulation was performed with maximal care and hygiene.

At the end of the reperfusion, rats were anaesthetized by i.p. injection of pentobarbital sodium (El-Gomhoreya Co., Egypt), in a dose of 40 mg/kg [27].

Then, a midline abdominal incision was made, and the abdominal aorta was exposed and cannulated. The blood was collected from the aorta into two tubes, a heparinized tube and serum clot activator tube with gel and then separated to plasma or serum and was stored at −80°C for later determination of biochemical assays.

After blood collection, animals were euthanized by intraperitoneal injection of overdose of pentobarbital sodium (El-Gomhoreya Co., Egypt), in a dose of 200 mg/kg.

Then, the liver was carefully dissected, and the left lobe of the liver was fixed in 10% buffered formalin solution for subsequent histopathological examination. Animal remains disposal occurred by incineration.

Biochemical analysis

- Determination of serum levels of alanine transferase (ALT) and aspartate transferase (AST) according to Henry [28] and Tietz [29], by the kinetic method optimized in accordance with I.F.C.C [30]., using BioMed-GPT kits supplied by Egy-Chem for Lab Technology, Egypt.
- Determination of the plasma level of nitrite according to Montgomery and Dymock [31], using the colorimetric kit supplied by Bio-diagnostic, Egypt.
- Determination of plasma level of malondialdehyde (MDA) according to Satoh [32] and Ohkawa et al. [33] using the colorimetric kit supplied by Bio-diagnostic, Egypt.
- Determination of the plasma level of total antioxidant capacity (TAC) according to Koracevic et al. [34], using colorimetric kit supplied by Bio-diagnostic, Egypt.
- Determination of the plasma level of tumor necrosis factor-alpha (TNF-α) by an enzyme immunoassay (ELISA) technique (Stat Fax 2100, Awareness Technology Inc, USA), using Rat TNF-α ELISA kits supplied by RayBio® tech, Inc., USA (Catalog: ELR-TNFa) according to the manufacturer instructions.

Histological examination of the liver tissue

The dissected specimens from the left lobe of the liver were fixed with 10% formalin solution immediately after removal (for at least 1 week) and were subjected to dehydration in ascending grades of alcohol, cleared in xylol, impregnated in pure soft paraffin, and embedded in hard paraffin [35]. Sections (8 μm) were cut and stained with hematoxylin and eosin (H&E). For microscopic examination, a microscope (Leica, DM2500) was used, and the images were taken at the Histology and Cell Biology Department, Faculty of Medicine, Ain Shams University, using a Canon EOS 1100D Digital SLR camera at 10 (ocular) × 40 (object lens) magnification. The liver histopathological changes were scored based on Suzuki et al. [36].

Statistical analysis

All statistical data, statistical significance, and correlations were performed by using the Statistical Program for Social Science (SPSS) statistical package (SPSS Inc.) version 20.0. One-way ANOVA was used to test for differences among the studied groups followed by LSD (least significant difference) to find inter-groupal significance. Results were expressed as mean and ± standard error of the mean and considered significant at a level $P<0.05$.

Results

Changes in serum levels of alanine transferase (ALT) and aspartate transferase (AST) and plasma level of nitrite (Table 1 and Fig. 1)

As compared to the sham group, the hepatic IR group resulted in a significant increase in the serum levels of ALT and AST. L-Arg + IR, Ex + IR, and Oxy + IR groups showed a significant decrease in the serum levels of ALT and AST compared to the hepatic IR group, but were significantly increased compared to sham group. L-Arg + IR, Ex + IR, and Oxy + IR groups exhibited statistically insignificant changes in the serum levels of ALT and AST when compared to each other.

Combined Ex + Oxy + IR group showed a significant reduction in serum levels of ALT and AST as compared to hepatic IR, L-Arg + IR, and Ex + IR groups. However, when compared to the sham group, the ALT level was significantly elevated, but the AST level was insignificantly changed.

As compared to the sham group, the hepatic IR group showed a significant decrease in the plasma level of nitrite. All treated groups—L-Arg+ IR, Ex+ IR, Oxy + IR, and combined Ex + Oxy + IR groups, showed a significant increase in the plasma level of nitrite as compared to the hepatic IR group. In L-Arg + IR group, the plasma level of nitrite showed a insignificant changes as compared to sham group. Both Oxy + IR and combined Ex + Oxy + IR groups showed statistically insignificant changes in the plasma level of nitrite as compared to the Ex + IR group, whereas in Ex + IR, Oxy + IR, and combined Ex + Oxy + IR groups, the nitrite level was significantly reduced compared to both the L-Arg + IR and sham groups.

Changes in plasma levels of malondialdehyde (MDA), total antioxidant capacity (TAC), and tumor necrosis factor-alpha (TNF-α) (Table 2 and Fig. 2)

As compared to the sham group, the hepatic IR group showed a significant increase in the plasma levels of MDA and TNF-α, but significant decrease in the plasma level of TAC.

Compared to the IR group, all the treated groups—L-Arg + IR, Ex + IR, Oxy + IR, and combined Ex + Oxy + IR groups, the plasma levels of MDA and TNF-α were significantly decreased, whereas the plasma level of TAC was significantly increased.

Table 1 Changes in the serum levels of alanine transferase (ALT) and aspartate transferase (AST), and the plasma level of nitrite in the different studied groups

Parameters groups	ALT U/ml	AST U/ml	Nitrite µmol/g
Sham-operated control	15.30 ± 0.955	21.30 ± 1.484	10.94 ± 0.596
Hepatic ischemia-reperfusion	51.70 ± 3.134 [a]	62.70 ± 4.475 [a]	2.879 ± 0.477 [a]
L-arginine-treated hepatic ischemia-reperfusion	28.00 ± 1.308 [a, b]	32.30 ± 1.274 [a, b]	11.32 ± 0.886 [b]
Exercise-trained hepatic ischemia reperfusion	26.70 ± 1.023 [a, b]	31.0 ± 2.056 [a, b]	6.240 ± 0.644 [a, b, c]
Oxytocin-treated hepatic ischemia-reperfusion	25.00 ± 1.528 [a, b]	31.30 ± 1.521 [a, b]	5.240 ± 0.578 [a, b, c]
Exercise-trained and oxytocin-treated hepatic ischemia-reperfusion	20.50 ± 1.500 [a, b, c, d]	22.20 ± 1.705 [b, c, d]	7.790 ± 0.484 [a, b, c]

Results are expressed as mean ±SEM and calculated by LSD at $P<0.05$
[a]Significance from the sham-operated control group
[b]Significance from the hepatic ischemia-reperfusion group
[c]Significance from the L-arginine hepatic ischemia-reperfusion group
[d]Significance from the exercise-trained hepatic ischemia-reperfusion group

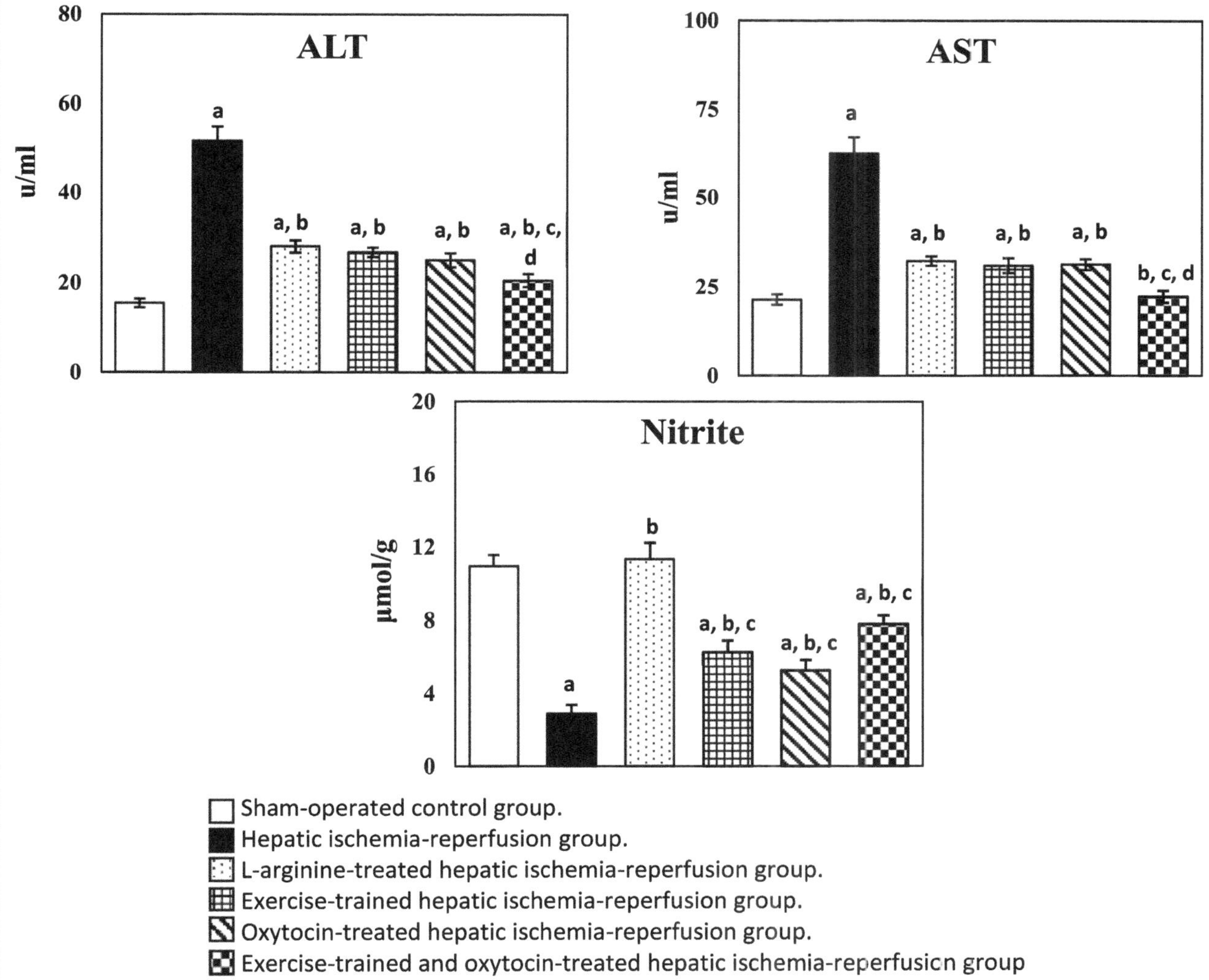

Fig. 1 Serum levels of alanine transferase (ALT), aspartate transferase (AST), and plasma level of the nitrite in the different studied groups. **a** Significance from the sham-operated control group calculated by LSD at $P<0.05$. **b** Significance from the hepatic ischemia-reperfusion group calculated by LSD at $P<0.05$. **c** Significance from the L-arginine-treated hepatic ischemia-reperfusion group calculated by LSD at $P<0.05$. **d** Significance from the exercise-trained hepatic ischemia-reperfusion group calculated by LSD at $P<0.05$

Table 2 Changes in the plasma levels of malondialdehyde (MDA), total antioxidant capacity (TAC), and tumor necrosis factor-alpha (TNF-α) in the different studied groups

Parameters groups	MDA nmol/g	TAC mM/L	TNF-α pg/ml
Sham-operated control	25.94 ± 3.237	80.48 ± 5.427	56.43 ± 3.662
Hepatic ischemia-reperfusion	110.6 ± 5.978 [a]	28.38 ± 2.584 [a]	145.2 ± 4.727 [a]
L-arginine-treated hepatic ischemia-reperfusion	67.70 ± 5.666 [a, b]	66.54 ± 3.784 [a, b]	96.24 ± 2.282 [a, b]
Exercise-trained hepatic ischemia reperfusion	56.08 ± 4.002 [a, b]	70.16 ± 3.938 [b]	85.52 ± 3.995 [a, b, c]
Oxytocin-treated hepatic ischemia-reperfusion	63.00 ± 4.567 [a, b]	65.30 ± 3.711 [a, b]	77.51 ± 2.721 [a, b, c]
Exercise-trained and oxytocin-treated hepatic ischemia-reperfusion	40.96 ± 4.334 [a, b, c, d]	76.77 ± 3.853 [b]	73.68 ± 3.612 [a, b, c, d]

Results are expressed as mean ±SEM and calculated by LSD at P<0.05
[a]Significance from the sham-operated control group
[b]Significance from the hepatic ischemia-reperfusion group
[c]Significance from the L-arginine hepatic ischemia-reperfusion group
[d]Significance from the exercise-trained hepatic ischemia-reperfusion group

However, in all studied treated groups, the plasma levels of MDA and TNF-α were still significantly higher compared to the sham group, whereas the plasma level of TAC was significantly decreased as compared to the sham group. Moreover, all the treated groups showed significantly lower plasma level of TAC except for Ex + IR and combined Ex + Oxy + IR groups which showed non-significant changes in TAC level.

Compared to the L-Arg + IR group, Ex + IR, and Oxy + IR groups showed a significant reduction in the plasma level of TNF-α with insignificant changes in the plasma levels of MDA and TAC, while the combined Ex + Oxy + IR group showed a significant reduction in the plasma levels of both MDA and TNF-α with non-significant change in the plasma level of TAC.

Compared to the Ex + IR group, the Oxy + IR group did not show any significant changes in the plasma levels of MDA, TAC, and TNF-α, while the combination of exercise and Oxy showed significantly lower plasma levels of MDA and TNF-α, but the plasma level of TAC exhibited an insignificant change.

Correlations between liver function parameters and other parameters (Fig. 3)

In correlation studies, the results were obtained from pooling of the different studied groups.

The serum levels of ALT and AST showed significant positive correlations with the plasma levels of MDA and TNF-α, but significant negative correlations with the plasma levels of TAC and nitrite.

Histopathological studies

Microscopic examination of the liver (Figs. 4 and 5)

The photomicrography of liver tissue of the sham-operated control group (Fig. 2a) showed that the liver was formed of acidophilic polyhedral hepatocytes having large central vesicular nuclei. The hepatocytes are arranged in irregular branching and anastomosing plates around a central vein (CV). The plates of hepatocytes are separated from each other by blood sinusoids (↑).

The photomicrography of the liver tissue of the hepatic IR group was shown in Fig. 4b, c. Figure 4b showed a wide area of hepatocyte vacuolization (▲), congestion of blood sinusoids (↑), and darkly stained pyknotic nuclei (P) in most of the hepatocytes. Figure 4 c showed wide area of focal hepatic necrosis (thick arrow) in which a number of adjacent hepatocytes are lost and replaced by inflammatory cells.

Photomicrography of the liver tissue of L-Arg group (Fig. 5a) showed dilatation and congestion of blood sinusoids (▲) in between hepatocytic cords. Some sporadic hepatocytes show condensed pyknotic nuclei (↑), whereas a small focal area of hepatocytic necrosis (thick arrow) is detected.

The photomicrography of the liver tissue of the Ex + IR group (Fig. 5b) showed dilatation and congestion of the blood sinusoids separating hepatocytes plates (▲). Focal areas of hepatocytes necrosis (thick arrow) in which the hepatocytes are replaced by inflammatory cells. Some hepatocytes show cytoplasmic vacuolization (↑).

Photomicrography of the liver tissue of the Oxy group (Fig. 5c) showed the focal area of hepatic necrosis (thick arrow) in which the hepatocytes are replaced by inflammatory cells. Some hepatocytes show vacuolation of their cytoplasm (V).

Photomicrography of the liver tissue of the combined Ex + Oxy group (Fig. 5d) showed a congestion of blood sinusoids (▲). A small focal area of hepatic necrosis (thick arrow) is detected where the hepatocytes are replaced by inflammatory cells.

Histopathological grading of the liver (Table 3)

As shown in Table 3, the histopathological grading for liver changes included three parameters: congestion, vacuolization, and necrosis. For all parameters, the

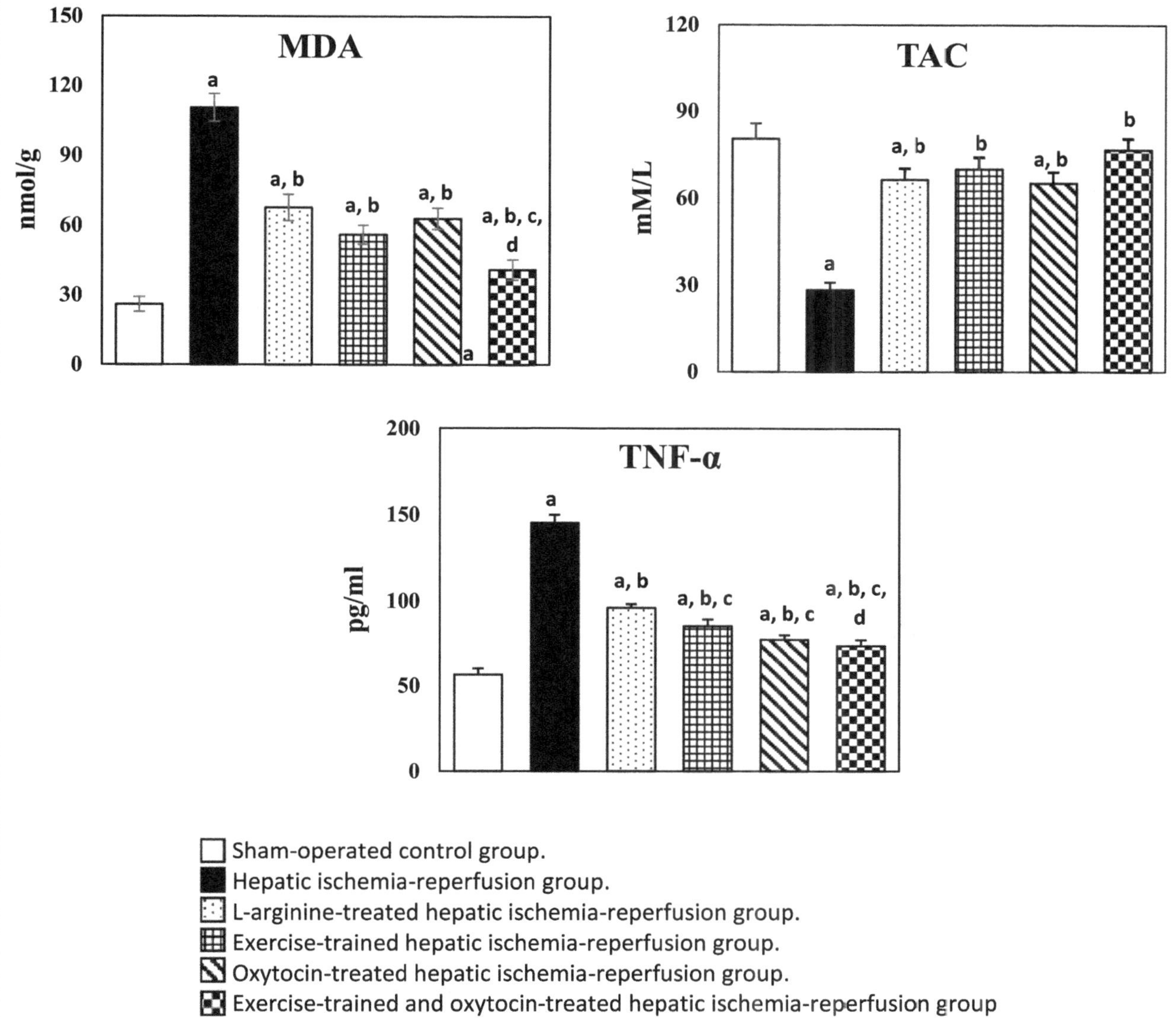

Fig. 2 Plasma levels of malondialdehyde (MDA), total antioxidant capacity (TAC), and tumor necrosis factor-alpha (TNF-α) in the different studied groups. **a** Significance from the sham-operated control group calculated by LSD at $P<0.05$. **b** The significance from the hepatic ischemia-reperfusion group calculated by LSD at $P<0.05$. **c** The significance from the L-arginine-treated hepatic ischemia-reperfusion group calculated by LSD at $P<0.05$. **d** The significance from the exercise-trained hepatic ischemia-reperfusion group calculated by LSD at $P<0.05$

hepatic IR group was the most affected and was graded for the highest scores in all parameters.

As regards congestion, the hepatic IR group was the most affected group followed by the L-Arg group and Oxy group as 65%, 55%, and 50%, respectively, of examined fields showed congestion in zones 2 and 3 of most lobules (score 3). On the other hand, the combined Ex + Oxy group scored 2 as 55% of the examined fields showed zone 3 sinusoidal congestion in some lobules. The least affected group by congestion was the Ex group, which scored 1 as 60% of the examined fields revealed scattered sinusoidal congestion.

Regarding hepatocellular vacuolization, the hepatic IR group was the most affected group in which 55% of the examined fields showed prominent clusters of hepatocellular vacuolization in most lobules (score 3). On the other hand, L-Arg, Ex, Oxy, and Ex + Oxy groups were all scored 1 but with variable percentages as 50%, 60%, 50%, and 60%, respectively, of the examined fields showed scattered cell vacuolization in most lobules or prominent cluster in one lobule.

Regarding the necrosis of the hepatocellular tissue, the hepatic IR group was the most affected group and the only group that scored 2, as 55% of the examined fields

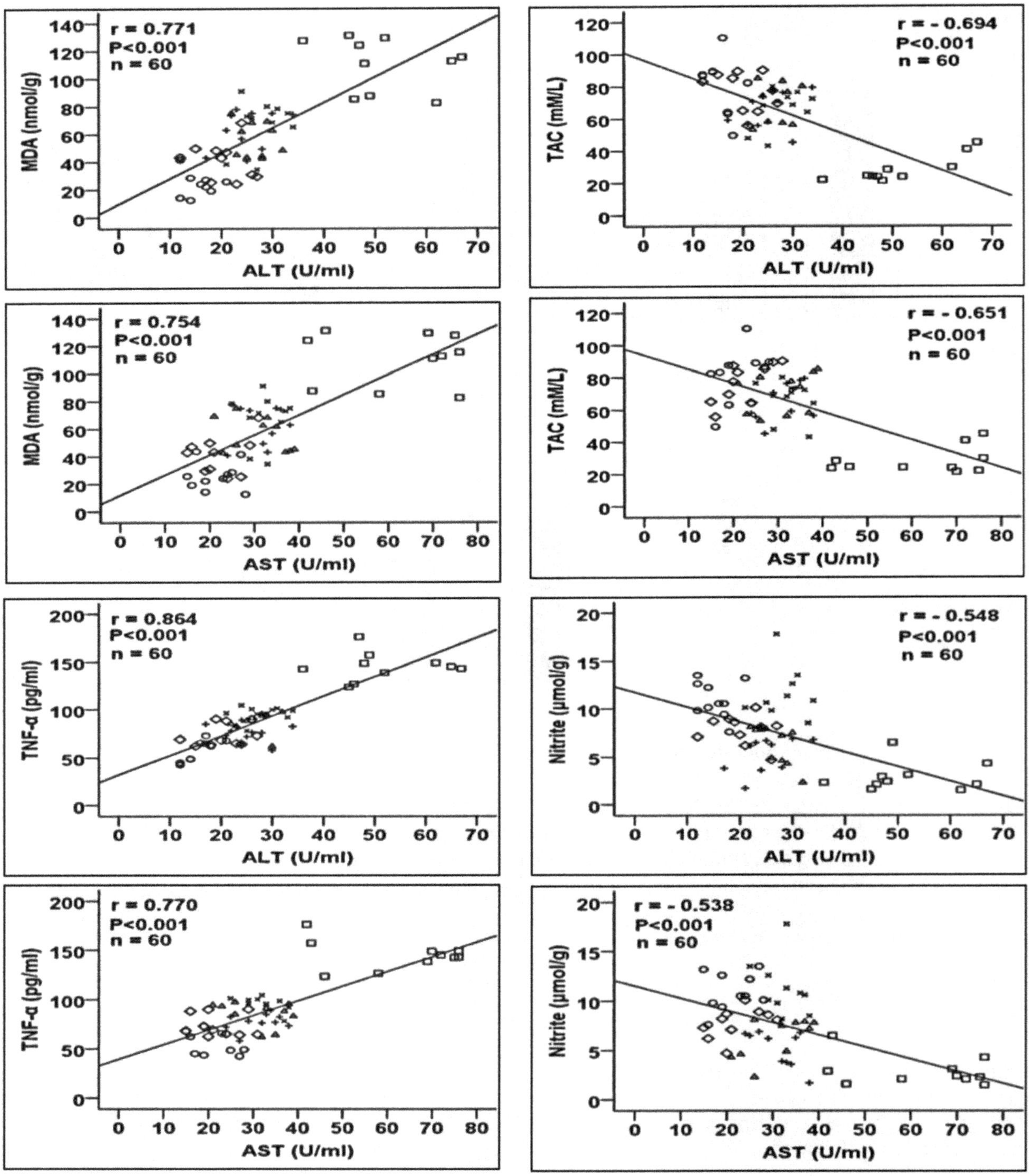

Fig. 3 Correlations between the serum levels of alanine transferase (ALT), aspartate transferase (AST), and plasma levels of malondialdehyde (MDA), total antioxidant capacity (TAC), tumor necrosis factor-alpha (TNF-α), and nitrite in the different studied groups. o Sham-operated control group. □ Hepatic ischemia-reperfusion group. x L-arginine-treated hepatic ischemia-reperfusion group. Δ Exercise-trained hepatic ischemia-reperfusion group. + Oxytocin-treated hepatic ischemia-reperfusion group. ◊ Exercise-trained and oxytocin-treated hepatic ischemia-reperfusion group

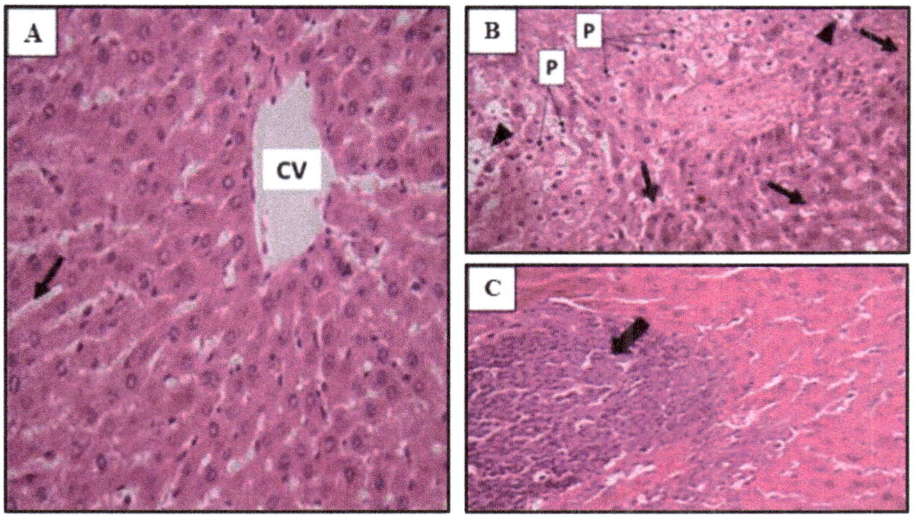

Fig. 4 Photomicrograph of liver tissue sections: **a** Sham-operated control group and **b, c** hepatic ischemia reperfusion group). (H&E X400)

showed less than 30% necrosis. On the other hand, L-Arg, Ex, Oxy, and Ex + Oxy groups, scored 1 as 45%, 50%, 55%, and 55%, respectively, of the examined fields in each group showed a single-cell necrosis in most lobules.

Discussion

In this work, hepatic ischemia was successfully induced by 70% occlusion for 30 min followed by 2 h reperfusion. Hepatic IR resulted in hepatic injury as proved by increased level of liver enzymes. Hepatic IR causes the disruption of the membrane stability of hepatocytes due to necrosis, cellular damage, and structural changes with release of large quantities of liver enzymes [37–39].

Moreover, a histopathological study showed a corrupted hepatic architecture in the form of hepatocyte vacuolization and necrosis, nuclear pyknosis, lymphocytic infiltration, and congestion of blood sinusoids. These findings agree with the results of previous studies by Peralta et al. [40], Serracino-Inglatt et al. [41], and Crockett et al. [42].

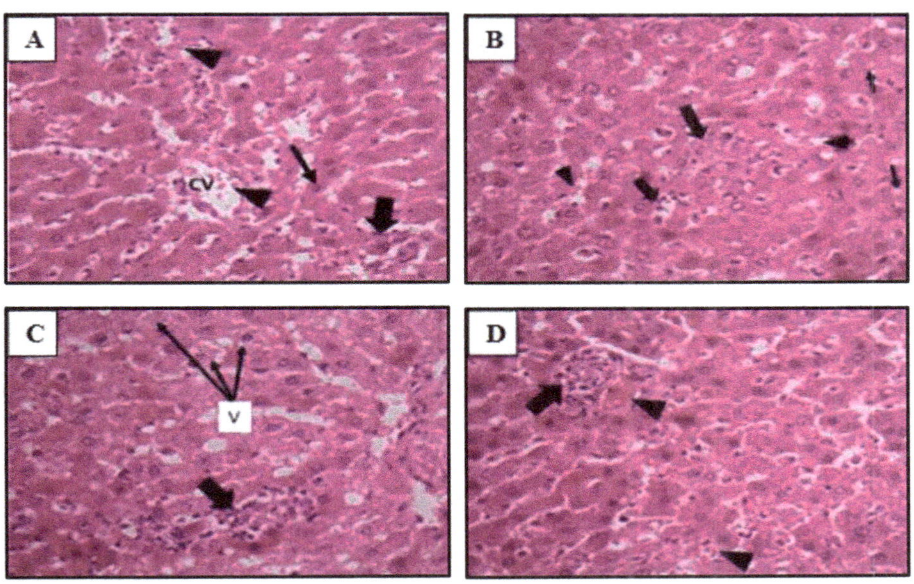

Fig. 5 Photomicrograph of liver tissue sections of **a** L-arginine-treated hepatic ischemia-reperfusion group, **b** exercise-trained hepatic ischemia-reperfusion group, **c** oxytocin-treated hepatic ischemia-reperfusion group, and **d** exercise-trained and oxytocin-treated hepatic ischemia-reperfusion group. (H&E X400)

Table 3 Liver histopathological scoring system showing number and frequency distribution (%) of each component examined in two different field sections in 10 rats (20 fields/group)

Component	Congestion[a]					Vacuolization[a]					Necrosis*				
Defined range Group	0	1	2	3	4	0	1	2	3	4	0	1	2	3	4
Sham-operated control group	16	3	1	0	0	19	1	0	0	0	18	2	0	0	0
	80%	15%	5%			95%	5%				90%	10%			
Hepatic ischemia-reperfusion group	2	2	3	13	0	3	1	5	11	0	1	4	11	4	0
	10%	10%	15%	65%		15%	5%	25%	55%		5%	20%	55%	20%	
L-arginine-treated hepatic ischemia-reperfusion group	2	3	4	11	0	2	10	5	3	0	4	9	4	3	0
	10%	15%	20%	55%		10%	50%	25%	15%		20%	45%	20%	15%	
Exercise-trained hepatic ischemia-reperfusion group	3	12	3	2	0	4	12	3	1	0	6	10	2	2	0
	15%	60%	15%	10%		20%	60%	15%	5%		30%	50%	10%	10%	
Oxytocin-treated hepatic ischemia-reperfusion group	2	4	4	10	0	2	10	4	4	0	4	11	3	2	0
	10%	20%	20%	50%		10%	50%	20%	20%		20%	55%	15%	10%	
Exercise-trained and oxytocin-treated hepatic ischemia-reperfusion group	3	3	11	3	0	3	12	3	2	0	6	11	2	1	0
	15%	15%	55%	15%		15%	60%	15%	10%		30%	55%	10%	5%	

In component: necrosis, the defined ranges indicate; 0= No damage; 1=Single cell necrosis; 2= less than 30% necrosis; 3= less than 60% necrosis; 4= more than 60% necrosis

[a]In components: Congestion and vacuolization, the defined ranges indicate; 0= No damage; 1=Minimal congestion, minimal vacuolization; 2= Mild congestion, mild vacuolization; 3= Moderate congestion, moderate vacuolization; 4= Severe congestion, severe vacuolization

The present hepatic functional and structural damage could be attributed to oxidative stress, increased ROS production, and lipid peroxidation associated with decreased antioxidant defense. This is proved by the increased plasma MDA and decreased plasma TAC. The decreased TAC could be explained by its over consumption to face the increased oxidative stress. Meanwhile, liver enzymes showed a significant positive correlation with MDA and a significant negative correlation with TAC.

This view is in line with previous reports which showed that reperfusion caused a generation of ROS that reacts with lipids in the cell membranes and initiate lipid peroxidation and is responsible for the IR injury [43, 44].

In addition, the initial stage of hepatic IR is reported to mediate the oxidative stress, the production of massive amounts of ROS, neutrophil activation, and its adherence to endothelial cells and release of proteases and finally induce death of hepatocyte [45].

In the current work, a significant positive correlation between the plasma levels of MDA and TNF-α is observed which could be explained by the ability of ROS to induce an inflammatory response via cellular signaling [46, 47]. In addition to the significant increase in the plasma level of TNF-α following hepatic IR and its significant positive correlations with liver enzymes in this study, it denotes that TNF-α could be involved as an underlying mechanism in the current hepatic dysfunction and structural damage [48].

Other studies demonstrated that IR results in increased gene expression of both nuclear factor kappa B (NF-kβ) and Toll-like receptor 4 (a protein involved in both innate and adaptive immune system response), which constantly increased TNF-α leading to liver damage [38, 49].

TNF-α has been reported to induce inflammation by several mechanisms. It interacts with other inflammatory cytokines and chemokines and activates the production of ROS [50]. In addition, TNF-α upregulates the expression of intercellular adhesion molecule-1 and vascular cell adhesion molecule-1 on endothelial cells, activating the transcription factor; NF-kβ resulting in the production of inflammatory mediators as TNF-α, interleukins (IL); IL-1-B, IL-6, inducible nitric oxide synthase, and cyclo-oxygenase with amplification of the process of inflammation [51–53].

The decreased plasma level of nitrite observed in hepatic IR rats provides an additional explanation for the observed hepatic functional and structural damage. This deduced from significant increase in the serum levels of ALT and AST and their significant negative correlations with the plasma level of nitrite.

In line with this, Taha et al. [54] reported that IR injury is associated with a remarkable decrease in the bioavailability of NO, which represents an important initiating event in the pathophysiology of post-ischemic injury in a variety of different tissues, including the liver.

Diminished NO levels within liver during IR was found to be derived from both decreased production due to downregulation of endothelial nitric oxide synthase (eNOS) with hepatic IR, and increased scavenging by the elevated levels of ROS produced during reperfusion [1, 55, 56]. This scavenging causes the formation of peroxynitrite, the free radical, that rapidly reacts with all components such as proteins, lipids, and DNA further damaging the cell [57].

Insufficient NO production was assumed to be the main cause for vasoconstriction during reperfusion period, sinusoidal narrowing, and reduction of microcirculatory blood flow [58, 59]. Moreover, hepatic IR injury was attributed to an imbalance in the ratio of endothelin (ET) to NO, with an increase in the plasma levels of ET and a concomitant fall in the plasma levels of NO in the first few hours of reperfusion [53].

The significant negative correlation exerted between the plasma nitrite and plasma MDA in the current work suggests that the oxidative stress could be implicated in reduction of nitrite plasma level.

Pretreatment with L-Arg attenuated hepatic IR injury as evidenced by decreased liver enzymes and hepatic damage. Hepatocytes had regression of necrosis, vacuolization, and nuclear pyknosis.

In this study, the favorable effects of L-Arg on hepatic functional and structural alterations could be attributed to the increased NO level deduced from the significant increase in the plasma level of nitrite by L-Arg treatment so that it reached the control values and the associated significant negative correlations existed between plasma level of nitrite and serum levels of ALT and AST.

This is in consistence with other studies, in which pretreatment with L-Arg resulted in activation of NO synthesis, increased concentrations of NO stable metabolites nitrite, and nitrate anions in both the blood and liver tissue and suppression of increased ALT and AST activities [60]. In addition, the activation of eNOS and the production of NO by this enzyme was found to increase liver graft preservation and improve liver function after reperfusion [61, 62].

The beneficial effects of the modulation of L-Arg/NO pathway was attributed before to the increase in NO bioavailability that acts by promoting microvasculature vasodilatation, opposing vasoconstriction mediated by ET, inhibition of platelet aggregation, and adhesion, as well as the reduction of interaction between leukocytes and endothelial surface resulting in the reduction of the inflammatory activity, and inhibiting caspases to prevent apoptosis, in addition to the superoxide scavenging property and detoxification of ROS following L-Arg use [63, 64].

It seems that L-Arg mediates its protective effect in hepatic IR in the present study not only through NO, but also has direct antioxidant effect deduced from the significant decrease in the plasma level of MDA and the significant increase in the plasma level of TAC. This assumption is supported by the significant negative correlations existed between nitrite and MDA, as well as the significant positive correlation between nitrite and TAC. In line with our assumption, in a rat model of carbon tetrachloride-induced hepatotoxicity, pre- and post-treatment with L-Arg decreased the hepatic MDA content and enhanced the hepatic antioxidant enzymes; these results were attributed either to NO ability to function as scavenger or to the antioxidant effects of L-Arg itself [65].

The other protective mechanisms of L-Arg could be attributed to its anti-inflammatory mechanism. This is deduced from the suppression of TNF-α plasma level by treatment as well as the significant negative correlation between plasma levels of nitrite and TNF-α.

In agreement, NO was reported to inhibit pro-inflammatory cytokines, including TNF-α, IL-1B, IL-1α, and IL-12, which may induce inflammatory cascade during liver IR injury [8, 54].

The exercise model encountered in this study was in the form of chronic moderate swimming exercise, 2 h daily and 6 days/week for 4 weeks. This exercise training ameliorated hepatic injury and dysfunction induced by hepatic IR, as revealed by a significant decrease in the serum levels of ALT and AST and the plasma levels of MDA and TNF-α, but a significant increase in TAC and nitrite levels. Also, an improvement of hepatic morphology was demonstrated by the decreased score of necrosis, vacuolization, and congestion compared to hepatic IR group.

These findings denote that exercise training abrogated hepatic functional and structural impairment induced by hepatic IR. These results are consistent with previous studies [21, 66, 67].

Exercise training exerts more powerful anti-inflammatory and antioxidant defense effects than L-Arg with less hepatocellular injury. This is evidenced by significant decrease in plasma TNF-α and the increase in plasma TAC that reached control values and better regression of scores of vascular congestion, hepatocyte necrosis, and vacuolization. Meanwhile, the serum levels of ALT and AST and plasma levels of nitrite and MDA were insignificantly changed.

The current proposed anti-inflammatory role of exercise training is supported by other studies [66, 68–70]. Similarly, Dallak et al. [71] showed that swim exercise for 60 min three times per week, for 4 weeks, reduced the serum levels of inflammatory biomarker, TNF-α in a rat model of high fat diet, via reduction in visceral fat mass with a subsequent decrease in adipokine release.

The decrease in final body weight and BW % change recorded in the Ex + IR group (unpublished data) compared to the IR, L-Arg – IR, and sham groups could provide possible explanation for the reduction of plasma TNF-α. The adipose tissue was found to be able to produce inflammatory cytokines such as TNF-α and IL-6 and several potent chemo-attractant cytokines [72]. The accumulation of monocytes as macrophages in the adipose tissue is thought to be a major source of increased systemic concentrations of inflammatory cytokines [73].

Opposite to our work, the intense exercise was found to induce muscle microtraumas, increase the release of inflammatory cytokines into the bloodstream [74, 75], and lead to tissue damage with increased production of ROS and inflammatory mediators [76, 77] induce hepatic inflammation through inflammatory cell infiltration in rats [78]. This contradiction could result from the use of different intensities and durations of exercise models other than the model used in the current study.

Exercise training in the present work had protective effect not only through anti-inflammatory mechanisms but also had antioxidant effect. Other studies showed that regular exercise enhance hepatic antioxidant capacity, redox status, reduced the hepatic MDA level which reflect lipid peroxidation [66, 67, 79, 80].

On the contrary to the present results, severe exercise was found to mediate an oxidative effect and to increase the hepatic MDA levels. The authors assumed that intense exercise increases oxygen consumption and may produce an imbalance between ROS and antioxidants, inducing oxidative stress [76].

Compared to L-Arg treatment, moderate intensity exercise did not differ significantly as regards the serum levels of ALT and AST and the plasma levels of MDA and TAC but showed only a significant decrease in the plasma levels of TNF-α and nitrite which indicated that the hepatoprotective effect of moderate intensity exercise was largely dependent of its anti-inflammatory effects and only dependent partly on increasing NO.

Compared to hepatic IR, Oxy pretreatment in the Oxy + IR group resulted in improvement of hepatic dysfunction which was observed from the significant reduction in the serum levels of ALT and AST, plasma levels of MDA and TNF-α together with significant increase in TAC and nitrite and alleviated IR histopathological injury. However, such improvements did not reach the control levels. These results are in agreement of other studies [81–83].

The beneficial effect of Oxy against hepatic IR could be attributed to suppression of oxidative stress as confirmed by the significant decrease in plasma level MDA and the significant increase in the plasma level of TAC. In addition to its anti-inflammatory effect as seen by decrease in plasma TNF-α.

The antioxidative effect of Oxy was attributed to its ability to break lipid peroxidation chain [82, 84, 85]. While its anti-inflammatory effect was mediated by reduction of the serum TNF-α, inhibition of neutrophils migration and neutrophil-derived pro-inflammatory cytokines, parenchymal injury, and tissue inflammation [81].

Also, the increased plasma level of nitrite upon Oxy treatment in the Oxy + IR group compared to the hepatic IR group, could be a third mechanism by which Oxy can produce hepatoprotection during IR.

However, the Oxy + IR group did not differ from the L-Arg + IR group regarding the serum levels of ALT and AST and the plasma levels of MDA and TAC but only showed a significant reduction in the plasma levels of TNF-α and nitrite which indicated that hepatoprotective effect Oxy was mediated mainly through its anti-inflammatory effect of but less on its NO producing effect.

Combination of both exercise training and Oxy pretreatment in the Ex + Oxy + IR group resulted in the attenuation of the hepatic damage caused by hepatic IR evidenced by the significant decrease in serum levels of ALT and AST, and plasma levels of MDA and TNF-α together with a significant elevation in the plasma levels of TAC and nitrite and histopathological improvement.

On comparison with L-Arg, combination of both exercise and Oxy in this study displayed more pronounced hepatoprotection evidenced by the significant decrease in the serum levels of ALT and AST together with recession of histopathological injury, to a greater extent than in L-Arg. Such superiority of combined treatment over L-Arg could be attributed to their more prominent antioxidant and anti-inflammatory effects but not due to their NO-enhancing effect as the plasma levels of MDA, TNF-α, and nitrite were significantly lower than in L-Arg-treated group.

Compared to exercise only group (Ex + IR), the combination of exercise and Oxy in the Ex + Oxy + IR group exerted additive effects which offered more hepatoprotection where the levels of ALT, AST, TNF-α, and MDA were significantly lowered indicating dampening of the inflammatory response and lipid peroxidation which is independent on NO as its level did not differ significantly in both groups.

Conclusion

Hepatic IR impaired functional and structural integrity of the liver. Pretreatment with L-Arg, Oxy, and exercise training abrogated hepatic functional and structural impairment induced by IR. Exercise training exerts more powerful anti-inflammatory and antioxidant defense effects than L-Arg, whereas Oxy acts as more powerful anti-inflammatory agent, however, a less powerful NO-inducing agent than L-Arg. Combination of both exercise and Oxy displayed more pronounced hepatoprotection on comparison with L-Arg on hepatic structural and functional changes induced by hepatic IR and such superiority of combined treatment over L-Arg could be attributed to their more prominent antioxidant and anti-inflammatory effects but not due to their NO-enhancing effect.

Abbreviations

ALT: Alanine transferase; ANOVA: Analysis of variance; AST: Aspartate transferase; ELISA: Enzyme immunoassay; ET: Endothelin; eNOS: Endothelial nitric oxide synthase; Ex + IR group: Exercise-trained hepatic ischemia-reperfusion group; Ex + Oxy + IR group: Exercise-trained and oxytocin-treated hepatic ischemia-reperfusion group; H&E: Hematoxylin and eosin; IL: Interleukin; IR group: Hepatic ischemia-reperfusion group; IR: Ischemia reperfusion; KCs: Kupffer cells; L-Arg + IR group: L-arginine-treated hepatic ischemia-reperfusion group; L-Arg: L-arginine; LSD: Least significant difference; MASRI: The Faculty of Medicine, Ain Shams University Research Institute; MDA: Malondialdehyde; NF-kβ: Nuclear factor kappa B; NO: Nitric oxide; NOS: Nitric oxide synthase; Oxy + IR group: Oxytocin-treated hepatic ischemia-reperfusion group; Oxy: Oxytocin; ROS: Reactive oxygen species; Sham group: Sham-operated control; TAC: Total antioxidant capacity; TNF-α: Tumor necrosis factor-α

Acknowledgements
I would like to thank Dr. Laila Ahmed Rashed, Professor of Medical Biochemistry and Molecular Biology, Faculty of Medicine, Cairo University, for her contribution in the biochemical studies.

Authors' contributions
AE was responsible for the manuscript elaboration and for conducting the project and worked on all of its stages. DA.S. and DA assisted in animal handling and in the discussions regarding the results. WB assisted in the histological procedures and result interpretation. BE revised the manuscript. MA is the main investigator who planned, designed, and supervised the project. The authors approved the final manuscript.

Declarations

Ethics approval and consent to participate
The study protocol was approved by the Research Ethical Committee of Faculty of Medicine, Ain Shams University (FMASU, MD 100/2018).

Competing interests
The authors declare that they have no competing interests.

Author details
[1]Physiology Department, Faculty of Medicine, Ain Shams University, Cairo, Egypt. [2]Histology Department, Faculty of Medicine, Ain Shams University, Cairo, Egypt.

References
1. Peralta C, Jiménez-Castro MB, Gracia-Sancho J (2013) Hepatic ischemia and reperfusion injury: effects on the liver sinusoidal milieu. J Hepatol. 59(5): 1094–1106. https://doi.org/10.1016/j.jhep.2013.06.017
2. Costa CCC, Pereira NG, Machado ALM, Dórea MA, Cruz RMMD, Silva RC, Domingues RJS, Yasojima EY (2019) Splenic ischemic preconditioning attenuates oxidative stress induced by hepatic ischemia-reperfusion in rats. Acta Cir Bras. 34(7):e201900707. https://doi.org/10.1590/s0102-865020190070000007
3. Jaeschke H (2003) Molecular mechanisms of hepatic ischemia-reperfusion injury and preconditioning. Am J Physiol Gastrointest Liver Physiol. 284(1): G15–G26. https://doi.org/10.1152/ajpgi.00342.2002
4. Douzinas EE, Livaditi O, Tasoulis MK, Prigouris P, Bakos D, Goutas N, Vlachodimitropoulos D, Andrianakis I, Betrosian A, Tsoukalas GD (2012) Nitrosative and oxidative stresses contribute to post-ischemic liver injury following severe hemorrhagic shock: the role of hypoxemic resuscitation. PLoS One. 7(3):e32968. https://doi.org/10.1371/journal.pone.0032968
5. van Riel WG, van Golen RF, Reiniers MJ, Heger M, van Gulik TM (2016) How much ischemia can the liver tolerate during resection? Hepatobiliary Surg Nutr. 5(1):58–71. https://doi.org/10.3978/j.issn.2304-3881.2015.07.05
6. Wang W, Wu L, Li J, Ji J, Chen K, Yu Q, Li S, Feng J, Liu T, Zhang J, Chen J, Zhou Y, Mao Y, Wang F, Dai W, Fan X, Guo C, Wu J (2019) Alleviation of hepatic ischemia reperfusion injury by oleanolic acid pretreating via reducing HMGB1 release and inhibiting apoptosis and autophagy. Mediators Inflamm. 2019:3240713–3240710. https://doi.org/10.1155/2019/3240713
7. Montalvo-Jave EE, Escalante-Tattersfield T, Ortega-Salgado JA, Piña E, Geller DA (2008) Factors in the pathophysiology of the liver ischemia-reperfusion injury. J Surg Res. 147(1):153–159. https://doi.org/10.1016/j.jss.2007.06.015
8. Guan LY, Fu PY, Li PD, Li ZN, Liu HY, Xin MG, Li W (2014) Mechanisms of hepatic ischemia-reperfusion injury and protective effects of nitric oxide. World J Gastrointest Surg. 6(7):122–128. https://doi.org/10.4240/wjgs.v6.i7.122
9. Jiang WW, Kong LB, Li GQ, Wang XH (2009) Expression of iNOS in early injury in a rat model of small-for-size liver transplantation. Hepatobiliary Pancreat Dis Int. 8(2):146–151. 19357027
10. Lucas ML, Rhoden CR, Rhoden EL, Zettler CG, Mattos AA (2015) Effects of L-arginine and L-NAME on ischemia-reperfusion in rat liver. Acta Cir Bras. 30(5):345–352. https://doi.org/10.1590/S0102-865020150050000006
11. Seo DY, Lee SR, Kim N, Ko KS, Rhee BD, Han J (2014) Humanized animal exercise model for clinical implication. Pflugers Arch. 466(9):1673–1687. https://doi.org/10.1007/s00424-014-1496-0
12. Orci LA, Gariani K, Oldani G, Delaune V, Morel P, Toso C (2016) Exercise-based interventions for nonalcoholic fatty liver disease: a meta-analysis and meta-regression. Clin Gastroenterol Hepatol. 14(10):1398–1411. https://doi.org/10.1016/j.cgh.2016.04.036
13. Jakicic JM, Rogers RJ, Davis KK, Collins KA (2018) Role of physical activity and exercise in treating patients with overweight and obesity. Clin Chem. 64(1):99–107. https://doi.org/10.1373/clinchem.2017.272443
14. Mastorakos G, Pavlatou M (2005) Exercise as a stress model and the interplay between the hypothalamus-pituitary-adrenal and the hypothalamus-pituitary-thyroid axes. Horm Metab Res. 37(9):577–584. https://doi.org/10.1055/s-2005-870426
15. Pillon Barcelos R, Bresciani G, Rodriguez-Miguelez P, Cuevas MJ, Soares FA, Barbosa NV, González-Gallego J (2016) Diclofenac pretreatment effects on the toll-like receptor 4/nuclear factor kappa B-mediated inflammatory response to eccentric exercise in rat liver. Life Sci. 148:247–253. https://doi.org/10.1016/j.lfs.2016.02.006
16. Pillon Barcelos R, Freire Royes LF, Gonzalez-Gallego J, Bresciani G (2017) Oxidative stress and inflammation: liver responses and adaptations to acute and regular exercise. Free Radic Res. 51(2):222–236. https://doi.org/10.1080/10715762.2017.1291942
17. Viero C, Shibuya I, Kitamura N, Verkhratsky A, Fujihara H, Katoh A, Ueta Y, Zingg HH, Chvatal A, Sykova E, Dayanithi G (2010) REVIEW: Oxytocin: crossing the bridge between basic science and pharmacotherapy. CNS Neurosci Ther. 16(5):e138–e156. https://doi.org/10.1111/j.1755-5949.2010.00185.x
18. Ondrejcakova M, Bakos J, Garafova A, Kovacs L, Kvetnansky R, Jezova D (2010) Neuroendocrine and cardiovascular parameters during simulation of stress-induced rise in circulating oxytocin in the rat. Stress. 13(4):314–322. https://doi.org/10.3109/10253891003596822
19. Uvnäs Moberg K, Handlin L, Kendall-Tackett K, Petersson M (2019) Oxytocin is a principal hormone that exerts part of its effects by active fragments. Med Hypotheses. 133:109394. https://doi.org/10.1016/j.mehy.2019.109394
20. Tas Hekimoglu A, Toprak G, Akkoc H, Evliyaoglu O, Ozekinci S, Kelle I (2013) Oxytocin ameliorates remote liver injury induced by renal ischemia-reperfusion in rats. Korean J Physiol Pharmacol. 17(2):169–173. https://doi.org/10.4196/kjpp.2013.17.2.169
21. Shibamoto T, Kuda Y, Tanida M, Wang M, Kurata Y (2015) Exercise attenuates ischemia-reperfusion injury of nonalcoholic fatty liver in OLETF rat. Gastroenterol Pancreatol Liver Disord. 2(2):1–6. https://doi.org/10.15226/2374-815X/2/2/00132
22. Chattopadhyay P, Verma N, Verma A, Kamboj T, Khan NA, Wahi AK (2008) L-arginine protects from pringle manoeuvre of ischemia-reperfusion induced liver injury. Biol Pharm Bull. 31(5):890–892. https://doi.org/10.1248/bpb.31.890
23. Abd-Allah AB, Megahed AAM, Gomaa RS, Hussein SFE (2013) Effect of moderate intensity exercise on serum visfatin level in male rat model of

obesity. AAMJ. 10(4):20–42 http://www.aamj.eg.net/inner/jarticle.aspx?aid=2045
24. Mostafa D, Khaleel E, Ahmed G (2015) Mechanism of action of oxytocin as cardioprotection in rat model of myocardial infarction. IOSR J Dent Med Sci. 14:25–36 https://www.iosrjournals.org/iosr-jdms/papers/Vol14-issue10/Version-1/E0141012536.pdf
25. Manna I, Jana K, Samanta PK (2004) Effect of different intensities of swimming exercise on testicular oxidative stress and reproductive dysfunction in mature male albino Wistar rats. Indian J Exp Biol. 42(8):816–822 PMID: 15573534
26. Ara C, Kirimlioglu H, Karabulut AB, Coban S, Ay S, Harputluoglu M, Kirimlioglu V, Yilmaz S (2005) Protective effect of resveratrol against oxidative stress in cholestasis. J Surg Res. 127(2):112–117. https://doi.org/10.1016/j.jss.2005.01.024
27. Barnes CD, Etherington LG (1964) Drug dosage in laboratory animals, a handbook. Berkeley (& Los Angeles): Univ. Calif. Press. Cambridge Univ. Press, London, p 41 (302)
28. Henry RJ (1964) Clinical chemistry, principles and techniques, vol 1964. New York: Hoeber Medical, Harper-Row; 2021. p 190
29. Tietz NW (1976) Fundamentals of clinical chemistry. W.B. Saunders Co., Philadelphia
30. Provisional recommendations on IFCC methods for the measurement of catalytic concentrations of enzymes Part 2 (1977) IFCC method for aspartate aminotransferase. J Clin Chem Clin Biochem. 15(1):39–51 PMID: 190335
31. Montgomery HAC, Dymock JF (1961) the determination of nitrite in water. Analyst. 86:414–416
32. Satoh K (1978) Serum lipid peroxide in cerebrovascular disorders determined by a new colorimetric method. Clin Chim Acta. 90(1):37–43. https://doi.org/10.1016/0009-8981(78)90081-5
33. Ohkawa H, Ohishi N, Yagi K (1979) Assay for lipid peroxides in animal tissues by thiobarbituric acid reaction. Anal Biochem. 95(2):351–358. https://doi.org/10.1016/0003-2697(79)90738-3
34. Koracevic D, Koracevic G, Djordjevic V, Andrejevic S, Cosic V (2001) Method for the measurement of antioxidant activity in human fluids. J Clin Pathol. 54(5):356–361. https://doi.org/10.1136/jcp.54.5.356
35. Bancroft JD, Gamble M (2008) Theory and practice of histological techniques, 6th edn. Elsevier, Churchill Livingstone China
36. Suzuki S, Toledo-Pereyra LH, Rodriguez FJ, Cejalvo D (1993) Neutrophil infiltration as an important factor in liver ischemia and reperfusion injury. Modulating effects of FK506 and cyclosporine. Transplantation. 55(6):1265–1272. https://doi.org/10.1097/00007890-199306000-00011
37. Mard SA, Akbari G, Dianat M, Mansouri E (2017) Protective effects of crocin and zinc sulfate on hepatic ischemia-reperfusion injury in rats: a comparative experimental model study. Biomed Pharmacother. 96:48–55. https://doi.org/10.1016/j.biopha.2017.09.123
38. Kamel EO, Hassanein EHM, Ahmed MA, Ali FEM (2020) Perindopril ameliorates hepatic ischemia reperfusion injury via regulation of NF-κB-p65/TLR-4, JAK1/STAT-3, Nrf-2, and PI3K/Akt/mTOR signaling pathways. Anat Rec (Hoboken). 303(7):1935–1949. https://doi.org/10.1002/ar.24292
39. Xia H, Liu Z, Liang W, Zeng X, Yang Y, Chen P, Zhong Z, Ye Q (2020) Vagus nerve stimulation alleviates hepatic ischemia and reperfusion injury by regulating glutathione production and transformation. Oxid Med Cell Longev. 2020:1079129–1079115. https://doi.org/10.1155/2020/1079129
40. Peralta C, Fernández L, Panés J, Prats N, Sans M, Piqué JM, Gelpí E, Roselló-Catafau J (2001) Preconditioning protects against systemic disorders associated with hepatic ischemia-reperfusion through blockade of tumor necrosis factor-induced P-selectin up-regulation in the rat. Hepatology. 33(1):100–113. https://doi.org/10.1053/jhep.2001.20529
41. Serracino-Inglott F, Virlos IT, Habib NA, Williamson RC, Mathie RT (2002) Adenosine preconditioning attenuates hepatic reperfusion injury in the rat by preventing the down-regulation of endothelial nitric oxide synthase. BMC Gastroenterol. 2(1):22. https://doi.org/10.1186/1471-230x-2-22
42. Crockett ET, Galligan JJ, Uhal BD, Harkema J, Roth R, Pandya K (2006) Protection of early phase hepatic ischemia-reperfusion injury by cholinergic agonists. BMC Clin Pathol. 6(1):3. https://doi.org/10.1186/1472-6890-6-3
43. Vardanian AJ, Busuttil RW, Kupiec-Weglinski JW (2008) Molecular mediators of liver ischemia and reperfusion injury: a brief review. Mol Med. 14(5-6):337–345. https://doi.org/10.2119/2007-00134
44. Abu-Amara M, Yang SY, Tapuria N, Fuller B, Davidson B, Seifalian A (2010) Liver ischemia/reperfusion injury: processes in inflammatory networks--a review. Liver Transpl. 16(9):1016–1032. https://doi.org/10.1002/lt.22117
45. Nastos C, Kalimeris K, Papoutsidakis N, Tasoulis MK, Lykoudis PM, Theodoraki K, Nastou D, Smyrniotis V, Arkadopoulos N (2014) Global consequences of liver ischemia/reperfusion injury. Oxid Med Cell Longev. 2014:906965–906913. https://doi.org/10.1155/2014/906965
46. Espinosa-Diez C, Miguel V, Mennerich D, Kietzmann T, Sánchez-Pérez P, Cadenas S, Lamas S (2015) Antioxidant responses and cellular adjustments to oxidative stress. Redox Biol. 6:183–197. https://doi.org/10.1016/j.redox.2015.07.008
47. Granger DN, Kvietys PR (2015) Reperfusion injury and reactive oxygen species: the evolution of a concept. Redox Biol. 6:524–551. https://doi.org/10.1016/j.redox.2015.08.020
48. Siriussawakul A, Zaky A, Lang JD (2010) Role of nitric oxide in hepatic ischemia-reperfusion injury. World J Gastroenterol. 16(48):6079–6086. https://doi.org/10.3748/wjg.v16.i48.6079
49. Mahmoud MF, Gamal S, El-Fayoumi HM (2014) Limonin attenuates hepatocellular injury following liver ischemia and reperfusion in rats via toll-like receptor dependent pathway. Eur J Pharmacol. 740:676–6782. https://doi.org/10.1016/j.ejphar.2014.06.010
50. Koh WU, Kim J, Lee J, Song GW, Hwang GS, Tak E, Song JG (2019) Remote ischemic preconditioning and diazoxide protect from hepatic ischemic reperfusion injury by inhibiting HMGB1-induced TLR4/MyD88/NF-κB signaling. Int J Mol Sci. 20(23):5899. https://doi.org/10.3390/ijms20235899
51. Moniruzzaman M, Ghosal I, Das D, Chakraborty SB (2018) Melatonin ameliorates H_2O_2-induced oxidative stress through modulation of Erk/Akt/NFkB pathway. Biol Res. 51(1):17. https://doi.org/10.1186/s40659-018-0168-5
52. Tang F, Wang Y, Hemmings BA, Rüegg C, Xue G (2018) PKB/Akt-dependent regulation of inflammation in cancer. Semin Cancer Biol. 48:62–69. https://doi.org/10.1016/j.semcancer.2017.04.018
53. Rampes S, Ma D (2019) Hepatic ischemia-reperfusion injury in liver transplant setting: mechanisms and protective strategies. J Biomed Res. 33(4):221–234. https://doi.org/10.7555/JBR.32.20180087
54. Taha MO, Caricati-Neto A, Ferreira RM, Simões Mde J, Monteiro HP, Fagundes DJ (2012) L-arginine in the ischemic phase protects against liver ischemia-reperfusion injury. Acta Cir Bras 27(9):616–623. https://doi.org/10.1590/s0102-86502012000900005
55. Tarsi AK, Ansari M, Ghazi-Khansari M, Keramatipour M, Ebrahimi A, Emamgholipour S, Joybari SV (2012) Melatonin inhibits endothelin-1 and induces endothelial nitric oxide synthase genes expression throughout hepatic ischemia/reperfusion in rats. Afr J Biotechnol. 11(58):12222–12228. https://doi.org/10.5897/AJB12.1577
56. Ghanaat K, Valizadeh-Dizajeykan A, Malekzadeh-Shafaroudi M, Khonakdar-Tarsi A (2016) Effect of dexamethasone on the endothelin-1 (ET-1) and endothelial nitric oxide synthase (eNOS) genes expression during hepatic warm ischemia/reperfusion in rat. Res Mol Med (RMM) 4(4):8–14 URL: http://rmm.mazums.ac.ir/article-1-216-en.html
57. Hide D, Ortega-Ribera M, Garcia-Pagan JC, Peralta C, Bosch J, Gracia-Sancho J (2016) Effects of warm ischemia and reperfusion on the liver microcirculatory phenotype of rats: underlying mechanisms and pharmacological therapy. Sci Rep. 6(1):22107. https://doi.org/10.1038/srep22107
58. Klune JR, Tsung A (2010) Molecular biology of liver ischemia/reperfusion injury: established mechanisms and recent advancements. Surg Clin North Am. 90(4):665–677. https://doi.org/10.1016/j.suc.2010.04.003
59. Bektas S, Karakaya K, Can M, Bahadir B, Guven B, Erdogan N, Ozdamar SO (2016) The effects of tadalafil and pentoxifylline on apoptosis and nitric oxide synthase in liver ischemia/reperfusion injury. Kaohsiung J Med Sci. 32(7):339–347. https://doi.org/10.1016/j.kjms.2016.05.005
60. Oleshchuk OM, Posokhova KA, Мудра AY (2014) L-arginine, but not L-name protects against liver injury induced by experimental ischemia-reperfusion. Int J Med Med Res 1(1). https://doi.org/10.11603/ijmmr.2413-6077.2015.1.2820
61. Zaouali MA, Ben Abdennebi H, Padrissa-Altés S, Alfany-Fernandez I, Rimola A, Roselló-Catafau J (2011) How Institut Georges Lopez preservation solution protects nonsteatotic and steatotic livers against ischemia-reperfusion injury. Transplant Proc. 43(1):77–79. https://doi.org/10.1016/j.transproceed.2010.12.026
62. Tabka D, Bejaoui M, Javellaud J, Roselló-Catafau J, Achard JM, Abdennebi HB (2015) Effects of Institut Georges Lopez-1 and Celsior preservation solutions on liver graft injury. World J Gastroenterol. 21(14):4159–4168. https://doi.org/10.3748/wjg.v21.i14.4159
63. Katsumi H, Nishikawa M, Yamashita F, Hashida M (2008) Prevention of hepatic ischemia/reperfusion injury by prolonged delivery of nitric oxide to

the circulating blood in mice. Transplantation. 85(2):264–269. https://doi.org/10.1097/TP.0b013e31815e902b
64. Abu-Amara M, Yang SY, Seifalian A, Davidson B, Fuller B (2012) The nitric oxide pathway--evidence and mechanisms for protection against liver ischaemia reperfusion injury. Liver Int. 32(4):531–543. https://doi.org/10.1111/j.1478-3231.2012.02755.x
65. Al-Dalaen S, Alzyoud J, Al-Qtaitat A (2016) The effects of L-arginine in modulating liver antioxidant biomarkers within carbon tetrachloride induced hepatotoxicity: experimental study in rats. Biomed Pharmacol J 9(1):293–298. https://doi.org/10.13005/bpj/938
66. El-Saka M, Madi N, Abou Fard G (2014) Effect of moderate and severe swimming exercise on hepatic injury and apoptosis induced by renal ischemia reperfusion in male albino rats. Bull Egypt Soc Physiol Sci 34(2): 160–175. https://doi.org/10.21608/besps.2014.34789
67. Silva RN, Bueno PG, Avó LR, Nonaka KO, Selistre-Araújo HS, Leal AM (2014) Effect of physical training on liver expression of activin A and follistatin in a nonalcoholic fatty liver disease model in rats. Braz J Med Biol Res. 47(9):746–752. https://doi.org/10.1590/1414-431x20143869
68. Huang CC, Chiang WD, Huang WC, Huang CY, Hsu MC, Lin WT (2013) Hepatoprotective effects of swimming exercise against d-galactose-induced senescence rat model. Evid Based Complement Alternat Med. 2013:275431–275439. https://doi.org/10.1155/2013/275431
69. Rodriguez-Miguelez P, Fernandez-Gonzalo R, Almar M, Mejías Y, Rivas A, de Paz JA, Cuevas MJ, González-Gallego J (2014) Role of Toll-like receptor 2 and 4 signaling pathways on the inflammatory response to resistance training in elderly subjects. Age (Dordr). 36(6):9734. https://doi.org/10.1007/s11357-014-9734-0
70. Gjevestad GO, Holven KB, Ulven SM (2015) Effects of exercise on gene expression of inflammatory markers in human peripheral blood cells: a systematic review. Curr Cardiovasc Risk Rep. 9(7):34. https://doi.org/10.1007/s12170-015-0463-4
71. Dallak MA, Bin-Jaliah I, Albawardi A, Haidara MA, Sakr HF, Eid RA, Hassan WN, Al-Ani B (2018) Swim exercise training ameliorates hepatocyte ultrastructural alterations in rats fed on a high fat and sugar diet. Ultrastruct Pathol. 42(2):155–161. https://doi.org/10.1080/01913123.2017.1422581
72. Shanely RA, Nieman DC, Henson DA, Jin F, Knab AM, Sha W (2013) Inflammation and oxidative stress are lower in physically fit and active adults. Scand J Med Sci Sports. 23(2):215–223. https://doi.org/10.1111/j.1600-0838.2011.01373.x
73. Gleeson M, Bishop NC, Stensel DJ, Lindley MR, Mastana SS, Nimmo MA (2011) The anti-inflammatory effects of exercise: mechanisms and implications for the prevention and treatment of disease. Nat Rev Immunol. 11(9):607–615. https://doi.org/10.1038/nri3041
74. Liburt NR, Adams AA, Betancourt A, Horohov DW, McKeever KH (2010) Exercise-induced increases in inflammatory cytokines in muscle and blood of horses. Equine Vet J Suppl (38):280–288. https://doi.org/10.1111/j.2042-3306.2010.00275.x
75. Bernecker C, Scherr J, Schinner S, Braun S, Scherbaum WA, Halle M (2013) Evidence for an exercise induced increase of TNF-α and IL-6 in marathon runners. Scand J Med Sci Sports. 23(2):207–214. https://doi.org/10.1111/j.1600-0838.2011.01372.x
76. Xu J, Li Y (2012) Effects of salidroside on exhaustive exercise-induced oxidative stress in rats. Mol Med Rep. 6(5):1195–1198. https://doi.org/10.3892/mmr.2012.1060
77. Korivi M, Chen CT, Yu SH, Ye W, Cheng IS, Chang JS, Kuo CH, Hou CW (2019) Seaweed supplementation enhances maximal muscular strength and attenuates resistance exercise-induced oxidative stress in rats. Evid Based Complement Alternat Med. 2019:3528932–3528939. https://doi.org/10.1155/2019/3528932
78. Praphatsorn P, Thong-Ngam D, Kulaputana O, Klaikeaw N (2010) Effects of intense exercise on biochemical and histological changes in rat liver and pancreas. Asian Biomed. 4(4):619–625. https://doi.org/10.2478/abm-2010-0078
79. Hoene M, Weigert C (2010) The stress response of the liver to physical exercise. Exerc Immunol Rev. 16:163–183 PMID: 20839498. http://eir-isei.de/2010/eir-2010-163-article.pdf
80. Lima FD, Stamm DN, Della-Pace ID, Dobrachinski F, de Carvalho NR, Royes LF, Soares FA, Rocha JB, González-Gallego J, Bresciani G (2013) Swimming training induces liver mitochondrial adaptations to oxidative stress in rats submitted to repeated exhaustive swimming bouts. PLoS One. 8(2):e55668. https://doi.org/10.1371/journal.pone.0055668
81. Düşünceli F, Işeri SO, Ercan F, Gedik N, Yeğen C, Yeğen BC (2008) Oxytocin alleviates hepatic ischemia-reperfusion injury in rats. Peptides. 29(7):1216–1222. https://doi.org/10.1016/j.peptides.2008.02.010
82. Welch MG, Anwar M, Chang CY, Gross KJ, Ruggiero DA, Tamir H, Gershon MD (2010) Combined administration of secretin and oxytocin inhibits chronic colitis and associated activation of forebrain neurons. Neurogastroenterol Motil. 22(6):654–e202. https://doi.org/10.1111/j.1365-2982.2010.01477.x
83. Saad AH, Nazmy WH, Ibrahim HM, Hussien A (2013) Oxytocin induced protection against non-alcoholic fatty liver disease in rats. Minia J Med Res (MJMR). 24(2):33–40 https://www.minia.edu.eg/med/Files/june2013pdf/6.%201219.pdf
84. Işeri SO, Sener G, Sağlam B, Gedik N, Ercan F, Yeğen BC (2005) Oxytocin ameliorates oxidative colonic inflammation by a neutrophil-dependent mechanism. Peptides. 26(3):483–491. https://doi.org/10.1016/j.peptides.2004.10.005
85. Elberry AA, Refaie SM, Kamel M, Ali T, Darwish H, Ashour O (2013) Oxytocin ameliorates cisplatin-induced nephrotoxicity in Wistar rats. Ann Saudi Med 33(1):57–62. https://doi.org/10.5144/0256-4947.2013.57

Permissions

All chapters in this book were first published by Springer; hereby published with permission under the Creative Commons Attribution License or equivalent. Every chapter published in this book has been scrutinized by our experts. Their significance has been extensively debated. The topics covered herein carry significant findings which will fuel the growth of the discipline. They may even be implemented as practical applications or may be referred to as a beginning point for another development.

The contributors of this book come from diverse backgrounds, making this book a truly international effort. This book will bring forth new frontiers with its revolutionizing research information and detailed analysis of the nascent developments around the world.

We would like to thank all the contributing authors for lending their expertise to make the book truly unique. They have played a crucial role in the development of this book. Without their invaluable contributions this book wouldn't have been possible. They have made vital efforts to compile up to date information on the varied aspects of this subject to make this book a valuable addition to the collection of many professionals and students.

This book was conceptualized with the vision of imparting up-to-date information and advanced data in this field. To ensure the same, a matchless editorial board was set up. Every individual on the board went through rigorous rounds of assessment to prove their worth. After which they invested a large part of their time researching and compiling the most relevant data for our readers.

The editorial board has been involved in producing this book since its inception. They have spent rigorous hours researching and exploring the diverse topics which have resulted in the successful publishing of this book. They have passed on their knowledge of decades through this book. To expedite this challenging task, the publisher supported the team at every step. A small team of assistant editors was also appointed to further simplify the editing procedure and attain best results for the readers.

Apart from the editorial board, the designing team has also invested a significant amount of their time in understanding the subject and creating the most relevant covers. They scrutinized every image to scout for the most suitable representation of the subject and create an appropriate cover for the book.

The publishing team has been an ardent support to the editorial, designing and production team. Their endless efforts to recruit the best for this project, has resulted in the accomplishment of this book. They are a veteran in the field of academics and their pool of knowledge is as vast as their experience in printing. Their expertise and guidance has proved useful at every step. Their uncompromising quality standards have made this book an exceptional effort. Their encouragement from time to time has been an inspiration for everyone.

The publisher and the editorial board hope that this book will prove to be a valuable piece of knowledge for researchers, students, practitioners and scholars across the globe.

List of Contributors

Ghada M. Galal, Ahmad Abudeif and Asmaa Naser Mohammad
Department of Tropical Medicine and Gastroenterology, Sohag University Hospital, Sohag, Egypt

Nagwa Sayed Ahmed
Medical Biochemistry, Sohag Faculty of Medicine, Sohag University Hospital, Sohag, Egypt

Nahed Fathallah Fahmy and Abeer Sheneef
Microbiology and Immunology, Sohag Faculty of Medicine, Sohag University Hospital, Sohag, Egypt

Elsayed Mostafa Ali
Clinical Oncology Department, Sohag Faculty of Medicine, Sohag University Hospital, Sohag, Egypt

Usama M. Abdelaal
Department of Internal Medicine, Sohag University, Sohag, Egypt

Akash Roy, Sunil Taneja, Arka De, Ajay K. Duseja and Virendra Singh
Department of Hepatology, Post Graduate Institute of Medical Education and Research (PGIMER), Chandigarh, India

Ashim Das
Department of Pathology, Post Graduate Institute of Medical Education and Research (PGIMER), Chandigarh, India

Aliasgar Hatimbhai Vohra, Apeksha Suhas Joshi, Hitarthi Swetang Vyas and Ranjitsinh Vijaysinh Devkar
Division of Metabolic Physiology and Endocrinology, Department of Zoology, Faculty of Science, The Maharaja Sayajirao University of Baroda, Vadodara, Gujarat 390002, India

Kapil Kumar Upadhyay
Department of Internal Medicine, Division of Gastroenterology & Hepatology, University of Michigan Medical School, Ann Arbor, Michigan, USA

Jaymesh Thadani
Total Potential Cells (P) Ltd., 1st floor Parimal Majumdar Wada, Pratap road, Raopura, Vadodara, Gujarat 390001, India

Ashraf Khalil, Manar Obada and Hala El-Said
Department of Biochemistry and Molecular Diagnostics, National Liver Institute, Menoufia University, Shebeen El kom, Egypt

Azza Elsheashaey and F. F. Mohamed Bayomy
Department of Biochemistry and Molecular Diagnostics, National Liver Institute, Menoufia University, Shebeen El kom, Egypt
Department of Zoology, Faculty of Science, Menoufia University, Shebeen El kom, Egypt; Misr University for Science and Technology (MUST), 6th of October City, Giza, Egypt

Eman Abdelsameea
Department of Hepatology and Gastroenterology, National Liver Institute, Menoufia University, Shebeen El kom, Egypt

Asmaa Ali, Mona Hasan, Shaimaa Hamed and Amir Elhamy
Theodor Bilharz Institute, Kornish Elnil, Embaba, Giza, Egypt

Nehal Mohamed Bahgat Gamil
Medical Physiology Department, Faculty of Medicine, Ain Shams University, Cairo, Egypt
Histology and Cell Biology Department, Faculty of Medicine, Ain Shams University, Cairo, Egypt

Sahar Mohamed El Agaty, Gehan Khalaf Megahed, Rania Salah Mansour and Marwa Saad Abdel-Latif
Medical Physiology Department, Faculty of Medicine, Ain Shams University, Cairo, Egypt

Dina Sweed and Asmaa Mosbeh
Pathology Department, National Liver Institute, Menofia University, Shibin El Kom 32511, Egypt

Esraa A. Khalifa
Radiology Department, Faculty of Medicine, Menofia University, Shibin El Kom, Egypt

Heba Abdallah
Clinical Pathology Department, National Liver Institute, Menofia University, Shibin El Kom, Egypt

Heba Moaz
Microbiology Department, Faculty of Medicine, Menofia University, Shibin El Kom, Egypt

Inas Moaz
Epidemiology and Preventive Medicine Department, Menofia University, Shibin El Kom, Egypt

Shimaa Abdelsattar
Clinical Biochemistry, and Molecular Diagnostics Department, National Liver Institute, Menofia University, Shibin El Kom, Egypt

Nadine Abdel-Rahman
Ohio State College of Medicine, Columbus, OH, USA

Hussein A. Elmahdy
Biochemistry Department, Faculty of Science, Cairo University, Giza, Egypt

Eman Sweed
Clinical Pharmacology Department, Faculty of Medicine, Menofia University, Shibin El Kom, Egypt

Haitham A. Azeem
Department of Internal Medicine, Assiut College of Medicine, Al-Azhar University, Assiut, Egypt

Ashraf M. Alkabeer
Department of Internal Medicine, Assiut College of Medicine, Al-Azhar University, Assiut, Egypt

Ali Sobhy Mohammed
Department of Clinical Pathology, Assiut College of Medicine, Al-Azhar University, Assiut, Egypt

Amira Ahmed Hussein
Department of Internal Medicine, Al-Sebaia Central Hospital, Aswan, Egypt

Hany Said Abd Elbaset
HPB Surgery and Liver Transplantation, Ain Shams University, Cairo, Egypt

Ahmad Mohammad Sultan
GI Surgery, Liver Transplantation Unit, Gastrointestinal Surgical Center, Mansoura University, Mansoura, Egypt

Iman Fawzy Montasser
Tropical Medicine and Gastroenterology, Ain Shams University, Cairo, Egypt

Hossam E. M. Soliman
Professor of HPB Surgery and Liver Transplantation, National Liver Institute, Menoufia University, Menuofia, Egypt

Mohamed Elayashy
Anesthesia, Intensive Care and Pain Management, Cairo University, Cairo, Egypt

Rehab Elsayed Elsafty, Abdallah Ahmed Elsawy, Ahmed Fawzy Selim and Atef Mohamed Taha
Department of Internal Medicine, Faculty of Medicine, Tanta University, Tanta, Egypt

Rasha Eletreby, Zeinab Abdellatif, Yasmine Gaber, Ahmed Ramadan and Yasmin Saad
Endemic Medicine and Hepatology Department, Cairo University, Cairo, Egypt

Mohamed Said
Endemic Medicine, Hepatogastroenterology, Liver Transplantation Unit, Kasr Al-Ainy Hospital, Faculty of Medicine, Cairo University, Cairo, Egypt

Naglaa Ahmad
Internal Medicine Department, Endocrine Section, Faculty of Medicine, Cairo University, Cairo, Egypt

Hany Khattab
Pathology Department, Faculty of Medicine, Cairo University, Cairo, Egypt

Rachida Laamiri, Sahla Sellami, Nahla Kechiche, Mongi Mekki and Mohsen Belghith
Pediatric Surgery Department, University Hospital, University of Monastir, Monastir, Tunisia

Mabrouk Abdelaali
Imagery Department, University Hospital, University of Monastir, Monastir, Tunisia

Azza Abd El-rahman Saab, Eman Saleh El-hadidi, Maram Saeed Abd El-baki Shararah and Heba Hassan Aly
Clinical Pathology Department, Faculty of Medicine, Ain Shams University, Cairo, Egypt

Maha Mohsen Hussein
Internal Medicine, Hepatology and Gastroenterology Department, Faculty of Medicine, Ain Shams University, Cairo, Egypt

Ebtisam Boushi, Khaled Cheha, Noha Hedar, Rasha Almokdad and Mohammed Waleed Alassi
Gastroenterology department, Damascus Hospital, Damascus, Syria

Ameer Kakaje
Faculty of medicine, Damascus University, Damascus, Syria
University Hospital Geelong, Barwon Health, Victoria, Australia

Abeer Awad Abdellatif, Mohamad Sherif Mogawer, Ahmed Abdel-Ghani, Amany Abdel-Maqsod and Mona El-Amir
Hepatogastroenterology, Liver Transplantation Unit, Internal Medicine Department, Kasr Al-Aini Hospitals, Cairo University, Kasr Al-Aini Street, Cairo PO: 11451, Egypt

Mostafa El- Shazli, Ayman Salah, Doaa A. Mansour and Ahmed Nabil
Department of General Surgery, Liver Transplantation Unit, Kasr Al-Ainy Hospital, Faculty of Medicine, Cairo University, Cairo, Egypt

Hanaa El-Karaksy, Karim Hosny, Engy A. Mogahed and Noha A. Yasin
Pediatrics Department, Liver Transplantation Unit, Cairo University, Cairo, Egypt

Naglaa Zayed
Endemic Medicine Department, Liver Transplantation unit, Kasr Al-Ainy Hospital, Faculty of Medicine, Cairo University, Cairo, Egypt

Hadeel Gamal Eldeen
Endemic Hepatology and Gastroenterology, Liver Transplantation Unit, Kasr Al-Ainy Hospital, Faculty of Medicine, Cairo University, Cairo, Egypt

Ayman M. A. Osman
General & HPB Surgery, Department of General Surgery, Unit of Hepatobiliary Surgery, Liver Transplantation Unit, Kasr Al-Ainy Hospital, Faculty of Medicine, Cairo University, Cairo, Egypt

H. Naguib
Internal Medicine, Hepatobiliary Unit, Department of Internal Medicine, Faculty of Medicine, Alexandria University, 17 Champollion Street, El Messallah, Alexandria 21131, Egypt

H. Kassab
Internal Medicine, Diabetes and Metabolism Unit, Department of Internal Medicine, Faculty of Medicine, Alexandria University, Alexandria, Egypt

Lerine B. El Shazli and Asmaa W. Abdelaziz
Pediatrics Department, Faculty of Medicine, Ain Shams University, Cairo, Egypt

Dina A. Ragab
Clinical Pathology Department, Faculty of Medicine, Ain Shams University, Cairo, Egypt

Karim A. Abdelhady
Ministry of health, Cairo, Egypt

Chidiebere Emmanuel Ugwu and Stephen Monday Suru
Department of Human Biochemistry, Faculty of Basic Medical Sciences, College of Health Sciences, Nnamdi Azikiwe University (Nnewi Campus), Nnewi, Anambra State, Nigeria

Ghalia Mohamed Kanawati and Iqbal Hassan Al-Khateeb
Pharmacological and Diagnostic Research Centre, Faculty of Pharmacy, Al-Ahliyya Amman University, Amman 19328, Jordan

Yasser Ibrahim Kandil
Pharmacological and Diagnostic Research Centre, Faculty of Pharmacy, Al-Ahliyya Amman University, Amman 19328, Jordan
Biochemistry and Molecular Biology Department, Faculty of Pharmacy, Al-Azhar University, Cairo 11884, Egypt

Hanan Mohamed Nafeh, Ahmad Farooq Alsayed Hasanain, Mohamed A. Mekky and Ahmed Medhat Nasr
Department of Tropical Medicine and Gastroenterology, Faculty of Medicine, Assiut University, Assiut, Egypt

Nahed A. Makhlouf
Tropical Medicine and Gastroenterology, Medical Team of Liver Transplantation at Al-Rajhi Liver Hospital, Faculty of Medicine, Assiut University, Assiut, Egypt

Mohamed Farouk
Assiut Center for Management of Viral Hepatitis, Assiut 71515, Egypt

Mohamed Ahmed El-Mokhtar and Helal F. Hetta
Department of Microbiology and Immunology, Faculty of Medicine, Assiut University, Assiut, Egypt

Mohamed Alboraie
Department of Internal Medicine, Al-Azhar University, Cairo, Egypt

Hussein ELamin
Assiut Center for Management of Viral Hepatitis, Assiut 71515, Egypt
Department of Internal Medicine, Faculty of Medicine, Assiut University, Assiut, Egypt

Yasser Hamada and Hassan El-Garem
Endemic Medicine Department, Faculty of Medicine, Cairo University, Cairo, Egypt

Ibrahim Emam and Rabab Maher
Student Hospital, Cairo University Hospitals, Cairo, Egypt

Debashis Chowdhury
Department of Gastroenterology and Hepatology, Chattogram Maa O Shishu Hospital (CMOSH) Medical College, Chattogram, Bangladesh

Farhana Mahmood
Department of Medicine, Chattogram Maa O Shishu Hospital (CMOSH) Medical College, Chattogram, Bangladesh

Cathryn Edwards
Office of the President, British Society of Gastroenterology, St Andrew's Place, London, UK

Simon D. Taylor-Robinson
Department of Surgery and Cancer, Imperial College London, St Mary's Hospital Campus, London, UK

Osama Elbahr, Ahmad Kamal, Ayman Alsebaey, Mohamed Amin, Mohamed Abbasy, Ahmad Edris, Ali Nada, Alyaa Sabry, Sameh Afiffy and Abd El-Aleem Helal
Hepatology and Gastroenterology Department, National Liver Institute, Menoufia University, Shebin Alkawm, Menoufia, Egypt

Mohamad Abd El-aziz
Internal medicine department, Alexandria University, Alexandria, Egypt

Abd El-naser Gad-Allah
Internal Medicine Department, Menoufia University, One, Meleeg Road, National liver Institute, Shebin Alkawm, Menoufia, Egypt

Afaf Y. M. Younes, Sherief Abd-Elsalam and Mona A. H. Shehata
Department of Tropical Medicine and Infectious Diseases, Faculty of Medicine, Tanta University, Elbahr Street, Tanta 35111, Egypt

Gehan F. Attia
Department of Clinical Pathology, Faculty of Medicine, Tanta University, Tanta, Egypt

Amr H. ELKady, Bataa M. Elkafoury, Dalia A. Saad, Doaa M. Abd el-Wahed and Mona A. Ahmed
Physiology Department, Faculty of Medicine, Ain Shams University, Cairo, Egypt

Walaa Baher
Histology Department, Faculty of Medicine, Ain Shams University, Cairo, Egypt

Index